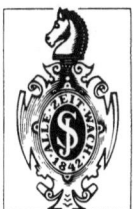

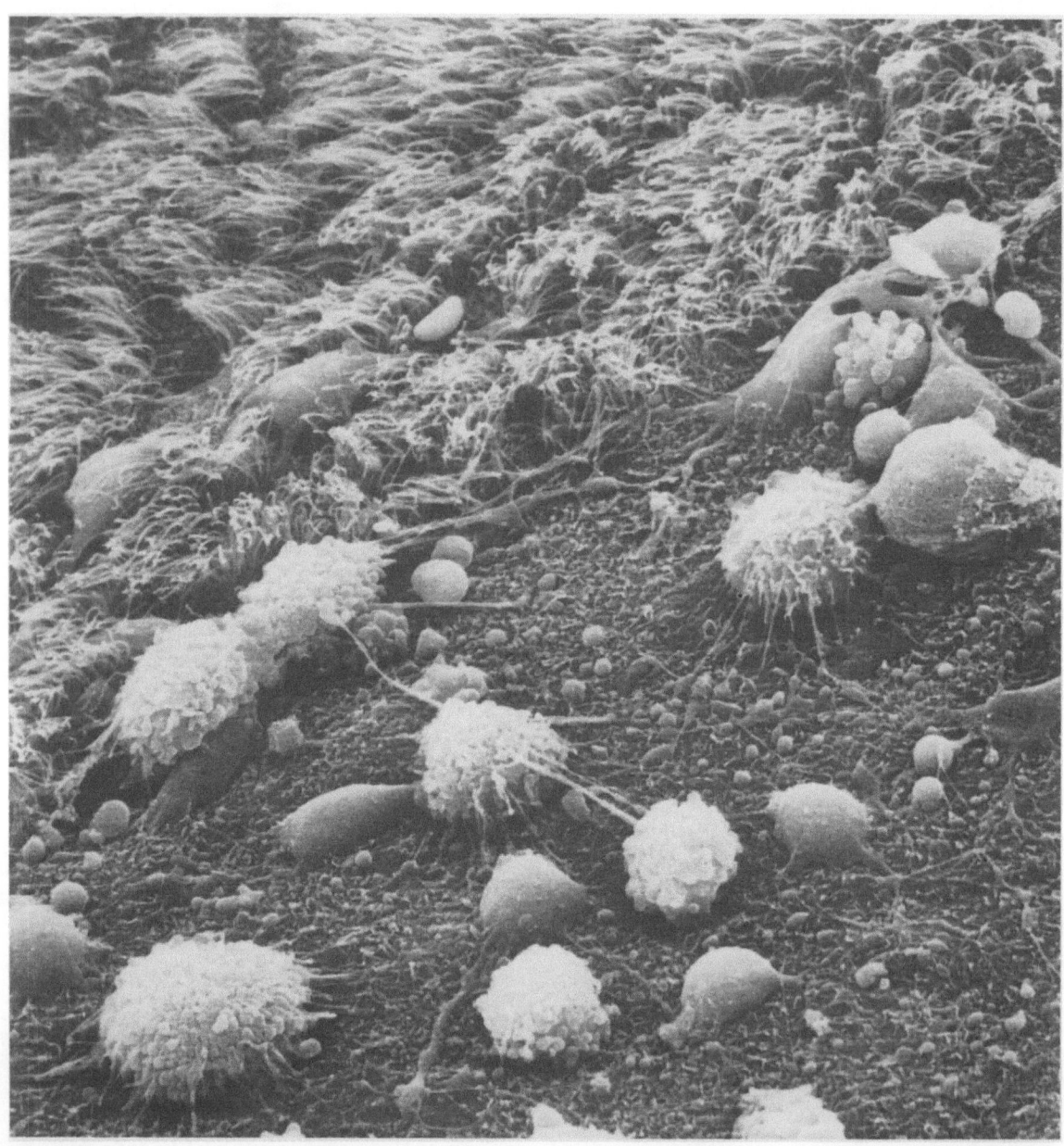

Frontispiece A scanning electron micrograph of the ventricular lining in hydrocephalus. Cilia of normal ependyma are seen at the top left and stretched non-ciliated ependyma is seen at bottom right. Supra-ependymal macrophages are seen clinging to the surface of the abnormal ependyma. (Magnification ×2880.)

R. O. Weller   M. Swash
D. L. McLellan   C. L. Scholtz

Clinical
Neuropathology

With 209 Figures

Springer-Verlag
Berlin Heidelberg New York 1983

Roy O. Weller, BSc, MD, PhD, FRCPath

Professor of Neuropathology, University of Southampton
and Consultant Neuropathologist, Wessex Regional Neurological Centre,
Southampton, England

Michael Swash, MD, FRCP, MRCPath

Consultant Neurologist, The London Hospital and St Mark's Hospital, London
and Senior Lecturer in Neuropathology, the London Hospital Medical College,
London, England

D. Lindsay McLellan, MA, MB, PhD, FRCP

Senior Lecturer in Neurology, University of Southampton
and Consultant Neurologist, Wessex Regional Neurological Centre,
Southampton, England

Carl L. Scholtz, MB, MSc, FRCPA

Senior Lecturer in Neuropathology, The London Hospital Medical College
and Consultant Neuropathologist, The London Hospital, London,
England

ISBN-13: 978-1-4471-1337-9   e-ISBN-13: 978-1-4471-1335-5
DOI: 10.107/978-1-4471-1335-5

Library of Congress Cataloging in Publication Data
Main entry under title:
Clinical neuropathology.
Includes bibliographies and index. 1. Nervous system—Diseases. I. Weller, Roy O. [DNLM:
1. Nervous system diseases—Pathology. WL 100 C6435] RC347.C53 1982 616.8′047 82-10309

BAS Printers Limited, Over Wallop, Hampshire

2128/3916 543210

Preface

Although most textbooks of neurology contain a certain amount of pathological information, neuropathology has often been treated in isolation. However, neuropathology has a close relationship to clinical neurology, neurosurgery and neuroradiology. Thus, advances in the rapidity and accuracy of pathological diagnosis have often led to changes in clinical management and, recently, improvements in clinical diagnosis, particularly CT scanning, have brought about a change in emphasis in the practice of neuropathology. In this textbook we have sought to present a widely based account of neuropathology in combination with information from clinical experience. We chose this approach in order to emphasize the close interrelation between clinician and pathologist. The book grew out of a course organised jointly by two neurologists and two neuropathologists from the Departments of Neuropathology and Neurology of The London Hospital and The University of Southampton. It is hoped that the book will be useful not only to pathologists, neurologists, neurosurgeons, and neuroradiologists, but also to general physicians.

In a period of rapid advance in knowledge it is important to recognise how changes in the clinical and laboratory disciplines overlap. In order to make the most of consultations with pathologist colleagues the clinician must know what skills and techniques are available in the laboratory, and similarly, the pathologist must keep abreast of changes in clinical practice. In the past the clinician and pathologist have often been slow to appreciate advances in each other's fields. We have therefore allowed relatively more space for areas in which substantial recent advances have been made, for example, in the understanding of pituitary tumours, and in biochemical aspects of nervous system disease. Subjects of considerable practical importance, for example, head injuries, tumours, infections, cerebrovascular disease, hereditary and neonatal disorders, and diseases of muscle and nerve have also been emphasised, and those principles underlying clinical management which are important for the neuropathologist, confronted with the problems posed by his clinical colleagues, have been described in some detail. The general anatomical and histological concepts, the interpretation of neurological signs and symptoms, and the basic pathological reactions of the nervous system, are discussed in introductory chapters in order to set the scene for the subsequent material. The historical background to the development of neuropathology and clinical neurology provides considerable insight into the directions taken in research in more recent years and we therefore thought it important to provide a historical account of clinical neuropathology. As a general principle it has been our policy to emphasize concepts rather than to maintain an excessive concern for the detailed accounts of all the lesser variations in the neuropathology of rare diseases and we hope that a proper perspective of the role of neuropathology in clinical practice is thus evident. Since the book is not intended to provide a complete review of all aspects of this enormous subject we have restricted references to a few pertinent approaches to the literature. These may be found at the end of each chapter. Only in the two chapters dealing with biochemical aspects of nervous disease is an attempt made to provide a fuller documentation of sources. We hope that this book will be used not only by residents and registrars in pathology and the neurological disciplines but also by students and their teachers.

London and Southampton
October 1982

R. O. Weller   M. Swash
D. L. McLellan   C. L. Scholtz

Acknowledgements

We wish to thank everyone who has helped in the production of this book. In particular, we express our gratitude to the participants of the Clinical Neuropathology course held in Southampton from whom we acquired some insight into the construction of the book. Our medical and scientific colleagues in London and Southampton have given their valuable criticism and practical help in preparing material for publication. We are indebted to Dr John Mitchell for Figs 2.5, 2.7 and 2.9, Mr Raymond Griffin for Fig. 9.8, Dr Peter Cook for Fig. 7.5, Dr Brian Lake for Fig. 13.1, the Department of Medical Illustration, Institute of Child Health, London, for Figs. 12.3, 12.6 and 13.2, and to the Royal College of Physicians, London for permission to publish Fig. 1.1.

The manuscript was very efficiently and untiringly typed by Miss Mandy Collins, Miss Karen Earnshaw, Miss Angela O'Sullivan and Mrs Linda Self at the London Hospital Medical College and by Mrs Olive Huber in Pathology, University of Southampton. We are grateful to Mr Frank Wallis' help in proof reading and, especially, in the preparation of the index.

List of Contributors

Jason Brice, MB, FRCS
Consultant Neurosurgeon
Wessex Regional Neurological Centre
Southampton SO9 4XY

Barbara E. Clayton, PhD, MD, FRCP, FRCPath
Professor of Chemical Pathology and
    Human Metabolism
University of Southampton
Consultant Chemical Pathologist
Southampton General Hospital SO9 4XY

John S. Garfield, MA, MChir, FRCP, FRCS
Consultant Neurosurgeon
Wessex Regional Neurological Centre
Southampton SO9 4XY

Elizabeth T. Houang, MB, MRCPath
Senior Lecturer in Microbiology
Consultant Microbiologist, The
London Hospital Medical College
London E1 2AD

Nicholas F. Lawton, MD, FRCP
Senior Lecturer in Neurology
Consultant Neurologist
Wessex Regional Neurological Centre
Southampton SO9 4XY

D. Lindsay McLellan, MA, MB, PhD, FRCP
Senior Lecturer in Neurology
University of Southampton
Consultant Neurologist
Wessex Regional Neurological Centre
Southampton SO9 4XY

Marie M. Ogilvie, BSc, MD
Senior Lecturer in Medical Virology
University of Southampton
Consultant Virologist
Southampton General Hospital SO9 4XY

John D. Pickard, MA, MB, MChir, FRCS
Senior Lecturer in Neurosurgery
University of Southampton
Consultant Neurosurgeon
Wessex Regional Neurological Centre
Southampton SO9 4XY

Peter J. Roberts, BSc, PhD
Lecturer in Pharmacology
Nuffield Foundation Science Research
Fellow
University of Southampton SO9 3TU

Carl L. Scholtz, MB, MSc, FRCPA
Senior Lecturer in Neuropathology
Consultant Neuropathologist
The London Hospital Medical College
London E1 2AD

Michael Swash, MD, FRCP, MRCPath
Consultant Neurologist, The London
Hospital and St Mark's Hospital,
London E1 1BB
Senior Lecturer in Neuropathology
The London Hospital Medical College
London E1 2AD

Roy O. Weller, BSc, MD, PhD, FRCPath
Professor of Neuropathology
University of Southampton
Consultant Neuropathologist
Wessex Regional Neurological Centre
Southampton SO9 4XY

Paul D. Whiteman, MSc, MD
Clinical Research Physician
Wellcome Research Laboratories,
Beckenham, Kent
Visiting Lecturer in Chemical Pathology
and Human Metabolism
University of Southampton
Southampton SO9 4XY

Contents

Chapter 1

Development of Neurology and Neuropathology

Advances in neuropathology have, for the most part, followed the introduction and exploitation of anatomical, histological and, more recently, biochemical techniques. Neuropathology developed more or less independently from clinical neurology but the two disciplines are, in many respects, interdependent and changing concepts in the one have often led to advances in the other. Progress in clinical neurology was limited at first by the absence of a clear concept of the function of the nervous system and its constituent parts. The various ideas of nervous function developed in successive cultures have gradually led to a more generally accepted classification of neurological disorders, and of the functional deficits caused by disease of the nervous system. In the modern era, understanding of neurological disorders has been derived not from philosophy, as in earlier times, but from the natural sciences. Something of the difficulties experienced in previous centuries in neurology may be made more apparent by a consideration of the acknowledged problems in the contemporary classification of psychiatric disorders.

Early concepts of neurological structure and function

Although dissections of animal brains were performed by Aristotle (384–322 BC), Galen (129–199 AD) and other Greek philosopher-biologists, anatomi-cal studies on human brains were rare until the Renaissance in Europe. Andreas Vesalius (1514–1564) wrote one of the first comprehensive anatomical studies of the human brain in his book, *De Humani Corporis Fabrica*, published in Basle in 1543 (Fig. 1.1). Little was known of the physiological significance of many of the structures within the brain at the time and most anatomical terms for various parts of the brain were related more to their shape and their implied connection with Greek or Roman mythology than to their functional significance. For example, the hippocampus may well have resembled the shape of a Roman horse-racing field to some, or the horn of plenty (Ammon's horn) to others. Similarly, the names of the caudate nucleus and the lentiform nucleus are based upon their shape and not upon any functional correlates. Confusion inevitably arises when the same tract passes through several differently named structures: for example, the corticospinal fibres pass through the internal capsule, the cerebral peduncles and the pyramids in various parts of their course.

In the Arab world, studies of human anatomy were accompanied by the investigation of brain anatomy by dissection, an approach which, unlike that in Europe during the same period, from about 900 to 1400 AD, was not dominated by rigid Galenic doctrines. For example, the optic chiasm, the cerebral ventricles and the membranous coverings of the brain were illustrated in Islamic writings as early as the 11th century. Indeed, the cerebral

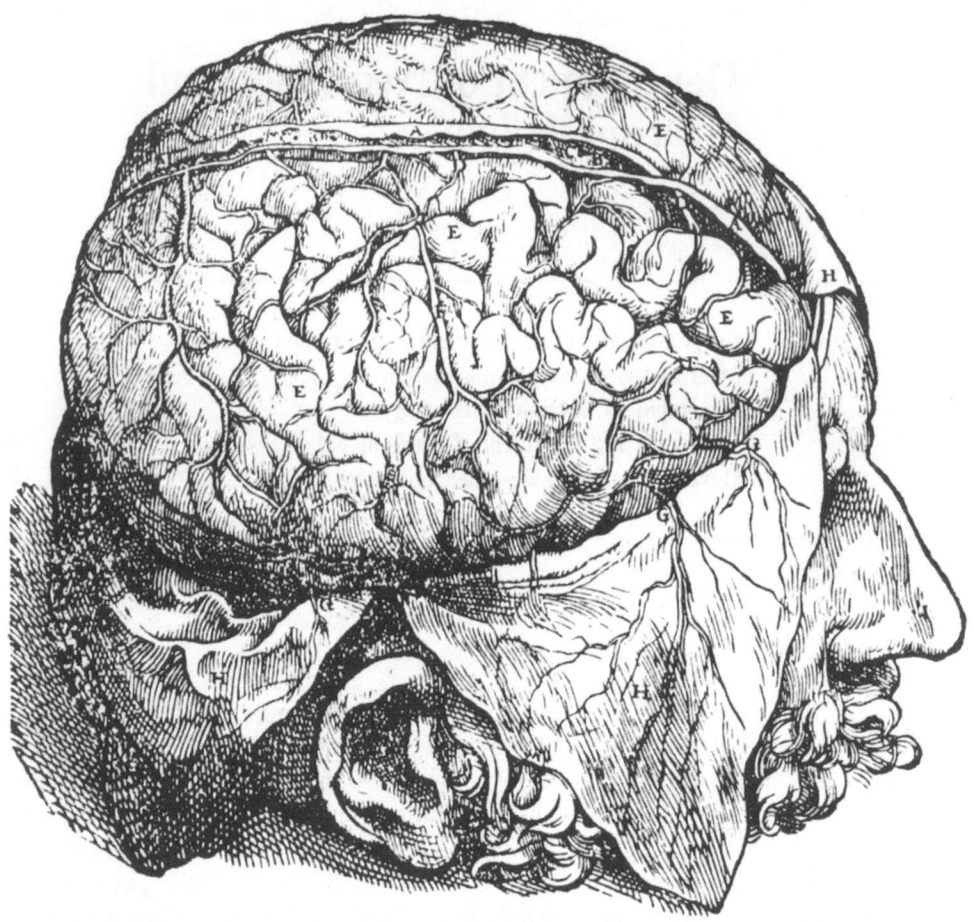

Fig. 1.1. The cerebral convolutions displayed by dissection, and drawn by Vesalius (1543) in *De Humani Corporis Fabrica*. The drawing is the first firmly representational illustration of the cerebral convolutions. Previously, drawings of the brain were greatly influenced by the established views of the artist as to the function of the brain. (Reproduced by kind permission of the Librarian of The Royal College of Physicians.)

convolutions were known to the ancient Egyptians, although they were not generally recognised until Vesalius' work in the 16th century, and the cerebral ventricles were known to the ancient Greeks.

The 17th century was a period of renewed freedom of thought and marks the foundation of modern studies of the brain. Descartes in his book *De Homine* (1662) evolved a theory of brain function which led to the development of the concept of reflex action, first clearly expressed by Marshall Hall (1790–1851), and later extended in a series of studies, fundamental to modern neurology and neurophysiology, by Sherrington (1857–1952). Descartes, however, thought of the ventricles as key structures between the sense organs and the pineal gland, a concept that owed its origins to the medieval view of the ventricles as the seat of the soul. Sylvius (1614–1672), in the course of his anatomical work on the cerebral convolutions,

proposed that the cerebral hemispheres themselves were the major functional unit of the brain. Thomas Willis extended this concept in his *Cerebri Anatome* (1664), a book with anatomical illustrations by Christopher Wren, to include sensory, motor and memory functions of the brain. Willis, himself a practising physician, described the anastomotic circle of vessels at the base of the brain and the clinical features of stroke and of other disorders, including epidemic fevers, asthma and diabetes mellitus.

These early attempts to correlate structure and function in the brain were followed by more detailed descriptions of cerebral anatomy, for example, by Steno (1638–1686), Santorini (1681–1737) and by Soemmering (1755–1830), who introduced the classification of the cranial nerves used today. However, recognition of the constancy of the pattern of the cerebral gyri and thus the application of names to the various gyri was delayed until the early years of the 19th century. At this time, interest in localisation of cerebral function developed rapidly in response to the phrenological concepts of Gall (1758–1818) and Spurzheim (1770–1832).

Gall named 27 mental faculties and localised them in different 'organs' or 'centres' which were mapped, at first, on the surface of the skull but later, by inference, on the gyri themselves. Phrenology soon assumed great importance in medical practice. It was not challenged by experiment until 1824 when Flourens (1794–1867) showed, both by electrical stimulation and by limited cerebral excisions, that although various functions could be localised in various parts of the brain, most of the cerebral cortex was inexcitable. These experiments mark the beginning of the modern era of research on cortical function and, in addition, illustrate the controversy between localisationist and equipotentialist doctrines which persisted until modern times, culminating in the 20th century in the pscyhoanatomical experiments of Lashley (1890–1958).

Microscopy of the nervous system

With the introduction of the microscope, structural elements in the central and peripheral nervous systems could be studied in more detail. Leeuwenhoek (1632–1723), working in Holland, was probably the first to describe myelinated fibres. Improvements in embedding techniques and in the staining of cells in the early part of the 19th century led to the description of large neurons and other structures. Purkinje (1787–1869), for example, not only described the large neurons in the cerebellum that bear his name but also described the axis cylinder (axon). Purkinje's observations probably owed their accuracy to his use of one of the first compound microscopes.

Other important early advances in the understanding of the structure of the nervous system took place in Berlin in the late 1830s. Theodore Schwann (1839) published a treatise on the microscopical structure of plant and animal cells which contains a brief description of the cells in the peripheral nerves that now bear his name. The complexity of the nervous system, however, meant that it was many years before even a basic understanding of many neuronal structures was obtained. An early step was taken by Remak (1815–1865) in 1838, also working in Berlin, when he put forward the concept that nerve fibres (axons) were extensions of ganglion cells (neurons); later (in 1844), Remak described the six cellular layers of the cerebral cortex.

Many other important studies were made in this period, such as the description of the large neurons of the motor cortex by Betz (1874), of the visual cortex and the cellular constituents of the grey matter by Baillarger (1840) and by the German school of histologists including Meynert and von Kolliker. These discoveries were of fundamental importance in later developments. On these anatomical foundations physiological studies could be designed and functional correlations made, in relation both to experimental work in animals, and to the effects of brain lesions in man. Furthermore, once an understanding of the anatomical relationships of the major components of the brain had been achieved, the way was clear for the development of the concept of susceptibility of related systems of neurons and their connections to disease processes, as in the familial cerebellar degenerations (Friedreich (1825–1882), motor neuron disease (Charcot 1825–1893), and Parkinson's disease (Parkinson 1755–1824).

Development of clinical neurology

Flourens' concept of the inexcitability of the cerebral cortex was challenged by Fritsch (1838–1927) and Hitzig (1838–1907) who observed, during the Prussian–Danish war of 1870, that stimulation of the cerebral cortex on one side could evoke movements of the opposite side of the body. This observation was taken up by Goltz (1834–1902), who not only investigated hemiparesis resulting from cerebral extirpation but also made fundamental observations on decerebration and brain stem function. Ferrier (1843–1928) clearly enunciated the experimental evidence for localisation of motor and sensory functions in the brain in his book, *The Functions of the Brain* (1876). At the same time Hughlings Jackson (1835–1911) correlated clinical observations with pathological studies and was able to investigate the clinical features and causation of epilepsy and initiate studies of motor control in man. In 1861 Broca (1824–1880) pointed out that speech was probably functionally localised in the left frontotemporal region, and by the end of the 19th century this observation had become especially important as representing the best example of lateralisation of function within the brain.

The spinal cord itself was shown to contain specialised and lateralised organisation of function by Brown-Séquard (1817–1894), who showed the existence of sensory pathways other than the posterior columns in his observations on experimental hemisection of the spinal cord published in 1846.

Diagnosis and treatment of neurological disease

The complex observations of function and structure in the central and peripheral nervous system, and the concepts that arose from them encouraged new approaches to diagnosis and treatment of diseases of the nervous system. Gowers (1845–1915), Brown-Séquard and Jackson in London and Charcot in Paris were particularly active in this approach. The opening of the National Hospital for Nervous Diseases, Queen Square, in London in 1860 marked the beginning of this phase of rapid advance in clinical studies. Epilepsy became better understood, and syphilitic and vascular diseases of the nervous system were investigated. Gowers and Horsley (1857–1910) diagnosed, localised and successfully removed a spinal tumour in 1886, and Godlee and Barnett attempted the removal of a cerebral tumour in 1884. Horsley described spinal meningitis as a pyogenic infection of the meninges in 1887, and Quincke (1842–1891) introduced the technique of lumbar puncture in 1891. Lumbar puncture was used at first for relief of hydrocephalus but later its importance in the diagnosis of other diseases, especially meningitis and syphilis, was recognised.

In the American Civil War, Weir Mitchell (1829–1914) made important observations on peripheral nerve injuries and causalgia. The First World War led to better understanding of cortical function, especially of speech (Head 1861–1940), vision (Holmes 1876–1964), and sensation (Head), and to major advances in treatment, especially of wounds and so, also, of tumours. Advances in neurosurgery were led by two American surgeons, Dandy (1886–1940) and Cushing (1864–1939). Advances in medical aspects of the treatment of neurological disease progressed more slowly, but have accelerated more recently since the introduction of new pharmacological approaches. These include more effective anticonvulsant drugs, antibiotics, synthetic vitamins, methods for the control of cerebral oedema, and neurotransmitter therapy, e.g. L-dopa for Parkinson's disease.

Development of modern neuropathology

Modern neuropathology probably began with the classic descriptions of axonal degeneration and regeneration by Augustus Waller in the 1850s. He observed the granular appearance and breakdown of myelin sheaths in the distal ends of severed glossopharyngeal and hypoglossal nerves of the frog. Later, Waller also described regeneration of peripheral nerve fibres in the frog tongue. With the introduction of osmic acid as a histological stain in the 1870s, knowledge of the anatomical and pathological features of peripheral nerves was quickly extended. Ranvier (1878) produced a superbly illustrated treatise on the histology of the nervous system (Fig. 1.2); he is particularly remembered for his preparations of teased nerve fibres and motor end-plates, and for his descriptions of the nodes of Ranvier. Using similar techniques, Gombault (1880) described segmental demyelination in peripheral nerves. The measurement of nerve conduction velocities in man was first performed by du Bois Reymond (1818–1896) and Helmholtz (1821–1894) as long ago as 1850, but was not used in clinical practice until after the Second World War, when advances in electronics made it a more readily practicable procedure.

In parallel with the light-microscope descriptions of peripheral nerve diseases, many of the gross morbid anatomical appearances of lesions within the brain were described in the mid- and late 19th century. Cruveilhier, for example, described the appearances of multiple sclerosis in 1835 and this was followed by the carefully documented clinical and pathological accounts of the disease by Charcot in the 1870s. Cerebral tumours, abscesses, tuberculomas and gummas were also well recognised in the latter part of the 19th century but at this time their pathology and relationship to each other were only partly understood.

Advances in histological techniques for the study of the central nervous system (CNS) in the late 19th century led to a significant improvement in the understanding of anatomical and pathological features of the brain. Nissl (1892) introduced a stain for neurons in which the ribonucleoprotein (RNP) of the endoplasmic reticulum stained a beautiful purple colour. Using this technique, Nissl described the effect of chromatolysis, which he observed in neuron cell bodies following axon section. Nissl's stain has continued to be widely used particularly on large celloidin and paraffin sections of brain for

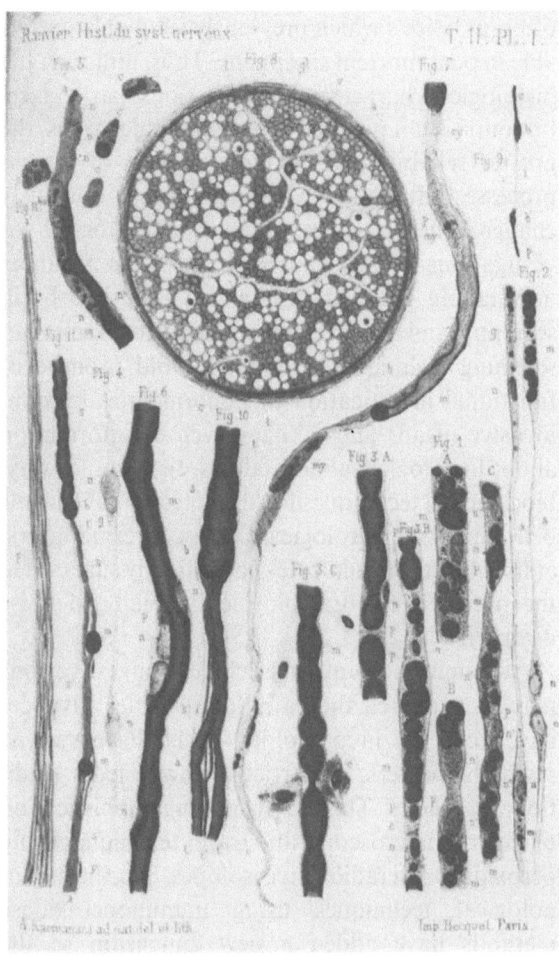

Fig. 1.2. A plate of illustrations reproduced from Ranvier's *Leçons sur l'Histologie du Système Nerveux* published in Paris in 1878. Axonal (wallerian) degeneration is seen in a cross-section of nerve and in teased fibres.

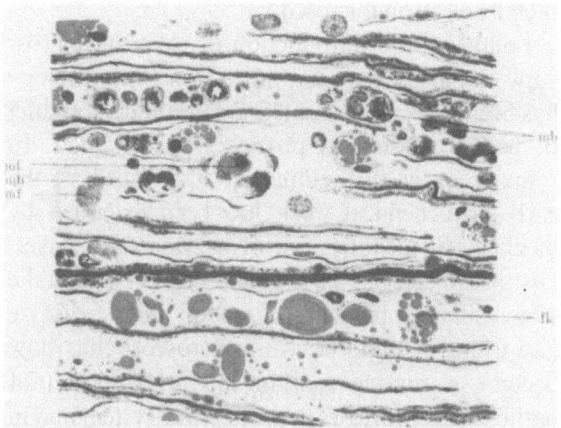

Fig. 1.3. Drawing from Spielmeyer's *Histopathologie des Nerven-systems* (1922). Fresh plaque of multiple sclerosis in longitudinal section. Bielschowsky silver and scharlach R. There is general loss of axons. There is poor staining and irregular thickening of several axis cylinders (myelin sheaths) in the lower half of the illustration. Myelin debris (*mb*) and lipid droplets (*mf* and *fk*) are prominent.

detecting changes in neuronal distribution and foci of neuronal loss.

Perhaps even more significant that Nissl's contribution was the introduction of metal impregnation techniques (Fig. 1.3) by Golgi (1881) whereby a small proportion of neurons are stained by a dense precipitate which outlines single cells. It was upon this technique that Ramón y Cajal (1852–1934) based much of his work on the structure of the nervous system and established the neuronal theory. Until this time there had been fierce argument about the relationship between individual neurons. Although Sherrington, in the 1890s, introduced the concept of synaptic transmission on the basis of physiological data, the nervous system was still widely believed to be a reticular system with no gaps between the neurons. Ramón y Cajal did

much to show that the nervous system consisted of separate neurons; however, confirmation of the presence of synapses and the nature of the neuronal cell membrane was delayed until the introduction of transmission electron microscopy in the 1950s. Ramón y Cajal's pupil, Hortega (1882–1945) described oligodendroglia and microglia in the 1920s.

In addition to the introduction of specific stains for neurons, techniques for the detection of other specific elements in the nervous system, e.g. microglial cells (Hortega), reactive astrocytes (Holzer and PTAH), and degenerating myelin (Marchi), were introduced to the study of pathology in the first half of the 20th century. A wide range of pathological changes was described during this time in the brains of patients dying with a variety of neurological diseases. In many instances, the basic pathology and aetiology of the disease process was ill understood, so that eponymous terms were often used. Such terms abound in neurology and neuropathology, e.g. Alzheimer's disease, Creutzfeldt–Jakob disease etc., although in some cases diseases have been renamed when the cause of a disorder or its functional defect have become apparent.

In the 20th century interest in molecular biology led to proposals for a bimolecular lipid structure for cell membranes by Gerter and Grendell (1926) and by Davson and Danielli (1930s). Schmidt and Bear (1939) used the results of their polarised light studies to carry these models further and to propose a lamellated structure for myelin; their results were confirmed a few years later by x-ray diffraction and then by electron microscopy.

Following the introduction of electron microscopy and histochemistry, much of neuropathology has been re-examined and a greater understanding of basic pathological processes has resulted. In some cases, as in the lipid storage disorders, the early histochemical work has been extended by biochemical identification of enzyme deficiencies. Histochemistry has played an important part in the diagnosis and characterisation of muscle disease (see Chap. 17) and electron microscopy has now become a routine tool in the investigation of pathological processes in the nervous system and in the diagnosis of neurological disease. A combination of electron microscopy and the use of radioactive tracers has greatly enlarged the body of knowledge concerning axoplasmic flow. Such data have recently been utilised in the investigation of toxic neuropathies (Chap. 16).

Other techniques are now widely employed in the study of the nervous system, for example formalin-induced fluorescence (FIF) techniques introduced for the identification of catecholaminergic tracts by Falck and others in the 1960s. New methods for visualisation of neurotransmitters and the immunocytochemical localisation of cell-specific proteins in cells in the CNS are now available. Tissue culture has been extensively used for many years to study tumours and normal cells derived from the CNS. This technique has been particularly useful in the evaluation of chemotherapeutic agents in the treatment of tumours and in the study of those functional aspects of cells which are difficult to investigate in the intact tissue.

Neuropathology continues to change with the introduction of new techniques both in pathology and in neurology. Computerised axial tomography (CT) of the brain (Hounsfield 1971) and more recently nuclear magnetic resonance (NMR) can often now reveal the gross anatomical appearances of brain lesions which previously were only detectable in post-mortem specimens. Thus, although the histological characterisation of lesions, particularly tumours, is not possible by radiographic means, the greater reliability of in vivo detection of disease processes afforded by CT scanning has obviously changed the relevance of gross pathological investigations of post-mortem brains. The advances now taking place in dynamic radionuclide brain scanning, and the development of positron emission scanning techniques and NMR hold promise of functional investigation of abnormalities by non-invasive means and perhaps even of information about histological abnormalities. In a similar way, biochemical techniques for the detection of enzyme deficiencies in neurological disease by examination of fibroblasts or leukocytes have already superseded the need for cerebral biopsies in many of these disorders.

Although non-invasive clinical investigations may have altered the pathologist's role, advances have occurred in pathology which have swayed research workers, in particular, away from traditional methods. There is increasing sophistication of electron microscopic and tracer techniques using peroxidase and radioactive isotopes. Specific immunological techniques using immunoperoxidase methods have added a new dimension to the detection of specific proteins within the nervous system. The boundaries between the different disciplines of histological pathology, immunology, physiology, biochemistry, and molecular biology are becoming increasingly blurred as our knowledge of disease processes increases and better techniques become available for the study of the nervous system.

Chapter 2

Functional Histology and Anatomy of the Central Nervous System

Any appreciation of the pathology of the nervous system must be based upon an understanding of the anatomical and functional complexity of the brain. The detailed anatomy of pathways and neuronal groups in the brain is well expounded in larger texts but there are a number of general principles in the organisation of the CNS which can be stated here as an introduction to neuropathology.

Histology of the brain

A histological section of the cerebral cortex stained with the routine haematoxylin and eosin (H&E) technique shows little of the complexity of the cellular organisation of the brain (Fig. 2.1). It does demonstrate, however, the distribution of *neurons*, the *glial* and *vascular endothelial nuclei* and how the cells are spatially related within the tissue. Although much of the cerebral cortex appears histologically similar, other areas of the brain show different patterns of organisation. The marked difference in size between anatomically closely related neurons can be seen particularly clearly in the cerebellar cortex (Fig. 2.2), where large *Purkinje cells* are

closely related to the very small *granule cell neurons*. White matter throughout the CNS is composed mainly of *axons*, their *myelin sheaths, oligodendroglial cells* and *astrocytes* (Fig. 2.3).

Despite the anatomical variations, cellular elements exhibit the same broad relationships to each other throughout the brain and spinal cord. Figure 2.4 shows, in diagrammatic form, a neuron in the cerebral cortex with an extensive dendritic network and its axon passing into the white matter. Oligodendroglial cells both in the cortex and in the white matter myelinate the axons in the CNS and, as shown in Fig. 2.4, internodes on different axons are myelinated by the same oligodendroglial cell. Astrocytes have many processes which form the enclosing layer of 'glia limitans' separating the neural elements of the brain not only from the arachnoid but also from blood vessels within the brain. During development of the nervous system, astrocyte processes play an important role in guiding neuronal migration. This is especially seen in the cerebellum where the developing neurons on the outer aspects of the cerebellar folia migrate along the radially disposed astrocyte processes towards the Purkinje cell and internal granule cell

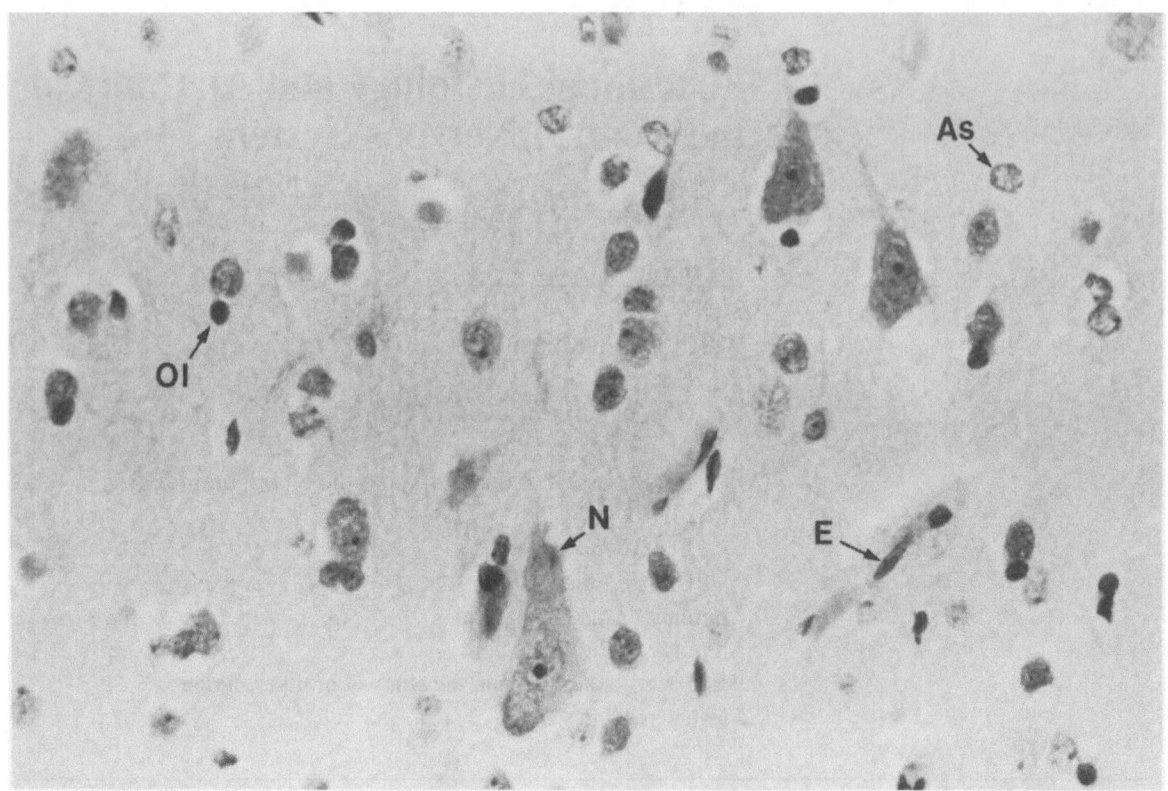

Fig. 2.1. Normal cerebral cortex. Neuron (*N*), oligodendrocyte (*Ol*), astrocyte (*As*), capillary endothelial cell (*E*). (H & E ×440)

layers. Astrocytes of the cerebellar cortex maintain their radial orientation in the cerebellar cortex throughout life; this pattern is most easily seen following damage to the cerebellum (see Chap. 4, Fig. 4.11). The internal, ventricular surfaces of the brain are lined by cuboidal or columnar *ependymal cells* which are usually ciliated. Within the ventricles are the *choroid plexuses*, which are vascular invaginations coated by modified ependymal cells. Cerebrospinal fluid (CSF) produced by the plexuses circulates through the ventricular system into the subarachnoid space before re-entering the blood largely through the arachnoid granulations.

Neurons

An adequate picture of the structural and functional attributes of neurons is only possible by the use of multiple histological and biochemical techniques. H&E- or Nissl-stained sections (see Chap. 4, Fig. 4.5) can be used to demonstrate the many large neurons in the CNS, each with a vesicular nucleus, a prominent nucleolus and coarsely granular cytoplasm. The coarse *Nissl*

granules in the neuronal cytoplasm are rich in RNA and represent stacks of rough-surfaced endoplasmic reticulum and intervening groups of polyribosomes. This high level of RNA in the cytoplasm suggests continuous and active protein synthesis which is probably necessary to maintain the often vast dendritic tree or very long axon. Cerebral cortex stained by the Golgi technique (Fig. 2.5) shows the complexity of dendritic arborisation of single neurons. Axons are well demonstrated by silver techniques, e.g. Palmgren, Bodian and Glees (see Chap. 4, Fig. 4.4).

Since the early work of Paul Weiss, it has been realised that various substances and cell organelles are transported by *axoplasmic* and *dendritic flow*. The *fast phase* of axoplasmic flow at 400–450 mm per day appears to be through cisternae of a smooth endoplasmic reticulum; this phase is probably concerned with the transport of neurotransmitters and enzymes from the neuron cell body along the axon, and with the transport of material for the renewal of axon and synaptic vesicle membrane. A similar system of smooth endoplasmic reticulum is involved in the retrograde axoplasmic flow of

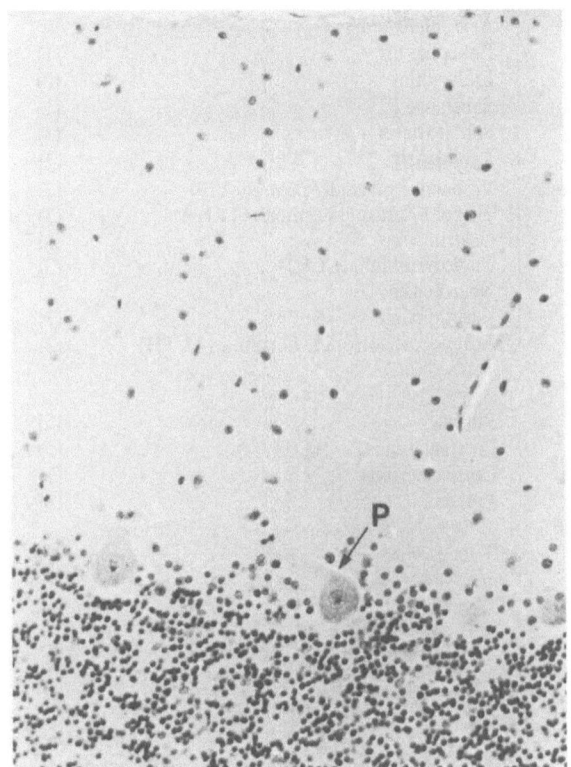

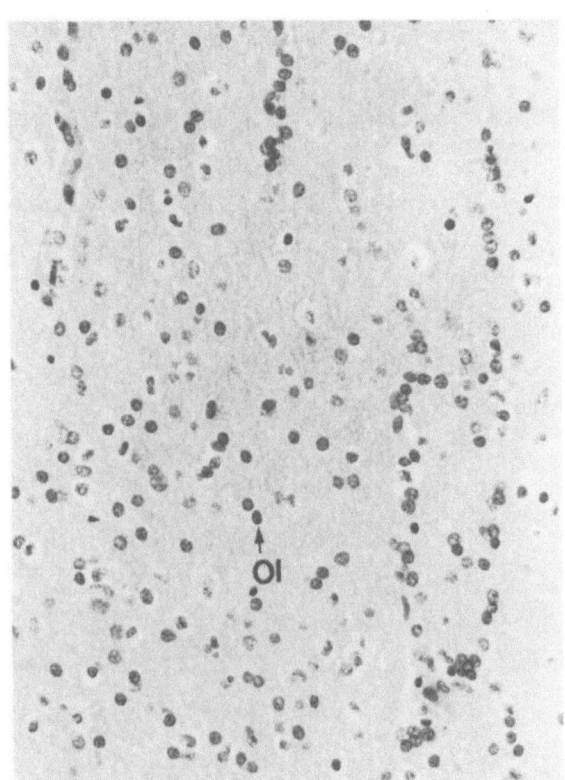

Fig. 2.2. Cerebellar cortex. Purkinje cells (*P*). Molecular layer (*above*), granule cells (*below*). (H & E ×270)

Fig. 2.3. White matter. Oligodendrocytes (*Ol*). (H & E ×270)

material from the periphery towards the cell body; viruses and tetanus toxin are transported in this way. The *slow phase* of axoplasmic flow is concerned with the transport of axonal proteins at a rate of only a few millimetres per day. The exact mechanism of the slow phase of axoplasmic flow is unclear. It may be associated with the longitudinally orientated microtubules and neurofilaments which are present in axons and dendrites (Figs. 2.8, 2.9).

Neurotransmitters

Neurotransmitters produced by the neuron are transported along axons to the *boutons terminaux* which form *synapses* on neuronal cell bodies or on dendrites within the CNS (Fig. 2.6). The boutons contain synaptic vesicles in which the *neurotransmitter* is stored, at least in the case of acetylcholine and the biogenic amines. In catecholaminergic fibres, the synaptic vesicles usually have a dense osmiophilic core, but in other neurons the contents of synaptic vesicles are unstained in electron micrographs (Fig. 2.6). With the arrival of a nerve

impulse at the bouton, there is an influx of calcium ions which induces the release of transmitter into the synaptic gap. This release occurs following fusion of the synaptic vesicles with the presynaptic membrane. Transmitter molecules bind to specific receptor proteins in the postsynaptic membrane and induce a series of reactions that may result either in depolarisation of the postsynaptic membrane and the generation of a nerve impulse, or in the stimulation of the adenylate or guanylate cyclase system with long-term effects upon the receiving neuron. In addition to *excitatory* transmitters, there are *inhibitory* transmitters in the brain, the commonest of which is gamma aminobutyric acid (GABA), an amino acid that is not incorporated into proteins. The histological or histochemical identification of transmitters themselves is rather restricted, but the formalin-induced fluorescence (FIF) technique does allow catecholamines, such as noradrenaline (norepinephrine) and dopamine, to be identified within neurons and their processes (Fig. 2.7).

A list of proposed transmitters and neuromodulators in the mammalian CNS is seen in Table 2.1.

Table 2.1. Proposed neurotransmitters and 'neuromodulators' in the mammalian CNS

	'Classic' transmitters			*Neuromodulators*	
	Acetylcholine	(1)		Enkephalins	(1)
	Noradrenaline	(1)		Endorphins	(2)
	Dopamine	(1)		Substance P	(1)
Amines	Serotonin	(1)		Somatostatin	(3)
	Adrenaline	(3)		Angiotensin	(3)
	Octopamine	(3)	Peptides	Vasoactive intestinal peptide (VIP)	(3)
	Histamine	(3)		Thyroid-releasing hormone (TRH)	(3)
	Tryptamine	(3)		Gastrin	(3)
				Cholecystokinin (CCK)	(3)
				Neurotensin	(3)
	Gamma aminobutyric acid	(1)		Vasopressin	(3)
	(GABA)			Adrenocorticotrophic hormone (ACTH)	(3)
	Glutamate	(3)			
Amino acids	Aspartate	(3)			
	Taurine	(3)		Purines	(3)
	Glycine (spinal cord)	(1)	Miscellaneous	Prostaglandins	(2)
	Cysteine sulphinate	(3)		Corticosteroids	(3)
				Prolactin	(3)

(1) Established   (2) Probable   (3) Proposed

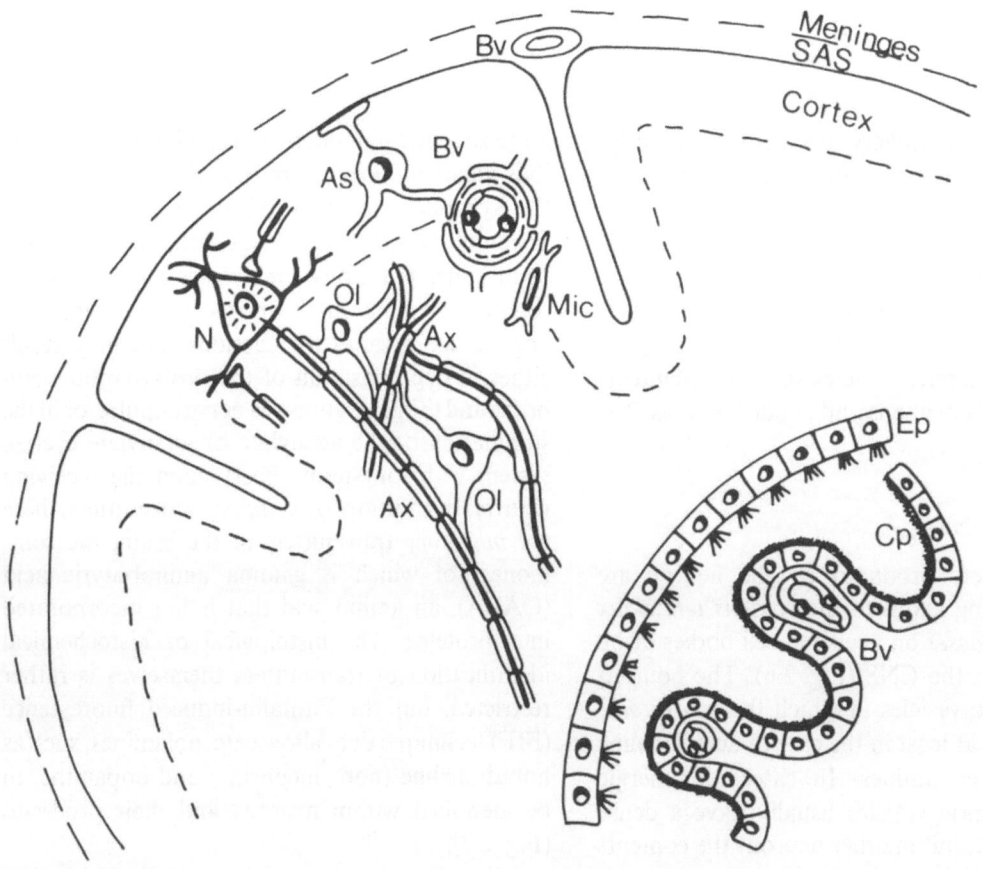

Fig. 2.4. Diagram of cell relationships in the brain. Neuron (*N*), axons (*Ax*), astrocyte (*As*), oligodendrocyte (*Ol*), microglia (*Mic*), ependyma (*Ep*), choroid plexus (*Cp*), blood vessels (*Bv*), subarachnoid space (*SAS*)

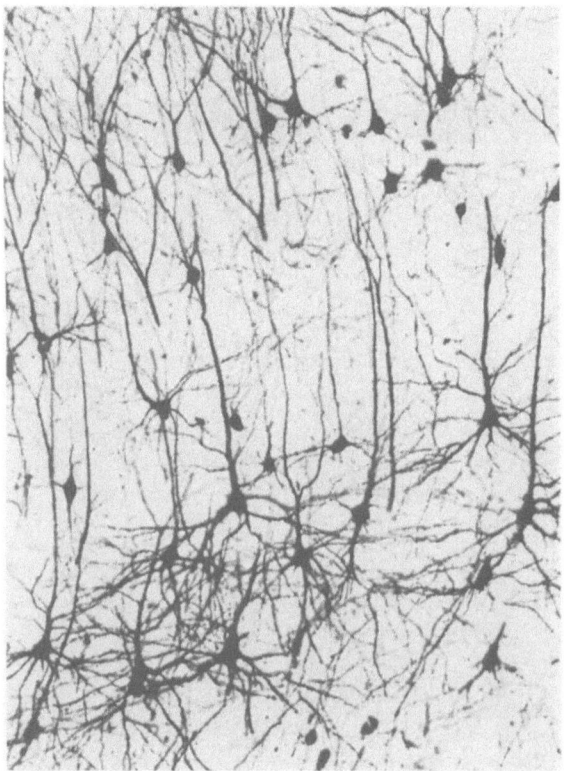

Fig. 2.5. Neurons and dendrites in cat cerebral cortex. (Golgi technique × 120)

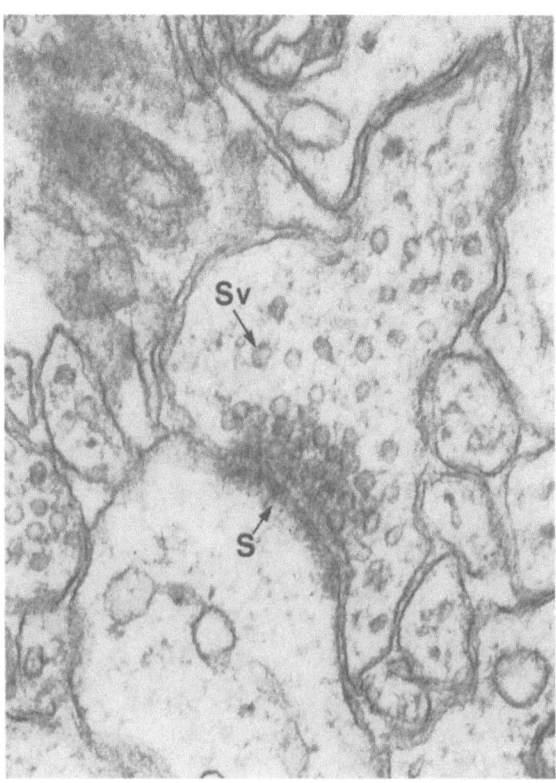

Fig. 2.6. Synapse (*S*). Synaptic vesicles (*Sv*) in presynaptic bouton. (EM × 34000)

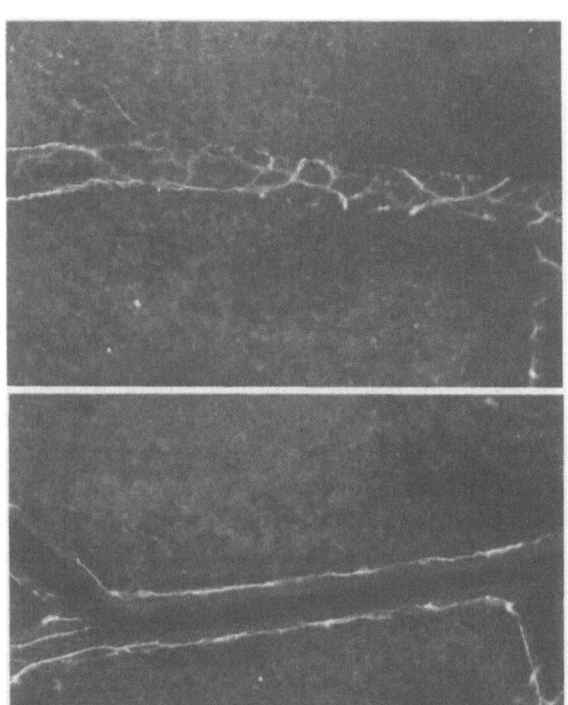

There are several criteria which need to be satisfied before a substance can be clearly defined as a transmitter. *Peptides* may not be true transmitters but rather *neuromodulators* which are packaged within a presynaptic cell and released concurrently with a transmitter from the same nerve terminal.

To be identified as a *transmitter* a substance must be present in a neuron with the relevant synthetic machinery and must be released by a selective calcium-dependent exocytosis mechanism. The transmitter should interact with a specific postsynaptic *receptor* and produce effects identical to those elicited by physiological stimulation of the presynaptic input. A specific and rapid mechanism for terminating the effect of the transmitter should be present so that the transmitter is either degraded by enzymes or taken up into the pre- or postsynaptic elements and glial cells. Very few substances meet all the criteria as the specific receptors of many of the proposed transmitters have not been identified.

◀ **Fig. 2.7.** Noradrenaline in nerve plexus around cerebral artery in rat. The artery is photographed in different planes of focus to show the plexus of nerve in the adventitia. [Formalin-induced fluorescence (FIF) × 75]

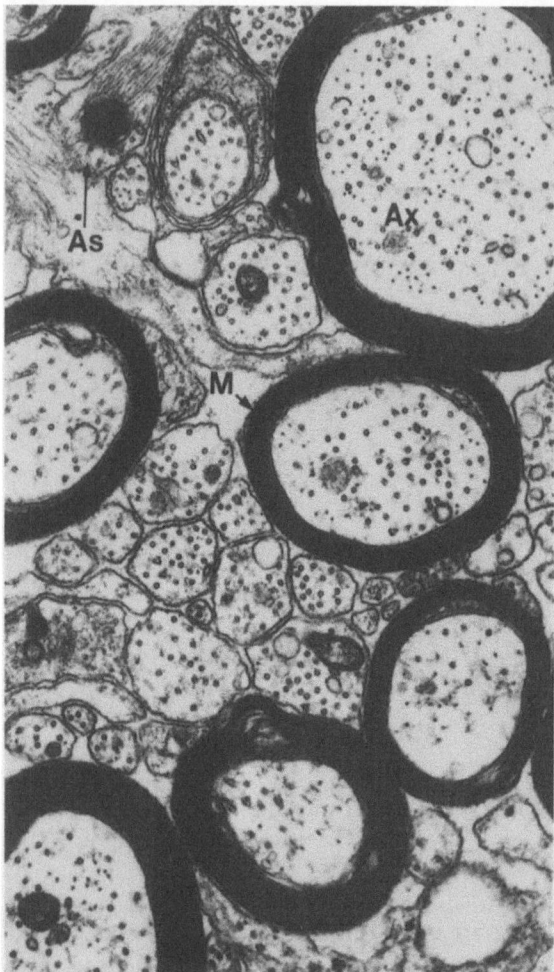

Fig. 2.8. White matter in a young dog. Astrocyte process (*As*), myelin sheath (*M*). Some axons are not yet myelinated. Numerous neurotubules and filaments cut in transverse section in axons (*Ax*). (Em × 18 000)

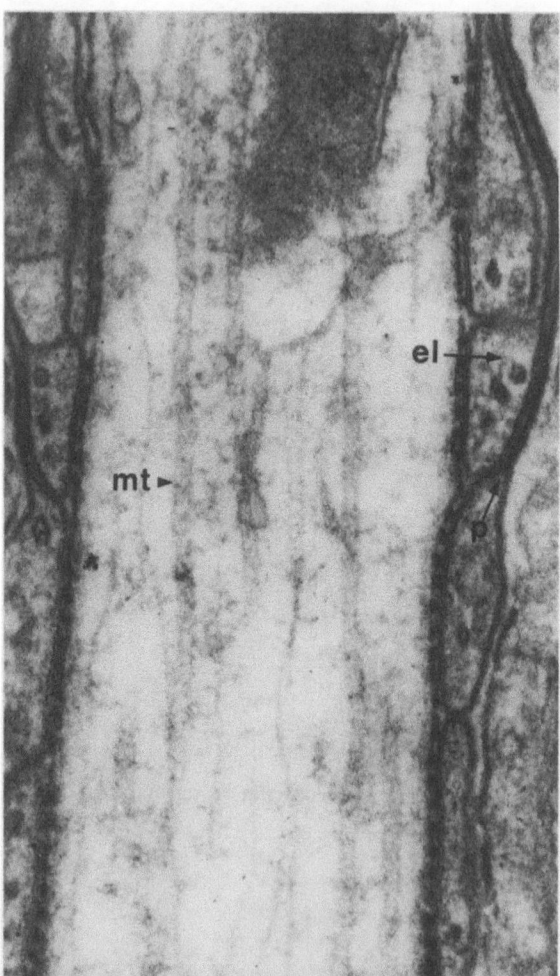

Fig. 2.9. Part of node of Ranvier in CNS. Axon contains neurotubules (*mt*) cut in longitudinal section. Myelin end loops (*el*) at node. Myelin period line (*p*). (EM × 112 000)

Oligodendrocytes

In H&E-stained paraffin sections, oligodendrocytes are detectable by their small, dark nuclei which are about the size and density of a lymphocyte; little can be seen of their cytoplasm. Although these cells are prominent in the white matter between the myelinated fibres (Fig. 2.3), they are also seen within the cortex, often closely associated with neurons (Fig. 2.1). The processes of oligodendrocytes may be demonstrated by light microscopy using a Hortega or Weil–Davenport stain; in electron micrographs these cells are marked by their relatively dense cytoplasm, and by clumping of nuclear chromatin beneath the nuclear envelope.

Microtubules are often detectable within oligodendrocyte cytoplasm but glial fibrillary acidic protein fibrils, similar to those found in astrocytes, are not present in oligodendrocytes.

Myelin

In the CNS, myelin is formed around axons by compaction of oligodendrocyte cell membrane (Fig. 2.8); the resulting lamellated structure has a periodicity of approximately 12 nm. A major dense period line is formed where the cytoplasmic aspects of the cell membranes fuse (Fig. 2.9) whereas the interperiod line, which is often discontinuous, results from the fusion of the outer aspects of the oligodendrocyte membrane. Cholesterol, phospholipids and cerebroside form the major lipid components of myelin and are located within the white areas within the myelin lamellae that are unstained by osmium. Protein forms some 50% of the bulk of myelin and consists of the Folch–Lees *proteolipid* and *myelin basic protein*. Proteolipid is mainly associated with the lipid component of myelin whereas the 18400-dalton myelin basic protein appears to be located within the period line. Much research has been concentrated upon myelin basic protein as its injection, together with Freund's adjuvant, causes experimental allergic encephalomyelitis in animals. This experimental disease has been used as a model for the study of multiple sclerosis. Myelin basic protein is also present in oligodendroglial cells; it has been used as a marker in immunoperoxidase studies to show how oligodendrocytes myelinate several internodes belonging to different nerve fibres.

The gaps between oligodendrocytes along the length of an axon form the *nodes of Ranvier*; myelin sheaths on either side of the node form end loops of cytoplasm and attachment zones between the sheath and the axon (Fig. 2.9). Conduction of nerve impulses along myelinated fibres occurs in a saltatory manner; the impulse, or wave of membrane depolarisation, jumps from one node of Ranvier to the next. Myelin acts as an insulator and prevents excitation of the axon cell membrane except where there are gaps in the sheaths at the nodes of Ranvier. Increased permeability of the excited membrane at the node to sodium ions causes ionic currents to flow to the next node and the current to flow in the reverse direction in the extracellular fluid. When the current density reaches the threshold level, depolarisation initiates similar permeability changes at the next node of Ranvier. As the flow of ions through the cytoplasm is much more rapid than the spread of the wave of depolarisation along the cell membrane, higher conduction velocities are reached by *saltatory conduction*. A similar pattern of nodes of Ranvier is seen between sequential Schwann cells ensheathing myelinated peripheral nerve fibres (see Chap. 16) but there are some ultrastructural differences.

Astrocytes

In Fig. 2.1, where the section of normal cortex has been stained by H&E, only the nuclei of astrocytes are identifiable but they can be differentiated from the smaller, densely stained oligodendrocyte nuclei. A more complete picture of an astrocyte and its numerous processes can be obtained by using a Cajal gold sublimate technique (Fig. 2.10). Anatomically, astrocytes seem to play

an important role in separating neural tissue from non-neural elements. The surface of the brain is composed of several layers of astrocyte processes which are separated from the arachnoid by a basement membrane. Similarly, even the smallest capillary in the brain is surrounded by astrocyte processes, which are in turn separated from the endothelial cells and pericytes by a basement membrane. The close association of astrocyte processes to blood vessels can be seen in Fig. 2.10. Electron microscopy of normal cortex shows a number of astrocyte processes between the myriad of dendritic profiles of the neuropil. Astrocyte processes can also be seen in white matter distributed between the myelinated fibres, where they can be identified by their intracellular 9-nm-diameter glial fibrils (Fig. 2.8). Few microtubules are present in astrocyte cytoplasm.

Glial fibrillary acidic protein (GFAP) is a major component of the intracellular 9-nm filaments, which increase in number when astrocytes become hypertrophic and reactive in response to brain tissue damage. Antibodies to GFAP can be used in immunofluorescence and immunoperoxidase techniques to identify astrocytes especially within damaged brain and within astrocytic tumours (Fig. 2.11). The Holzer and PTAH techniques are two long-established histological stains which can be used to detect reactive astrocytes in paraffin sections; both these techniques probably depend upon the increase in GFAP for their demonstration of astrocyte processes.

In postnatal life, astrocytes appear to be concerned with the control of the extracellular space in the brain so that when there is an excess of fluid or protein, these substances are imbibed by astrocytes. These cells also play an important role in brain injury as they are the major scar-forming cell of the CNS (see Chap. 4).

Blood vessels of the brain, and the blood–brain barrier

The blood supply of the brain is derived from the vertebral and internal carotid arteries which pass into the subarachnoid space as they enter the intracranial cavity. Similarly, the major arteries supplying the brain stem, cerebellum and cerebral hemispheres are also located in the subarachnoid space from which they perforate the surface of the brain. The Virchow–Robin space, seen around the larger arteries as they enter the brain, represents an extension of the subarachnoid space. This space is

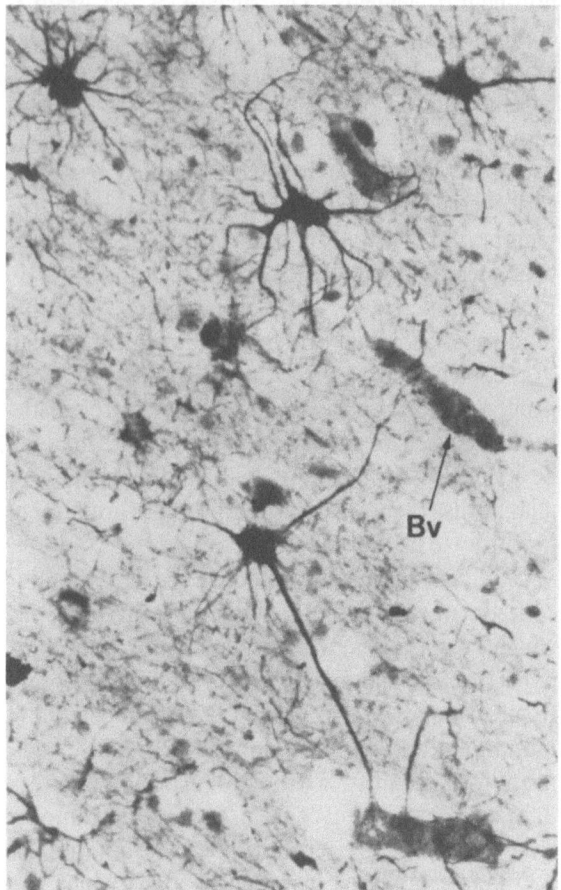

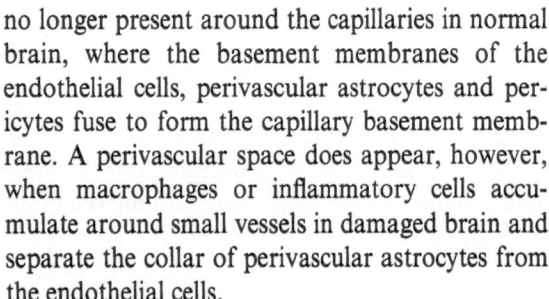

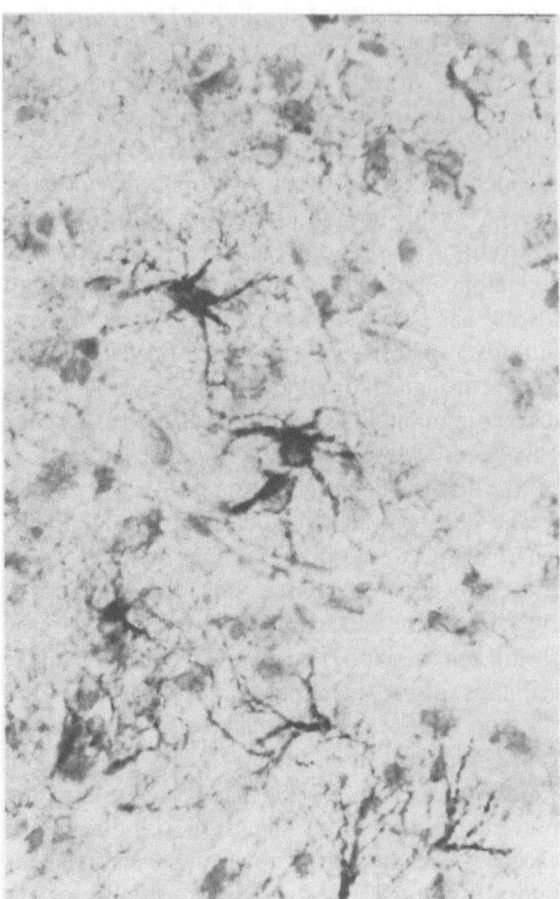

Fig. 2.10. Astrocytes stained by Cajal technique. Blood vessels (*Bv*). (× 500)

Fig. 2.11. Astrocytes stained for glial fibrillary acidic protein (GFAP) by immunoperoxidase (PAP) technique. (× 500)

no longer present around the capillaries in normal brain, where the basement membranes of the endothelial cells, perivascular astrocytes and pericytes fuse to form the capillary basement membrane. A perivascular space does appear, however, when macrophages or inflammatory cells accumulate around small vessels in damaged brain and separate the collar of perivascular astrocytes from the endothelial cells.

Capillaries throughout most of the brain differ from those in other parts of the body. The endothelial cells have a thicker layer of cytoplasm and relatively few microvillous processes on their luminal surfaces. There are very few pinocytotic vesicles within the cells and no fenestrae; furthermore, tight junctions (zonulae occludentes) between adjacent endothelial cells prevent the passage of proteins and other substances from the blood into the extracellular space of the brain. The brain capillaries, therefore, are thought to be the major site of the *blood–brain barrier*.

Microglia

Microglial cells are often difficult to identify in H&E-stained sections of normal brain. They may be detectable by the use of the Hortega silver technique, where they are seen as very small cells with an elongated rod-shaped nucleus and a small number of processes. During the early stages of tissue reaction following brain damage, however, microglial cells increase in number and phagocytose tissue debris (see Chap. 4). Recent studies suggest that microglia are derived from blood monocytes. Electron microscopy has shown that microglial cells have densely staining cytoplasm and few organelles except for the occasional lysosome.

Ependyma

The ventricular system of the brain and the central canal of the spinal cord are lined by cuboidal or columnar ependymal epithelium . Cilia and microvilli arise from the surface of most ependymal cells (Figs. 2.12, 2.13). In the adult human brain, breaks in the ependymal lining of the ventricles may be seen and, in the adult spinal cord, the central canal is often no longer patent and may only be represented by an irregular cluster of ependymal cells. In some regions of the hypothalamus, ependymal cells (tanycytes) have long processes extending to adjacent intracerebral blood vessels. The exact role of the cilia on the ventricular surface of the ependyma is not fully understood but synchronised waves of cilial action have been observed in the fourth ventricle which may play a role in the circulation of the CSF. Cilia also appear to be used as anchorage sites for supra-ependymal macrophages.

There are gap-junctions between adjacent ependymal cells which allow protein tracers to flow from the ventricular CSF into the extracellular space of the brain. It appears, therefore, that the ependyma is not a barrier to the percolation of CSF into the extracellular fluid of the brain, neither does it seem to prevent drainage of extracellular fluid from the brain into the ventricles.

Choroid plexus

The choroid plexuses are vascular structures in the lateral, third and fourth ventricles where the majority of the CSF is produced. Blood vessels within the plexus are separated from the ventricular lumen by loose connective tissue and by a layer of choroid plexus epithelium (Fig. 2.14). Although similar in structure to ependymal cells, the surface of the choroid plexus epithelium is not ciliated (Fig. 2.15).

CSF differs in composition from the blood, particularly with its low protein, and there is a definite barrier to the entry of certain substances to the CSF. In the normal brain, CSF passes through the ventricular system, and from the fourth ventricle into the subarachnoid space and its cisterns at the base of the brain. Thereafter most of the CSF spreads through the subarachnoid space over the vertex of the brain and passes back into the blood of the superior sagittal sinus by a bulk-flow mechanism involving vesicular transport across the cells lining the arachnoid villi.

Anatomy of the human brain

Full reviews of the anatomy of the human brain are to be found in a number of works referred to at the end of the chapter. This section on neuroanatomy will be restricted to a superficial view of the growth and structure of the CNS and to a short account of the phylogenetic development of the vertebrate brain which the reader may find helpful as a basis for understanding the relative positions of important structures in the human brain.

During *fetal life*, the brain develops as a series of vesicles expanding from the cranial end of the neural tube. By *20 weeks in utero*, the human brain has its basic shape and the cerebral hemispheres, cerebellum and brain stem are recognisable. But at this time, only the largest fissures such as the lateral fissures and the sagittal fissure, are visible on the surface of the cerebral hemispheres. Over the next 20 weeks until birth, the brain increases in weight and the other major fissures and sulci on the cerebral hemispheres develop.

At *birth* the brain weighs approximately 400 g and the major surface landmarks are present. One of the last developmental events before birth is closure of the lateral fissure so that the insula on the lateral aspect of the hemisphere is buried under the lips of frontal and temporal lobe. The cortex is still immature at birth and most of the future white matter in the cerebral hemispheres is not yet myelinated. At the lateral angles of the lateral ventricles there is a remnant of the *germinal plate*, from which neurons have migrated into the cerebral cortex. Similarly the germinal layer of the cerebellar cortex, the external granular layer, is still present on the surface of the cerebellar folia at birth and usually remains for the first $1\frac{1}{2}$–2 years of postnatal life (see Chap. 11).

A substantial increase in the size of the brain occurs during the *first year* of life and much of the white matter becomes myelinated. In general, it is the phylogenetically older parts of the brain which tend to become myelinated before more newly acquired tracts. The brain has almost reached its adult size by the end of the *second year* but it is largest at the end of the *second decade* when it weighs between 1200 and 1300 g. Thereafter, the brain decreases in weight so that in many older people, particularly those over 70 years of age, the brain may weigh less than 1100 g. Loss of brain weight may be accentuated by disease processes, particularly cerebral infarction, and by the changes accompanying presenile and senile dementia.

The *major anatomical divisions* of the brain are depicted in a specimen cut in the midsagittal plane (Fig. 2.16). Complex gyral patterns are seen on the medial surfaces of the frontal, parietal and occipital

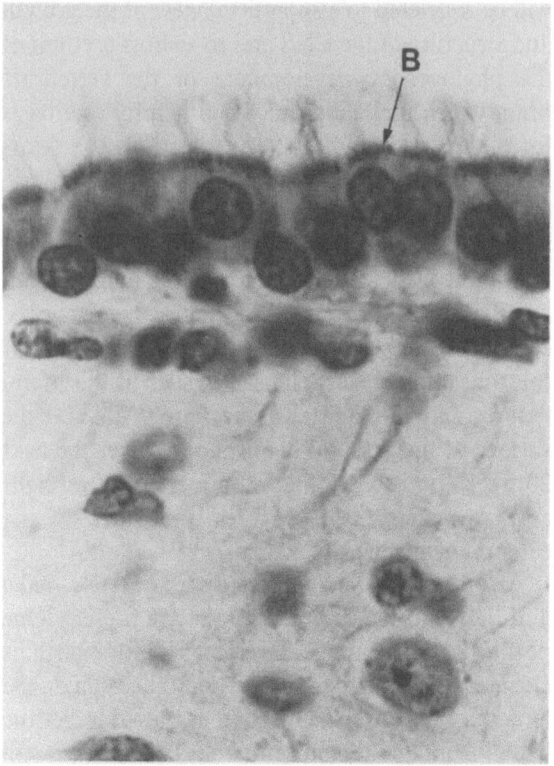

Fig. 2.12. Ependyma with cilia and basal bodies (blepharoplasts) (*B*) on surface. (PTAH × 1300)

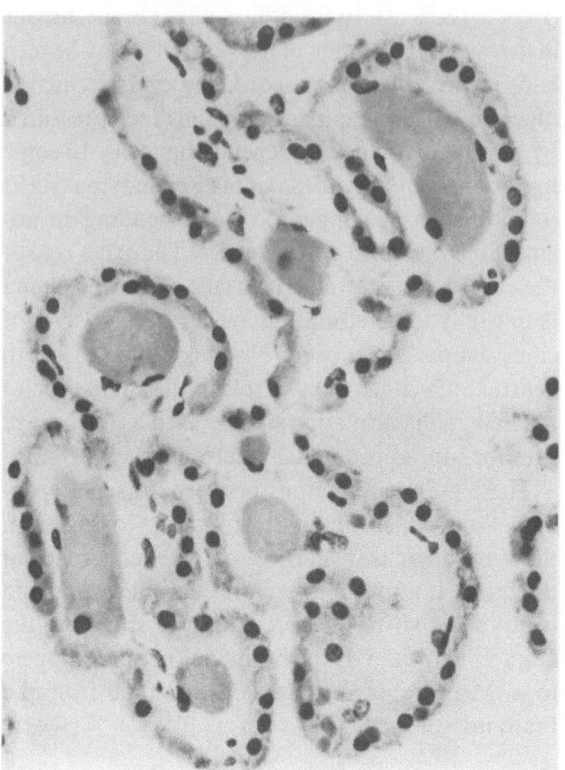

Fig. 2.14. Tufts of choroid plexus. (H & E × 390)

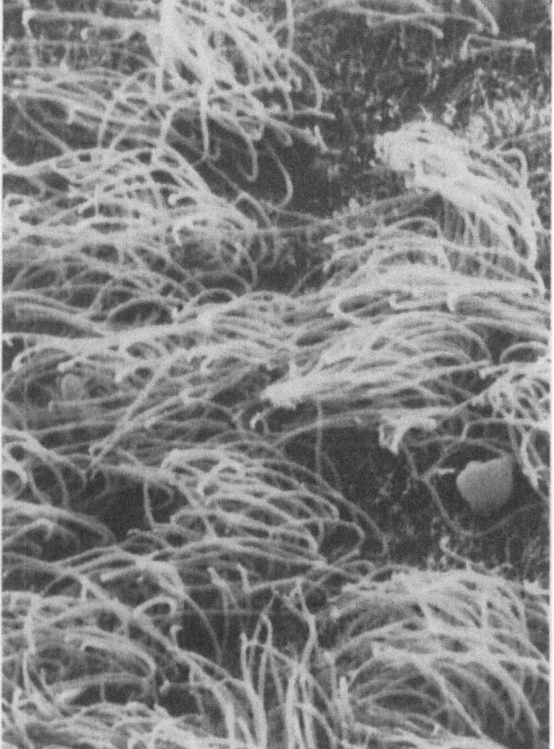

Fig. 2.13. Ependymal surface showing cilia and microvilli. (SEM × 4800)

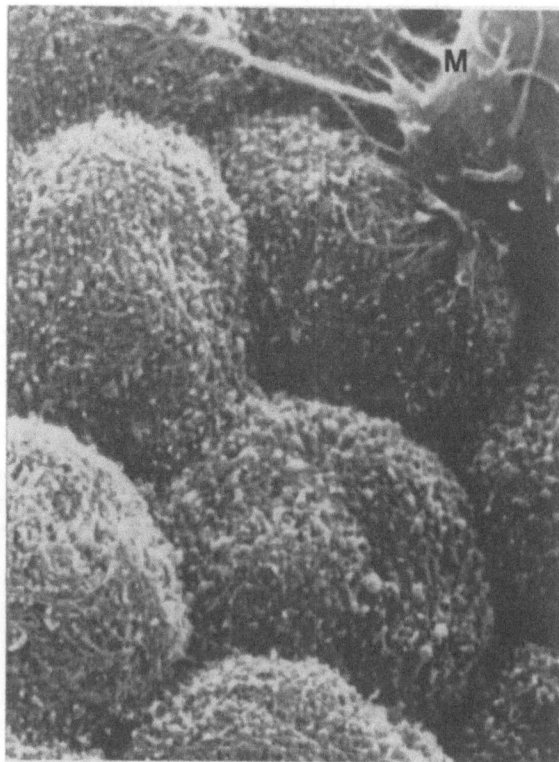

Fig. 2.15. Choroid plexus surface. Adherent macrophage (*M*). (SEM × 4300)

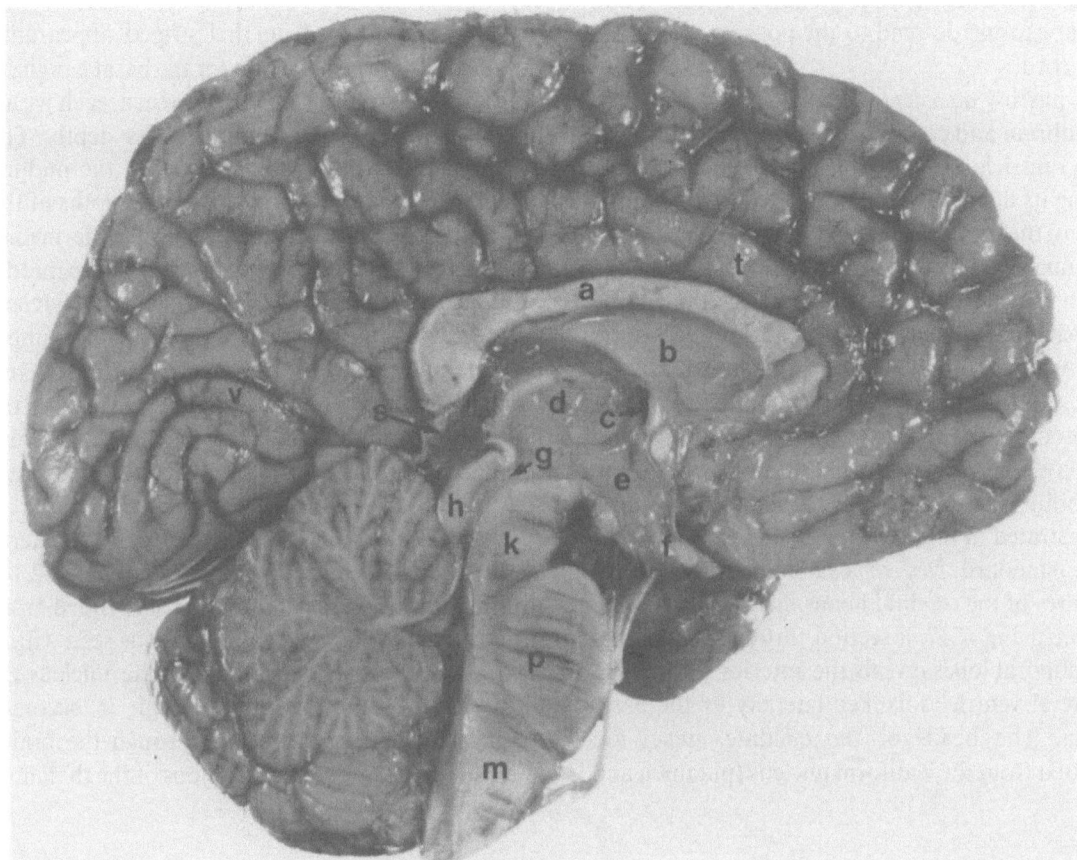

Fig. 2.16. Normal brain cut in the midline sagittal plane. *a*, corpus callosum; *b*, septum pellucidum; *c*, interventricular foramen of Monro; *d*, thalamus; *e*, hypothalamus; *f*, optic chiasma; *g*, aqueduct of Sylvius; *h*, colliculi (corpora quadrigemina); *k*, midbrain; *m*, medulla; *p*, pons; *s*, pineal; *t*, cingulate gyrus; *v*, visual cortex.

lobes and the tip of the temporal lobe is observed as it extends forwards just below the frontal lobe. The cingulate gyrus extends along the medial surface of the hemisphere immediately above the large inter-cerebral commissural tract, the corpus callosum; the anterior commissure is also seen. Prominently displayed on the medial surface of the occipital lobe is the calcarine fissure where the visual cortex is located. Further forward, the triangular sheet of septum pellucidum extends down from the corpus callosum and separates the anterior parts of the lateral ventricles. In the lower edge of the septum is the fornix, which is a long arching tract running from the hippocampus in the temporal lobe to the mammillary bodies in the posterior part of the hypothalamus. The fornix on each side forms the anterior border of the foramen of Monro, which connects the lateral ventricle and the third ventricle. Just behind the foramen is the thalamus bulging into the third ventricle; the hypothalamus can be seen below and anterior to the thalamus with the

optic chiasm in front, the pituitary stalk in the floor, and the mammillary bodies posteriorly. Groups of neurons regulating pituitary function and auto-nomic function reside in the hypothalamus. The third ventricle represents the terminal part of the primitive neural tube and the midline structures such as the thalamus and hypothalamus constitute the *diencephalon*. During development, the cerebral hemispheres arise from vesicles which grow out from the diencephalon and constitute the pro-sencephalon. From these vesicles, the cerebral cortex and *basal ganglia* (caudate nucleus and lentiform nucleus) develop.

Nestling below the posterior end of the corpus callosum is the pineal and below the pineal are the corpora quadrigemina (superior and inferior col-liculi or *tectum* of the midbrain). The aqueduct of Sylvius lies posteriorly in the midbrain and is surrounded by grey matter which includes the third and fourth cranial nerve nuclei. Anteriorly in the midbrain are the red nuclei, substantia nigra, part of the reticular formation and the cerebral peduncles through which tracts from the cerebral cortex and internal capsule descend to the pons, medulla and spinal cord.

The narrow *aqueduct* of Sylvius passes through the midbrain and connects the third ventricle to the fourth ventricle. In front of the fourth ventricle and forming its floor is the hind brain, consisting of the *pons* and the more caudally placed *medulla*. Cranial nerve nuclei are situated in the grey matter of the floor of the fourth ventricle whereas the ascending and descending tracts run in the more anterior portions of the brain stem. All the cranial nerves, except the fourth nerve, pass out of the anterior surface of the *brain stem* (midbrain, pons and medulla). The cerebellum is an outgrowth of the hind brain and its delicate folial pattern is well demonstrated in sagittal section (Fig. 2.16).

One standard way of examining the internal structures of the cerebral hemispheres is by *coronal section*. In Fig. 2.17, a section through the frontal and temporal lobes reveals the anterior portions of the lateral ventricles flanked laterally by the basal ganglia. The heads of the caudate nuclei are separated from the lentiform nucleus (putamen and

globus pallidus) by the anterior limb of the internal capsule but they are connected by strands of grey matter; it is probably from this 'striped' appearance that the term *corpus striatum* for the basal ganglia is derived. Two large fissures are also seen, each with a major cerebral artery running in its depth. The anterior cerebral arteries run back in the midline just above the corpus callosum in the depths of the sagittal fissure; their branches supply the medial aspects of the hemispheres. Branches of the middle cerebral arteries fan out from the lateral (Sylvian) fissures on to the surface of the brain to supply the lateral aspects of the cerebral hemispheres. Branches from arteries of the circle of Willis at the base of the brain and from the major cerebral arteries perforate the brain and supply the central structures of the hemispheres.

An *enlarged coronal section* of the hemispheres taken through a more posterior plane (Fig. 2.18) shows the fornices in the midline suspended from the corpus callosum. Choroid plexus is seen within each lateral ventricle and the caudate nucleus on both sides is still present although it becomes smaller as it passes backward through the brain. Some of the major nuclear divisions of the thalamus

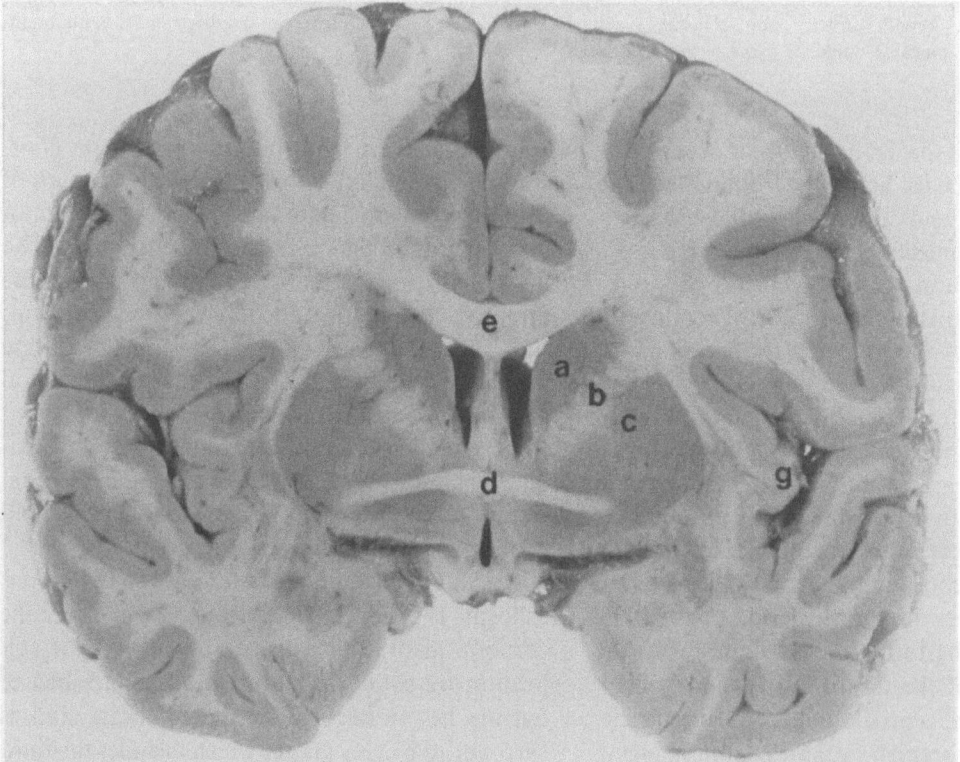

Fig. 2.17. Normal brain: coronal section. *a*, head of caudate nucleus; *b*, internal capsule (anterior, limb); *c*, lentiform nucleus (putamen laterally, globus pallidus medially); *d*, anterior commissure; *e*, corpus callosum; *g*, insula in depth of lateral fissure.

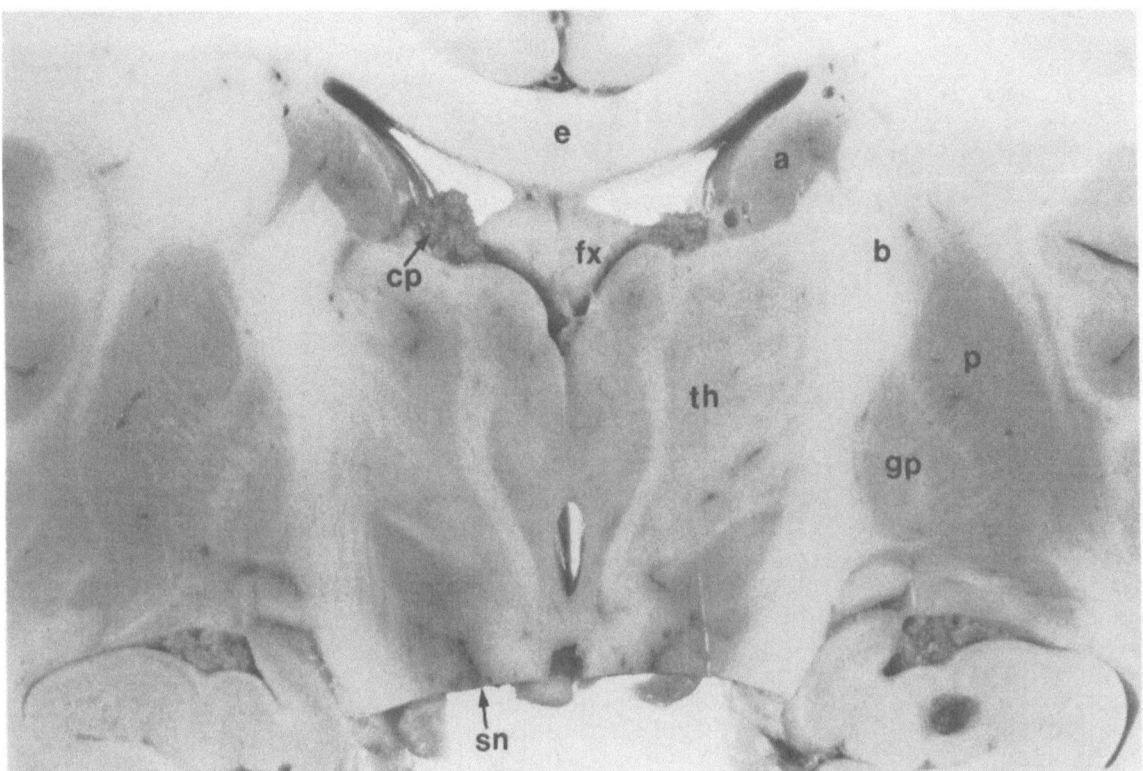

Fig. 2.18. Normal brain cut in coronal plane through the thalamic region. *a*, caudate nucleus; *b*, internal capsule; *cp*, choroid plexus in lateral ventricle; *e*, corpus callosum; *fx*, fornix; *gp*, globus pallidus; *p*, putamen; *sn*, substantia nigra in amputated midbrain; *th*, thalamus.

can be discerned; the mammillothalamic tract is prominent as it terminates in a well-demarcated anterior thalamic nucleus. Subthalamic nuclei, including a fragment of the substantia nigra, are separated from the lentiform nuclei by the internal capsule which enters the cerebral peduncles below.

With the widespread use of computerised axial tomography (CT scans), an understanding of the anatomical arrangements of cerebral structures in the *horizontal plane* has become more important (Fig. 2.19). In many ways, it is easier to visualise brain structures in this plane as there is a more extensive view of the ventricles, basal ganglia, thalamus and internal capsule. The lentiform nucleus actually appears as a 'lens-shaped' structure in this plane, and the *V*-shape of the internal capsule with its anterior and posterior limbs and genu can be appreciated.

Anatomy of the spinal cord

The spinal cord in man is approximately 45 cm long; it extends from the first cervical vertebra to the second lumbar vertebra and is attached at its lower end by the filum terminale to the first coccygeal segment of the spine. Enclosed in a dural sleeve, the spinal cord and cauda equina are covered by a thin layer of arachnoid. Although the cord tends to taper towards its lower end, it has two noticeable expansions, one in the cervical region and the other in the lumbosacral region; both are related to innervation of the limbs. The cervical enlargement extends from C3 to T2 with a maximum circumference of approximately 38 mm at C6. In the lumbosacral region, the enlargement of the cord extends from L1 to S3; thereafter the cord rapidly dwindles in size to form the conus medullaris.

The *anterior surface* of the cord can be recognised by the presence of a single longitudinal anterior spinal artery and by the discrete anterior roots arising from each segment of the cord. On the *posterior surface*, there is a plexus of tortuous veins particularly on the lower part of the cord; the two major posterior spinal arteries are less prominent than the anterior spinal artery. The posterior spinal roots are inserted as multiple rootlets into the dorsal

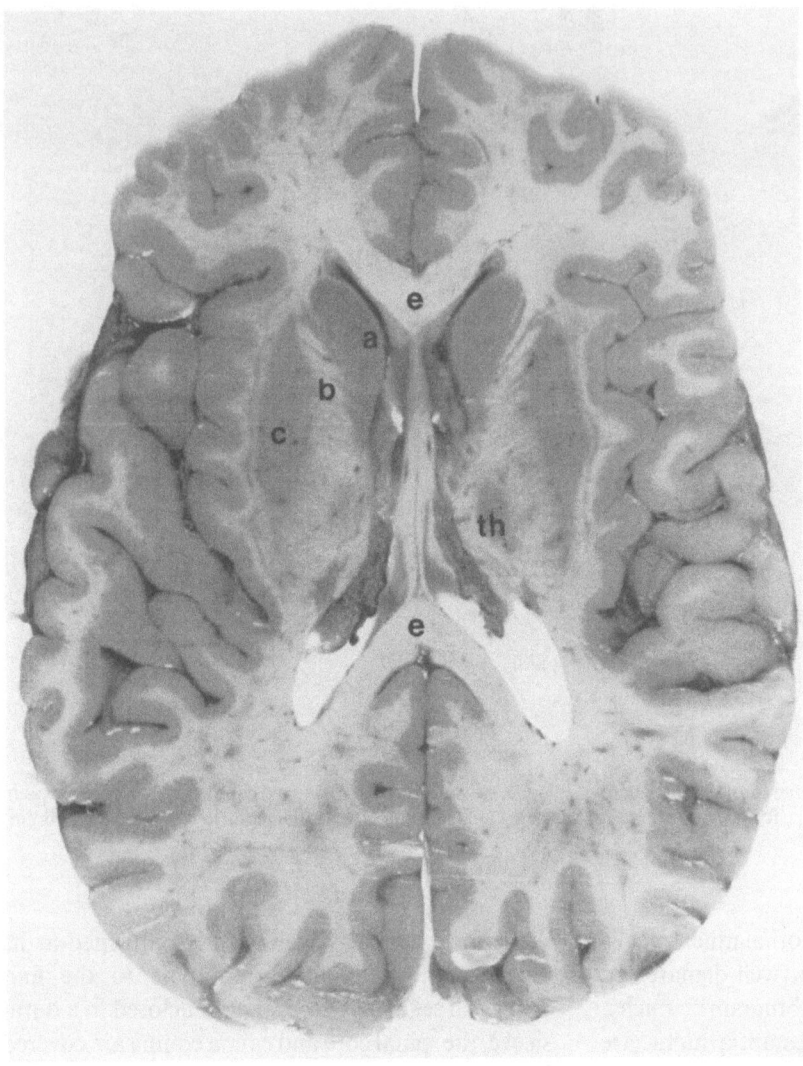

Fig. 2.19. Normal brain cut in horizontal plane. *a*, caudate nucleus; *b*, internal capsule; *c*, lentiform nucleus; *e*, corpus callosum; *th*, thalamus (superior extremity).

aspect of the spinal cord. In the cervical region, they form a continuous line of insertion down to the first thoracic root. The latter is the lowest large dorsal root of the cervical enlargement and can thus be used as an anatomical landmark for the first thoracic segment of the cord. As the spinal cord is shorter than the spine, the neural segments are not at the same level as the corresponding bony segments. For example, in the cervical region the C6 spinal vertebra is opposite C7 cord segment. In the upper thoracic region, the cord is two segments lower than its corresponding vertebral level, whereas in the lower thoracic region the cord is three segments lower than its vertebral level, e.g. T11 spinal vertebra is opposite the third lumbar cord segment. An appreciation of such an anatomical arrangement may be important when assessing spinal injuries.

When the spinal cord is cut in *cross-section*, the *H*-shaped central grey matter is seen to vary in size and shape according to the level at which the cord is sectioned. The *dorsal horns* of grey matter are enlarged in the cervical and lumbosacral regions in association with the numerous sensory fibres entering the cord from the arms and legs. Enlargement of the ventral horns of grey matter in the cervical and lumbosacral regions is even more marked due to the large number of anterior horn cells supplying muscles in the limbs. *Anterior horn cells* are grouped in longitudinal columns within the cord; the more medial groups extend throughout the length of the cord and innervate axial muscles. The lateral group of anterior horn cells innervate limb muscles and so they are only prominent in the cervical and lumbosacral enlargements. Within the lateral group of anterior horn cells, the more distal limb muscles are innervated by the more dorsally disposed anterior horn cells (Fig. 2.20). Within

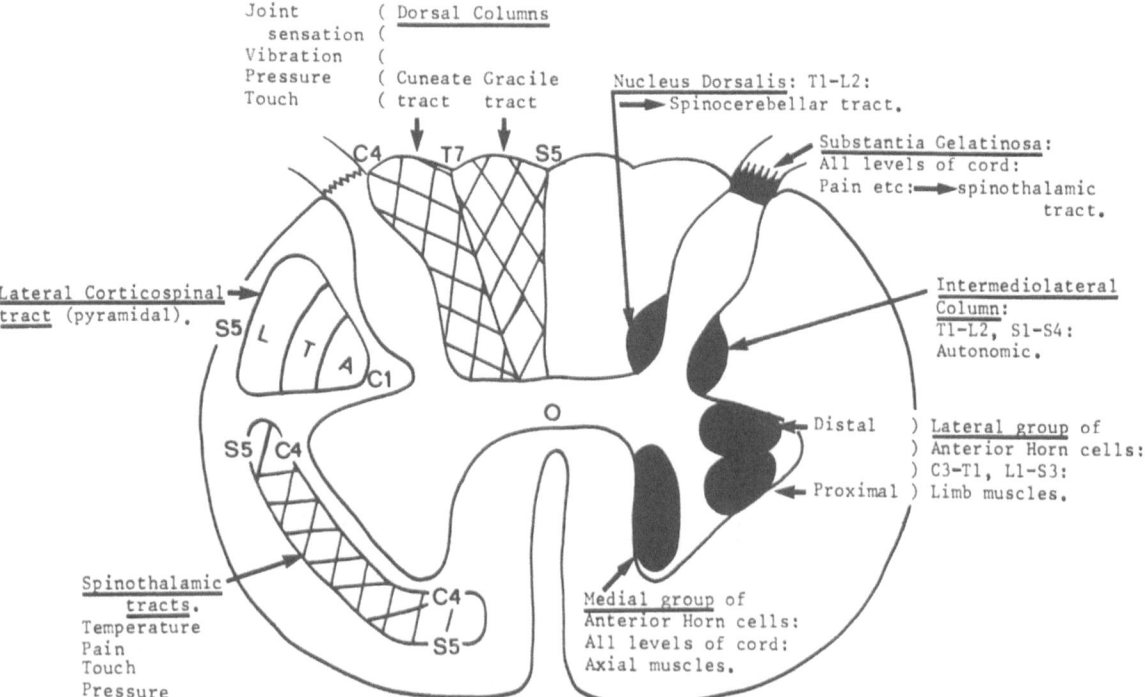

Fig. 2.20. Spinal cord. Diagram to show the main anatomical arrangement of neuronal groups (columns) in the anterior horns of grey matter (*right of figure*) and of fibres within long, white matter tracts (*left of figure*). Lateral corticospinal tract: fibres to leg (*L*), trunk (*T*) and arm (*A*). Dorsal columns: joint sensation here includes some input from muscle spindles. The anterior corticospinal tracts, spinocerebellar tracts and other ascending pathways have been omitted from the diagram.

these columns of anterior horn cells, the neurons innervating individual muscles are in discrete groups arranged longitudinally within the cord.

Anterior horn motor neurons receive *connections* from many neural pathways. For example there are direct monosynaptic terminals from proprioceptive dorsal roots in the same or neighbouring segments in addition to connections through interneurons in the dorsal horn. A few direct monosynaptic terminals from the vestibulospinal and corticospinal tracts also end on the anterior horn cells, but these connections are mainly mediated through interneurons within the central grey matter.

Two other prominent columns of neurons are seen in the grey matter on each side of the cord. The *intermediolateral column* extends from C8 to L3 and from S2 to S4; this group of neurons contains preganglionic, *autonomic* neurons, which are sympathetic in the thoracic region and parasympathetic in the sacral region. The other column is the *nucleus dorsalis of Clarke* (Clarke's column) which extends from C8 to L3–4; neurons in this column send axons to the spinocerebellar tracts.

The *white matter* of the cord progressively increases in bulk from the sacral to cervical regions.

Fibres from the dorsal roots associated with joint sensation, vibration, pressure and touch, enter the dorsal columns and are pushed medially by fibres entering at segments higher up the cord. Thus the *gracile tracts* carry fibres from segments S5 to T7 and the *cuneate tracts* contain mainly fibres entering the cord in the cervical region. There is considerable anatomical and functional subdivision in the *spinothalamic tracts* (Fig. 2.20) in which the fibres associated with temperature, pain, touch and pressure from the lower parts of the opposite side of the body are more superficially placed than those arising from the cervical region. A similar disposition is seen in the *lateral corticospinal tracts*, in which the fibres supplying motor neurons innervating the arm muscles are sited medially, whereas the fibres destined for the sacral region are placed more laterally. It is thought that descending fibres associated with higher control of *bladder* function are also in the lateral white matter of the cord just in front of the lateral corticospinal tracts. Ascending fibres associated with bladder function are probably in the more superficial part of the lateral white matter columns.

The *blood supply* of the spinal cord is derived

from longitudinal anastomosing vessels on the anterior and posterior aspects of the cord. There is a single anterior spinal artery which receives branches from the intercostal and lumbar arteries; they reach the anterior spinal artery along the anterior roots. Large contributions to the anterior spinal artery are derived from the vertebral arteries above, and large radicular arteries in the lower cervical and lower thoracic regions. Branches of the anterior spinal artery penetrate the central regions of the spinal cord and supply some two-thirds of the cord including the anterior horns of grey matter. A corona of vessels derived from the posterior spinal arteries supplies the superficial parts of the cord through penetrating branches.

Basic neuroanatomy from the study of brain evolution

The general concept of the organisation of the human brain is most easily understood from a study of its phylogenetic development. It is upon this general plan that a more detailed understanding of the functional anatomy can be built.

In *primitive chordates* there is segmental innervation; intersegmental tracts then develop and the medulla at the front end of the spinal cord develops as a co-ordination centre. From a very early stage in the evolution of the vertebrate nervous system there is crossing of long tracts. It has been suggested that when there is an insult to the front of the body on one side, the crossed long tracts enable the animal to take rapid evasive action by contracting the muscles on the other side of the body.

From the primitive neural tube of the chordate nervous system, the vertebrate brain has developed above and in front of the medulla with the interposition of co-ordination and association centres between the sensory input and the motor outflow tracts. In can further be said that most of the evolution of the vertebrate brain has been due to enlargement of *dorsal* areas of grey matter associated with the primary somatic functions of *smell*, *vision* and *balance*. Ventral areas of grey matter, such as the medulla and the hypothalamus, which contain visceral co-ordination centres, have, on the other hand, remained comparatively small.

It is thought that in the early stages of evolution of the vertebrate brain, the *hind brain* acted as a co-ordination centre between the sensory input from the spinal cord and its motor activity; the *cerebel-*

lum developed on the dorsal aspect of the hind brain as a co-ordination centre important for balance (Fig. 2.21a). Further forward, the *midbrain* became the main visual centre with the enlargement of the tectum (superior colliculi) in the dorsal aspect of the midbrain. At the front of the brain, just behind the olfactory bulbs, the *cerebral hemispheres* developed as outgrowths of the forebrain and were initially concerned with smell.

The first steps in the progressive forward translocation of co-ordinating centres were taken in *lower vertebrates* when the *tectum* became a dominant co-ordinating centre (Fig. 2.21b) receiving connections from the cerebellum (balance), from the eye (vision) and from the cerebral hemispheres (smell). At a later stage, co-ordination of motor function was partially taken over by the *corpus striatum* (basal ganglia) in the centre of the cerebral hemispheres (Fig. 2.21c); this region thus received information from the spinal cord, cerebellum and tectum through the thalamus, and directly from the primitive olfactory cerebrum. The forward progression of the co-ordinating centres to the *cerebral cortex* eventually reaches its peak in mammals as sensory inputs from the spinal cord, cerebellum and tectum are relayed by the thalamus to the cerebral cortex (Fig. 2.21d). Motor fibres passing from the cerebral cortex through the corticospinal tracts to anterior horn cells in the spinal cord play an important part in voluntary movement, particularly in fine discriminatory movements of the digits. Similar motor connections are made with the brain stem nuclei. Despite the forward progression of the control centres in the brain, many patterns of movement probably continue to be generated in the phylogenetically older structures of the spinal cord and midbrain under the modifying influence of the basal ganglia and descending bulbospinal pathways. Phylogenetically older parts of the brain also influence the output of the cerebral hemispheres through the action of the reticular formation.

In addition to the alterations in basic structure of the brain that have taken place during vertebrate evolution, changes have also occurred in the later stages of evolution of the human brain which make its anatomy very different from that of non-primate mammals. The change in shape of the brain is due largely to the *differential expansion* of the newer areas of the cerebral hemispheres. Figure 2.22 shows how the tortuous circular pathway of the limbic system, and the strange shape of the caudate nucleus develop in the human brain. Fibres pass from the hippocampus to the hypothalamus by a

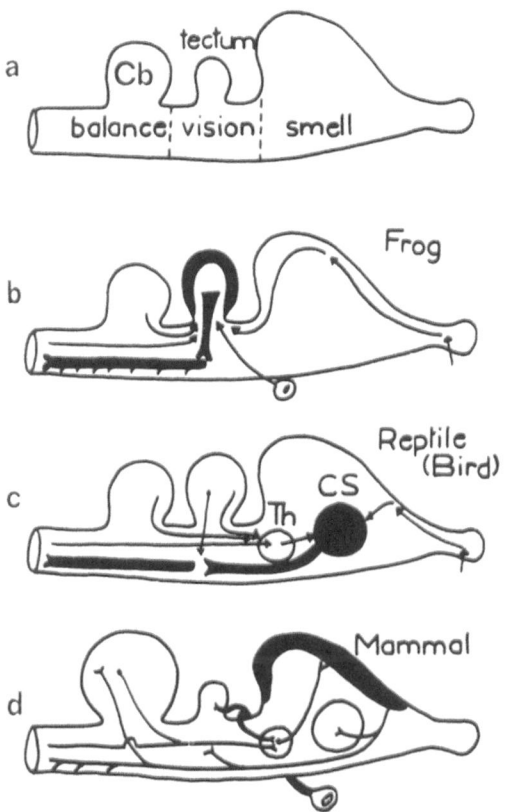

Fig. 2.21. Diagram to show evolution of the vertebrate brain. For explanation see text.
a Primitive organisation. *Cb*, cerebellum
b Frog brain
c Reptile and bird brain. *CS*, corpus striatum or basal ganglia; *Th*, thalamus
d Mammalian brain

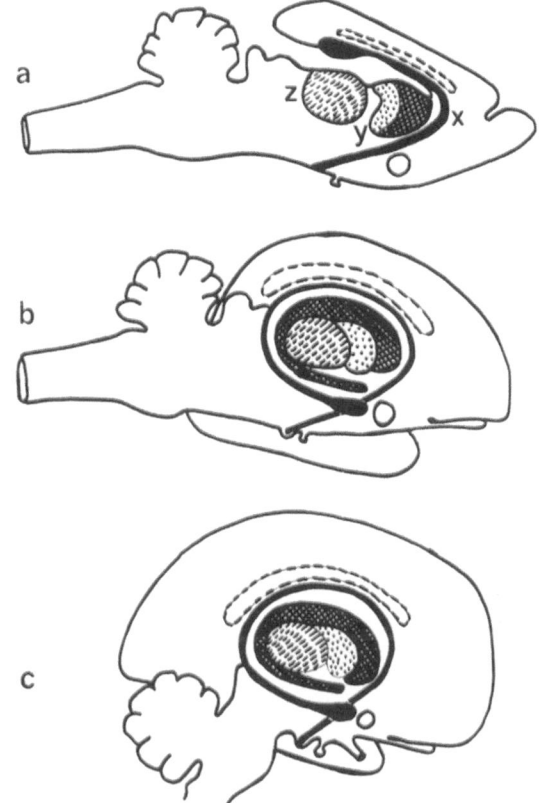

Fig. 2.22. Diagram to show development of limbic system and caudate nucleus in human brain (see text).
a Rodent brain. *x*, fornix connecting hippocampus to hypothalamus; *y*, corpus striatum—future caudate nucleus anteriorly and lentiform nucleus posteriorly; *z*, thalamus.
b Arcuate elongation of fornix and caudate nucleus with enlargement of cerebral hemisphere and development of temporal lobe.
c Rearrangement of brain stem to represent human brain.

comparatively short route in primitive mammalian brains but, as the cerebral hemispheres enlarged during primate evolution, the hippocampus was displaced along a *C*-shaped pathway to become part of the temporal lobe (Figs 2.22b, c). Similarly, the tail of the caudate nucleus became elongated so that the shape of both the hippocampo-hypothalamic tract (fornix) and the caudate nucleus reflects the pathway of migration during phylogenetic development.

Further reading

Brodal A (1981) Neurological anatomy in relation to clinical medicine, 3rd edn. Oxford University Press, Oxford
Cox G (1977) Neuropathological techniques. In: Bancroft J D, Stevens A (eds) Theory and practice of histological techniques. Churchill Livingstone, Edinburgh, London, New York, p 249

Eng L F (1980) Brain-related antigens. In: Thomas D G T, Graham D I (eds) Brain tumours: scientific basis, clinical investigation and current therapy. Butterworths, London, p 109
Iverson L L (1979) The chemistry of the brain. Sci Amer 241:118
Norton W T (1977) Isolation and characterization of myelin. In: Morell P (ed) Myelin. Plenum, New York, p 161
Olsson Y, Kristensson K (1979) Recent application of tracer techniques to neuropathology with particular reference to vascular permeability and axoplasmic flow. In: Smith W T, Cavanagh J B (eds) Recent advances in neuropathology. Churchill Livingstone, Edinburgh, London, New York, p 1
Peters A, Palay S, Webster H de F (1976) The fine structure of the nervous system: the neurons and supporting cells. Saunders, London, Philadelphia
Romer A S (1970) The vertebrate body, 4th edn. Saunders, London, Philadelphia, p 477
Schwartz J H (1980) The transport of substances in nerve cells. Sci Amer 242:122
Sternberger L A (1979) Immunocytochemistry, 2nd edn. Wiley, Chichester, New York
Williams P L, Warwick R (1980) Gray's Anatomy, 36th edn. Churchill Livingstone, Edinburgh, London, New York

Chapter 3

The Interpretation of Neurological Symptoms and Signs

The clinical diagnosis of neurological disease requires a particularly detailed analysis of patients' symptoms. This is partly because the nervous system is a communications system with direct access to consciousness, so that the patient is in a unique position to monitor his own disorder. Clinical diagnosis becomes very difficult in the presence of dysphasia, confusion or dementia. Another reason is that useful biochemical and histological information about the function of neurons is rarely available, in contrast to the wealth of data used in the assessment of diseases of other organs, such as the lungs, liver or kidneys. The failure of neurons in the CNS to regenerate means that delay in making a precise diagnosis can worsen the eventual outcome; the clinician often cannot afford to watch how an illness progresses before intervening.

The clinical diagnosis is established in about four out of five cases on the basis of the patient's history. There are two important components to diagnosis. The *symptoms and signs* help to locate the site of the pathology. The *time course of the symptoms* and the age of the patient suggest the nature of the pathology.

Such information is used to try to place the patient's illness into one of four broad structural groups. The *first* group is the largest and includes focal lesions, such as tumours or the effects of trauma, that damage all the various structural elements in a circumscribed part of the nervous system. The lesions may be single or multiple. The *second* group includes conditions which cause widespread or diffuse pathological changes such as presenile dementia or encephalitis; such processes may be hard to distinguish clinically from the effects of multiple discrete lesions. The *third* group comprises system disorders such as motor neuron disease or parkinsonism, in which the damage is confined to specific neuronal systems that traverse a number of different anatomical regions of the brain and intermingle with unaffected structures. The *fourth* group includes conditions secondary to systemic disorders, such as toxaemia, biochemical disorders, or cardiac failure, in which there is usually no structural abnormality of the nervous system.

This chapter briefly reviews those aspects of clinical diagnosis that are of special relevance to the pathologist and indicates the areas in which the clinician is likely to be mistaken.

Clinical localisation of brain disorders

Focal lesions

A focal lesion in the brain gives rise to appropriate focal signs if a region with a clearly defined function is damaged. For example, a lesion of the motor cortex causes paralysis of voluntary movement in the appropriate limb. The impairment of function may be due to destruction of normal tissue, in which case function is permanently lost. Some loss of function may be due to potentially reversible factors such as oedema, distortion, raised intracranial pressure or ischaemia, which can affect a larger volume of brain tissue than the provoking lesion itself.

By distorting intracranial structures, a mass can produce signs of impaired function in areas some distance away. One example of this is the temporal lobe tumour that causes herniation of the parahippo-campal gyrus on the medial aspect of the temporal lobe through the opening in the tentorium cerebelli (transtentorial herniation; see Chap. 4) compressing the third cranial nerve and causing diplopia. A second example is the deficit caused by cerebral arterial spasm following subarachnoid haemorrhage. Focal neurological deficit after subarachnoid haemorrhage is more often due to cerebral ischaemia than to haematoma and the part of the brain affected by vasospasm may be some distance away from the site of the haemorrhage, or even in a different vascular territory.

The time course of the development of symptoms helps to distinguish infarction or haemorrhage (sudden onset) from neoplasia (gradual onset). Infective lesions such as an abscess are usually accompanied by systemic signs of infection. Degenerative diseases usually run an insidious course. The age of the patient helps to restrict the possible diagnosis in a particular case; cranial arteritis, for example, is virtually unknown under the age of 55 years.

Synopsis of regional functions in the cerebral hemispheres

Impaired function on one side of the body is generally due to a lesion in the contralateral cerebral hemisphere, especially if the face is also involved. Formal loss of power with 'upper motor neuron' signs in lesions of motor cortex, and profound sensory loss in lesions of sensory cortex are usually easy to diagnose and will not be elaborated here, except to point out that homonymous hemianopia due to a lesion of the contralateral optic radiations or visual cortex is often undetected by the patient provided macular vision is spared. Even with a complete homonymous hemianopia, the patient may notice only that he keeps colliding with objects on one side.

Frontal lobe syndromes

Lesions of the frontal lobe are associated with changes in personality, usually in the direction of disinhibition, euphoria, increased appetite and lack of foresight and judgement. Sometimes a frontal lobe tumour presents as progressive dementia without other focal symptoms; careful assessment supported by psychometric testing may identify circumscribed functions that are normal, casting doubt on the diagnosis of a generalised degenerative process. Dementia is further discussed in Chap. 15. Features suggesting parkinsonism may further complicate the clinical picture and presumably result from the combined effects of destruction of the frontal lobes and distortion of the premotor cortex and its connections with the basal ganglia. Damage to the hypothalamus may disrupt temperature control, either increase or abolish the appetite and give rise to various metabolic disturbances, notably hyponatraemia.

Temporal lobe syndromes

Unilateral lesions of the temporal lobe, especially of the non-dominant temporal lobe, often produce little clinical deficit apart from epilepsy. Speech functions are vulnerable in dominant temporal lobe lesions and *bilateral* lesions may have catastrophic effects upon memory. The cerebral localisation of *speech* is complex. There are two principal areas: Wernicke's area 40 in the supramarginal gyrus and Broca's area 44 in the posterior part of the frontal lobe near the Sylvian fissure. The arcuate fibres connecting these areas run through the dominant temporal lobe.

Wernicke's area is the principal receptive station for speech, processing the input from auditory and visual association areas of the cortex of both hemispheres. Focal lesions here cause dyslexia and receptive dysphasia in which the patient cannot understand speech and his spontaneous speech is plentiful but jumbled and full of paraphasic errors. Focal lesions in Broca's area impair the patient's spoken speech and writing, but comprehension of written and spoken speech is retained. In practice, most patients have a mixture of *receptive* and *expressive* dysphasia that reflects the location and extent of their particular lesion.

Parietal lobe syndrome

The non-dominant parietal lobe is specifically concerned with the appreciation of three-dimensional space. If it is damaged the patient may lose his way, even in his own house. Concepts of personal space and shape are lost so that he is unable to draw and cannot complete constructional tasks or dress himself.

Association areas: agnosia

Damage to cortical association areas responsible for the interpretation of primary sensation produces subtle but disabling effects that may never-

theless be quite impossible for a clinician to detect if the patient is confused, dysphasic or demented. *Agnosia* is the failure to interpret the meaning of sensation when threshold stimuli can be shown to reach consciousness. Sensory input may be ignored by consciousness when a similar input is concurrently presented to the normal side; this is referred to as *sensory inattention* or *suppression* and occurs when sensory association areas or projections to them are damaged. The clinician may specify precisely the deficit that is present by the use of related terms such as *astereognosis*; more detailed clinical texts should be consulted for further discussion of this intriguing subject.

Visual agnosia is due to damage to association areas of the visual cortex and is rarely detected in practice, provided that the other occipital lobe retains its connections with the speech centres in the dominant temporal lobe.

Thalamic syndrome

Sensory loss combined with painful dysaesthesiae and spontaneous pain in the appropriate region of the body constitutes the *thalamic pain syndrome*; it results from damage to the sensory nuclei of the thalamus. The commonest cause is a stroke which also causes an upper motor neuron lesion; the history and the motor signs help to differentiate such sensory disturbances from those of painful peripheral neuropathies.

Apraxia

Apraxia is most simply regarded as a motor disorder equivalent to agnosia. Movements cannot be performed in response to stimuli that would normally evoke them, even though there is no formal motor or sensory loss and the patient is alert, comprehends normally and is motivated to respond. Frequently the patient is observed to achieve parts of the movements, or even the whole movement spontaneously, which confirms that the failure to respond to appropriate stimuli is not due to paralysis. Apraxia can result from damage to motor association areas. *Dressing apraxia* is a term used by some clinicians to indicate difficulty in dressing in patients in whom non-dominant parietal lobe lesions cause loss of three-dimensional comprehension; this is really a form of agnosia. Apraxia is seen also in lesions of the speech centres or of the connections between Broca's area and the motor association cortex, which prevent the translation of linguistic ideation into movement.

Silent areas

Certain sites in the brain have been termed clinically 'silent areas' in which an enlarging mass may declare itself only by raising the intracranial pressure. These so-called silent areas are reviewed in more detail in relation to tumours in Chap. 7. They are the non-dominant temporal lobe, the corpus callosum, the frontal lobes, the thalamus, the pineal region, the vermis of the cerebellum and the third ventricle. These are important parts of the brain with well-defined functions, but even careful clinical technique may fail to demonstrate any neurological deficit.

Disorders of the cerebellum and basal ganglia

A number of symptoms help to localise a lesion in the basal ganglia or cerebellum and their connections.

Ataxia

Ataxia denotes poor co-ordination due to inappropriate timing and intensity of muscle activation associated with damage to the ipsilateral cerebellar hemisphere or its connections. Lesions of the vermis may greatly impair balance in the standing position and give rise to ataxia of the trunk which is out of proportion to the ataxia seen in the limbs once the trunk is supported on a couch.

Intention tremor is an irregular tremor, particularly affecting the postural muscles of the limb; it is accentuated whenever precise movements are attempted and is also a feature of damage to the ipsilateral cerebellar hemisphere or its connections. When the superior cerebellar peduncle or its crossed projection to the thalamus is damaged, the intention tremor is often very severe and ballistic in character.

Nystagmus occurs when the cerebellum and particularly the pathways between the cerebellum and the oculomotor nuclei are damaged. It is seen also in lesions of the vestibular pathways and their connections to the oculomotor nuclei.

Parkinsonism

Bilateral resting or postural tremor, cog-wheel rigidity, chorea and athetosis are usually due to degenerative conditions affecting specific neuronal pathways. When such symptoms are entirely *unilateral*, however, a focal lesion may be present in the contralateral basal ganglia. Parkinsonism is a syndrome of which the pathognomonic clinical feature is bradykinesia. In most cases some or all of the other features of the syndrome are also present, namely rigidity, resting or postural tremor, a flexed posture and disordered autonomic control of sebum secretion and blood pressure. Clinically, idiopathic parkinsonism is often unilateral in its early stages. In postencephalitic parkinsonism, postural and autonomic disorders tend to be prominent and there may be signs of impaired upper motor neuron, cerebellar or intellectual function. A reversible form of parkinsonism may be caused by phenothiazine drugs that interrupt dopaminergic transmission. Parkinsonism appears to be associated with disinhibition of cholinergic neurons in the corpus striatum which eventually project to the thalamus. Such disinhibition is usually caused by damage to the inhibitory dopaminergic pathways from the substantia nigra, putamen and globus pallidus.

Chorea, athetosis and ballism

Chorea and athetosis are particularly associated with damage to the contralateral caudate nucleus and putamen. Clinically and pharmacologically these movements are the reverse of parkinsonism.

The term *chorea* is applied to involuntary, rapid, irregular jerking movements that are usually of small amplitude and may resemble fidgeting or tics. The latter movements are characterised by their repetitive and stereotyped form, whereas chorea produces many different rapid movements occurring at random in the limbs, trunk or face. Sometimes chorea is mistaken for tremor, which is stereotyped and regularly repeated, or for myoclonus, which is stereotyped, irregular and tends to occur synchronously in more than one limb. The term 'choreiform movement' is rarely used by neurologists and it usually indicates that the clinician is uncertain of his categorisation.

Athetosis is a more writhing, prolonged, involuntary movement, often accompanied by intermittent dystonia (see below), and also by chorea. The term 'chorea-athetosis' denotes a combination of chorea and athetosis. Chorea confined to the face, lips and tongue is referred to as *orofacial dyskinesia* and is usually caused, paradoxically, by prolonged treatment with phenothiazine drugs. Dopaminergic drugs used to treat parkinsonism may produce temporary chorea which may, in this instance, coexist with the refractory signs of the patient's parkinsonism.

Ballism or ballistic involuntary movements of large amplitude affecting proximal segments of the limb (often in practice accompanied by dystonic posturing and fragments of athetosis) classically result from damage to the contralateral sub-thalamic nucleus.

Other tremors

Tremors at rest (resting tremor) or on attempting to maintain the position of a limb (postural or action tremor) occur not only in parkinsonism but also in a number of ill-understood degenerative conditions, notably in familial or idiopathic tremor, which are discussed further in Chap. 14. *Asterixis* or 'flap' is an irregular and variable form of action tremor associated with metabolic disturbances such as hepatic failure and hypercapnia rather than with structural brain disease. Intention tremor is discussed above, under the heading of ataxia, with which it is clinically associated.

Abnormalities of muscle tone

Traditionally, increased muscle tone is categorised as either rigidity or spasticity. *Rigidity* is associated with basal ganglia disease and *spasticity* with lesions of upper motor neuron pathways in the hemisphere, brain stem or spinal cord. In some patients, particularly when both pyramidal and extra-pyramidal systems are involved, muscle tone may not be easy to characterise clinically. In this case the posture adopted by the patient is often helpful in diagnosis and this is discussed below in the section on coma.

One of the most severe extrapyramidal diseases is *dystonia musculorum deformans* or torsion dystonia, in which there may be powerful co-contraction of antagonistic muscle groups in a limb. This leads to severe postural deformities that may be associated with bizarre tremors or involuntary movements resembling athetosis. In general, the degree of disability in extrapyramidal diseases correlates rather poorly with the amount of visible neuronal destruction in the basal ganglia. This dissociation is most remarkable in torsion dystonia, in which the brain usually appears normal at autopsy.

Therapeutic lesions

Lesions in the ventrolateral nucleus of the thalamus, produced either intentionally by stereotactic surgery or fortuitously by disease, may prevent or abolish the expression of chorea, athetosis, most forms of tremor and ballistic movements in the contralateral limbs. The fact that a second lesion can abolish the worst clinical consequences of a primary lesion may partly explain the poor correlation between the extent of the pathological findings and the severity of clinical disability in extrapyramidal disease.

Clinical effects of lesions of the midbrain, pons and medulla

Brain stem lesions usually produce a combination of deficits due to interruption of tracts passing through the brain stem and disruption of cranial nerve nuclei. Disorders of individual cranial nerve functions help to locate the level of the lesion. In addition, there is usually bilateral impairment of sensory and motor function, including cerebellar function, in the limbs.

Lesions in the *midbrain* often cause double vision by disrupting conjugate eye movements and may impair control of the pupils. Lesions in the *pons* affect facial movement and hearing. Cerebellar signs are prominent and there may be pupillary constriction. Respiration may become irregular or 'central neurogenic hyperventilation' may occur, lowering the arterial pCO_2 and inducing cerebral vasoconstriction. Damage to the *medulla* may cause hiccup, vomiting, dizziness, yawning, and disturbance of speaking and swallowing mechanisms (dysarthria and dysphagia). It may also interrupt vasomotor and respiratory mechanisms and be responsible for death by causing arterial hypotension and respiratory arrest.

Involvement of the *reticular formation* reduces the level of consciousness and coma is usual in acute focal lesions of the midbrain and pons, whether or not intracranial pressure is raised. The patterns of brain stem dysfunction associated with coma are discussed in more detail below.

Interaction between focal and generalised effects of intracranial lesions

The foregoing account of the localisation of clinical disorders is greatly simplified. In a particular case, the clinical features may be confusing or appear contradictory, but experience does help to identify those features likely to be of greatest pathological significance.

Certain symptom complexes reflect the interaction between different pathological processes going on simultaneously within the skull and they will be considered in this section. They are alteration in the state of consciousness, epilepsy, headache and raised intracranial pressure.

Altered states of consciousness

Discussion of this subject is complicated by the mixture of lay and technical terms that tend to be used idiosyncratically by different clinicians. The terminology used here is adopted from the monograph by Plum and Posner (1980).

In assessing a patient's state of consciousness, a crucial distinction is made between his state of arousal and the content of his consciousness. Broadly speaking, the *state of arousal* is determined by the midbrain reticular formation and its projections to the cerebral hemispheres, provided that the cerebral cortex itself has not been damaged so extensively that no evidence of consciousness can be detected. The *content of consciousness* may diminish and become distorted when arousal is reduced, but in normal states of wakefulness the content of consciousness can indicate the site of dysfunction in the cerebral hemispheres.

Behaviour and the mental state can be distorted by psychological factors but the borderline between normal and abnormal here is empirical. Certain patterns of abnormality in the content of consciousness are aggregated into psychiatric syndromes such as *schizophrenia* or *mania*, identified empirically as recurring patterns of symptoms with a restricted range of presentation and natural history. Localised organic disease of the brain sometimes causes similar disturbances, but the established psychiatric syndromes are sufficiently coherent to enable experienced psychiatrists to identify patients suffering from organic diseases of the cerebral hemispheres.

Assessment is made more difficult when the patient is in a state of psychic withdrawal resembling a disorder of arousal. A further difficulty for the clinician is that metabolic disturbances and drugs can act differentially upon the level of arousal and the content of consciousness. Electroencephalography (EEG) can be very helpful in determining whether a patient has structural or metabolic disease.

States of arousal

The terms commonly used to describe the state of consciousness are normal, confusion, delirium, stupor and coma. *Delirium* differs from the other terms in that it refers more to the content of consciousness than to the state of arousal. Delirium implies disorientation, fear, irritability and usually hallucinations; it can be defined as a state of disordered mentation associated with clouding of consciousness. The state of arousal may be increased or diminished. In dementia, arousal is unimpaired.

Stupor is unresponsiveness from which the patient can be aroused by vigorous stimulation. In *coma*, there is no sign of consciousness even in response to sensory stimuli.

Lesions of the cerebral hemispheres do not cause serious impairment of arousal unless they are very large, multiple or diffuse; in practice such lesions are nearly always due to head injury or hypoxia. In patients with coma, lesions are found much more commonly in the posterior basal diencephalon or the adjacent midbrain as far caudal as the mid pons. There may, of course, be lesions in both of these parts of the brain and it may be possible for the clinician to demonstrate this by careful examination.

Coma produced by supratentorial lesions

Raised intracranial pressure alone is seldom sufficient to impair consciousness until levels approaching the diastolic blood pressure are reached. Coma from supratentorial masses is caused by damage to the reticular midbrain structures associated with downward compression of the diencephalon and the adjoining midbrain through the tentorial opening. Two clinical and pathological patterns are recognised. The first is central herniation in which displacement of the brain stem occurs in a more or less caudal direction (Chap. 4). The second occurs with herniation of the uncus and parahippocampal gyrus of the temporal lobe, which is pushed medially and downwards over the medial edge of the tentorium by an expanding lesion in the temporal lobe or in the adjacent frontal or parietal lobes. When this happens the midbrain is pushed against the opposite edge of the tentorial opening compressing the contralateral third nerve and the ipsilateral posterior cerebral artery.

Central transtentorial herniation tends to give rise to a characteristic clinical sequence of events.

After a period of increasing confusion, the level of arousal falls. Respiration is interrupted by deep sighs or yawning, and may become periodic ('Cheyne–Stokes respiration'). The pupils become constricted and the patient passes into stupor. Conjugate eye movements can still be demonstrated at this stage. Usually the limbs contralateral to the expanding lesion show increased muscle tone but later increased tone is found in all four limbs and both plantar responses become extensor. At this stage 'decorticate posturing' can be demonstrated in response to painful stimuli. The *'decorticate posture'* consists of flexion and adduction of the arm, wrist and fingers, with extension, plantar flexion and internal rotation of the lower limb. It indicates dysfunction at a level higher than the internal capsule or rostral cerebral peduncle. As the process of central herniation continues, this gives way to the *'decerebrate posture'* characterised by opisthotonos, clenching of the teeth and extension, adduction and hyperpronation of the arms with stronger extension and plantar flexion of the lower limbs. The decerebrate posture is usually due to lesions in the midbrain. At this stage the pupils enlarge, conjugate eye movements and corneal reflexes are lost and the respiration becomes faster and deeper—'central neurogenic hyperventilation'. As the effects of brain stem compression spread to involve the lower pons and medulla, respiration becomes rapid, shallow and irregular. The limbs become flaccid, the pupils return to near normal size but do not react to light, and finally, respiration and blood pressure fail and brain stem death occurs.

Uncal and parahippocampal gyral herniation produces a sequence of clinical changes that in the early stages differs from the effects of central herniation. The ipsilateral pupil enlarges and responds sluggishly to light. This sign may be present for some time before further progression occurs, but once the pupil fully dilates and a full third nerve palsy develops, deterioration is often very rapid. The patient lapses into coma over the course of a few hours and because the uncus has compressed the cerebral peduncle against the opposite edge of the tentorium, hemiplegia may develop in the limbs ipsilateral to the expanding lesion. From this stage deterioration proceeds as in central herniation.

Coma from subtentorial expanding lesions is usually preceded by headache, meningism and signs of lower brain stem dysfunction.

To some extent the time course of these events reflects the rate at which herniation is occurring; it is accelerated considerably if the escape of CSF from the lateral ventricles is obstructed. An exceedingly rapid progression from the early signs of herniation to death may occur in a sudden, large intracerebral haemorrhage, or after ill-timed lumbar puncture.

Coma caused by metabolic disorders is not usually accompanied by focal neurological deficits. All functions in the hemispheres and brain stem are depressed concurrently. Rarely, the developing sequence of signs seen in central tentorial herniation may occur, including 'decerebration', but these signs are reversed when the metabolic disturbance is corrected. Hepatic coma is a well-documented example.

Abnormally increased alertness: the 'diencephalic syndrome'

Rarely, lesions in the midline diencephalon can cause increased arousal and alertness even when other evidence suggests that intracranial pressure is raised. This apparently paradoxical combination is usually seen in children, suggesting that the clinical effects of such lesions partly reflect the stage of maturation of the brain.

Discrepancies between apparent state of arousal and content of consciousness

Once the pathological process causing coma has ceased to progress, some recovery in the state of arousal often occurs. Usually it is easy to assess the content of consciousness, but there are three well-delineated syndromes in which there is a discrepancy between the apparent state of arousal and the content of consciousness.

The locked-in syndrome

The motor and sensory tracts connecting the limbs to the cerebral hemispheres pass through the brain stem and if they are damaged by a lesion in the central portion of the lower pons, all voluntary movement apart from blinking and vertical eye movement may be lost, although consciousness remains relatively undisturbed. This condition has been designated the 'locked-in' syndrome. The precise level and content of consciousness is difficult to ascertain and varies from patient to patient. Nevertheless, some patients have been able to communicate using a type of morse code, and in a few cases complex mental activity may be possible.

Akinetic mutism and persistent vegetative state

Brain stem function may recover in a patient in whom the projections from the reticular formation to the cortex, or the cerebral cortex itself, have been destroyed. Under these circumstances, the eyes may open and appear to follow objects in the room, giving the spurious impression that consciousness has returned.

In *akinetic mutism*, the cortex is substantially intact; the patient retains cycles of 'sleep' and 'wakefulness', giving the appearance of vigilance but making little or no noise or movement. Clinical examination shows little or no evidence of damage to descending motor pathways. In their examination of the causes of this syndrome, Plum and Posner concluded that

> Akinetic mutism can arise early in the course of three types of lesions, all of which largely interfere with reticular-cortical integration but largely spare corticospinal pathways: subacute communicating hydrocephalus; large, bilateral, basal-medial, frontal lobe lesions involving the orbital complex, septal area, and cingulate gyri; and tiny (and probably incomplete) lesions interrupting the reticular formation of the posterior diencephalon and adjacent mid brain.

The *persistent vegetative state* is a condition in which the patient is motionless and shows no evidence of any conscious activity over a period of many weeks or months. This syndrome is usually due to widespread cortical damage from head injury or hypoxia and implies that consciousness has been irretrievably lost. The term 'persistent vegetative state' delineates the prognosis without making claims as to the precise underlying pathology.

Epilepsy

According to its aetiology, epilepsy is classified into *idiopathic* and *secondary* forms. Uncomplicated idiopathic or 'primary generalised' epilepsy is not associated with pathological abnormalities. This type of epilepsy is regarded as a constitutional variant and its clinical expression is grand mal; in children true petit mal may occur also. These attacks occur without warning and display no focal features.

Focal epilepsy is almost always due to focal pathology in the cerebral hemisphere though the lesion may be very small and in most cases is not progressive. Lesions of the inferior surface of the temporal lobes and the frontal lobes are much more likely to cause epilepsy than lesions of the occipital pole, which is the least 'epileptogenic' area of the cerebral cortex. The commonest clinical variety of focal epilepsy is temporal lobe epilepsy, possibly because the hippocampus is particularly sensitive to hypoxic damage in the neonate. Such damage may occur during the process of birth. If the neonate has idiopathic epilepsy, focal hippocampal damage may also occur as a result of hypoxia during a grand mal seizure in the neonatal period and the child then grows up with clinical and electroencephalographic evidence of a combination of idiopathic and focal, temporal lobe epilepsy.

The clinical features of an epileptic attack arising from a focus may help to locate the focus. The classic *Jacksonian* attack due to a focus in the hand area in the motor cortex starts with twitching in the thumb which gradually spreads to involve the whole limb and culminates in a generalised convulsion. *Temporal* lobe attacks are well-known phenomena because of the bizarre auras that may occur. The *aura* is the part of the attack that the patient can remember (or thinks he can remember) afterwards. Olfactory hallucinations, distortion of vision and hearing, *déjà vu* sensations and compulsive visions may occur. Attacks deriving from a *parietal* lobe may be ushered in by sensory hallucinations in which part of the body seems to develop a bizarre shape or posture; when the *occipital* cortex is involved visual hallucinations may occur. These phenomena are by no means invariable in focal epilepsy. A clinical attack may consist only of the aura, or the combination of aura and generalised convulsion, or may mimic a grand mal attack. Some clinicians refer to all minor attacks in which generalised convulsions have not occurred as 'petit mal' but in adults such transient episodes are, of course, minor focal attacks. Even when the attack itself has no distinguishing focal features, transient abnormalities during the phase of recovery after the convulsion can betray its focal origin. Thus, a transient hemiparesis ('Todd's paresis') is strong evidence for a focal lesion in the contralateral hemisphere; aggressive behaviour during recovery suggests a temporal lobe focus, and so on.

A number of physiological events occur during grand mal seizures that may provoke pathological changes in the brain. The part of the brain involved in the paroxysmal activity shows a great increase in its metabolic rate, accentuating the effects of any pre-existing hypoxia or metabolic disorder. At the same time, the consumption of oxygen declines in areas of the hemisphere not involved in the paroxysmal activity. A number of autonomic changes occur, notably hypertension and tachycardia. But prolonged attacks may cause severe hypotension, thus adding the effects of impaired perfusion to those of hypoxia. Such changes are particularly likely to occur when cerebral vascular autoregulation is impaired, when intracerebral pressure is raised, or when fever has raised the metabolic rate of the brain, as in encephalitis.

There are a few rare forms of epilepsy such as myoclonic epilepsy that are sometimes due to specific degenerative conditions, especially in childhood. Physiological evidence suggests that many cases of myoclonic epilepsy are associated with abnormalities of the brain stem reticular formation.

Finally, and of importance to both clinician and pathologist, generalised seizures may be provoked by a variety of metabolic disorders, notably hypoglycaemia, hypocalcaemia, hyponatraemia and hepatic or renal failure.

Pathological implications

From the pathologist's point of view, the occurrence of epilepsy should lead to the identification of a focal lesion if the attacks were focal, or if a focus was found on the electroencephalogram. Static or slowly progressive lesions of the temporal or frontal cortex are particularly liable to cause epilepsy. Epilepsy starting after the age of 25 years is more likely to be due to acquired or progressive disease. Non-focal attacks could be due to a systemic toxic or metabolic disorder. Prolonged seizures and status epilepticus may be accompanied by hypoxia and under-perfusion of the brain, possible accentuating the effects of the primary pathology and causing further pathological changes such as loss of neurons from the hippocampus (Ammon's Horn sclerosis or mesial temporal sclerosis) and the cerebellum.

Headache

Contrary to popular belief, headache is an unhelpful symptom in the diagnosis of most intracranial lesions. The proximal portions of the intracranial vessels and the venous sinuses are the usual source of intracranial pain. Pain arising in supratentorial structures is referred to the eyes, forehead or temple. Pain produced by distortion of meninges and blood vessels of the posterior fossa is referred to the C2 dermatomes, running backwards from the vertex of the skull to the top of the neck.

Headache associated with raised intracranial pressure is classically worse on waking up in the morning and tends to ease off after the patient has been up and about for a few hours. It is accentuated by coughing, stooping or straining, presumably because the rise in venous pressure is transmitted to the intracranial vessels. Associated symptoms of confusion, drowsiness or vomiting are often present.

Raised intracranial pressure

The sequence of events in herniation through the tentorial opening is described above in the section on coma. A mass lesion causes intracranial pressure to rise when enlargement of the mass can no longer be accommodated by the expulsion of CSF. The open skull sutures of the neonate and the atrophied brain of the elderly subject may delay the time at which such decompensation occurs. Lesions in the posterior fossa cause intracranial pressure to rise at a much earlier stage of their development than do supratentorial lesions, because they obstruct the free egress of CSF from the ventricular system. The only clinical sign of chronically raised intracranial pressure may be progressive visual failure, due to optic nerve ischaemia, of which the patient is often unaware. Clinical assessment of patients with acutely raised intracranial pressure can be very difficult because evidence that would help to localise the cause may be obscured by the effects of transtentorial herniation, notably confusion and drowsiness.

Raised intracranial pressure is accompanied by reflex arterial hypertension which maintains perfusion of the brain with blood. The normal autoregulation of the cerebral circulation may become disturbed in such circumstances, so that a modest fall in arterial blood pressure gives rise to severe cerebral ischaemia or infarction. An increase in the metabolic demands of the tissue, by pyrexia or epileptic seizures, also increases the risk of infarction.

In summary, both the clinical and the pathological consequences of a focal lesion of the brain may crucially be altered by the patient's general condition and in particular by impairment of respiratory or circulatory function, by the development of metabolic disorders, by epilepsy and by raised intracranial pressure.

Spinal cord lesions

Correlation of clinical and pathological findings in disease of the spinal cord is easier than in diseases of the brain. A space-occupying lesion in the spinal canal often causes signs of dysfunction of nerve roots at about the same level. When there are no root signs as a guide, the lesion may be located several segments higher than the signs of cord dysfunction suggest.

Extrinsic lesions

The first symptoms of an extrinsic lesion compressing the spinal cord are weakness and clumsiness of the legs. Weakness of hip flexion and of dorsiflexion of the feet are typical features. Signs and symptoms of an upper motor neuron disturbance (weakness, brisk tendon reflexes and spasticity) spread proximally as the lesion enlarges. The symptoms are normally bilateral. Bladder control is usually affected at a late stage, a fact of some interest since the thinly myelinated descending tracts subserving voluntary control are located close to the lateral corticospinal tracts. Sensory deficits, usually in the form of sensory loss, appear later and are always more mild than the motor deficits until paraplegia is severe. Autonomic dysfunction, apart from sphincter control, is rarely symptomatic.

Intrinsic lesions

An enlarging, space-occupying, intrinsic lesion of the spinal cord classically evolves in a different way from an extrinsic lesion. If the anterior horns of the grey matter are involved, the muscles innervated by that segment show signs of denervation, namely weakness, wasting and fasciculation. The spinothalamic tract fibres subserving pain and temperature sensation decussate at or near the segment of their entry into the cord, and are therefore damaged at an early stage; upper motor neuron signs in the legs do not develop until later. When the lesion is confined to one side of the cord and extends into the ipsilateral dorsal columns mediating light touch and proprioception, these modalities, together with motor function and autonomic function, are impaired below the lesion on the same side of the body, while pain and temperature sensation is lost below the lesion on the opposite side of the body (Brown–Séquard syndrome). Intrinsic lesions are more likely than extrinsic lesions to produce pain or paraesthesiae. Paraesthesiae are spontaneously arising inappropriate sensations, usually likened to feelings of warmth or pins and needles and they are referred to the parts of the body served by the damaged fibres.

Damage to spinocerebellar tracts might be expected to produce cerebellar ataxia, but in practice ataxia is rarely prominent in diseases that are restricted to the spinal cord. A disorder of movement that superficially resembles cerebellar ataxia can occur if proprioceptive input is lost. Such 'sensory ataxia' is dramatically accentuated when the patient closes his eyes, because this removes the visual information necessary to monitor the position of the limbs.

Romberg introduced the clinical test of asking a patient to stand upright and close his eyes. Patients with impaired proprioception who fall over when their eyes are shut are said to 'show Rombergism' or to have a 'positive Romberg sign'.

Pain

In contrast to its poor localising value in intracerebral disease, pain is a useful localising sign in spinal cord disease, especially when it has a squeezing, girdle-like quality. This generally indicates damage to the posterior columns or nerve roots at that segmental level. Intrinsic or extrinsic lesions, especially in the cervical cord, where most movement occurs, may be associated with *Lhermitte's sign*. Lhermitte's sign is a symptom consisting of a sudden shooting, tingling, shock-like sensation running down the centre of the back into the legs on voluntary flexion of the neck. It was originally described as a helpful sign in multiple sclerosis, which it is, but it occurs also in other inflammatory or space-occupying lesions affecting the posterior columns in the cervical spinal cord. Burning pain may be an intractable feature of some patients with partial spinothalamic tract lesions.

Radiology

Plain radiographs of the spine can show bone erosion, collapse, spondylosis, listhesis and abnormalities of the disc spaces. Calcification or the outline of a soft-tissue paraspinal mass may be seen and the anteroposterior diameter of the bony spinal canal can be assessed. A myelogram is mandatory when space-occupying or compressive lesions of the spinal cord or spinal nerve roots are suspected. Water-soluble contrast material injected into the subarachnoid space not only allows the identification of various areas of expansion or compression of the cord but also helps to delineate the meningeal root pockets and sometimes the roots themselves as they pass across the spinal canal.

Peripheral nerve disease

Diseases of the peripheral nerve are characterised by muscle weakness and wasting, disturbance or loss of sensation especially distally in the limbs, and occasionally autonomic disturbances according to which groups of neurons or nerve fibres are involved. A more detailed account of the various types of neuropathy is given in Chap. 16.

The symptoms and signs of peripheral nerve disease can be used to place the patient's condition in four overlapping classifications. The *first* of these is based upon the regional distribution of the disorder, that is whether lesions are located distally, proximally or diffusely. *Second*, the anatomical pattern of the disorder can be classified as generalised polyneuropathy, polyradiculopathy, mononeuritis multiplex or mononeuritis. *Third*, the type of fibre predominantly involved can be deduced from the modalities of function that have been affected. Further investigation (particularly electromyography) may be needed to confirm this. *Fourth*, the time course of the neuropathy designates it as acute, subacute, chronic, relapsing or progressive. The predominant pathological changes can be identified by electromyography followed by biopsy, distinguishing segmental demyelination from axonal degeneration.

Symptoms

The symptoms of peripheral neuropathy depend upon the population of nerve fibres affected. Characteristically the symptoms and signs are worse distally than proximally and this can help in distinguishing a neuropathy from a myopathy.

Motor symptoms

The motor symptoms are weakness and wasting; foot drop is an early sign and if the hands are affected the patient may first become aware of his neuropathy while dressing or handling keys or tools. Fasciculation may be seen in muscles close to the skin, particularly the calf muscles, quadriceps, biceps and deltoid muscles, and especially if the neuropathy is advancing fairly rapidly. Fasciculation is due to denervation hypersensitivity of recently denervated motor units which fire spontaneously. When the muscle has been subject to concurrent denervation and re-innervation, some of the re-innervating motor units are larger than normal. If they subsequently become denervated

their fasciculations may appear particularly prominent. Fasciculation is often difficult to detect in peripheral neuropathies, but is a particular feature of anterior horn cell disorders, especially motor neuron disease.

Sensory symptoms

The sensory symptoms of peripheral neuropathy are due mainly to a loss of afferent or incoming impulses in sensory neurons. If the neuropathy is insidious in onset the patient may be unaware of sensory loss until sensation is tested; this applies particularly to the modalities of pain and vibration. By contrast, patients often have symptoms of altered light touch sensation before it can be detected by formal clinical testing. Light touch, proprioception and vibration sense are mediated by rapidly conducting myelinated fibres; the smaller fibres serve pain and temperature sensation and autonomic function. Some pathological processes affect one type of fibre more than the other, so that careful analysis of the modalities of sensation that have been lost can help to narrow the differential diagnosis.

The quality of residual sensation may be abnormal. Usually the abnormal sensation is unpleasant, even painful, so that a piece of cotton wool feels like sandpaper, a cluster of needles or a burning object. This dysaesthetic sensation occurs in the presence of *reduced* input from the periphery. Specifically, there is reduced light touch sensation mediated by rapidly conducting, well-myelinated fibres. Normally, this input is thought to modulate the physiological 'gates' in the spinal cord and midbrain, controlling the transmission of impulses to the thalamus and higher centres in which pain is appreciated. The absence of such modulating activity may thus disinhibit activity in central pain pathways.

Paraesthesiae are sensations, usually likened to 'pins and needles', occurring in the absence of any external stimulus. They may arise acutely, for example as a result of transient ischaemia in a limb, but when chronic and persistent are usually due to peripheral neuropathy. After traumatic lesions of peripheral nerves, movement of the nerve may evoke a barrage of impulses in the sensory fibres, especially when a neuroma has formed at the site of the injury.

Autonomic disturbances

Autonomic dysfunction in peripheral neuropathy is usually asymptomatic. Postural hypotension, tachycardia, impotence, incontinence or retention or urine or faeces, and lack of sweating and piloerection may occur. Denervated skin often looks thin, shiny and hairless and may be prone to excessive trauma because of the absence of pain. These changes are compounded by abnormalities in the blood vessels themselves, as for example in diabetes or collagen diseases, which further delay healing of wounds and predispose to ulceration.

Distribution of symptoms and signs

The differentiation of polyneuropathy from radiculopathy, mononeuritis or mononeuritis multiplex requires a knowledge of basic neuroanatomy. If specific nerve roots are involved the reflexes mediated by them become sluggish or disappear and the appropriate muscles become weak and wasted. The pattern of cutaneous sensory loss is of the greatest help in differentiating lesions of the roots from lesions of the plexuses or peripheral nerves.

Radiculopathies may involve only the anterior (motor) or posterior (sensory) spinal roots. Since the cell bodies of the motor nerves lie in the anterior horn of the grey matter of the cord, a lesion there can produce denervation without causing any disturbance of sensation as, for example, in poliomyelitis. Vascular or neoplastic lesions of the anterior spinal cord cause denervation at that segmental level with signs of cord dysfunction below it. A combination of cord and peripheral nerve signs occur in intervertebral disc disease when local roots become trapped at the level of the cord compression. Upper and lower motor neuron signs coexist in motor neuron disease, in subacute combined degeneration of the cord with peripheral neuropathy due to vitamin B_{12} deficiency and, rarely, in association with intraspinal vascular malformations.

Investigation of peripheral neuropathy

The clinical features outlined above, which are discussed further in Chap. 16, are of considerable help in narrowing the differential diagnosis. In addition, many neuropathies are associated with systemic disease such as diabetes, malabsorption, cancer and collagen diseases. If myopathy cannot be excluded on these grounds, measurement of the serum creatine kinase is helpful for it is normal or only slightly raised in motor neuropathies.

Electromyography

Electromyography is a valuable diagnostic tool and should always be performed before considering muscle or nerve biopsy. Denervated muscle fibres and motor units have electrical characteristics that can be detected by a needle electrode inserted into the muscle; this enables the precise distribution of denervation to be established. It may identify denervation in small areas of muscle, for example in paraspinal muscle, identifying the affected spinal roots. Myotonia and the myopathies create different and distinctive changes in the behaviour of motor unit potentials.

The second type of information provided by electromyography is the maximal conduction velocity in the fibres of a mixed peripheral nerve. Axonal neuropathies often leave some of the fastest conducting fibres undamaged so that there may be little or no change in the recorded conduction velocity. By contrast, in demyelinating neuropathies the fast-conducting fibres are involved, so that the maximal conduction velocity for the peripheral nerve as a whole is reduced. Focal slowing of conduction occurs over regions of segmental demyelination even if conduction is not blocked.

Electromyographic methods can also detect the amplitude and rate of conduction of sensory volleys by measuring the compound action potential induced in the nerve by transcutaneous electrical stimulation. From these data the integrity and range of conduction rates in sensory fibres can be deduced. Evoked potentials can also be detected over the brachial plexus and the cervical spinal cord, thus locating the site of proximal focal nerve lesions.

In certain circumstances, the electromyogram may fail to make a distinction between axonal and demyelinating neuropathy, as when there is gross loss of motor axons which reduces the maximal conduction velocity or abolishes the response to peripheral nerve stimulation. In some neuropathies the motor unit potentials may resemble those found in a myopathy; this is particularly likely to occur in chronic neuropathies such as Charcot–Marie–Tooth syndrome (peroneal muscular atrophy) in which the disorder is only very slowly progressive.

Autonomic system

Autonomic neuropathies may be investigated by careful testing of autonomic functions, notably control of blood pressure, pulse rate, sweating and bladder. This may help to confirm that autonomic failure is due to peripheral nerve disease but it does not provide direct information about pathogenesis. These tests can usually distinguish between preganglionic and postganglionic nerve involvement, and specific involvement of afferent autonomic pathways (as for example from baroreceptors) can be identified by exclusion provided that efferent activity is unimpaired.

Correlation of clinical findings, electromyography and biopsy

In most cases the diagnosis of peripheral neuropathy can be made unequivocally on clinical grounds as described above. Electromyography is useful in further delineating difficult cases and in providing evidence of recovery before it is clinically evident. In some cases nerve biopsy is helpful as an aid to diagnosis and as evidence of the extent of nerve damage.

Formerly, nerve biopsy was required to diagnose metabolic disorders such as metachromatic leukodystrophy, but these conditions can now be diagnosed on the basis of enzymatic tests on blood leukocytes or on skin biopsies (Chap. 13). Amyloid neuropathy is an unusual but important diagnosis that normally requires nerve biopsy. There are some specific and rare disorders of peripheral myelin (discussed in Chap. 16) which have pathognomonic histological appearances, but even in these cases the diagnosis is usually established by careful clinical, electromyographic and biochemical screening. Muscle biopsy is often of more value than nerve biopsy in neuropathies; the uses of nerve and muscle biopsy are discussed further in Chaps. 16 and 17.

Conclusion

Difficulties in clinical diagnosis in the acutely ill patient are most frequently encountered in disorders of the brain. Congenital disorders such as dystrophies and neurogenic muscular atrophies tend to run a much more insidious course but can pose equally difficult dilemmas to the clinician. Detailed clinical information is essential for a realistic interpretation of the pathological findings of autopsy or biopsy. The flow of information prior to biopsy should not, however, be all in one direction. A sound grasp of the principles of clinical diagnosis is valuable to the pathologist in helping the clinician to decide on the best strategy for reaching a diagnosis.

Further reading

Bradley W G (1974) Disorders of peripheral nerves. Blackwell, Oxford, pp 286–290

Lance J W, McLeod J G (1980) A physiological approach to clinical neurology, 3rd edn. Butterworths, London

Mason A S, Swash M (1980) Hutchison's clinical methods, 17th edn. Baillière Tindall, London

Patten J (1977) Neurological differential diagnosis. Harold Starke, London

Plum F, Posner J B (1980) The diagnosis of stupor and coma, 3rd edn. Davis, Philadelphia

Swash M, Schwartz M S (1981) Neuromuscular diseases: a practical approach to diagnosis and management. Springer-Verlag, Berlin Heidelberg New York

Chapter 4

General Pathology of the Central Nervous System

Many parallels can be drawn between pathological reactions in the CNS and those occurring elsewhere in the body. Acute pyogenic and granulomatous *inflammation* are both seen in the brain as in other organs and atherosclerosis affects the cerebral blood vessels as it involves the medium-sized arteries in other parts of the body. Occlusion of arteries will result in *infarction* both in the brain and in systemic organs like the heart and kidney. As in other organs, viruses, bacteria, fungi, protozoan and metazoan parasites, may affect the CNS, although these organisms may show some specificity for the brain or spinal cord. The CNS is a common site for metastatic tumours and both well- and poorly differentiated primary *tumours* occur in the brain. *Metabolic disorders* and *ageing* processes also have well-recognised effects upon CNS structure and function.

Certain problems are inherent in the study of the pathology of the CNS. Lesions in the brain are often difficult to examine as there is no equivalent of the diagnostic laparotomy for lesions in the abdomen and the complications which may accompany cerebral biopsy often inhibit the use of this technique for obtaining a tissue diagnosis. The difficulties in obtaining a pathological diagnosis in many neurological diseases are to some extent reflected by the way in which neurological clinical examinations and electrophysiological investigations, such as EEG and visual evoked responses, have been developed for defining not only the anatomical site of brain lesions but also their possible pathology. Computerised axial tomography (CT scanning) has been especially valuable in this respect.

Two major aspects of the general pathology of the nervous system will be considered here. *First*, the reaction to disease processes shown by each of the individual cell types within the brain, and *second*, the secondary complications of pathological processes in the brain, especially the effects of space-occupying intracranial lesions.

Reactions of brain cells to disease processes

Neurons

Not only are neurons very sensitive to many of the insults that affect the brain but they are also irreplaceable. Except for a brief period in the cerebellum, neurons probably do not proliferate in postnatal life; if a neuron dies it cannot be replaced. Regeneration of neuronal processes in the CNS is poorly understood but it does not appear to be very effective in postnatal human brains. There is, however, some degree of *plasticity* within the brain whereby the territory of influence of lost neurons may be taken over by adjacent neurons terminating in the same area.

Hypoxia

Neurons are very sensitive to hypoxia and certain areas of the brain are more sensitive than others. For example, the pyramidal neurons in Sommer's sector (h_1) of the *hippocampus* (Fig. 4.1), together with the *Purkinje cells of the cerebellum*, are particularly sensitve to hypoxia. Long-standing epileptics, especially if poorly controlled, often show loss of neurons from the hippocampus and from the Purkinje cell layers of the cerebellum. Although less sensitive than the hippocampus, other neurons of the *cerebral cortex* may also be affected by hypoxia; neurons of the brain stem and spinal cord are less susceptible.

The earliest histological changes due to hypoxia can usually be detected in neurons after about 6 h. Affected cells lose their cytoplasmic organelles including the Nissl granules so that hypoxic neurons appear as brightly eosinophilic pink cells with pyknotic shrunken nuclei. Figure 4.2 shows an area of hypoxic hippocampus where some normal neurons remain; they can be distinguished by their normal granular (blue) cytoplasm, vesicular nucleus and prominent nucleolus. *Hypoxic neurons*, on the other hand, have homogeneous, pink cytoplasm and pyknotic nuclei. Rod-shaped microglial nuclei are prominent in this area of damaged brain. Eventually the hypoxic, dead neurons will be phagocytosed by microglia.

Neuronal damage in profound *hypoglycaemia* is similar to that seen in hypoxia; the cerebral cortex and hippocampus are most severely affected.

Axonal degeneration

Axons in the CNS may be damaged because the area through which they pass becomes infarcted, or they may be damaged by an intracerebral haemorrhage. Similarly, axons may be severed by trauma either from direct crushing, as in the spinal cord, or from shearing in the cerebral hemispheres. As tumours invade the white matter and the cortex, axons again may be damaged. The distal ends of axons in the CNS and in the peripheral nervous system may degenerate in toxic neuropathies as part of a 'dying-back' phenomenon (see Chap. 16).

The *sequence of events* following axonal severance in the CNS is expressed diagrammatically in Fig. 4.3. Following axonal transection, the cut ends of both the proximal and distal stumps swell due to the accumulation of neurofibrils, neurotubules, mitochondria and small lamellated lipid droplets (myelin figures). Such swelling probably occurs due to the continuance of axoplasmic flow in both orthograde and retrograde directions. *Axon balloons* such as those shown in Fig. 4.3B may be seen some 3–20 days after injury and may reach sizes in excess of 50 μm in length and 20 μm in diameter (Fig. 4.4). It is from the swellings at the distal ends of the proximal stumps that *regeneration* of fibres occurs in the peripheral nervous system (see Chap. 16) but little, if any, regeneration occurs in the CNS. The distal portion of the severed axon soon degenerates and the axon and myelin debris is phagocytosed by microglia and macrophages (Fig. 4.3C). Degenerating boutons terminaux can be detected in relation to the surface of the target neurons and their dendrites; they are shrunken and densely staining particularly in electron micrographs.

Degenerating axons can be detected histologically within the brain either by silver stains for axons (e.g. Glees and Marsland or Fink and Heimer) or by stains for myelin debris (Oil-Red-O or Marchi techniques (Fig. 4.12)). At a later stage, when all the myelin and axon debris has been removed from the tissue, degenerated tracts may be detected by loss of myelin staining (Fig. 4.5), or by the concentration of oligodendroglial cells which have remained in the tissue following degeneration of their axons. In addition to these features there is often an increase in astrocytes with *gliosis* of the degenerated tracts and an increase in the number of corpora amylacea, particularly in the long spinal tracts.

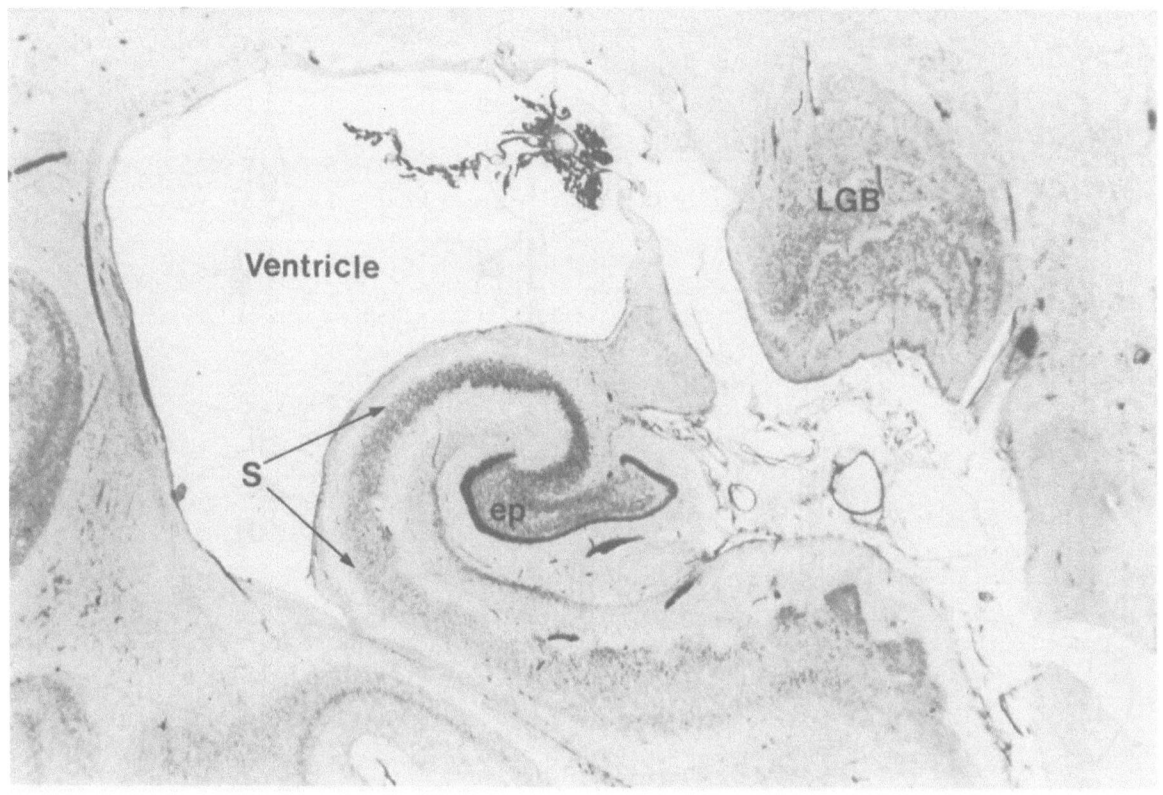

Fig. 4.1. Hippocampus: Sommer's sector (*S*); end plate (*ep*); the subiculum is between them. The hippocampus is divided into several areas: Sommer's sector is h_1, the end plate region is h_4 and h_5; the intervening band of pyramidal neurons is h_2 and h_3. Lateral geniculate body (*LGB*). Nissl stain × 1.5)

Chromatolysis

About 8 days after the axon has been sectioned, the phenomenon of chromatolysis may be seen in the parent neuron. Such changes are more likely if the axon is severed near the cell body. The cell soma swells and becomes almost spherical in shape (Figs. 4.3C, 4.6). The nucleus and nucleolus become eccentric and the clumps of endoplasmic reticulum and polyribosomes (Nissl granules) are no longer stainable in the cytoplasm except perhaps near the edge of the cell. It is this loss of colour from the centre of the swollen neuron that lends its name to the phenomenon of chromatolysis.

Although for many years following the original description of chromatolysis by Nissl in the 1890s this reaction to axonal section was thought to be degenerative in nature, recent studies have shown that there is, in fact, an increase in RNA within the cell and an increase in protein synthesis. It is therefore considered that the chromatolytic reaction is a *regenerative* phenomenon or, at least, is associated with regenerative activity. Soon after the

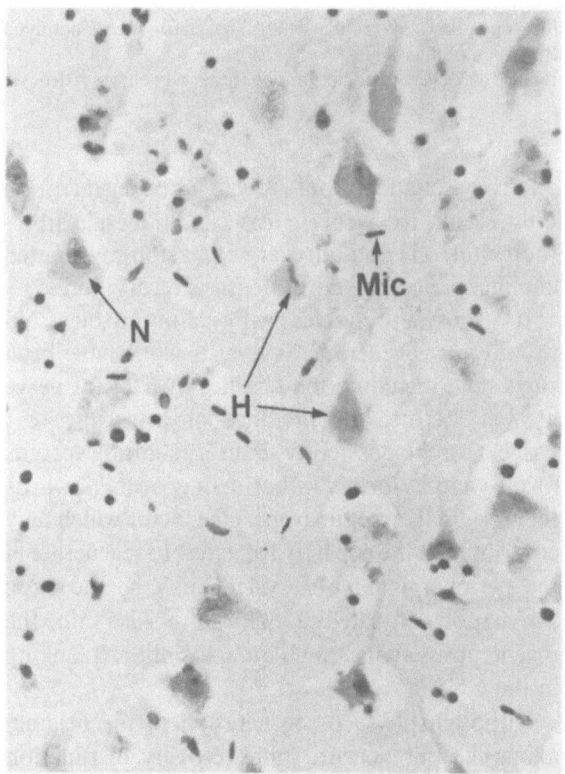

Fig. 4.2 Hippocampus in hypoxic brain. Normal neuron (*N*) and hypoxic neuron (*H*); microglia (*Mic*). (H & E × 300)

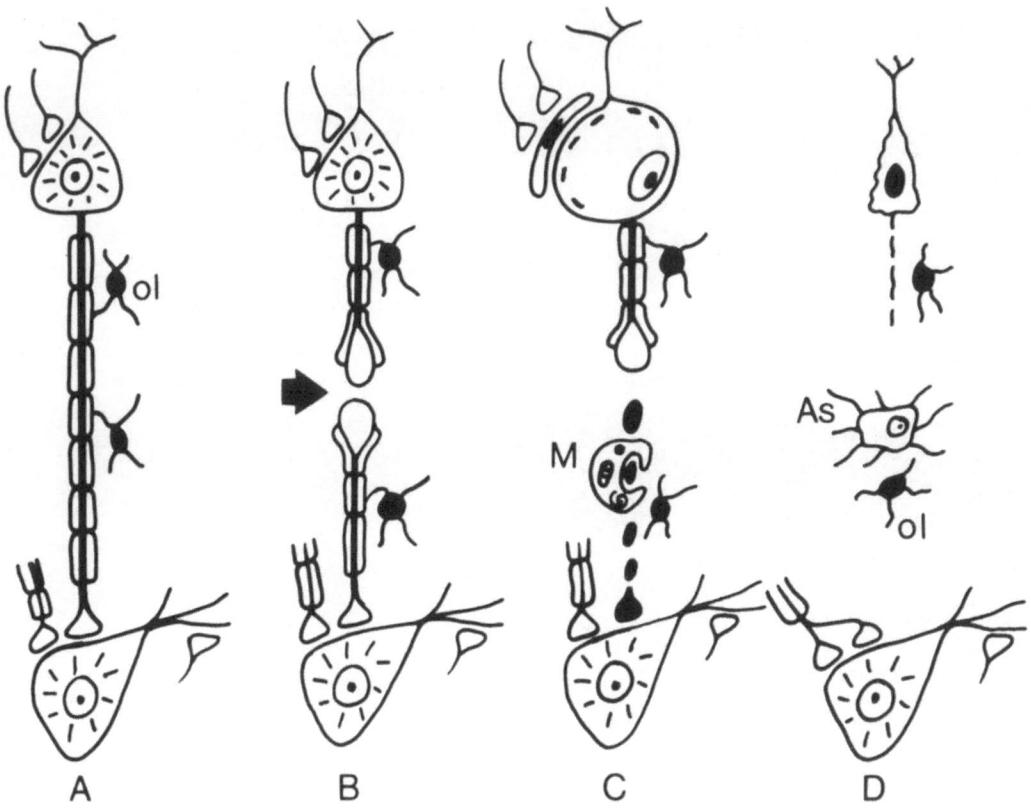

Fig. 4.3. Axonal degeneration in the CNS.
A Normal neuron. Oligodendrocyte (*ol*).
B Severed axon (*arrow*) with proximal and distal axon balloons.
C Fragmentation and phagocytosis of distal axon (axonal or wallerian degeneration). Macrophage (*M*). The neuron is chromatolytic and nerve terminals have been removed from its surface by the interposition of microglia.
D Failure of regeneration. Sprouts from adjacent terminal axons may replace the degenerated boutons on the target neuron. Astrocyte (*AS*).

axon is severed, afferent boutons terminaux become separated from the cell body surface by the interposition of microglial cells; the neuron is, in effect, deafferented.

Regeneration within the CNS is for the most part ineffective and the fate of the parent neurons is variable. It is known that in some cases the neurons eventually die and disappear and, in certain specific tracts like the visual pathways, the target neurons also degenerate. It is probable, however, that some neurons remain as deafferented cells.

Regeneration and recovery of function

Partial recovery of function following an intracerebral haemorrhage, cerebral infarct, or spinal cord injury, may be mainly due to the subsidence of oedema in the surrounding tracts. For, despite early axonal sprouting and regeneration of the CNS, growth in the majority of

axons ceases after about 2 weeks. True regeneration only seems to occur in catecholaminergic fibres (dopaminergic and adrenergic), in non-myelinated cholinergic axons and in neurosecretory fibres.

It is not entirely clear why axons in the CNS should not regenerate. Several reasons have been suggested, including the absence of relevant nerve growth factors, the presence of astrocytic scar tissue, and the possibility that regenerating sprouts form synapses locally rather than growing towards their original target neurons. One factor which may contribute to the capacity for axons to regenerate in the peripheral nervous system may be the close association of satellite Schwann cells with the regenerating axons. Such an association is lacking in the CNS.

Although physical regeneration of the original axons may not occur, some recovery of function may continue to appear in neurologically damaged patients for some time after the initial insult. An

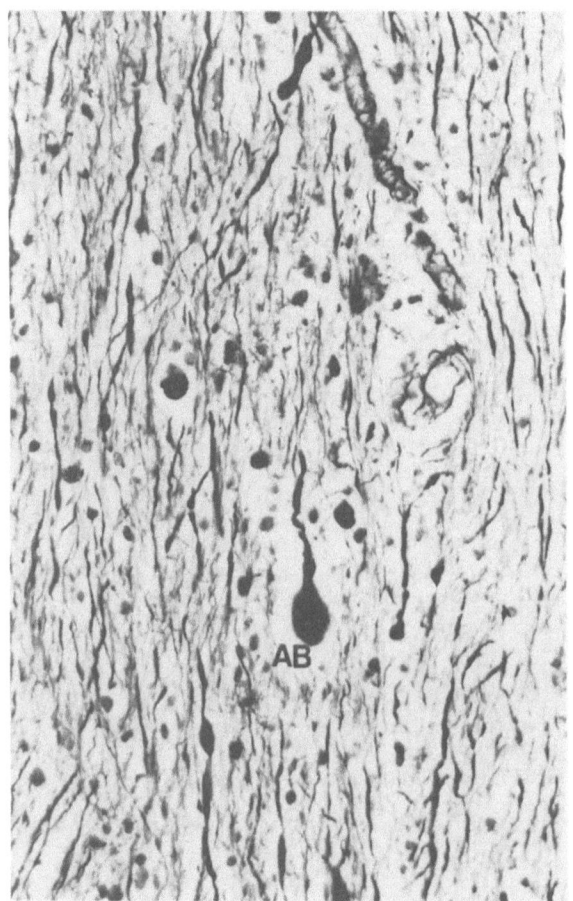

Fig. 4.4. Axon balloon (*AB*) in corpus callosum 5 days after the axon was damaged in a severe head injury. (Palmgren silver method × 300)

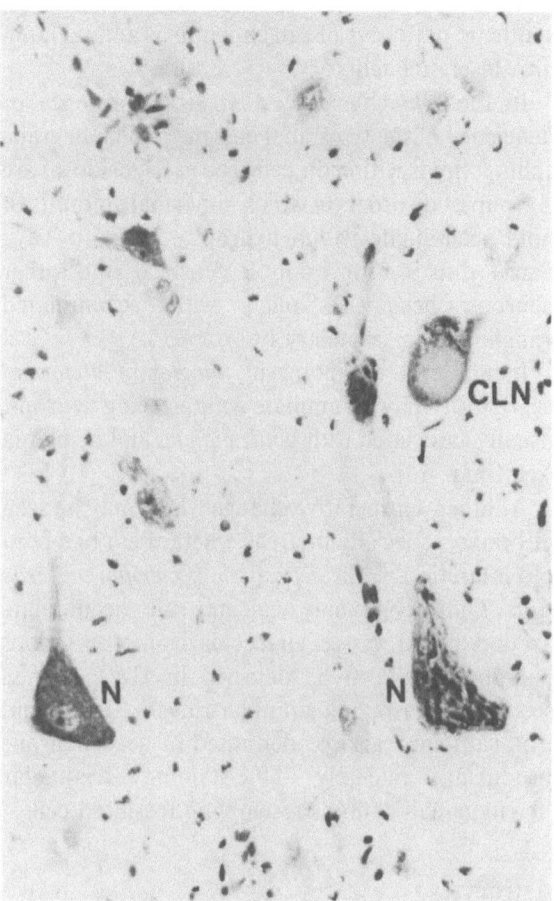

Fig. 4.6. Normal neurons (*N*), chromatolytic neuron (*CLN*). (Nissl stain of spinal cord × 300)

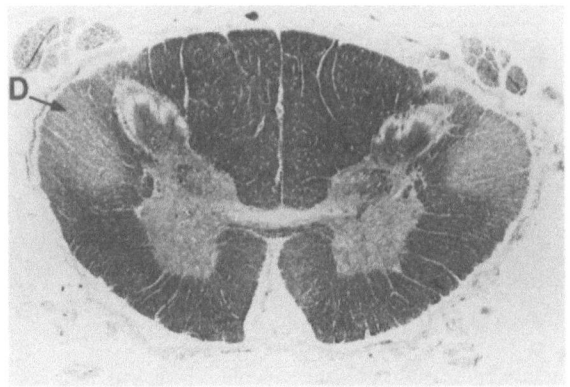

Fig. 4.5. Spinal cord in motor neuron disease showing loss of myelin staining in degenerate lateral corticospinal tracts (*D*). (Luxol-fast blue × 20)

important concept of *plasticity* has arisen from experiments in animals and may account for much of the adaptation that occurs following brain damage. It has been shown that when a target neuron becomes deafferented, or innervation is prevented, intact neurons innervating either those target neurons or adjacent neurons, form new contacts with the denervated neurons. In this way the receptive surface of the target neurons may again be covered by boutons terminaux (Fig. 4.3D).

Ageing and degenerative changes in neurons

In common with many long lived cells, neurons accumulate lipofuscin in their cytoplasm during life so that in older people brown-staining, PAS-positive, lipid-rich *lipofuscin* granules may be seen within the cytoplasm of many neurons throughout the brain. Electron microscopically, the secondary lysosomal nature of lipofuscin may be seen both in human neurons and in animal neurons. These granules are, in effect, waste products that accumulate throughout the life of the cell, and in some cases the accumulated material is quite specific. For example, in the substantia nigra and locus coeruleus, two dopaminergic nuclei in the brain, melanin accumulates within the cytoplasm of the neurons probably as a waste product, as the synthetic pathways of catecholamines and melanin are closely related.

In the *sphingolipidoses* there is an absence or deficiency of the lysosomal enzymes which degrade sphingolipids within the cell. The gangliosidoses are a group of disorders in which abnormal amounts of lipid accumulate within neurons so that in Tay–Sachs disease, for example, cortical and other neurons become swollen with accumulated ganglioside in secondary lysosomes.

In addition to lipofuscin, *tangles of abnormal neurofibrils* may accumulate within ageing neurons, usually associated with *senile plaques* and dementia (see Chap. 15).

Another degenerative change which may be seen in brains, especially in areas where there has been old infarction, is the *deposition of calcium and iron salts*. Quite commonly, calcium salts accumulate around blood vessels, particularly in the globus pallidus; they can be detected in H & E-stained sections as basophilic granular rings. Calcium and iron salts may also be deposited in dead neurons producing intensely blue-staining triangular 'ferruginated' neurons resembling fossilised cells.

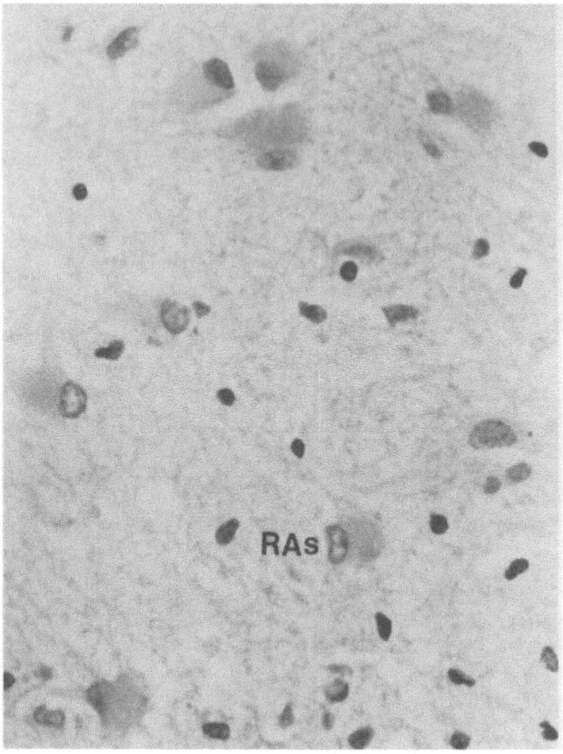

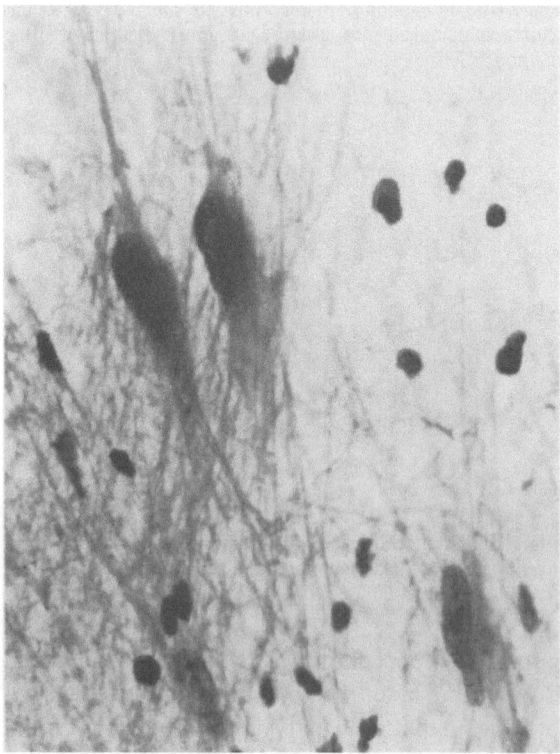

Fig. 4.7. Reactive astrocytes (*RAs*). (H & E × 530)

Astrocytes

One of the major roles of astrocytes in the normal brain appears to be the regulation of fluid and electrolytes in the extracellular space. In some diseases, particularly liver disease, astrocytes may be the first cells in the brain to show histological changes with enlargement, lobulation and pallor of nuclei (Alzheimer type 2 cells).

When there is *tissue damage* in the brain due, for example, to infarction or trauma, astrocytes in the surrounding tissue proliferate and then become enlarged or hypertrophic. Such *reactive astrocytes* can be detected in sections stained with H & E (Fig. 4.7) by their abundance of paranuclear cytoplasm and by their eccentric nuclei. When isolated in smear preparations (Fig. 4.8), the large number of fine processes extending from a reactive astrocyte can be seen. Similarly, astrocyte processes can be stained in paraffin sections by the Holzer technique and by PTAH, or in frozen sections by the Cajal technique (Fig. 4.9). One of the changes that occurs during this reactive phase is the appearance of large numbers of 9-nm glial fibrillary acidic protein (GFAP) fibrils within the cytoplasm; the GFAP nature of these fibrils can be verified by

Fig. 4.8. Reactive astrocytes in a smear preparation. (Toluidine blue × 700)

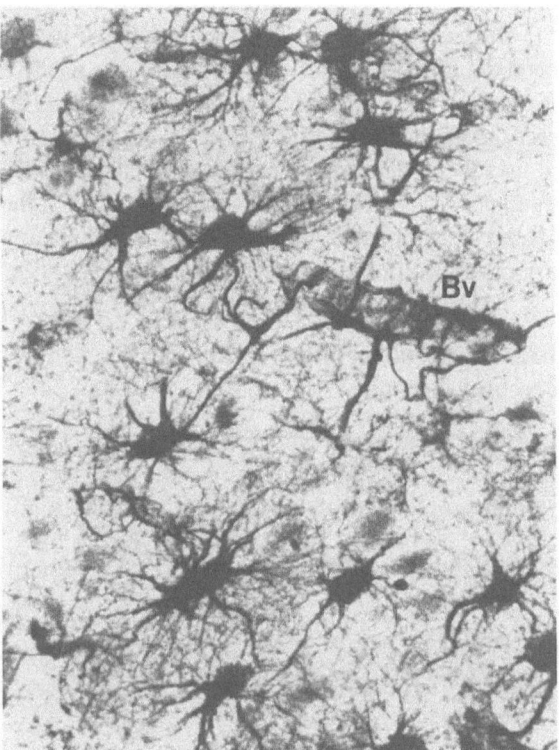

Fig. 4.9. Reactive astrocytes with long processes extending to blood vessels (*Bv*). (Cajal × 410) (*cf.* Fig. 2.10)

immunoperoxidase or by immunofluorescence techniques (Fig. 2.11). Glial scars formed around old infarcts, in areas of old trauma or in old multiple sclerosis plaques, are composed of a multitude of astrocytes and their processes containing GFAP.

The role of astrocytes in regulating the fluid, electrolyte, and protein balance of the extracellular space in the brain is particularly well demonstrated following brain damage when astrocytes imbibe fluid and protein from the extracellular compartment. The uptake of serum proteins extravasated from the blood can be detected in reactive astrocytes and a similar uptake can be seen in tumour astrocytes in the intact tissue and in culture. The imbibed protein appears to collect within lysosomes and is thus probably degraded by the astrocytes. *Corpora amylacea* also accumulate in areas of long-standing brain tissue damage; they are basophilic circular bodies which are probably derived or excreted from astrocytes.

Microglia

Microglia are uncommon and difficult to detect in H&E sections of normal brain but they may be visualised by silver techniques such as that devised by Hortega. Unlike other glial cells, microglia are not derived from neuro-ectoderm. Hortega originally proposed that microglia entered the brain during fetal life and then transformed into phagocytes when the brain was damaged. More recent autoradiographic and immunocytochemical studies, however, suggest that microglia are derived directly from peripheral blood monocytes.

Following brain damage, microglia are seen in H&E-stained sections as small, rod-shaped nuclei in and around areas of tissue destruction (Fig. 4.2); their scanty, short cytoplasmic processes may be stained by Hortega's silver carbonate method or by an immunocytochemical method for α-1-antitrypsin. The elongated rod-shape of the cells is uncharacteristic of blood monocytes and may be adopted initially as they migrate through relatively intact brain tissue. As the monocyte-microglia ingest lipid-rich tissue debris they become swollen foamy cells with a shape more characteristic of reactive macrophages. Such cells have been called 'compound granular corpuscles' or 'gitterzellen' in the past.

Reactions to brain tissue damage

Inflammation and repair

When brain tissue is damaged, for example by infarction, the sensitive neurons may die and all the other cellular elements within the tissue may also be destroyed. An acute inflammatory reaction ensues with the exudation of protein-rich fluid into the tissue from the surrounding blood vessels. Such *oedema* fluid is rapidly taken up by astrocyte processes in the cortex but in the white matter it may spread extensively through the extracellular space. During the first 12 h following brain infarction, both fluid and a small number of polymorphonuclear leukocytes can be found in the infarcted tissue especially near the edge of the lesion. During the next 24 h the amount of oedema fluid within the damaged area may increase and rod-shaped microglial cells proliferate in the surrounding tissue. By 3 days after the event, more monocyte-macrophages have entered the tissue from surrounding intact blood vessels. At this time, monocytes may be seen dividing in the perivascular spaces and subsequently their cytoplasm becomes full of lipid-rich material producing the typical foamy appearance in H&E sections. Astrocytes also proliferate in the intact tissue surrounding the area of damage so that as the dead tissue is removed, leaving a cystic space filled with fluid and foamy macrophages, a glial scar forms around the edge (Fig. 4.10). Fibrosis and collagen formation following brain tissue damage usually only occurs around abscesses or where the meninges are involved in the damage. Scars under other circumstances within the brain are formed from astrocytes and their processes (gliosis).

Although areas of infarction larger than about 0.5 mm in diameter in the brain eventually result in a cystic lesion surrounded by astrocytes, very small lesions may only be detectable as microscopic areas of astrocyte proliferation. Holzer or PTAH stains for astrocytes are particularly useful for detecting such small areas of infarction. In the cerebellum, *Bergmann astrocytes* in the cerebellar cortex retain

contact with the pial surface of the cerebellum, although their cell bodies are situated in and around the Purkinje cell layer. Following damage to the cerebellum, the parallel processes of reactive Bergmann glial cells are prominent, especially in sections stained with PTAH (Fig. 4.11); this feature is useful for detecting areas of cerebellar cortical damage. As myelin also stains blue with PTAH, the Holzer technique is more reliable for detecting astrocyte proliferation in white matter.

Breakdown of the blood–brain barrier, and cerebral oedema

In most regions of normal brain, there is a blood–brain barrier which prevents the entry of serum proteins, protein-bound dyes, and many

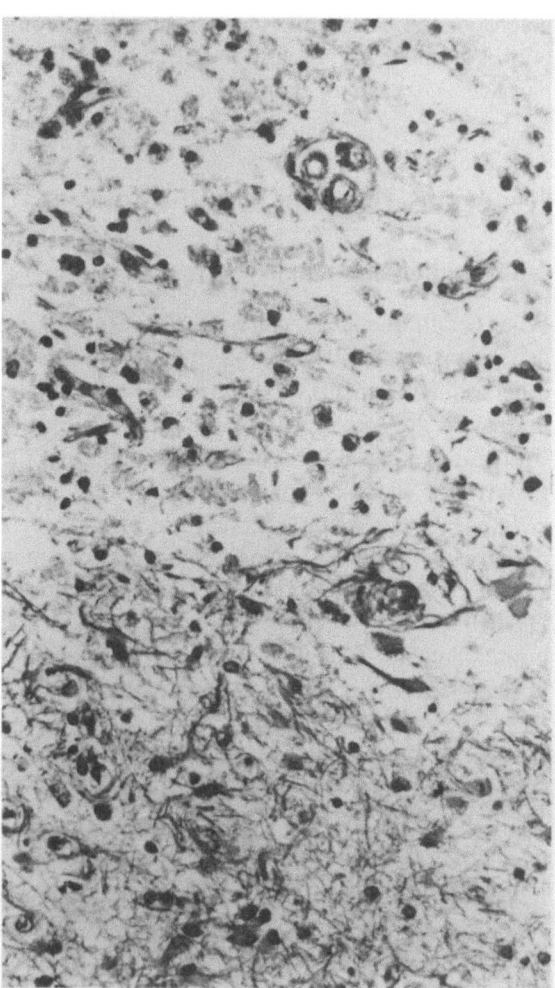

Fig. 4.10 Old cystic cerebral infarct. Cyst containing foamy macrophages (*top*); reactive astrocytes forming gliotic scar tissue (*bottom*). (PTAH × 280)

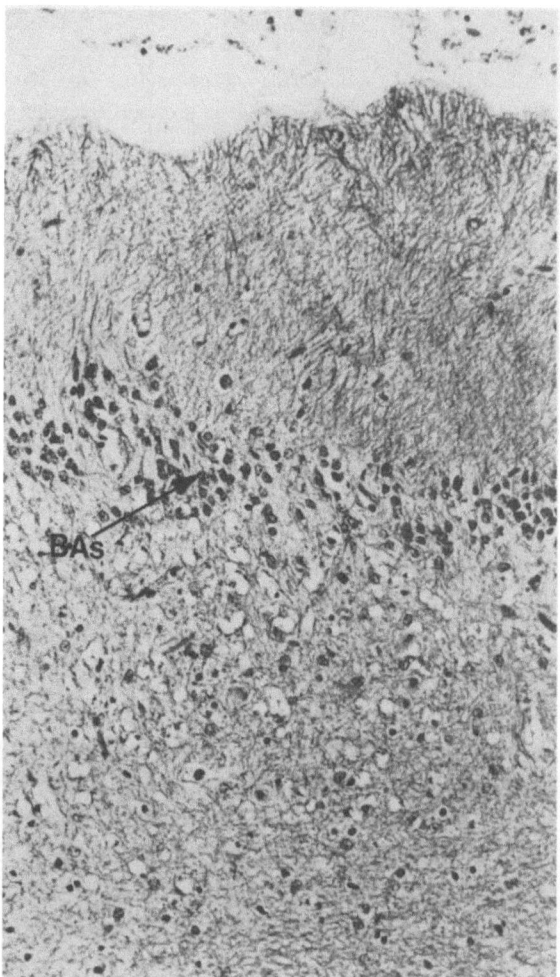

Fig. 4.11. Ischaemic, scarred cerebellar cortex showing proliferation of Bergmann astrocytes (*BAs*) and their prominent processes in the molecular layer. (PTAH × 200) (*cf.* Fig. 2.2.)

other substances into the brain tissue. Following tissue damage, there is breakdown of the blood–brain barrier with the entry of fluid and protein into the tissue; the oedema that ensues has been termed *vasogenic oedema* by Klatzo. Oedema also occurs around tumours where the blood vessels may be so different from those in normal brain that they do not impose a blood–brain barrier.

Clinically, breakdown of the blood–brain barrier can be detected in the early stages of infarction, around abscesses, and in tumours by radiographic or isotope techniques. Injection of aqueous iodinated contrast media such as meglumine iothalamate (Conray) allows regions of altered blood–brain barrier to be detected in CT scans as the radioopaque tracer leaks out of the blood to cause enhancement of the areas with a deficient blood–brain barrier (Chap. 5, Fig. 5.3). Similarly Technetium[99]-labelled serum albumin, when injected intravenously, will leak into areas of brain with a deficient blood–brain barrier; these areas can be detected by a gamma camera.

Much of the information about breakdown and re-establishment of the blood–brain barrier following brain tissue damage has been gathered from *experimental* studies. In histological investigations, leakage of protein from the blood into areas of damaged brain has been the main method of investigation. Evans blue, when injected into the blood, becomes bound to serum albumin so that areas of brain damage are stained blue due to the leakage of labelled protein from the blood. Similarly, fluorescein-labelled albumin can be used as a marker. By *immunoperoxidase* staining, the leakage of serum proteins themselves can be detected in areas in which the blood–brain barrier is altered. For electron microscopy, and for many light-microscope studies, an exogenous protein, horse-radish peroxidase, has been used to define the mechanisms of blood–brain barrier breakdown. Using this technique, it has been shown that the increased permeability of the vascular bed to proteins following brain damage is through their transport across the endothelial cells in pinocytotic vesicles rather than through separation of the intercellular junctions between endothelial cells. Fluid and proteins escaping through the altered blood–brain barrier are taken up by astrocytes both in the cortex and the white matter.

Histologically, the oedema caused by the breakdown of the blood–brain barrier differs in the cortex and white matter. In the *cortex*, the extracellular space initially remains small whereas astrocyte processes and particularly their perivascular end-feet swell up as they pinocytose the fluid that has escaped from the vessels. As the oedema becomes more severe, astrocyte processes may rupture and the tissue becomes disrupted. A different picture is seen in the *white matter*, in which oedema fluid spreads in the extracellular space between the myelinated nerve fibres; the white matter can therefore accommodate much more oedema fluid and is usually a more severely swollen part of the brain than the cortex. Some fluid may subsequently drain through the white matter into the CSF in the ventricles, and some is taken up by astrocytes in a similar way to that seen in the cortex.

The major outflow of protein and fluid from damaged vessels in an area of infarction or brain injury, occurs during the first 24 h. Fluid and protein also leaks from the preserved vessels in the tissues surrounding the area of injury. During the subsequent 1–2 weeks as capillaries regenerate into damaged tissue, the capillary blood–brain barrier becomes re-established. However, some leakage of fluid and protein may still occur from arterioles even 4 weeks after the injury.

The extent and time course of the oedema will vary according to the size of the lesion. Oedema fluid within the brain tissue may interfere with neural function; one example of this interference is seen in multiple sclerosis, in which some of the temporary neurological deficit that occurs in a relapse is probably due to oedema rather than to demyelination. Frequently, however, more significant complications arise from the sheer volume of the oedema fluid. Following infarction of a large area of the cerebral hemisphere, oedema of the damaged and surrounding tissue may cause problems through brain displacement (see p 52). Similarly, oedema of the spinal cord tissue within the confines of the spinal canal may result in further ischaemic damage due to compression of blood vessels.

Breakdown of myelin

Myelin is rich in phospholipids and cholesterol; electron microscopically it is seen as a lamellated structure surrounding axons (see Chap. 2). In the CNS myelin is formed by the compaction of oligodendroglial cell membrane whereas in the peripheral nervous system it is formed by Schwann cells. When myelin is broken down in pathological lesions within the brain and spinal cord, the lamellated myelin debris is taken up into macrophages where it is transformed into globules of ultrastructurally amorphous lipid. This structural transformation may take days or even weeks and is due mainly to the *esterification of cholesterol*, so that the amorphous droplets are to a large extent composed of cholesterol ester.

An understanding of the chemistry of myelin breakdown is useful when considering how to detect *myelin breakdown products* in tissue sections. The normal lamellar structure of myelin is birefringent in polarised light, but when the change to amorphous lipid droplets takes place, the birefringence is lost and the droplets become isotropic. Two of the main histochemical methods for detecting myelin breakdown products rely upon the different physical properties of normal myelin and the cholesterol ester breakdown products. Sudan stains, such as Oil-Red-O, have a greater solubility in cholesterol ester droplets than in normal myelin; macrophages laden with degenerate myelin products therefore are brightly stained with Sudan dyes whereas normal myelin is coloured only a dull red. Cholesterol esters in degenerating myelin are stained black by osmium in the Marchi technique (Fig. 4.12), which relies

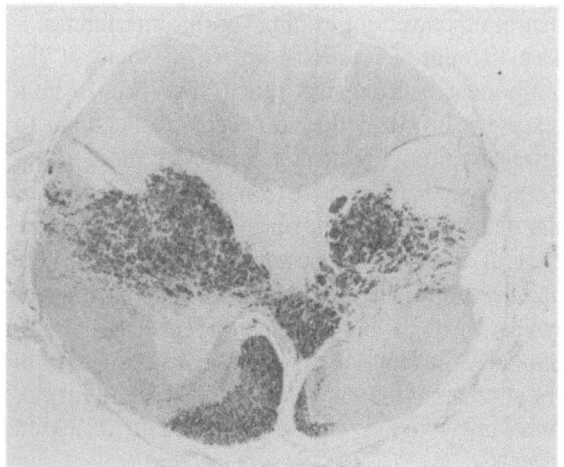

Fig. 4.12. Upper spinal cord showing degenerate myelin (*black*) in the decussation of the pyramids 3 months after an infarct in the pons. (Marchi × 6)

upon the osmiophilia of normal myelin being blocked by potassium chlorate or chromate. Triglycerides also stain black with the Marchi technique, but in practice there is little triglyceride in the CNS. One advantage of the Marchi technique is that, following the reaction, blocks of tissue may be embedded in paraffin and then sectioned.

Apart from the techniques that detect the degeneration products of myelin in the tissue, myelin loss may be observed through the lack of staining by myelin techniques such as Luxol-fast blue (Fig. 4.5) or Loyez techniques. In this way, degenerate tracts within the brain and spinal cord may be detected.

Degeneration of myelin in the CNS follows two major patterns: axonal degeneration and demyelination.

Axonal degeneration

When an axon is damaged, the portion distal to the site of injury degenerates and its myelin sheath is also broken down. Thus, following an infarct in the internal capsule or the pyramidal tracts in the pons, myelin degeneration may be detected in the corticospinal tracts below the lesion when the distal portions of the axons have degenerated (Fig. 4.12).

Demyelination

This term is normally reserved for pathological processes in which the myelin is destroyed and the *axons remain intact*. Demyelination is a feature of a number of CNS diseases. It occurs in *leukodystrophies* in which there is a defect in myelin formation and, in some cases, abnormal lipids accumulate within the white matter, e.g. metachromatic leukodystrophy (sulphatide lipidosis). Demyelination is prominent in *some viral infections*, especially in progressive multifocal leukoencephalopathy (see Chap. 9). *Allergic encephalomyelitis* is also characterised by demyelination but as part of a delayed hypersensitivity reaction. Various *toxins* such as chlorhexidine and triethyl tin cause a type of demyelination which is characterised, in the early stages, by the formation of large, fluid-filled vacuoles within myelin sheaths. Some *metabolic* and *nutritional diseases*, for example, subacute combined degeneration of the cord, may be characterised by demyelination.

In many of the diseases listed above, demyelination is only one of the features of the disorder, but in *multiple sclerosis* it is a major aspect of the disease.

Multiple sclerosis

A demyelinating disease which affects the brain and spinal cord, multiple sclerosis is commoner in Northern Europe and Switzerland than in the

United States, and is rare in Japan and in the Tropics. In general, the crude *prevalence* rate rises progressively upon moving away from the equator; thus, Boston, Massachusetts, has a higher prevalence rate than New Orleans and the highest prevalence in the world is in South East Norway and the Shetland Islands. Similarly, Hobart in Tasmania has a higher prevalence rate of multiple sclerosis than rural Western Australia. Individuals moving from a high to a low risk area after the age of 15 carry the high risk with them.

Some 60% of cases of multiple sclerosis occur between 20 and 40 years of age but many first present in their twenties. Women are more often affected than men; further the disease often presents earlier in women and may follow a more rapid course.

Clinical features

The clinical presentation and course of multiple sclerosis is very varied. Its onset is usually characterised by the sudden development of a single focal neurological deficit which then recovers. Subsequently, the disease follows an episodic course with different focal neurological defects appearing with each exacerbation; although recovery from the acute episodes usually occurs, it is incomplete and the neurological disability is cumulative and progressive. Commonly, the initial onset involves limb weakness, or visual disturbances including blindness, or focal numbness and paraesthesia. Patients with long-standing multiple sclerosis often exhibit ataxia, spasticity, motor weakness and bladder dysfunction.

Several *distinct clinical syndromes* are recognised. About 50% of patients with retrobulbar neuritis subsequently develop typical features of multiple sclerosis. In its early stages, multiple sclerosis often runs a relapsing and remitting course, especially in young adults. In older patients, particularly in women, a progressive paraplegia, often without other clinical manifestations, is a common form of the disease. After 7 or 8 years the relapsing form often changes gradually into the progressive form. Devic's disease is a rare syndrome in Europe and the United States but is commoner in the Far East. It consists of retrobulbar neuritis, which may be bilateral, followed by an acute transverse myelitis from which recovery is often incomplete.

The effects of demyelination can be detected *electrophysiologically* by measuring visual evoked response latencies or auditory evoked response latencies in patients with multiple sclerosis. Demyelinated segments of axons conduct impulses more slowly than the normally myelinated segments; this leads to delays in the latencies of the potentials generated in these structures.

Pathology

The pattern of disability presumably reflects the distribution of the plaques of demyelination throughout the nervous system. However, it is often difficult at post mortem to correlate the pathological findings completely with the clinical defects. Brains of patients dying with long-standing *multiple sclerosis* show varying numbers of grey, sclerotic plaques of gliosis ranging from a few millimetres in diameter to a centimetre or more. No site in the CNS appears to be exempt; plaques may involve white matter or grey matter. Periventricular plaques, however, are seen in many multiple sclerosis brains at post mortem (Fig. 4.13), and the spinal cord frequently contains plaques, particularly in the lateral columns of white matter. The optic nerves or chiasm may also be affected by plaque formation. Even in the gross brain specimen, the sharply defined borders of the multiple sclerosis plaque may be seen (Fig. 4.13) but are more easily demonstrated in myelin-stained sections. *Histologically*, chronic multiple sclerosis plaques appear as a mass of fibrous astrocytes and processes and, in those plaques which are many years old, very few axons survive. Oligodendroglial cells are also scarce or completely absent from the plaques.

A very different picture is seen in *active multiple sclerosis* plaques of recent origin. They appear as soft granular areas in the white matter. *Histologically*, there is disintegration of myelin but with preservation of many of the axons. Macrophages containing myelin breakdown products are prominent and there is widespread perivascular cuffing by lymphocytes and plasma cells (Fig. 4.14). It has been estimated that some 10% of the perivascular cells in active lesions are plasma cells. There is a striking loss of oligodendroglial cells from the multiple sclerosis plaques and there is little, if any, remyelination. Reactive astrocytes abound within the plaque (Fig. 4.15) and gradually the histological picture changes to a chronic multiple sclerosis plaque from which all the myelin debris has been removed and many of the axons have been lost. A tough, gliotic plaque composed almost entirely of astrocytes remains.

The exact *cause* of multiple sclerosis has not been

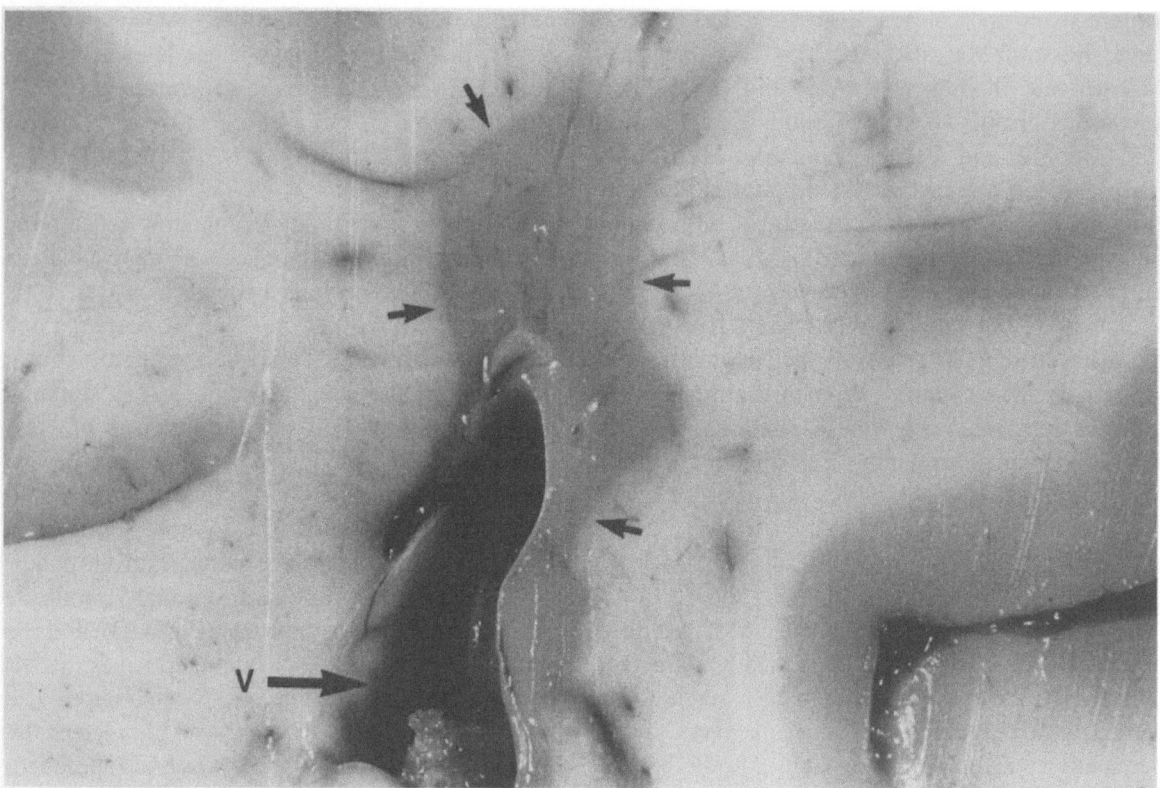

Fig. 4.13. Old grey gliotic multiple sclerosis plaque in the periventricular white matter. Its sharp border is outlined by *small arrows*. Ventricle (*V*).

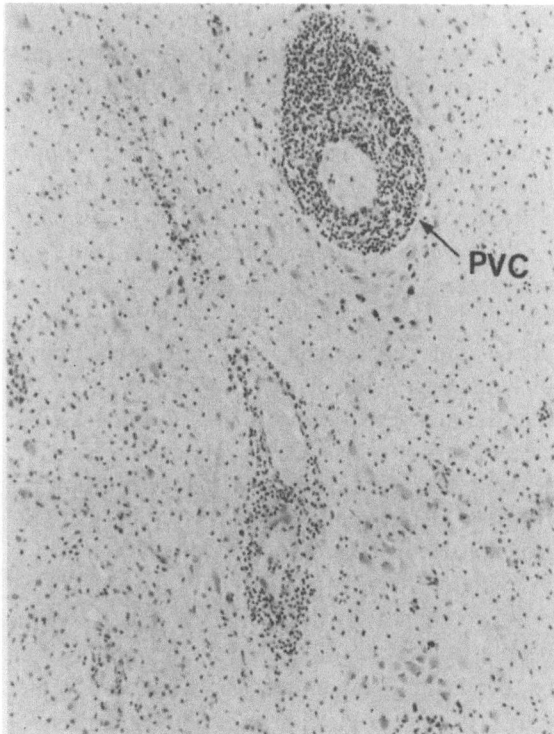

Fig. 4.14. Active multiple sclerosis plaque. Inflammatory cells form thick perivascular cuffs (*PVC*) but are also seen distributed within the tissue. (H & E × 100)

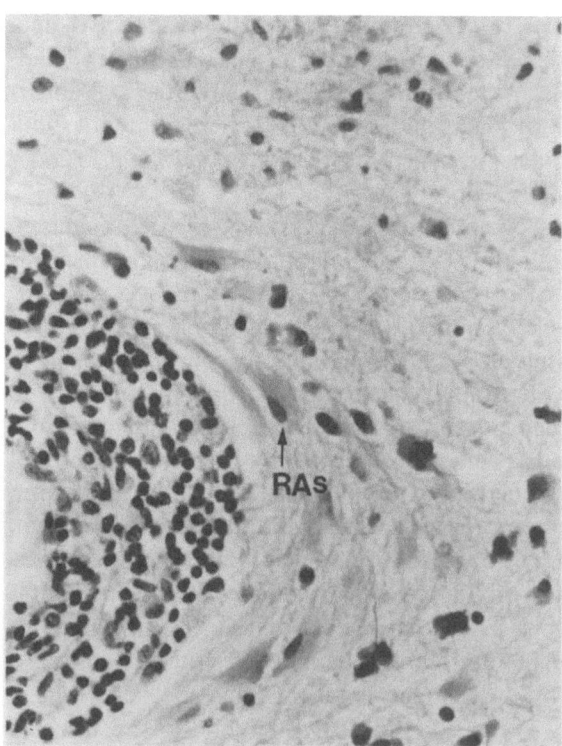

Fig. 4.15. Active multiple sclerosis plaque showing perivascular cuff of inflammatory cells (*left*) and reactive astrocytes (*RAs*). (H & E × 415)

elucidated, but there are several features which suggest that the disease may have an auto-immune pathogenesis. Perivascular accumulations of lymphocytes and plasma cells in the active lesions indicate that immune mechanisms are involved and oligoclonal bands of IgG in the CSF of 90% of patients with multiple sclerosis suggest that there is protracted antigenic stimulation in the CNS. Indeed, viral antibody titres are raised in the CSF, e.g. measles virus antibodies. Recent studies of chronic experimental allergic encephalomyelitis produced by the administration of myelin basic protein have shown many similarities between this disease and multiple sclerosis. Abnormalities in lymphocyte subsets, particularly a deficiency of suppressor T-cells, also suggest that immune responses are abnormal in multiple sclerosis. These features, together with the restriction of multiple sclerosis to certain geographical areas and the over-representation of B7 and DW2 histocompatibility antigens in multiple sclerosis patients of European races, suggest that a genetically determined defect in immunological response may play a role in the pathogenesis of the disease. The identity of the antigen or antigens involved remains uncertain.

The secondary effects of intracranial space-occupying lesions and cerebral oedema

In addition to their primary destructive effects, intracranial lesions may induce secondary complications due to their space-occupying nature. A rapid rise in the volume of the intracranial contents occurs with an intracerebral haemorrhage and following subdural or extradural haemorrhages. A similar, but often a less rapid increase in brain volume, accompanies the cerebral oedema induced by trauma, cerebral infarction or by a cerebral abscess. Raised intracranial pressure associated with gliomas and meningiomas may have a slow onset but infarction or haemorrhage within a glioma may induce a more rapid increase in intracranial pressure. There is a limited amount of CSF which can be displaced from the cranial cavity by an enlarging space-occupying lesion, and when this reserve capacity is exhausted, displacement of the brain occurs.

Figure 4.16 summarises the major patterns of brain displacement and points of herniation induced by space-occupying lesions. Sheets of dura

such as the *falx cerebri* and the *tentorium cerebelli* divide the cranial cavity into compartments. A space-occupying lesion in one cerebral hemisphere will displace the brain towards the opposite side and may cause herniation of the cingulate gyrus under the falx cerebri: *subfalcine herniation*.

A more significant complication occurs when there is downward and medial displacement of a hemisphere, resulting in herniation through the opening in the tentorium cerebelli. Under normal circumstances, the aperture in the tentorium cerebelli (Fig. 4.17) allows the brain stem, posterior cerebral arteries and various other structures to pass from the posterior fossa into the supratentorial region of the skull. The aperture has a bony anterior border and tough, rather sharp posterior lateral borders formed by the tentorium cerebelli. An expanding lesion in one hemisphere may cause the uncus and parahippocampal gyrus on the medial aspect of the temporal lobe, to herniate through the tentorial opening: *transtentorial herniation*.

There are several important effects of transtentorial herniation, some of which are fatal. One particularly severe complication is brain stem compression, which may be accompanied by haemorrhage and congestion of the midbrain (Fig. 4.18). The patient becomes comatose, probably due to damage to the brain stem reticular formation, and may die (see Chap. 3). A prominent groove may be made in the herniated parahippocampal gyrus by the free edge of the tentorium (Fig. 4.18). Branches of the posterior cerebral artery crossing the groove become compressed, resulting in infarction of the temporal lobe and occipital lobe cortex, including the visual cortex. If the patient survives, there may be a residual homonymous hemianopia. Third nerve compression with ophthalmoplegia and pupillary signs may be an early complication of transtentorial herniation.

Compression of the midbrain and transtentorial herniation may be detected in a CT scan, particularly if the subarachnoid space is outlined by Metrizamide contrast medium (Fig. 4.19).

Herniation of the *cerebellar tonsils* down through the foramen magnum is a major complication of enlarging lesions in the posterior fossa and cerebellum (Fig. 4.16). Plugging of the foramen magnum by the cerebellar tonsils interferes with the flow of CSF between the spinal and cranial cavities and may cause compression of the medulla. Hydrocephalus or fatal compression of the medulla may result.

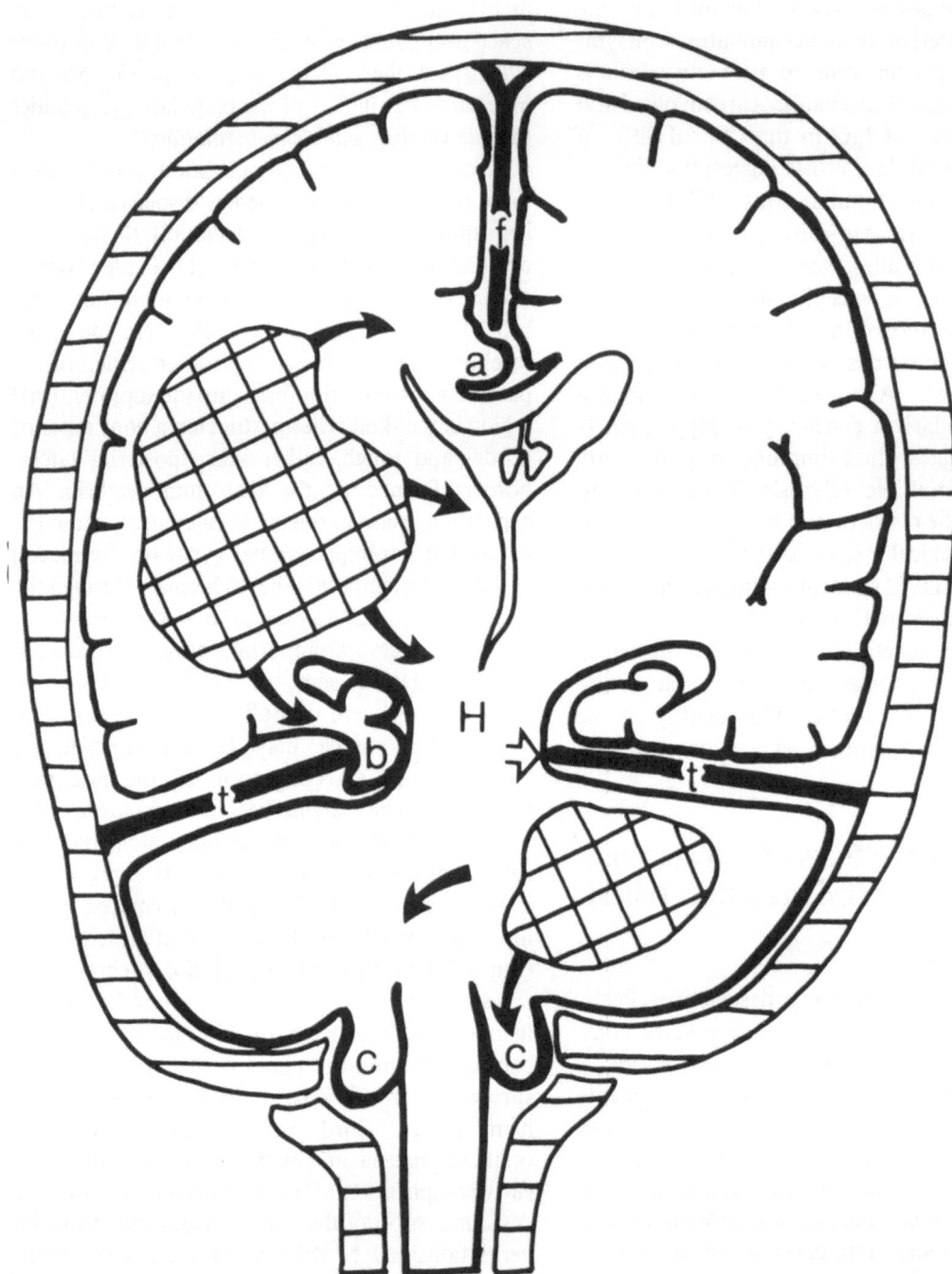

Fig. 4.16. Brain displacement and herniation induced by space-occupying lesions. A mass in the left cerebral hemisphere has caused displacement of midline structures to the right, and herniation of the cingulate gyrus (*a*) under the falx cerebri (*f*). Herniation of the uncus and parahippocampal gyrus (*b*) through the tentorial (*t*) aperture (transtentorial herniation) has compressed the midbrain and caused haemorrhage (*H*). The opposite cerebral peduncle has been damaged by pressure against the free edge of the tentorium (*open arrow*). A mass in the cerebellum has caused herniation of the tonsils (*c*) through the foramen magnum.

Hydrocephalus

If the circulation of CSF through the ventricular system is blocked, or the absorption of CSF from the subarachnoid space through the arachnoid villi is impaired, the cerebral ventricles dilate and hydrocephalus ensues. Ventricular dilatation may be detected on CT scans or at post mortem (Fig. 4.20). Not only are there many causes of hydrocephalus but there are also several different types.

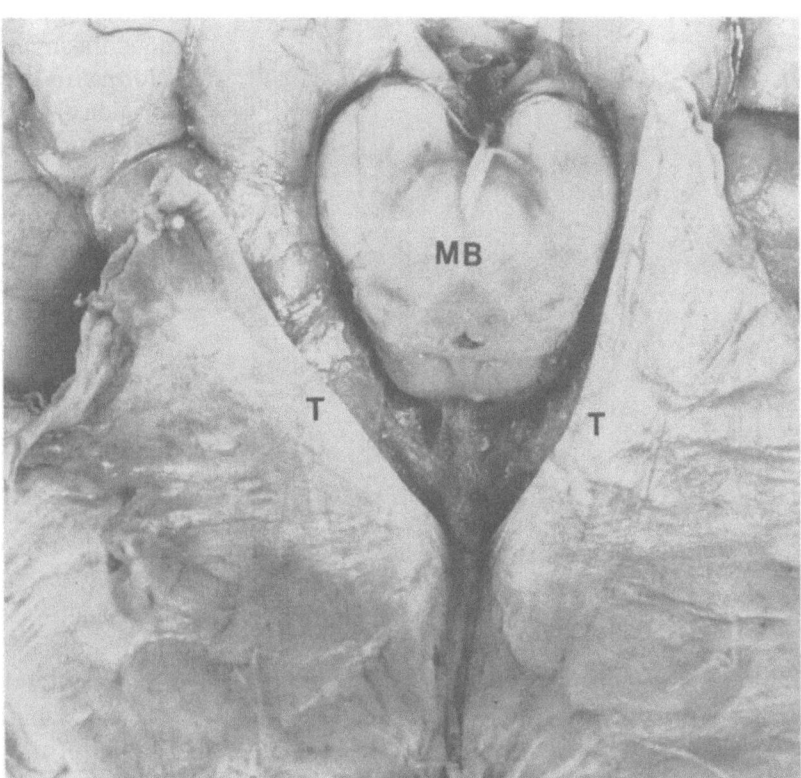

Fig. 4.17. Midbrain (*MB*) in a normal tentorial aperture. Anterior is to the top of the picture. Tentorium (*T*).

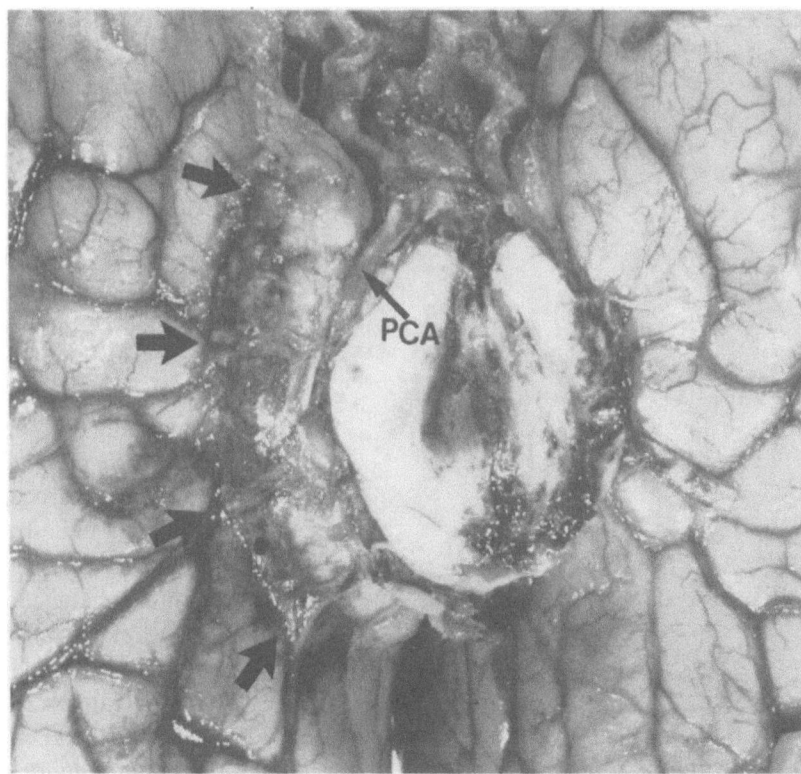

Fig. 4.18. Herniation of parahippocampal gyrus through the tentorial aperture. A groove (*large arrows*) has been formed by the free edge of the tentorium and branches of the posterior cerebral artery (*PCA*) are compressed as they cross the groove. The midbrain is compressed and haemorrhagic.

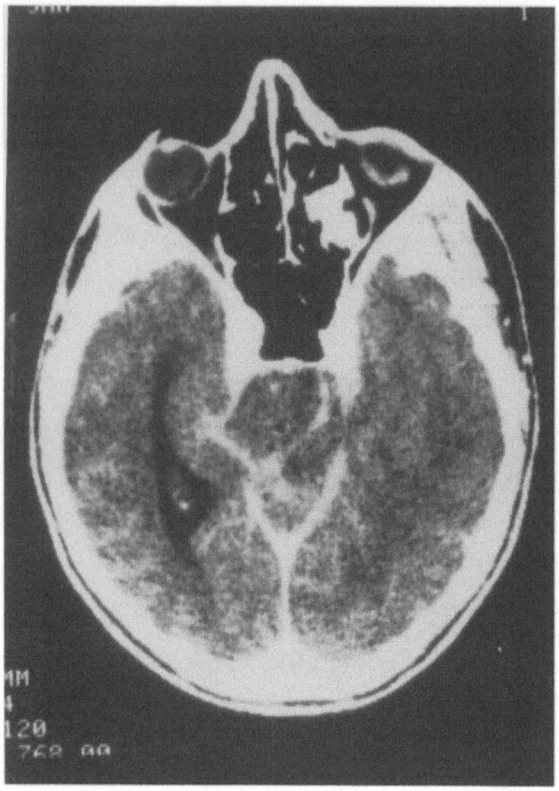

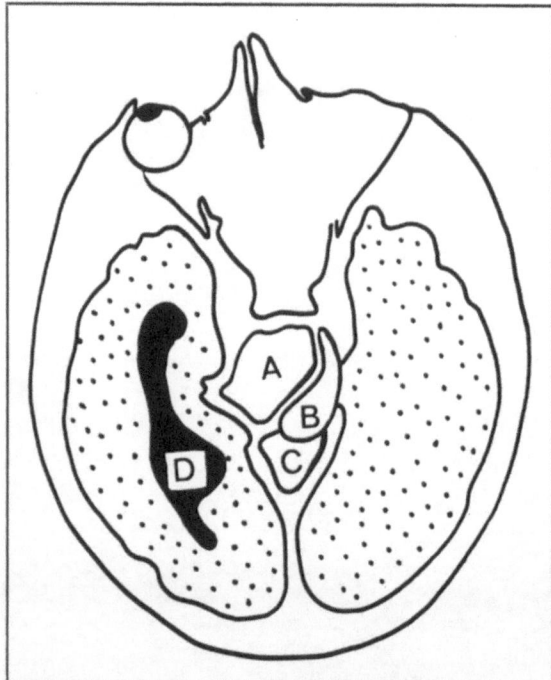

Fig. 4.19. Transtentorial herniation. CT scan showing parahippocampal herniation and midbrain compression. The subarachnoid space has been outlined (*in white*) by Metrizamide. *Key*: (*lower diagram*)
A, distorted midbrain; *B*, herniated parahippocampal gyrus; *C*, cerebellar vermis; *D*, dilated contralateral ventricle.

Obstruction of the outflow of the lateral ventricles, the third ventricle or the fourth ventricle by tumour, inflammation or congenital defects, results in *obstructive hydrocephalus*. When the defect in absorption of CSF is due to a block in the subarachnoid space or a defect in the arachnoid villi *communicating hydrocephalus* may result. Fibrosis of the arachnoid following meningitis or subarachnoid haemorrhage may obliterate the subarachnoid space and so cause communicating hydrocephalus.

When the block in CSF circulation is *acute*, the intracranial pressure may rise and unless a shunt is inserted into the ventricles, the patient may die. In infants the cranial sutures have not fused, and head enlargement may then accompany hydrocephalus.

In some cases, there is ventricular dilatation but without clear signs of raised intracranial pressure; some of these patients have *intermittently raised pressure hydrocephalus (IRPH)* or normal pressure hydrocephalus (see Chap. 15) and present with dementia, gait disturbances and incontinence. Amelioration of the neurological signs may follow ventricular shunting in this group of patients. Dilatation of the ventricles may also occur when there is loss of brain tissue in patients with Alzheimer's disease or multi-infarct dementia (see (Chap. 15). In these cases there is usually no defect in CSF absorption, the pressure is normal and this type of hydrocephalus is often referred to as *hydrocephalus ex vacuo*.

Effects of hydrocephalus upon the brain

CT scans taken during the *acute* stages of ventricular dilatation in hydrocephalus often show oedema of the periventricular white matter. Contrast medium injected into the hydrocephalic ventricles passes into the periventricular tissue, suggesting that the oedema is due to the infusion of CSF. *CSF oedema* has been observed histologically in acute hydrocephalus and is accompanied by damage and destruction to the axons and myelin in the periventricular tissue. In the later stages of hydrocephalus the oedema subsides, probably due to the establishment of alternative pathways of CSF drainage through the blood vessels in the periventricular tissue. In such cases, damage to the periventricular tissue may be reflected in the amount of *gliotic scarring* in the white matter.

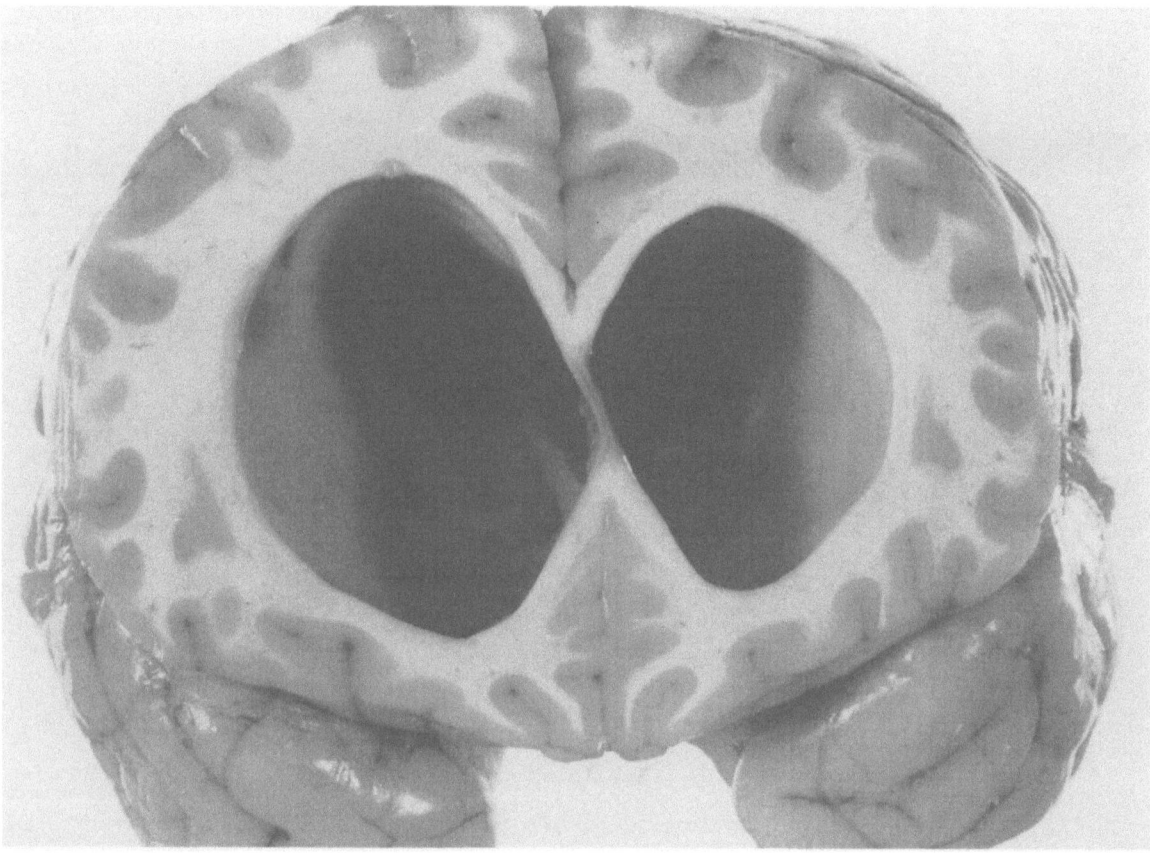

Fig. 4.20. Hydrocephalus following meningitis. There is gross dilatation of the lateral ventricles.

Further reading

General pathology

Berry M (1979) Regeneration in the central nervous system. In: Smith W T, Cavanagh J B (eds) Recent advances in neuropathology. Churchill Livingstone, Edinburgh, p. 67

Blackwood W, Corsellis J A N (eds) (1976) Greenfield's neuropathology, 3rd edn. Arnold, London

Bradbury M (1979) The concept of a blood–brain barrier. Wiley, Chichester, New York

Caine G D, Weller R O, Davis B E, Cox S (1980) Mechanisms of uptake and the fate of serum proteins and horseradish peroxidase in cultured human glioma cells. Acta Neuropathol (Berl) 52: 169

Devor M (1982) Plasticity in the adult nervous system. In: Illis L S, Glanville H H, Sedgwick E M (eds) Rehabilitation of the neurological patient. Blackwell Scientific, Oxford, London

Klatzo I (1979) Cerebral oedema and ischaemia. In: Smith W T, Cavanagh J B (eds) Recent advances in neuropathology. Churchill Livingstone, Edinburgh, p. 27

Tomlinson B E (1979) The ageing brain. In Smith W T, Cavanagh J B (eds). Recent advances in neuropathology. Churchill Livingstone, Edinburgh, p 129

Torvik A (1976) Central chromatolysis and the axon reaction. A reappraisal. Neuropathol Appl Neurobiol 2: 423

Weller R O, Mitchell J (1980) Cerebrospinal fluid edema and its sequelae in hydrocephalus. In: Cervós-Navarro J, Ferszt R (eds) Brain edema. Advances in neurology, vol. 28. Raven Press, New York, p 111.

Weller R O, Shulman K (1972) Infantile hydrocephalus: clinical histological and ultrastructural study of brain damage. J Neurosurg 36: 255

Multiple sclerosis

Acheson E D (1977) Epidemiology of multiple sclerosis. Br Med Bull 33: 9

Allen I V (1981) The pathology of multiple sclerosis—fact, fiction and hypothesis. Neuropathol Appl Neurobiol 7: 169

Cuzner M L (1980) Recent biochemical and immunological observations in multiple sclerosis, Neuropathol Appl Neurobiol 6: 405

Davison A N, Cuzner M L (eds) (1980) The suppression of experimental allergic encephalomyelitis and multiple sclerosis. Academic Press, London

Lumsden C E (1970) The neuropathology of multiple sclerosis. In: Vinken P J, Bruyn G W (eds) Handbook of clinical neurology, vol 9. North-Holland, Amsterdam, p 217

Tallis R C (1980) Some recent advances in the clinical aspects of multiple sclerosis. Neuropathol Appl Neurobiol 6: 325

Chapter 5

Cerebral Vascular Disease

Stroke

In the United Kingdom, and in other developed countries in which the population includes relatively large numbers of people older than 50 years, stroke is one of the commonest causes of disability and death. The term *stroke* is used to describe *a sudden event, due to vascular disease, in which paralysis or (other) disturbance of function in the CNS occurs*. It is thus a *clinical* term without a strictly defined meaning in pathology. Strokes are often referred to as cerebral vascular accidents, but, since there is always a cause, however difficult to understand or establish, this latter term is best avoided. Because the cause of a stroke is so frequently uncertain in clinical practice, clinicians and pathologists may use different classifications. While the pathologist can note the presence of *infarction* or *haemorrhage*, the two major subdivisions, the clinician can only consider which of these two lesions might be present. It is often difficult, therefore, to compare clinical and pathological data. However, clinical information about stroke syndromes can be helpful in understanding the underlying causation of these two major types of stroke. The advent of CT scanning has largely resolved this problem.

Clinical features

The clinical features of a stroke depend on the *location* of the lesion, on its *causation*, and on the presence of underlying *risk factors* (Table 5.1). A

Table 5.1. Risk factors in the pathogenesis of atherosclerosis[a]

Cigarette smoking
Hypertension
Diabetes mellitus
Hyperlipoproteinaemia
Obesity
Increasing age
Male sex
Low high-density lipoprotein level

[a]These risk factors for atherosclerosis are in general the same as those which delineate patients at risk of suffering stroke.

classification according to the site of the lesion can be attempted on the basis of the clinical features and from this the vascular territory in which the stroke has occurred can be inferred. This information provides a guide to the prognosis for functional recovery.

Strokes are often recurrent or multiple. *Recurrence* is more likely if certain underlying risk factors are present, such as diabetic or hypertensive vascular disease, or the presence of a site from which emboli might arise. Common examples of the latter include chronic valvular heart disease, myocardial infarction with endocardial damage, and atheromatous plaque at the bifurcation of the carotid artery in the neck. As a general rule the prognosis in a patient surviving the initial illness after an intracerebral haemorrhage is better than that following an infarct. Haemorrhages disrupt white matter without necessarily causing extensive destruction and, when the haemorrhage is absorbed, functional recovery may be excellent. Following a cerebral infarct, on the other hand, brain tissue has been destroyed and recovery is usually incomplete as it depends on the functional state of the remaining brain tissue.

The clinical features of a major stroke due to infarction or haemorrhage are similar. The patient suddenly develops hemiplegia and becomes drowsy or even comatose. Focal or generalised seizures may sometimes occur at the onset. Coma is associated with very large infarcts, and the prognosis both for survival and for recovery of function is poor. Death may occur within a few hours, as happens in about a third of patients with intracerebral haemorrhage, or the patient may die from a recurrent episode, brain shift with herniation and raised intracranial pressure, pneumonia or another infarction. Brain stem infarction can be recognised by the development of signs of focal brain stem dysfunction. Disturbances of ventilation and of circulatory control in such patients, and other signs of bilateral brain stem dysfunction carry a bad prognosis. Bilateral signs imply that the infarct is due to occlusion of the main trunk of the basilar artery rather than one of its branches.

Intracerebral haemorrhage, or haemorrhage into a cerebellar hemisphere produces a sudden, and therefore poorly compensated, space-occupying lesion with raised intracranial pressure and displacement of brain both caudally and to one side. These effects may be profound and difficult to control. In both cerebral haemorrhage and cerebral infarction, oedema may lead to further increases in intracranial pressure and thus to subsequent clinical deterioration. Signs of meningism may arise either as a result of haemorrhage tracking out of the brain into the ventricular or subarachnoid systems or from tentorial herniation consequent on the space-occupying effect of the infarct or haemorrhage (see Chap. 4). Lumbar puncture may reveal blood-stained CSF in haemorrhagic stroke, but as this procedure increases the risk of transtentorial or foramen magnum herniation it is probably best deferred.

Patients with subarachnoid haemorrhage may show signs of localised neurological disturbance. In this disorder, bleeding is limited almost entirely to the subarachnoid space; it is commonly due to rupture of an aneurysm or less commonly due to bleeding from a cerebral arteriovenous malformation, but also occurs in patients with a bleeding diathesis. However, in some patients with subarachnoid haemorrhage there may be an associated intracerebral or intraventricular haemorrhage, producing focal signs. Secondary cerebral ischaemia may also occur, with cerebral infarction and the late onset of focal neurological disturbances.

Clinical classification

Because of the difficulties in reaching a pathological diagnosis in patients with stroke syndromes, and the problem of categorising them by vascular territory, it is convenient to classify patients as suffering from *completed stroke, stroke in evolution* or *transient ischaemic attacks*. A completed stroke is a stroke in which there has been no progression of the neurological deficit in the previous few hours, or in which the clinical signs are such that it can confidently be predicted that there has been infarction in virtually the whole of a particular vascular territory, for example a middle cerebral artery territory. In such a patient it is not possible to modify the neurological deficit by treatment in the acute stage. *Stroke in evolution* is a term used to describe patients in whom the disability, whether due to intracerebral or subarachnoid haemorrhage, is continuing to evolve, either stepwise or gradually, during a period of minutes or hours. The term implies that it might be possible by suitable treatment to prevent further disability developing and also that an alternative diagnosis, for example, some other cause of progressive neurological deficit, should be entertained.

By *transient ischaemic attack* is meant a transient neurological disturbance of sudden onset lasting for less than 24 h. Since a transient episode lasting as long as this can be the result of small zones of infarction ('microinfarcts'), the term transient ischaemic attack (TIA) has been reserved by some clinicians for episodes of shorter duration, say only 2 h, but such a brief episode is difficult to distinguish from a focal seizure. Since recovery occurs after a transient ichaemic attack, it is implicit in the concept that the disorder is due to a transient disturbance of blood flow within the vascular territory affected. It was at first thought that this disturbance was due to spasm of arterioles or arteries in the affected part of the brain, but this suggestion has not been supported by the results of angiographic studies or by experimental work. The alternative and more acceptable explanation is that the disturbance in blood flow is usually due to embolism from a more proximal site in the arterial system.

It has been known for some years that some patients with transient ischaemic attacks subsequently develop completed strokes within the same vascular territory. It may be possible to prevent the development of strokes in such patients with appropriate treatment, for example anticoagulant drugs, or drugs which impair platelet function such as aspirin. The management of transient ischaemic attacks has therefore become increasingly important in the treatment and prevention of strokes.

Embolism and cerebral infarction

Cerebral infarction accounts for about 85% of patients with completed strokes, the remainder being due to haemorrhage. Embolism of the arterial tree is probably the major factor in the pathogenesis of these infarcts. Five types of emboli are recognised in the cerebral circulation:

Thrombus

Calcified material from degenerative changes in the mitral or aortic valves

Material derived from vegetations on these damaged heart valves

Cholesterol, often in crystalline form

Other atheromatous debris

Emboli consisting of formed thrombus may originate within the heart, especially in patients with uncontrolled atrial fibrillation or with mural thrombosis associated with subendocardial myocardial infarction. Such emboli may also form in relation to damaged valves on the left side of the heart and from thrombus forming on ulcerated atheromatous plaques in the great vessels, or in the carotid, vertebral or basilar arteries. Emboli of this type are usually relatively large and result in occlusion of large vessels, for example, the carotid, basilar or middle cerebral arteries, rather than smaller arteries. Such emboli are not usually visible in the retinal vessels, although these vessels may be empty and the retina infarcted when the ophthalmic artery is occluded by thrombus in the internal carotid artery. Emboli from thrombus formed within the heart or aorta are also likely to affect other organs, for example, the kidney, the gut or the skin. Emboli derived from vegetations on damaged valves on the left side of the heart consist of thrombus, which may contain bacteria in patients with infective endocarditis. In patients with infective endocarditis embolism of the brain is usually an event occurring in the context of a serious systemic illness, but it may be a presenting feature of the illness.

Cerebral emboli are often quite small but nevertheless often cause *cerebral infarction*. Most emboli are carotid in distribution, and left middle cerebral embolism predominates. Micro-thrombi arising from platelet/fibrin aggregates on ulcerated (complicated) atheromatous plaques are often so small that they may not produce clinically detectable effects in organs other than the brain. In the brain, however, even small zones of ischaemia in critical regions such as the brain stem, the left temporal lobe, or the internal capsule, may be immediately

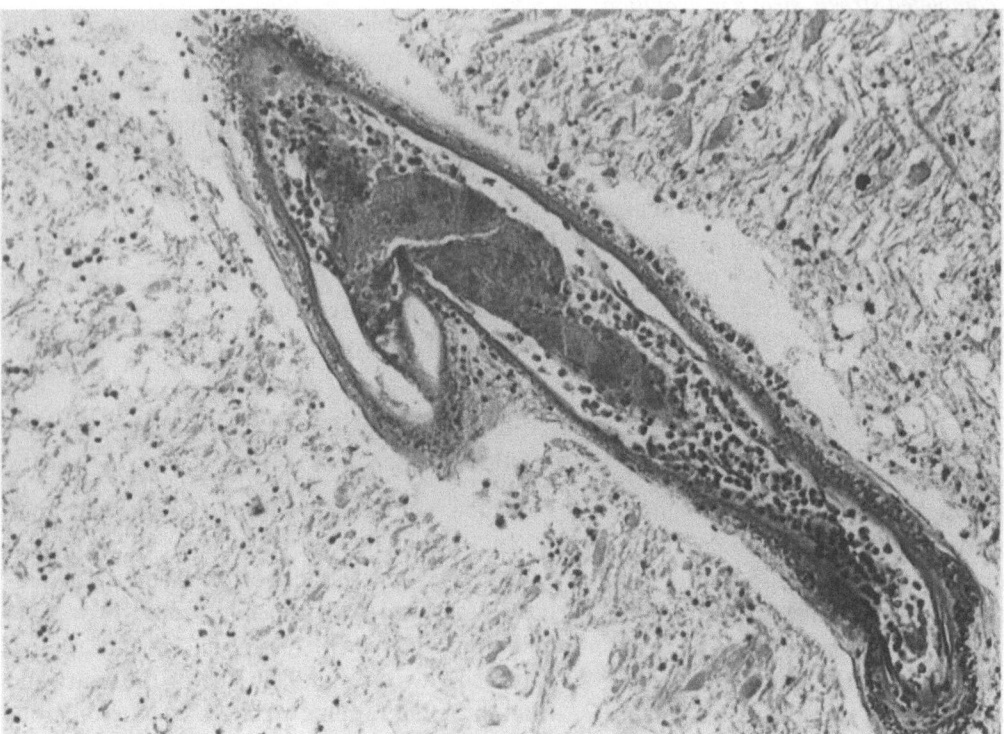

Fig. 5.1. Micro-thrombus. The lumen of the vessel contains a thrombus composed of fibrin and platelets. (H & E × 160)

obvious to the patient. Episodes of recurrent monocular blindness are thought to be due to embolism of this type. These emboli (Fig. 5.1) may be visible in the retina as grey amorphous material occluding retinal arteries and resulting in oedema, vascular spasm and slow blood flow, or even in a small patch of retinal infarction. Sometimes the syndrome of unilateral blindness and contralateral hemiplegia occurs, indicating that there have been emboli in the territory of the internal carotid artery involving the ophthalmic artery and the middle cerebral artery. Embolism by material rich in cholesterol crystals is probably relatively common, although rarely diagnosed. Its recognition depends upon the appearance of highly refractile material occluding retinal branch arterioles, often associated with episodes of monocular blindness.

Clinical studies in patients with presumed transient cerebral or retinal ischaemic attacks have suggested that structural cardiac abnormalities, especially valves damaged by calcific or rheumatic disease are potential sources of emboli. However, the detection rate for significant cardiac arrhythmias in 24-h monitoring studies is not very high and the incidence of symptomatic ischaemic heart disease is similar in patients and in controls. In a quarter of

patients investigated no cardiovascular abnormality can be detected.

Arterial occlusion

Primary thrombotic occlusion of intracranial arteries is often put forward as a cause of cerebral infarction. Angiography frequently shows occlusion of a middle cerebral artery, of the intracranial part of the internal carotid artery, or of the basilar artery. Although this may sometimes result from thrombosis occurring on atherosclerotic plaques in these vessels it is likely that a large proportion of such cases, perhaps as many as 80%, result from embolic occlusion rather than from primary thrombosis in situ. This concept has led to the recognition of the importance of extracranial vascular disease in the pathogenesis of ischaemic stroke. Atheromatous plaques are a particularly important source of emboli either from thrombus, or cholesterol-rich plaque contents. The aorta, the common carotid at its bifurcation where it forms the internal and external carotid arteries, and the basilar artery are particularly important sites of origin for these emboli. In about 20% of cases of embolic cerebral infarction the embolus originates in the heart. Embolism may thus lead to transient ischaemic attacks, or to completed stroke due to cerebral infarction. Indeed, in clinical practice, the importance of transient ischaemic attacks rests on their association with cerebral infarcts occurring at a later date in the same vascular territory. Nonetheless, it is important to recognise that even severe atheroma in large vessels is not necessarily associated with infarction. It is possible to maintain normal flow in arteries made tightly stenotic by atheroma; and emboli are not an inevitable consequence of atheromatous vascular disease.

The relative proportions of cholesterol esters, cholesterol, triglyceride and phospholipid in atheromatous plaques are probably important in determining the effects of atheromatous embolism on the cerebral circulation. Phospholipid has an emulsifying effect on lipid-based emboli, mainly consisting of cholesterol and its esters, and may therefore protect against vessel obstruction. A further important factor is the quantity of cholesterol contained in the embolus. Embolism by clusters of cholesterol crystals is a relatively innocuous occurrence, as shown by the observation of such emboli in the retinal vessels in patients with a history of transient ischaemic attacks, but without symptoms of retinal dysfunction. However, a massive shower of such emboli can produce cerebral infarction, presumably due to the simultaneous embolic occlusion of too great a proportion of the available arterial tree, with both pial and precapillary circulations becoming ischaemic during the critical period of hypoperfusion. Haemorrhage into an atherosclerotic plaque or dissection of a cerebral vessel is an uncommon cause of arterial occlusion. Rarely occlusion can result from a space-occupying lesion compressing a vessel.

Large and small vessel disease in cerebral infarction

Atherosclerosis affects larger muscular arteries such as the common carotid and vertebral artery outside the cranium, and the internal carotid, basilar, and anterior, middle and posterior cerebral arteries, and the circle of Willis itself, within the skull. The cerebellar arteries and smaller vessels such as the perforating arteries of the basal ganglia, and the circumferential arteries supplying the brain stem and spinal cord, are less affected. Atherosclerosis is particularly common in the elderly although young people may also be affected. Both genetic and environmental factors, particularly smoking and

dietary fat intake, may be important in its pathogenesis. The most important of these risk factors are listed in Table 5.1.

Fatty intimal streaks are common in young people and are probably of no clinical significance in themselves, being potentially reversible with dietary management. The atheromatous plaque itself is characterised by smooth muscle cell proliferation and migration into the intima. Lipids, especially cholesterol and cholesterol esters, accumulate within these cells and within macrophages. Destruction of the elastic lamina, and fibrosis of the vessel wall ultimately occurs. Atheromatous plaques assume clinical significance either when they obtrude into the lumen of a vessel so as almost to occlude it, as occurs in the internal carotid artery at its origin from the common carotid artery or, more commonly, when degenerative changes occur within the plaque leading to the formation of '*complicated plaques*'.

In complicated plaques, there is calcification and ulceration of the luminal surface of the plaque resulting in the release of atheromatous cholesterol-rich debris into the circulation. Thrombus formation on the luminal surface or haemorrhage into the plaque can occur secondarily. Thrombus on an ulcerated plaque, haemorrhage into the plaque, or the dissection of blood along the vessel wall, may occlude the affected artery. In larger vessels thrombosis more commonly results in partial occlusion of the vessel. This leads to increased turbulence in blood flow distal to the region and to the formation of moderate-sized emboli, arising from mural thrombus. Such emboli may be large enough to occlude a medium-sized intracerebral artery, such as the main stem of a middle cerebral artery, causing a major completed stroke. Ulcerated plaques may also be a source of micro-emboli composed of fibrin and platelets. Finally, in complicated atheromatous plaques, damage to the elastic lamina causes loss of elasticity of the vessel wall, and aneurysmal dilatation of the vessel.

Unlike atherosclerosis, *hypertension* and *diabetes mellitus* affect smaller vessels. Hypertensive disease results in hyaline change in the walls of small arteries with intimal and medial thickening, and a reduction of adaptive collateral flow in the arterial circulation. A similar thickening occurs in diabetes when mucopolysaccharide is deposited in the walls of small vessels. In addition, both these conditions are associated with more severe, and more rapidly progressive atherosclerosis affecting large muscular arteries.

If the hypertension has entered an accelerated phase fibrinoid necrosis of vessel walls is found. This is associated with zones of constriction and dilatation of arteries, indicating that autoregulation has failed. Localised zones of arterial dilatation occur because the arteries' ability to constrict in response to a very high intraluminal pressure has failed, and at these sites there is extravasation of protein, with vasogenic oedema. Later, fibrinoid necrosis and haemorrhage occur in the intima, or small perivascular haemorrhages may be seen. This is a serious and often fatal disorder.

Other forms of vascular disease, including syphilitic arteritis, polyarteritis nodosa, temporal (giant cell) arteritis, allergic angiitis, rheumatoid arteritis and septicaemia, leading to mycotic aneurysm, can involve the cerebral vessels, and cause infarction or, less commonly, haemorrhage. However, these are all uncommon when compared with the frequency of atherosclerotic and hypertensive large and small vessel disease. Primary involvement of veins, *cortical thrombophlebitis*, is a rare cause of haemorrhagic stroke, often presenting with sudden, persistent focal seizures and a rapidly deteriorating level of consciousness. It occurs in polycythaemia rubra vera and leukaemia, during pregnancy and to varying degrees with prolonged oral contraceptive use especially in women aged 30–40 years.

Thrombosis of the superior sagittal sinus and deep cerebral veins may occur spontaneously but is more commonly seen after cranial or other trauma, or in patients with bacterial meningitis or subdural empyema. It is usually fatal. Intracranial venous thrombosis due to extreme dehydration is rare; it occurs especially in infants. Disseminated intravascular coagulation syndrome may also lead to intracranial venous thrombosis.

Fibromuscular hyperplasia is a rare form of arterial disease recognised in many large arteries, especially in the renal and mesenteric arteries, which may also involve the carotid and cerebral arteries. It is usually limited to the cervical parts of these vascular territories, only rarely affecting intracranial arteries. It may present as transient ischaemic attacks, or as stroke, and is usually recognised by its characteristic angiographic appearance consisting of a 'string of beads' deformity—a succession of rings of moderately tight stenosis and dilatation of the arterial lumen in the affected portion of the vessel. It has been recognised principally among women, at any age. Histologically there are alternating zones of thickening and thinning of the media due to fibrosis,

and degeneration of the elastic lamina. The intimal layer is usually thickened. The outer muscular coat is often thinned in the dilated regions of the abnormal vessels.

Risk factors

Certain additional factors, listed in Table 5.2, are relevant in the causation of ischaemic stroke. Most

Table 5.2. Additional risk factors for stroke

Increased coagulability of blood, e.g. polycythaemia rubra vera
Leukaemia
Gastric carcinoma
Platelet disorders
Hyperviscosity, e.g. dehydration
Polycythaemia (of any cause)
Hypoxia
Recent cranial or other trauma
Emotional stress
Other forms of vascular disease, e.g. polyarteritis nodosa
Syphilitic vasculitis
Giant cell arteritis

of these are treatable, or even preventable but their recognition is not always easy without special investigation and they are usually discovered only after the patient has had a stroke or a transient ischaemic attack. Nonetheless, attention to these factors may diminish the risk of subsequent stroke. The importance of attempting correction of these underlying risk factors for stroke or atherosclerotic vascular disease has been demonstrated in epidemiological studies of stroke and transient ischaemic attacks in populations at risk.

Epidemiology

Careful prospective and retrospective studies have shown that about 85 % of strokes are due to cerebral infarction, the remainder being haemorrhages. In the past, the incidence of cerebral haemorrhage was thought to be very much higher than this, but this apparent change seems to have been due to inaccurate diagnosis in previous years. In a defined population the overall incidence of stroke is about 200/100 000 per year, but stroke is much commoner in the elderly than in younger people. In those older than 85 years, the annual incidence is about 5000/100 000 per year, whereas in the seventh decade it is about 400/100 000 per year. Further, mortality after a stroke is itself related to age. The mortality in stroke occurring in the fifth decade is about 10 %, but in the ninth decade it is about 60%. Morbidity is also usually greater in elderly patients with stroke, when compared with younger patients. Mortality in the 6 months after a stroke is twice as great in patients older than 70 years as in patients aged 30–60 years. Life expectancy tables in patients aged less than 60 years at the time of their stroke suggest that the excess mortality levels off within a few years of the stroke.

Survival rates in patients with strokes have been related to mean diastolic blood pressure. Patients with normal diastolic pressures have a survival rate of about 90% at 5 years, but patients with mean diastolic blood pressures of 120 mmHg have a survival rate at 5 years of only 60%.

Treatment

The blood pressure is raised in 50%–75% of all patients with stroke and there is evidence that reduction of blood pressure occurring in response to treatment with antihypertensive drugs improves the prognosis. Furthermore, effective antihypertensive treatment seems to increase the interval between the first and second stroke in those in whom a second stroke develops.

For many years, patients with *transient ischaemic attacks* (TIA) have been treated with anticoagulant drug therapy, but the evidence that it prevents a stroke is inconclusive in patients in whom the TIAs are in a carotid distribution. Correction of polycythaemia and of asymptomatic hyperlipidaemia may also prevent the progression of TIA to a stroke. In patients with completed stroke there is no evidence that anticoagulant drugs are effective in preventing further strokes. Similarly, treatment of hypercholesterolaemia in patients with cerebral vascular disease seems to have no effect on prognosis.

The results of treatment in patients with established strokes is disappointing but there is good evidence that strokes can be prevented by controlling hypertension, and by surgery for valvular heart disease or localised carotid atherosclerosis. The indications for extracranial-intracranial anastomoses, for example, between the superficial temporal artery and the middle cerebral artery, remain controversial. Nevertheless, refractory transient ischaemic attacks in the presence of carotid occlusion or inaccessible carotid or middle cerebral stenoses may benefit from such an operation.

Vascular territories and infarction

In the presence of severe stenotic or complicated atherosclerosis, certain regions of the brain are at risk of infarction, especially when the atherosclerosis is associated with hypertension or with diabetes mellitus.

The *cerebral hemispheres* are largely supplied by branches from the internal carotid artery, and the *brain stem* and *cerebellum* by branches of the vertebro-basilar system. The basilar artery also supplies the occipital lobes and the inferior surface of both temporal lobes by its posterior cerebral branches. In addition, perforating branches of the basilar artery supply the pulvinar of the thalamus and, in some patients, more anterior thalamic nuclei. The anterior and middle cerebral arteries are branches of the internal carotid artery. Anastomoses between these vessels occur at several sites.

The *circle of Willis* is a ring-like vascular anastomosis between the two carotid arteries and the basilar artery, situated at the base of the brain. The anterior communicating artery interconnects the two anterior cerebral vessels and the two posterior communicating arteries interconnect the internal carotid arteries with the basilar artery. The posterior cerebral arteries are the terminal branches of the basilar artery, and their perfusion is usually from the basilar circulation. In about 10% of patients, however, perfusion of the posterior cerebral arteries is derived from the internal carotid circulation via the posterior communicating arteries. The circle of Willis allows anastomotic blood flow from one carotid system into the other or into the basilar circulation and vice versa in relation to physiological stresses, such as that induced by turning the neck or by forced neck extension, in which reduction in blood flow can occur in the carotid or basilar circulations. This physiological role of the circle of Willis is also important in establishing collateral flow in patients with occlusive disease of the carotid or vertebral arteries.

Anastomoses also occur between the circulations of the major branches of the carotid and basilar arteries. For example, leptomeningeal anastomoses between the anterior cerebral and middle cerebral circulations at the convexity of each hemisphere, and deep anastomoses within the frontal white matter are important. Similar anastomoses occur between adjacent circulations elsewhere within the brain, especially between the posterior and middle cerebral arteries in the temporal and parietal lobes, and between the basilar and carotid circulations in the thalamus, and in the white matter of the posterior part of the internal capsule. In addition, the branches of the basilar artery, supplying the brain stem and cerebellar hemispheres, have well-developed anastomotic circulations at the extremes of their vascular territories. Within the brain stem itself, anastomoses are present between the circulations of the deep perforating vessels, and the short and long circumferential branches of the basilar artery. In the spinal cord an identical pattern of vascularisation occurs, the perforating, short-circumferential and long-circumferential vessels forming anastomoses within the substance of the spinal cord.

Finally, *potential anastomotic circulations* exist between the internal and external carotid territories in the scalp vessels, in the face, and in the bones at the base of the skull. These are sometimes important in patients with long-standing atheromatous stenosis of the carotid circulation in the neck, and can often be demonstrated by angiography. Anastomoses between the vertebral circulation in the neck and the subclavian territory also occur and are sometimes important, as in the *subclavian steal syndrome*. In patients with subclavian artery stenosis, blood may be diverted from the vertebro-basilar circulation into the subclavian circulation when muscular work of the arm increases the metabolic demand in the limb so that blood flows via these anastomoses into the arm rather than up the basilar circulation to the brain stem. The patient complains of symptoms of brain stem ischaemia when the arm is exercised. This syndrome is very rare.

A number of *anomalies* have been described in the circle of Willis, for example, congenital failure of development of the anterior or posterior communicating arteries. These may be important in the development of symptoms in patients with advanced atherosclerotic stenosis of the internal carotid or basilar arteries. For example, absence of this anastomotic circulation in a patient with severe stenosis of an internal carotid artery may place one hemisphere normally perfused by the disordered internal carotid circulation at risk if no anastomoses can be developed. The posterior cerebral artery territories are particularly vulnerable if, in the presence of severe vertebro-basilar atherosclerosis, the posterior cerebral vessels cannot be perfused via a posterior communicating artery from the internal carotid circulation.

In normal subjects the *leptomeningeal anastomoses* cannot easily be demonstrated. They are best seen at angiography in patients with stenotic disease of the large vessels of the neck, and are particularly well developed in children in whom internal carotid artery thrombosis has resulted in the hemisphere perfused by the damaged carotid artery being entirely dependent for its vascularisation on its collateral circulation. Sometimes in such patients, a leash of moderately large vessels extends into the ischaemic hemisphere from deep perforating branches of the basilar circulation, and extends over the convexity of the hemisphere from the posterior cerebral circulation, so perfusing the middle cerebral territory.

Physiological aspects of the cerebral circulation

Blood flow–metabolism coupling

In the normal brain, following activation of an area of cortex or white matter pathway, either physiologically or by epilepsy, there is an appropriate increase in cerebral blood flow (CBF) to meet the increased metabolic demand. As the energy requirements for cerebral tissue are derived almost exclusively from the aerobic catabolism of glucose, there is a close association between the level of CBF and the level of glucose utilisation in every region of the CNS. However, the precise nature of how this coupling between CBF and metabolic activity is achieved remains obscure. The view that the chemical products of cerebral metabolism and neuronal activity (such as carbon dioxide, adenine nucleotides, hydrogen and potassium ions, prostaglandins and neurotransmitters) present in perivascular fluid were principally involved in the coupling has been popular for many years but no coherent view has yet emerged.

Thresholds

CBF in a normal man is about 50 ml/100 g per minute; it is higher in grey matter and lower in white matter. Global CBF falls with conditions producing a fall in cerebral oxidative metabolism such as general anaesthesia, decreasing conscious level and dementia. When CBF falls below about 25 ml/100 g per minute, mental confusion develops and, below about 18 ml/100 g per minute, EEG flattening occurs. Below 10 ml/100 g per minute, depletion of high-energy phosphates, membrane ion pump failure, efflux of cellular potassium, influx of sodium, calcium, chloride and water, and membrane depolarisation occur. With complete arrest of the cerebral circulation for longer than 5–10 min, irreversible cell damage begins. With incomplete ischaemia the degree of permanent damage is less predictable.

Carbon dioxide

The cerebral circulation is exquisitely sensitive to the vasodilating effect of carbon dioxide as $PaCO_2$ increases in the range 30–70 mmHg. This response of CBF to carbon dioxide is impaired with hypotension, lowered cerebral oxygen consumption, cerebral vasospasm and carotid ligation. The blood-brain barrier is freely permeable to carbon dioxide but not to hydrogen ions so that acute changes in plasma pH have no effect on CBF in the healthy brain provided $PaCO_2$ is held constant.

Oxygen

Hypoxia has little effect on CBF until PaO_2 falls below about 60 mmHg when there is a very great vasodilatation.

Arterial blood pressure and cerebral perfusion pressure

Cerebral perfusion pressure is defined as the mean arterial blood pressure minus the cerebral venous pressure, (cerebral venous pressure equals intracranial pressure). Over the approximate range 60–140 mmHg of mean arterial blood pressure, CBF remains relatively constant because the cerebral vessels constrict with hypertension and dilate with hypotension. Above and below these upper and lower limits of 'autoregulation', CBF increases and decreases respectively. Hence in patients with stenosis of the main extracranial or intracranial arteries this capacity for 'autoregulation' maintains a nearly normal blood flow to potentially ischaemic parts of the brain. When cerebral perfusion pressure falls as the result of increasing intracranial pressure, for example, with change in body posture, Valsalva manoeuvre, or a space-occupying lesion, CBF does not fall until cerebral perfusion pressure is less than 50 mmHg.

Above the upper 'breakthrough' point, acute hypertension provokes ballooning of segments of the cerebral arterioles (Byrom's sausage-string phenomenon) and then generalised vasodilatation

with breakdown of the blood–brain barrier, protein extravasation and oedema formation occur. With chronic hypertension, both the lower and upper limits of autoregulation are shifted upwards. Hence, over-enthusiastic reduction of blood pressure may precipitate cerebral infarction even though the absolute level to which the blood pressure has fallen may not normally be regarded as in the hypotensive range. If blood pressure is lowered gradually over some days, the autoregulatory curve may shift back toward normal, although clearly such management is not possible when the patient has hypertensive encephalopathy, eclampsia, left ventricular failure or aortic dissection.

Autoregulation is impaired following head injury, cerebral ischaemia, hypoxia, hypercapnia and subarachnoid haemorrhage. In such cases, the arterioles may behave as a passive tubular system so that blood flow changes according to changes in pressure. In this situation, the brain is susceptible to hypoxia from sudden reductions in blood pressure, and to oedema or haemorrhage in the presence of sudden increases in blood pressure.

Following severe ischaemia, there is a central area of necrosis, surrounded by a potentially viable ischaemic penumbra. Blood vessels in this zone lose their normal reactivity both to changes in arterial blood pressure and blood gases; they behave as if in a state of vasoparalysis. However, vasodilating factors such as hypercapnia will dilate normal blood vessels elsewhere in the brain, thereby *stealing* blood from the ischaemic zones. Attempts to induce 'inverse steal' by hyperventilation have not proved to be clinically useful in adequately controlled studies.

Autonomic innervation

Only the extraparenchymal cerebral arteries such as branches of the circle of Willis and arterioles in the subarachnoid space and pia are innervated by the cervical sympathetic (noradrenergic) nerves. Under resting conditions, neither cervical sympathectomy nor sympathetic stimulation has much effect on cerebral blood flow. Although the extraparenchymal vessels constrict slightly with sympathetic stimulation, the intracerebral vessels, which contribute over 50% of the cerebral vascular resistance can dilate and CBF does not change. When the intracerebral vessels are maximally dilated, as with hypercapnia or hypotension, then sympathetic stimulation will reduce CBF. *In summary* the extraparenchymal vessels can be influenced by the peripheral sympathetic system but the intracerebral vessels can usually compensate to maintain normal flow. The cerebral capillaries may receive a central noradrenergic innervation but its role and that of the cholinergic and peptidergic innervations remain subjects for much further study.

Viscosity and haematocrit

Whole blood viscosity increases with haematocrit. CBF is low in polycythaemia rubra vera and the incidence of cerebral ischaemia rises with increasing haematocrit in this condition. Venesection reverses these effects.

Cerebral infarcts

The size and location of cerebral infarcts vary. Their gross and microscopic appearances depend upon the presence or absence of haemorrhage in the lesion, and upon the time that has elapsed between infarction and histopathological examination.

Recent infarcts are often haemorrhagic, especially if they involve the central grey matter or cortex. In small areas of infarction or at the periphery of large infarcts, the cortex is often outlined by petechial haemorrhage (Fig. 5.2). The

underlying infarcted white matter, however, remains pale and it is frequently difficult to detect white matter infarction in the early stages. *Petechial haemorrhages* in the infarcted cortex are due to leakage of blood from damaged capillaries. During the initial stages of ischaemia, the capillary endothelial cells die, swell and burst so that when some blood flows through the capillaries again, it leaks into the tissue. It is thought that the 'reflow' is from collateral circulation from neighbouring preserved areas of the brain, or possibly from reflow through the vessels which were originally occluded by thrombus or embolus. There is some radiographic evidence of reflow through blocked vessels from sequential angiograms of patients with cerebral infarction. It is possible that fragmentation of occluding thrombus may occur in some cases soon after infarction so that large amounts of blood flow into the infarcted area. Removal of thrombus from

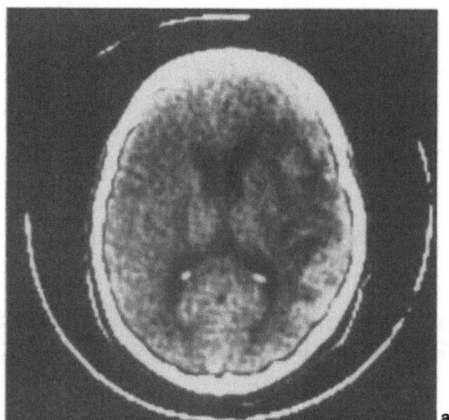

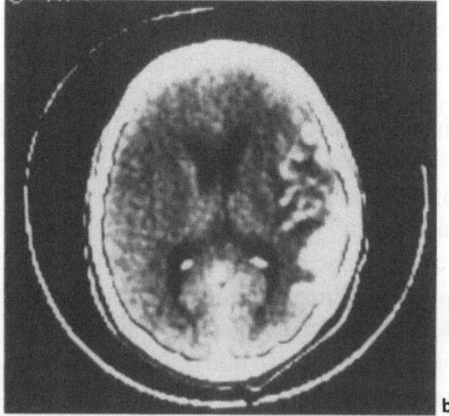

Fig. 5.3. CT scans. Cerebral infarction. **a** There is an area of low attenuation representing infarction and oedema in the right middle cerebral artery territory. The scan was made 5 days after infarction. **b** CT scan enhanced by intravenous contrast medium. There is enhancement in the infarcted area due to breakdown of the blood–brain barrier and increased permeability to the contrast medium.

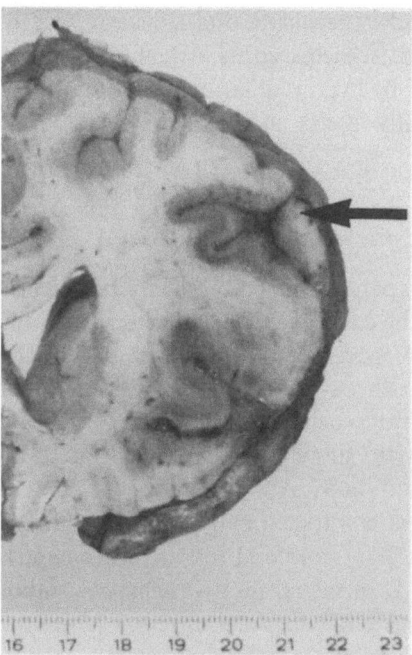

Fig. 5.2. Recent infarction in the middle cerebral artery territory. There is loss of demarcation of the cortex and white matter and petechial haemorrhages in the cortex (*arrow*).

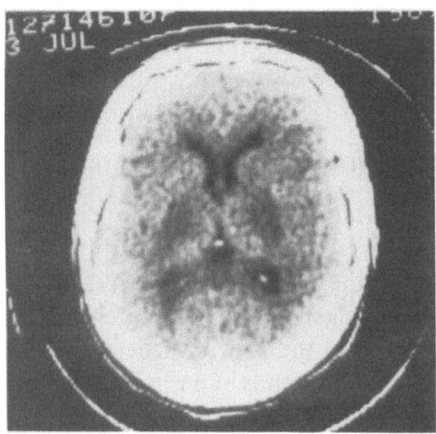

Fig. 5.4. CT scan showing recent bilateral infarction of the basal ganglia.

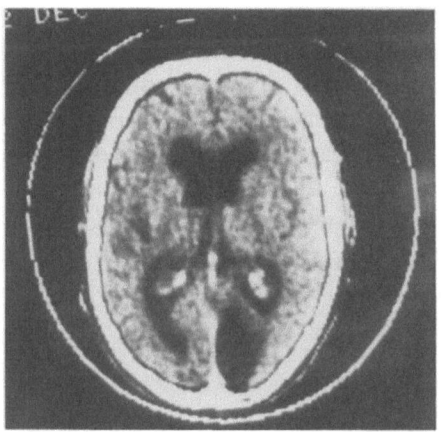

Fig. 5.5. CT scan showing an old cystic infarct in the right occipital lobe. The brain is atrophic with large ventricles.

vessels at a later stage may be due to the action of fibrinolysins.

After *2–3 days*, the dark red colour of the cortex imparted by the petechial haemorrhages starts to fade and the whole area of infarction becomes swollen and *oedematous* (Figs. 5.3, 5.4). The extent of infarction in the white matter can now be detected as it is oedematous, granular, friable and soft. Oedema extends beyond the edges of the infarct and if extensive, as in large infarcts, the brain swelling may cause transtentorial herniation, midbrain compression, and haemorrhage which may be fatal (see Chap. 4).

The oedema starts to subside after the first *7–10 days* and the infarcted tissue becomes very soft and almost liquid. If the area of infarction is small, it may become cystic (cystic malacia) within a few

weeks but it may be many months before the necrotic tissue is removed in the case of larger infarcts. Extensive infarcts involving much of the middle cerebral artery territory may show little reduction in tissue bulk even after 1 year; the white matter remains as a chalky-white, soft, granular mass covered by a convoluted ribbon of shrunken, yellow cortex. It may be *several years* before such an infarct evolves into a thin-walled cyst (Fig. 5.5) covered only by a thin coat of leptomeninges, and traversed by thin blood vessel trabeculae. Evidence of previous haemorrhage into the infarct may be seen in the form of orange blood pigment staining in the walls of the cyst.

Secondary changes may be observed in the brains of patients dying many years after a large infarct. If the middle cerebral artery territory is involved, the internal capsule, cerebral penduncle, and pyramidal tract on the same side may be shrunken and atrophic due to wallerian (axonal) degeneration following destruction of cortical neurons by the infarct (Fig. 5.6). The lateral ventricles may be

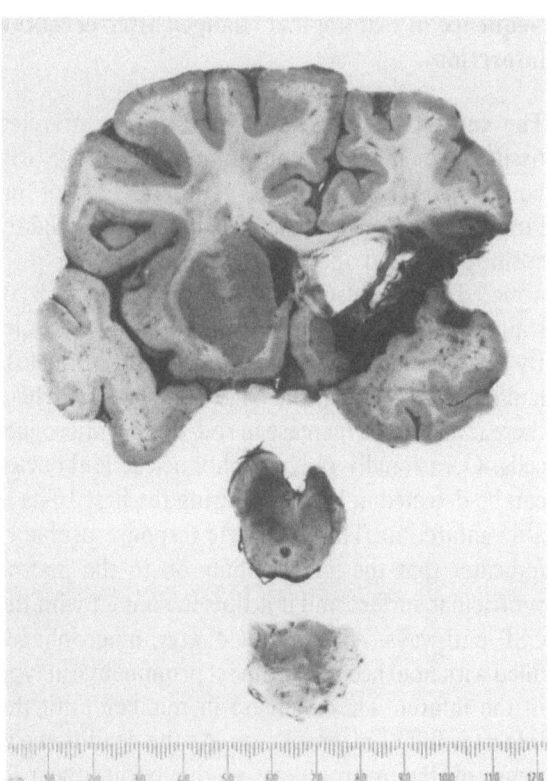

Fig. 5.6. Old infarction in the right middle cerebral artery territory. The coronal slice of cerebral hemisphere shows a cystic cavity and dilated lateral ventricles on the right. There is atrophy of the ipsilateral cerebral peduncle and right side of the pons.

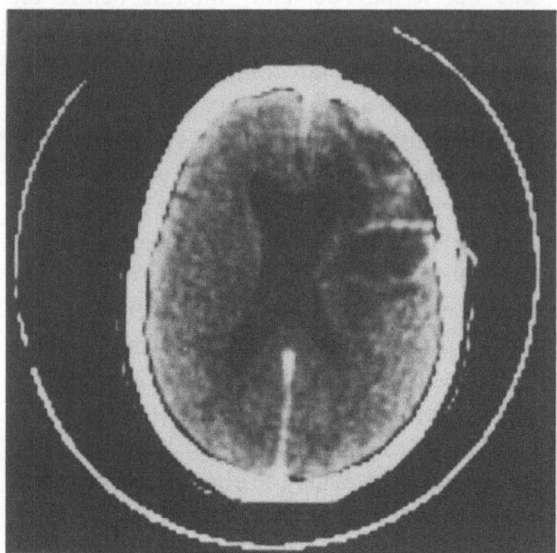

Fig. 5.7. CT scan after injection of contrast medium. There is a cystic area of old infarction in the right middle cerebral artery territory and enhancement around the main cavity. The ventricles are enlarged.

dilated, especially on the side of the infarct, to compensate for the loss of brain tissue (Fig. 5.7).

Sequence of histological changes after cerebral infarction

The earliest histological change in the infarcted tissue is seen in the neurons. Ischaemic changes can be recognised in neurons within *6–12 h* of infarction; the neuronal cytoplasm becomes brightly eosinophilic and the nucleus shrunken and pyknotic. There is usually also some reduction in staining intensity of the infarcted tissue as a whole. By *24 h*, there is a prominent polymorphonuclear leukocyte response at the edge of the infarct where there is also some increase in rod-shaped microglial cells. Occasionally polymorphonuclear leukocytes can be detected in the CSF during the first 10 days after infarction. This leukocyte response probably indicates that the infarct abuts on to the pial or ventricular surface and it is thus in contact with the CSF pathways. After about *4 days*, macrophages filled with lipid become the most prominent cell type in the infarct. They increase in number until the infarct is full of macrophages. As the dead tissue is removed, the macrophages gradually disappear to leave a cystic, fluid-filled cavity; this process may take many years depending on the size of the infarct. Small numbers of macrophages usually persist

within the cyst and within its walls. Astrocyte proliferation and hypertrophy is seen at the edge of an infarct within the first days and gradually a gliotic wall forms around the edge of the cystic infarct.

Blood flow changes after cerebral infarction

A feature of infarction during the period of resolution, that is from about 7 days to 3 months after infarction, is the increased vascularity found in a zone around the edges of the infarct, often more or less corresponding to the zone of oedema around the infarct. The latter extends into white matter, but usually spares adjacent grey matter (oedema from cerebral tumour or abscess involves both grey and white matter). Increased blood flow cannot be appreciated at histopathological examination but has been demonstrated in cerebral blood flow studies using a regional technique with radioactive xenon. In those studies it was called 'luxury perfusion' to emphasise its occurrence in the region of ischaemic infarction. It is often demonstrated in CT scan examinations of large cerebral infarcts, especially when studied about 1 month after infarction. This increased vascularity and oedema is accompanied by a local breakdown in the impermeability of the blood–brain barrier, and this is exemplified by the persistence of radioisotope in the region of resolving infarcts in radioisotope brain scans (Fig. 5.3b).

Lacunes

Small infarcts, or lacunes, up to about 15 mm in diameter, are commonly found in the deep central parts of the brain, especially in the putamen, thalamus, basis pontis and white matter of the cerebral hemispheres. They are probably due to occlusion of deep perforating arteries either by microemboli, or from hyalinisation of these vessels. Some may represent the final stage of resolution of tiny haemorrhages. These irregular cystic lacunes must be distinguished pathologically from the widening of perivascular spaces in senescent brains and from the smooth-walled cavities produced postmortem in brain tissue by gas-forming organisms.

Carotid artery territory infarction

The carotid artery supplies the *ophthalmic, anterior cerebral* and *middle cerebral* arteries. Occlusion of the internal carotid artery may occur suddenly or gradually, in association with atheroma at its origin from the common carotid artery in the neck. It may also occur as a sequel to trauma in the neck, dissection of the wall of the vessel or, rarely, in infancy it may occur in association with a febrile illness, especially with tonsillitis. Sudden complete occlusion of an internal carotid artery leads to massive infarction of most of the cerebral hemisphere on the same side, including frontal, anterior temporal and parietal lobes, and their deep white matter. Death follows in many such cases within a few hours, and in those that survive 12–36 h oedema leads to subfalcine and transtentorial herniation, which may itself be fatal. There is a dense contralateral hemiparesis with sensory loss and hemianopia.

This typical clinical syndrome does not always occur after carotid occlusion. Complete occlusion of the internal carotid artery may also be found unexpectedly and apparently without clinical complications in healthy subjects, even younger than 30 years, dying of unrelated causes, such as trauma. In these patients it is thought that the carotid occlusion may develop gradually from thrombosis associated with local atherosclerosis, so that an extensive and effective collateral circulation develops. This collateral circulation can sometimes be demonstrated angiographically, most characteristically in patients with autoimmune aortitis (Takayasu's disease) in whom a 'rete mirabile'—a leash of dilated collaterals—develops in the basal ganglia, so vascularising the ischaemic hemisphere from the basilar circulation.

Carotid stenosis is associated with recurrent emboli in the internal carotid circulation, causing ipsilateral episodes of transient monocular blindness and contralateral transient hemiparesis. These may culminate in completed retinal infarction, and in a stroke resulting from infarction of part or the whole of the middle cerebral artery territory. The anterior cerebral artery territory is less commonly involved.

The major part of the cerebral hemisphere is supplied by the *middle cerebral artery* through its five distal branches. Infarction in the whole territory of this artery produces a similar infarct to that seen with internal carotid artery thrombosis and, if the patient survives, disability is usually severe. Aphasia occurs in left middle cerebral territory infarction and left or right parietal lobe infarction causes severe perceptual deficits, including disorders of visuo-spatial orientation. Penetrating branches of the middle cerebral arteries supply the internal capsular white matter, the caudate and lenticular nuclei, and the anterior thalamus; infarction in the territory of these branches causes the familiar syndrome of motor hemiplegia, with prominent involvement of the arm, some degree of sensory loss and an incomplete hemianopia. The deep basal nuclei are usually involved in the infarct, but quite small lacunar lesions may occur, causing pure motor or sensory strokes.

The *anterior cerebral artery* supplies the orbital surface and tip of the frontal lobe, the entire mesial surface of the hemisphere to the parieto-occipital junction, most of the corpus callosum, and the anterior part of the caudate nucleus. Heubner's artery, a branch of the anterior cerebral artery, penetrates the anterior perforated substance, and supplies the anterior part of the anterior limb of the internal capsule. Infarction in this territory causes a hemiplegia mostly involving the leg and shoulder muscles. Complete anterior cerebral artery territory infarction is dominated by mental symptoms of frontal lobe dysfunction and incontinence. It is most frequently seen in patients with subarachnoid haemorrhage associated with aneurysms of the anterior cerebral or anterior communicating arteries.

Vertebro-basilar territory infarction

Infarction in the complete territory of this vessel, or in a major part of it, causes death from brain stem failure. Most of the clinical syndromes associated with vertebro-basilar disease therefore represent ischaemia or infarction in the territory of the major branches of the basilar artery.

The *posterior cerebral artery* is nearly always supplied by the basilar circulation. Infarction in this territory involves the upper midbrain and superior cerebellar peduncle, the posterior part of the internal capsule, the inferior and mesial surface of the temporal lobe, the splenium of the corpus callosum and the calcarine (visual) cortex of the occipital lobe and its white matter (Fig. 5.5). Most infarcts in this territory are partial. Hemianopia, quadrantanopia, or cortical blindness result from bilateral lesions involving the occipital regions. Contralateral hemiballismus is seen with infarction in or near the subthalamic nucleus; contralateral hemianaesthesia and hemianopia occurs with infarction of the thalamus and lateral geniculate body; oculomotor palsy with contralateral hemiparesis is characteristic of infarction of the third nerve and of the basis pedunculi. As in the case of middle cerebral artery infarction and its relation to disease of the internal carotid artery, infarction in the territory of the posterior cerebral artery is nearly always due to occlusion at a proximal site in the vertebro-basilar system, or due to embolism from this larger vessel. It may also occur in patients with supratentorial space-occupying lesions in whom transtentorial herniation results in occlusion of the ipsilateral posterior cerebral artery (see Chap. 4).

Syndromes of *superior cerebellar*, *anterior inferior cerebellar* and *posterior inferior cerebellar artery* territory infarction, involving cerebellar hemisphere, lower midbrain, pons and medulla are well recognised, but usually reflect embolism into these circulations, or occlusion of the basilar or of one vertebral artery rather than primary thrombosis of these vessels themselves. Aplasia of a vertebral artery is often found in patients with posterior inferior cerebellar artery territory infarction, the circulation of the latter territory on the side of the aplastic vessel being then especially vulnerable to episodes of hypotension or reduced flow in the remaining vertebral artery.

Both the posterior cerebral artery and the posterior inferior cerebellar arteries are vulnerable to compression in the presence of raised intracranial pressure and brain herniation associated with space-occupying lesions, the former becoming compressed at the tentorial edge and the latter in the foramen magnum. Infarction in the territories of these vessels may then occur, causing false localising signs.

Infarction of the major part of a cerebellar hemisphere is sometimes followed by oedematous swelling of the infarcted tissue in the subsequent 12–72 h, leading to progressive obtundation and the gradual development of lower cranial nerve palsies from compression on the side of the infarcted cerebellum. These clinical features are due to the secondary effects of swelling. They may progress to cause torsion of the brain stem, with the development of circulatory and respiratory disturbances, and so to death. This progressive syndrome can be relieved by surgical decompression of the posterior fossa, one of the very few stroke syndromes associated with infarction in which neurosurgical intervention is indicated in the acute stage of the disorder.

Boundary zone infarction

Infarction in the cerebral hemispheres in a zone between the territories supplied by the middle and posterior cerebral arteries or between the territories of the middle and anterior cerebral arteries is known as boundary zone infarction. Infarction occurs because of a failure of cerebral perfusion leading to critical reduction in blood flow in the terminal parts of the cerebral circulation. This is usually the result of a period of profound hypotension lasting longer than 10 min.

Macroscopically, there is infarction of the cortex in the depths of the sulci, sometimes with involvement of the underlying white matter (Fig. 5.8). The parieto-occipital area is infarcted initially, but, in severe cases, the zone of infarction may extend anteriorly over the superior surface of the hemisphere between the areas supplied by the middle and anterior cerebral arteries. In the posterior fossa the zones between the superior and inferior cerebellar arteries may also undergo boundary zone infarction during prolonged hypotension.

In patients with profound hypotension due to cardiorespiratory arrest, infarction may occur in all boundary zones more or less symmetrically but if there is marked focal stenotic vascular disease asymmetrical lesions may result, as can often be demonstrated clinically in survivors of this catastrophe.

The appearance of the infarction in the boundary zones depends on the time between infarction and death. Lindenberg referred to this typical watershed distribution of boundary zone cortical infarction as 'granular atrophy' when observed years after the event. Areas of congestion and softening in the depths of the sulci are often bilaterally symmetrical (Fig. 5.8). Microscopically the changes observed in boundary zone infarction are similar to those seen in infarction elsewhere in the brain. Eventually the cortex and underlying subcortical white matter becomes a soft yellow shrunken ribbon.

Death due to hypotensive brain damage

Very prolonged, severe hypotension or circulatory arrest results in a lesion more severe than boundary zone infarction. In such cases the whole cortical grey matter, and the deep grey nuclei, together with cerebellar and spinal grey matter, have been subjected to stagnant hypoxia during the period of hypotension or circulatory arrest. Not only are the boundary zones infarcted but the whole cortex undergoes laminar necrosis, with relative sparing of the underlying white matter and the most superficial layer of the cortex. This disorder is usually fatal within a few days, and it can be recognised only if survival occurs for a day or so since the laminar

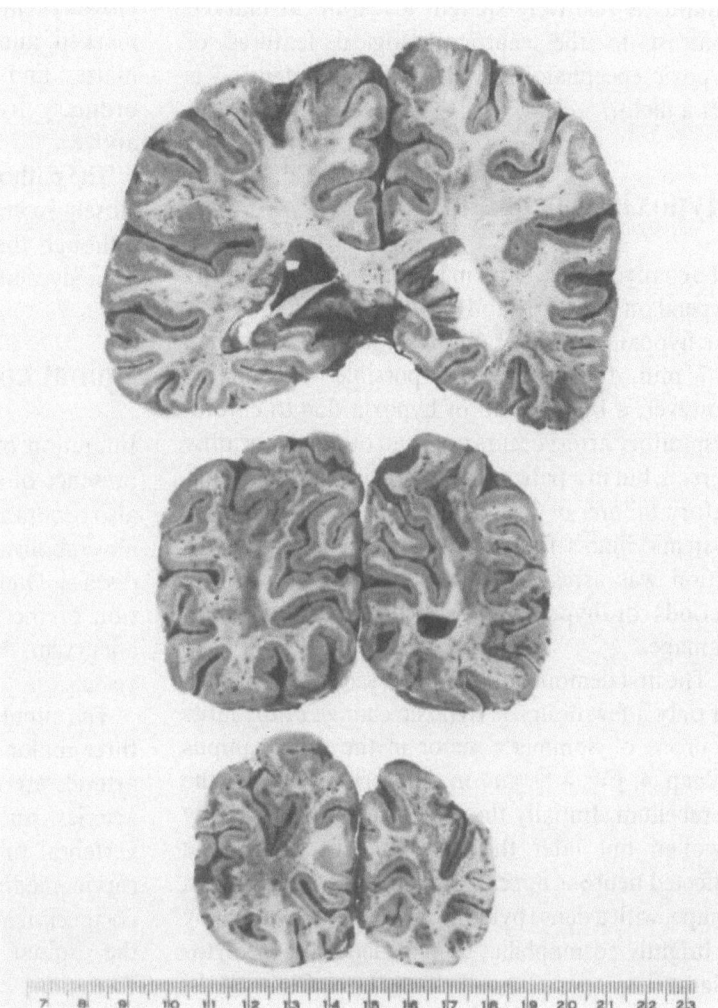

Fig. 5.8. Boundary zone infarction. **a** Recent infarction in the watershed areas between the middle, anterior and posterior cerebral artery territories. **b** Enlargement of the lower brain slices in Fig. 5.8a showing recent infarction in the grey matter in both hemispheres with haemorrhage into the infarcted cortex, especially in the depths of the sulci.

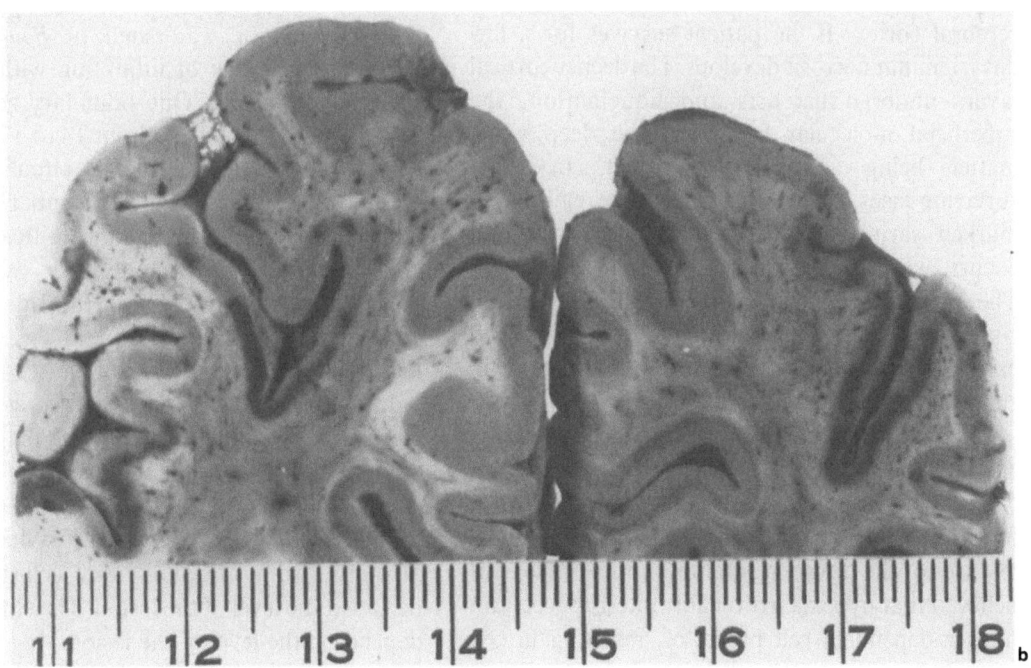

nature of the widespread cortical necrosis is obvious only as tissue breakdown occurs. Only the hippocampus is relatively spared, a feature in marked contrast to the neuropathological features of hypoxic encephalopathy, in which hypotension is not a factor.

Hypoxic encephalopathy

The changes in the brain in hypoxic encephalopathy depend on the *degree* and *duration* of the hypoxia. If the hypoxia is of brief duration, meaning less than 5–7 min, full recovery is possible. Frequently, however, a brief period of hypoxia due to cardiorespiratory arrest occurs not in an otherwise healthy person, but in a patient who has been in cardiorespiratory failure, or has been acidotic with a serious systemic illness for many hours before the circulation was arrested. In such patients quite brief periods of hypoxia may result in severe brain damage.

The first demonstrable change, seen after survival of only a few hours, is hypoxic change in the large neurons of Sommer's sector in the hippocampus (Chap. 4, Fig. 4.1), and in the Purkinje cells in the cerebellum. Initially these neurons appear slightly swollen but later they become shrunken. The affected neurons appear triangular and irregular in shape, with a dense pyknotic nucleus surrounded by a brightly eosinophilic, homogeneous, dense cytoplasm (homogenising cell change) (see Chap. 4). In patients surviving 12–24 h this hypoxic cell change may be found in neurons widely distributed in the cerebral cortex. If the patient survives for a few days, laminar necrosis develops. The deeper cortical layers undergo necrosis and liquefaction, the superficial molecular layer and the deep white matter being relatively unaffected. In longsurviving cases, gliosis develops in these regions and marked shrinkage of the brain and cerebellum occurs, with compensatory ventricular dilatation. The deep grey nuclei of the basal ganglia are similarly affected, accounting for the marked extrapyramidal features often noted clinically in survivors of hypoxic episodes.

In some patients with hypoxic encephalopathy, especially in the special instance of hypoxia due to carbon monoxide poisoning, there is a delay of a few hours, or even a day or so, before the clinical features of the disorder develop. In these cases it is believed that hypoxia irreversibly interrupts certain oxygen-dependent cell processes, resulting in cell

death a few days later when intracellular stores of the relevant metabolites have been exhausted. However, in carbon monoxide poisoning there is a marked, and specific, involvement of central white matter, and globus pallidus; features not found in ordinary hypoxic encephalopathy, as discussed above.

The pathology of *hypoglycaemic* encephalopathy closely resembles that of hypoxic encephalopathy, although the Purkinje cells are less vulnerable to hypoglycaemia than to hypoxia.

Spinal cord infarction

Infarction of the spinal cord is rare, except in the presence of spinal cord compression or trauma. It also occurs as part of the clinical syndrome of fat or air embolism and, as an isolated event, in caisson disease. One of the most frequent causes is dissection of the aorta or aortic surgery for repair of aneurysm, leading to occlusion of the radicular vessels.

The circulation of the spinal cord is derived from three major groups of vessels. The anterior spinal arteries are much larger than the posterior spinal arteries, and are supplied by branches from the vertebral arteries within the spinal canal at the cervicomedullary junction, by branches from the costocervical trunk, from radicular vessels entering the spinal canal through the intervertebral foramina, especially prominent in the thoracic region, and by a single major radicular branch at about T10, the artery of Adamkiewicz. There are thus two major watershed or *boundary zones*, particularly at risk of infarction with hypoxia or severe hypotension. One boundary zone is in the upper thoracic region at about T4 to T7 between the cervical and thoracic radicular circulations, and a second zone is in the upper lumbar segments in which the blood supply becomes critical if the artery of Adamkiewicz is occluded, for example, by a dissecting aneurysm of the aorta. Infarction of the cord in these zones causes paraplegia and sensory loss below the level of the lesion.

Infarction in the territory of the *anterior spinal arteries* causes infarction of the majority of the anterior half of the spinal cord, since these vessels supply the anterior two-thirds of the cord, with paraplegia and dissociated sensory loss. Muscular atrophy, from anterior horn cell involvement, occurs at the level of the lesion. The clinical features depend on the level of the lesion.

Posterior spinal artery territory infarction is very rare; it causes loss of posterior column function. This, and the other manifestations of spinal vascular disease discussed above, is usually due not to primary thrombosis of these small spinal arteries, but to severe vertebro-basilar or aortic atherosclerosis. However, syphilitic or autoimmune vasculitis, and mycotic vascular disease associated with tuberculous or pyogenic infection of the spinal canal and meninges may also cause spinal cord infarction. Compression of the cord, especially in patients with vertebral metastatic cancer, leads to infarction from compression of the cord's blood supply and so to irreversible paraplegia.

Venous infarction

Thrombosis is an uncommon event in veins or sinuses in the cranial cavity, or in spinal veins, but may occur as a localised phenomenon or as part of a widespread cortical thrombophlebitis. The superior longitudinal (sagittal) sinus and the lateral sinuses are the most commonly affected sinuses, but thrombosis of small veins may occur at any site on the cortical surface or in the spinal cord and it is this which results in infarction. Thrombosis of the sagittal sinus itself, if anteriorly located, may not cause cerebral infarction unless small cerebral veins themselves are involved. Venous thrombosis leads to stagnation of blood flow and so to cerebral infarction. The increased capillary pressure caused by the obstruction to blood flow is accompanied by petechial and subarachnoid haemorrhage and by cerebral oedema. Small, limited sites of venous thrombosis may be clinically apparent only as focal seizures with a minor neurological deficit, since collateral venous channels can accommodate flow round the obstructed vessels. However, thrombosis of a major vein, such as the vein of Labbe or the sagittal sinus, is a catastrophic event associated with recurrent seizures, dense hemiplegia or even quadriplegia and coma. Death often follows in a matter of hours.

Cerebral venous thrombosis is rarely a primary event; in most cases a cause can be discovered by clinical examination, or by further investigation (Table 5.3). Extreme dehydration, or malnutrition are rare causes in the developed world, and most cases result either from a complication of pregnancy or the puerperium, from blood dyscrasias accompanied by a thrombotic tendency, as part of a disseminated intravascular coagulopathy, or from

Table 5.3. Causes of cortical venous thrombosis

Dehydration and malnutrition, especially with fever
Tuberculous meningitis
Pyogenic subdural abscess
Otitis media and mastoiditis, especially with petrositis
Head injury
Blood dyscrasias, e.g. leukaemias
Pregnancy, abortion and oral contraceptives
Severe right-sided heart failure
As a remote manifestation of gastric neoplasm
Non-ketotic hyperglycaemic coma
Disseminated intravascular coagulation
Drug induced, e.g. epsilon-aminocaproic acid therapy for subarachnoid haemorrhage

intracranial or intraspinal sepsis. Trauma is also a relatively infrequent, although often unrecognised, cause of cortical thrombophlebitis. Although it was at first thought that most instances of stroke occurring in women treated with oral contraceptive drugs were due to thrombosis of cortical veins or venous sinuses, investigation has suggested that the majority of these strokes are due to occlusion, probably embolic, of small cerebral arteries. Sepsis, particularly in the mastoid process, tends to cause *lateral sinus thrombosis*. This may produce little or no clinical disturbance if the contralateral sinus is patent, but if the other sinus is congenitally absent (as in about 10%–20% of normal people) or the thrombus propagates to the vein of Galen, venous drainage of the thalamus and central parts of the limbic system is obstructed. Flaccid, quadriplegic coma then results, with hydrocephalus and extensive cerebral oedema.

Lateral sinus thrombosis itself, even if unilateral, may present as hydrocephalus of the communicating type. Because of its association with ear infection this is often called 'otitic hydrocephalus'. The hydrocephalus occurs because venous pressure in the sagittal sinus becomes increased, impairing CSF absorption. However hydrocephalus is not an inevitable sequel of such thrombosis.

The causes of *cavernous sinus thrombosis* are similar to those of thrombosis of other cerebral sinuses and veins, but blood dyscrasias and sepsis in the orbit are the most frequent causes. The onset is usually abrupt with complete ophthalmoplegia, exophthalmos and periorbital oedema, blindness and a fixed dilated pupil. The disorder is often fatal, especially if bilateral, because of the associated pituitary and hypothalamic infarction. In addition, the causative infection may be widespread and associated with fatal meningitis.

Thrombophlebitis is an almost invariable finding at the cortical margin of a cerebral abscess, whether otogenic or embolic. In the former case, the abscess is formed in the cortex adjacent to a region of dural penetration by the infection and the first stage of abscess formation is then septic cortical thrombophlebitis and infarction, often presenting as focal seizures. Septicaemia, particularly when associated with gram-negative organisms, may lead to intracranial venous thrombosis.

Spinal thrombophlebitis most commonly occurs in relation to tuberculous infection, as in Pott's paraplegia, when surface veins become involved in the granulomatous inflammation. Paraplegia then develops suddenly, but often incompletely, despite the chronicity of the infection and its associated vertebral deformity. Partially treated pyogenic meningitis may, similarly, be followed by paraplegia from thrombophlebitis.

Thrombosis of abnormal, dilated, spinal veins is a rare presenting feature of spinal arteriovenous malformations causing sudden neurological deficits, often without evidence of haemorrhage from the lesion. The diagnosis can be suspected clinically by the occurrence of pain at the onset of the neurological disorder but myelography or spinal angiography are required to demonstrate the angiomatous malformation.

Intracranial haemorrhage

Of the three major pathological types of intracranial haemorrhage two, *intracerebral* haemorrhage and *subarachnoid* haemorrhage, are common spontaneous events due to cerebral vascular disease or to bleeding disorders. The common sites of spontaneous intracranial haemorrhages are shown in Table 5.4. The third type of intracranial haemor-

Table 5.4. Common sites of hypertensive intracerebral haemorrhage

Putamen	55%
Cerebral cortex	15%
Thalamus	10%
Pons	10%
Cerebellar hemisphere	10%

rhage, *extradural* and *subdural* haemorrhage, is usually due to trauma although in patients with a haemorrhagic diathesis or in dehydrated infants such haemorrhages may rarely occur spontaneously. Traumatic haemorrhages, including extradural, subdural and intracerebral haemorrhages are discussed in Chap. 6.

Although cerebral infarction is much commoner than cerebral haemorrhage the mortality of the latter disorder is far greater than the former. In most post-mortem series in the past, deaths from cerebral haemorrhage exceeded deaths from cerebral infarction. This led to an undue emphasis on the supposed frequency of cerebral haemorrhage itself in epidemiological studies based on cases examined at autopsy. Nonetheless there is evidence that the incidence of cerebral haemorrhage has declined since the introduction of effective antihypertensive drugs, and now represents about 15% of all cases of stroke. Despite this, intracerebral haemorrhage is still the most common cause of sudden death in patients with cerebral vascular disease. Most patients with cerebral infarction survive the event itself, to die of other disorders, such as pneumonia, urinary tract infection, or other complications of their vascular disease.

Hypertensive cerebral and cerebellar haemorrhage

Haemorrhages may occur in many sites in the brain, but in hypertensive patients they are particularly likely to occur in the basal ganglia, especially the putamen (Table 5.4). In patients with intracerebral bleeding due to other causes, such as leukaemia, haemorrhage may occur in any location. Such haemorrhages may be spontaneous or induced by minor trauma. In hypertensive patients, *intracerebral* haemorrhage is a spontaneous event, usually causing deep coma with a dense hemiparesis from the onset. These signs indicate a mass lesion in the central white matter. Seizures may occur and, if blood enters the CSF via the ventricles or the subarachnoid space, neck stiffness and fever may develop so that other causes of meningeal irritation, especially pyogenic infection, must be considered in the differential diagnosis. The blood pressure is usually extremely high after the haemorrhage, a reflex response to the sudden rise in intracranial pressure. The pulse becomes slowed and respirations deep or Cheyne–Stokes in type. Signs of transtentorial herniation develop before death supervenes.

The clinical presentation of *brain stem* haemorrhage is similar, but the pupils are pinpoint from the onset and deterioration of brain stem function leads to death from cardiopulmonary failure within a few hours. In *cerebellar* haemorrhage, however, the patient may recover initially from the coma which usually develops at the onset of the haemorrhage, being left drowsy with a combination of cerebellar and corticospinal signs and lower cranial nerve palsies. Secondary oedematous swelling in the haemorrhage and surrounding brain tissue then leads to progressive displacement of the brain stem, with increasingly evident cranial nerve palsies, drowsiness and cardiopulmonary collapse. This progressive syndrome is similar to that which occurs after massive cerebellar hemisphere infarction, and neurosurgical evacuation of the cerebellar haemorrhage may be life saving. The results of surgical attempts to remove intracerebral haemorrhages acutely are less satisfactory. However, if the patient deteriorates after initially stabilizing, the mass of clot may be removed surgically.

Most intracerebral haemorrhages are large, often occupying most of a hemisphere when examined at autopsy (Fig. 5.9a). Occasionally smaller 'slit haemorrhages' may be found in the putamen or white matter orientated along fibre tracts in the deep central white matter. It is probable that resolution and absorption of such haemorrhages can occur, with clinical recovery. Large fatal haemorrhages often rupture into the lateral vent-

ricles, sometimes causing rupture of the anterior and posterior horns of the ventricles so that blood extends into the frontal and occipital white matter through these secondary breaches in the ventricular walls. Acute hydrocephalus may result, which is often fatal. It used to be thought that intraventricular haemorrhage, particularly when the third ventricle is involved, was uniformly fatal but CT scanning has shown that this is not the case. Massive cerebral haemorrhages cause sudden subfalcine and transtentorial herniation with marked deformation of the brain, often associated with uncal herniation, hippocampal and occipital infarction, and fatal brain stem compression with secondary haemorrhage (Fig. 5.9b). The remaining cerebral tissue is ischaemic and multiple areas of focal ischaemia and infarction may lead to massive oedema of the brain, affecting both white and grey matter.

In patients surviving the initial haemorrhage, absorption of the haematoma occurs. Macrophages invade the blood clot and eventually a cavity forms, filled with proteinaceous fluid and lined by a gliotic,

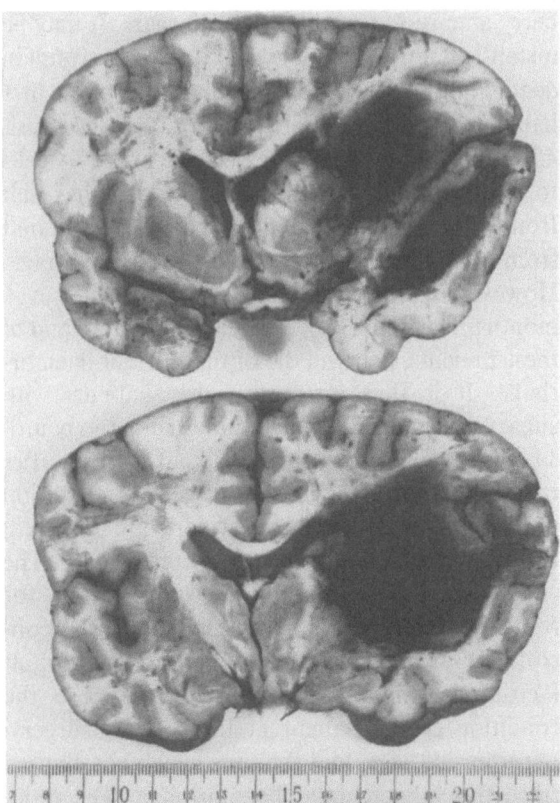 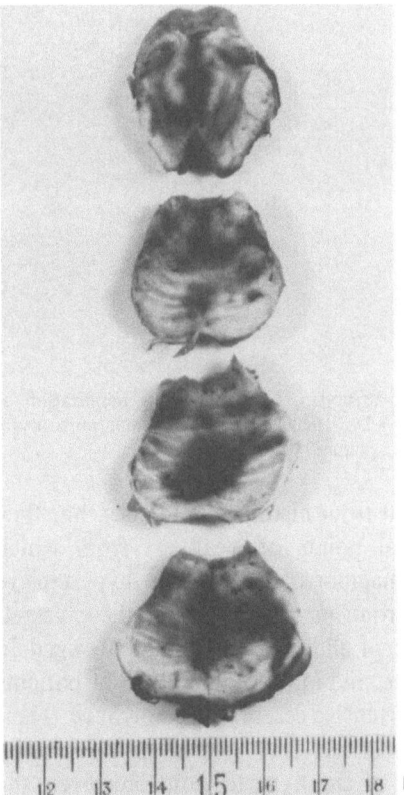

Fig. 5.9. Hypertensive intracerebral haemorrhage. **a** There is a large haematoma, mainly in the white matter, lateral to the basal ganglia, rupturing into the lateral ventricle. **b** Same case as Fig. 5.9a showing haemorrhage into the midbrain and pons, probably occurring as a result of brain displacement.

orange-brown, haemosiderin-stained wall. This may be virtually indistinguishable from the end-stage of cerebral infarction. Histological examination of the brain reveals hypertensive changes in vessels, including thickening of the intima and media of arteries and arterioles, with hyaline change. Occasionally fibrinoid necrosis of arterioles is seen particularly when hypertension is an accelerated (malignant) phase.

The *pathogenesis* of hypertensive cerebral haemorrhage is not entirely understood. Charcot and Bouchard, nearly a hundred years ago, described micro-aneurysms on the walls of small arteries in hypertensive patients, especially in the territory of the lenticulo-striate branches of the middle cerebral arteries. They termed these latter vessels the 'arteries of cerebral haemorrhage'. These microaneurysms have since been demonstrated by a number of other workers (Fig. 5.10) and it has

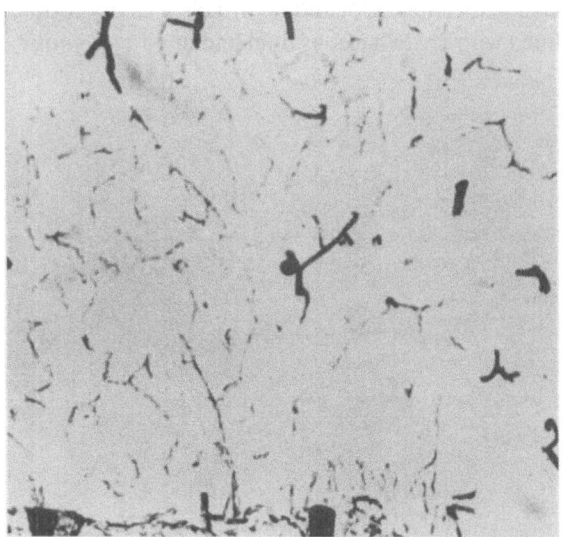

Fig. 5.10. Micro-aneurysm. Carbon-injected preparation of cerebral vessels in a hypertensive rat showing a micro-aneurysm in the centre of the picture.

been suggested from histological studies that they represent focal points of weakness from which intracerebral haemorrhages begin in hypertensive patients. Microaneurysms occur on these vessels in nearly 50% of all hypertensive patients aged 50 years and over, and in more than 90% of patients dying of hypertensive cerebral haemorrhage. Their size and number has been related to the severity and duration of the hypertension. However, the natural history of these microaneurysms is not known and their precise role in hypertensive haemorrhage is thus not certain. Similar abnorma-

lities have been reported on mesenteric vessels in hypertensive patients.

Spontaneous haemorrhage into the spinal cord, *haematomyelia*, is very rare. It is usually associated with trauma, haemophilia or with spinal arteriovenous malformations.

Subarachnoid haemorrhage

While subarachnoid haemorrhage is usually due to rupture of a berry aneurysm (Fig. 5.11), it may also occur from bleeding from an arteriovenous malformation. Other causes, such as mycotic aneurysm, hypertensive cerebral haemorrhage, bleeding diathesis, encephalitis, tumours or trauma are uncommon since in these disorders bleeding usually occurs primarily into the brain and involvement of the subarachnoid space is a secondary phenomenon.

Clinical features

Subarachnoid haemorrhage from berry aneurysm is a serious disorder, though uncommon (4/100000 per year). Its incidence increases with age: 50% of patients with subarachnoid haemorrhage due to berry aneurysm are older than 40 years. It may be instantly fatal, and as many as 25% of cases result in death immediately or within a few hours of the first haemorrhage. If untreated, apart from bed rest, 45% of hospitalised patients will die in the 8 weeks following the initial bleed; half of these deaths result from second or subsequent haemorrhages and half from complications of the first haemorrhage. However, of the survivors, 10% will die in the next 6 months. Thereafter, 4% per year will rebleed and of these patients, half will die of that further haemorrhage. It is thus imperative that patients with subarachnoid haemorrhage should undergo neurosurgical investigation and treatment as soon after the initial haemorrhage as their general condition permits. A third of the survivors are disabled, usually by hemiparesis, dementia or epilepsy. The choice of timing of surgical intervention for ruptured intracranial aneurysms has caused controversy for many years. The four most important factors determining surgical mortality are the condition of the patient at the time of surgery, hypertension, age, and the time which has elapsed since the subarachnoid haemorrhage. The more severely ill the patient and the earlier the operation, the greater is the risk from surgery. In *uncomplicated subarachnoid haemorrhage*, bleeding occurs

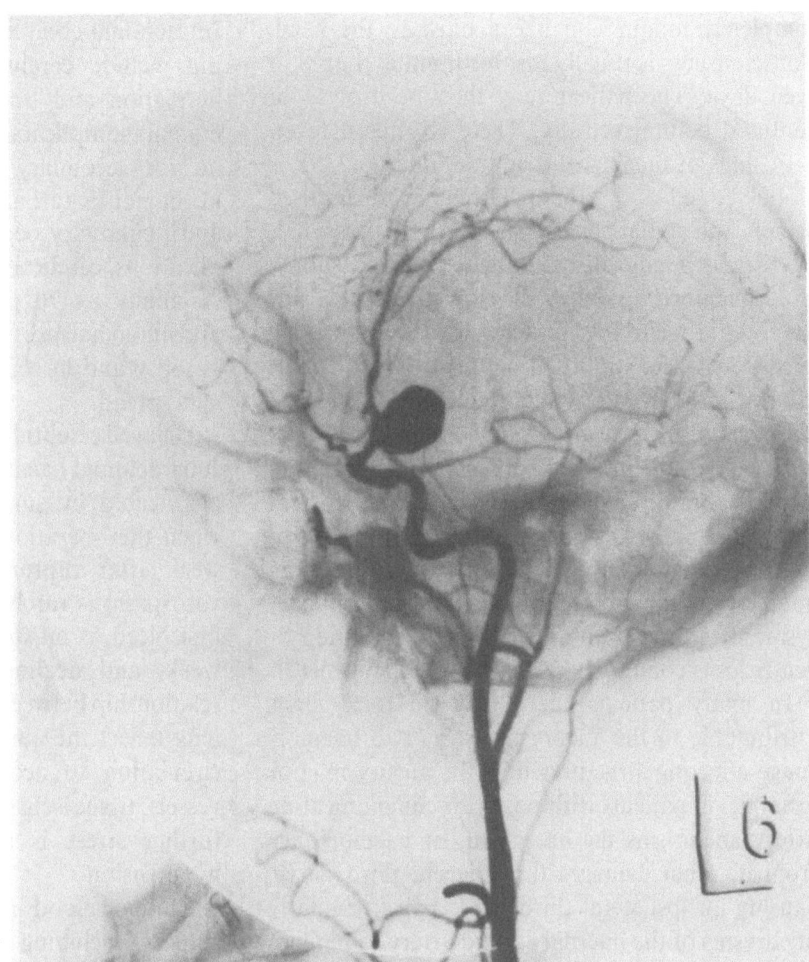

Fig. 5.11. Carotid angiogram demonstrating a large saccular berry aneurysm arising from the middle cerebral artery at its origin from the internal carotid artery. The middle cerebral artery is displaced upwards indicating that there is a haematoma in the temporal lobe.

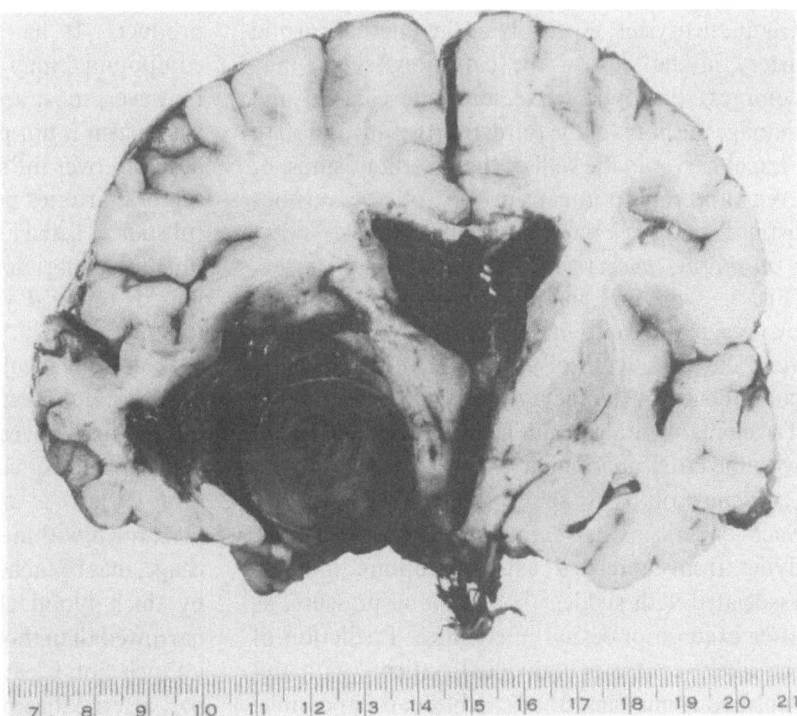

Fig. 5.12. A large berry aneurysm containing thrombus. There is recent haemorrhage around it extending in to the lateral ventricles. The haemorrhage has a space-occupying effect which has resulted in a shift of the brain to the right and subfalcine herniation.

only into the subarachnoid space. The patient may experience a sudden headache often described as completely unique and like a blow to the head. Consciousness is usually lost for minutes, hours or even days. The patient may then be drowsy or confused before recovery. There is often a fever, with signs of meningeal irritation, and the CSF is blood-stained and xanthochromic, with a raised protein and a mild pleocytosis. The CSF pressure is raised and papilloedema, with retinal and subhyaloid haemorrhages may develop in the next few days. Xanthochromia and a raised CSF protein may persist for up to 1 month after a single subarachnoid haemorrhage.

In *complicated subarachnoid haemorrhage* bleeding occurs both into the subarachnoid space and into the brain, so that focal signs or persistent confusion or drowsiness develop. This is particularly common in patients with bleeding from middle cerebral and anterior cerebral artery aneurysms. Rupture of an aneurysm into the brain or ventricles is commonly seen at autopsy (Fig. 5.12).

In many patients there may be focal signs attributable to the aneurysm itself or to haemorrhage affecting structures near the aneurysm. For example, in patients with posterior communicating artery aneurysms the aneurysm, or haemorrhage from it, often damages the adjacent third nerve, causing an ipsilateral third nerve palsy; similarly aneurysms of the internal carotid artery sometimes cause an ipsilateral Horner's syndrome from involvement of the intramural sympathetic fibres. Giant aneurysms, especially of the internal carotid artery in the wall of the cavernous sinus, may compress the optic nerve, or optic chiasm, and damage the fibres of the third, fourth, fifth and sixth cranial nerves in the wall of the cavernous sinus, or even rupture into it, causing a carotico-cavernous fistula, and thus a pulsating exophthalmus.

Fusiform aneurysms of the basilar artery (Fig. 5.13) are rare, but many cause hydrocephalus by invagination into the posterior part of the third ventricle, or a series of cranial nerve palsies from compression by the aneurysm in the posterior fossa. Trigeminal neuralgic pain has also been associated with the latter abnormality.

Rupture of berry aneurysms is not inevitable. Such aneurysms are sometimes found in people dying from unrelated causes. Rupture may be associated with sudden rises in blood pressure, as after exercise or sexual intercourse. Prediction of the likely course in individual patients with unruptured aneurysms, or after a bleed, is impossible.

Late complications

Intracranial complications of subarachnoid bleeding include cerebral infarction, hydrocephalus, herniation and brain stem haemorrhage. Extracranial complications of subarachnoid bleeding include secondary hypertension, electrolyte and hormonal disturbances, ECG changes, glycosuria and pulmonary oedema. Of the intracranial complications, cerebral infarction is the most common. As many as 70% of patients dying with subarachnoid haemorrhage show cerebral infarction at autopsy and in some patients this is massive and widespread.

Delayed cerebral ischaemia occurs naturally after subarachnoid haemorrhage but often appears to be aggravated by surgical intervention, particularly when the operation is performed during the first week after rupture of the aneurysm. Cerebral vasospasm is rarely seen prior to 3 days after the first bleed, is maximal around the end of the first week, and declines thereafter. The capricious relationship between spasm and neurological deficit may reflect the ability of the individual's cerebral circulation to accommodate to such narrowed vessels; tissue ischaemia may be exacerbated when a further stress is applied such as a period of hypotension.

Clotted blood releases many vasoactive substances, including serotonin, bradykinin, thromboxane A_2, adenine nucleotides, catecholamines, haemoglobin derivatives, and fibrin degradation products. It has been proposed that all these compounds may provoke cerebral vasospasm. However, most are released immediately, whereas vasospasm is not present initially but progressively develops over the succeeding days. Contractions of cerebral arteries produced in vitro by many of the substances listed above can be inhibited by appropriate blocking or inhibitory drugs. In contrast, human cerebral vasospasm is refractory to such therapy.

Prolonged incubation of clotted blood at 37°C, however, does result in the production of some ill-defined derivatives of haemoglobin which, in high concentrations, cause vasoconstriction. Furthermore, there is now evidence, from CT scans performed within 48 h of a subarachnoid haemorrhage, that branches of the circle of Willis enveloped by thick blood clot are more likely to become narrowed than those arteries surrounded by little or no such clot. Clearly there is a relationship between peri-arterial haematoma and subsequent arterial narrowing, but the relationship is not a simple one. Many neurosurgeons defer operation when vasospasm is marked. Post-mortem studies have shown that the cerebral arteries affected by blood in the subarachnoid space may subsequently develop thickened fibrotic walls.

Arterial spasm is usually most marked in the artery bearing the aneurysm which has bled, particularly in those parts of the vessel and its branches distal to the aneurysm. Vessel spasm, it should be noted, does not occur only in response to subarachnoid haemorrhage; it is often seen in angiograms of patients with pyogenic meningitis, particularly in vessels in the basal meninges.

Berry aneurysms

The incidence of aneurysms at various sites in patients presenting with subarachnoid haemorrhage is shown in Table 5.5. Multiple aneurysms are

Table 5.5 Sites of aneurysms in patients with subarachnoid haemorrhage

Middle cerebral artery	19%
Anterior cerebral and anterior communicating arteries	41%
Internal carotid and posterior communicating arteries	37%
Basilar artery circulation	3%

found in about 15% of patients with subarachnoid haemorrhage. The true incidence of multiple aneurysms may be greater than this, the figure depending on the completeness of angiography from case to case.

Although often termed berry aneurysms, saccular aneurysms of the cerebral arteries vary greatly in shape. They often take the form of a small, sausage-shaped sac, arising from the branch point of two cerebral arteries by a narrow neck, and pointing away from the origin. Sometimes aneurysms consist of an irregularly shaped sac, indicating multiple zones of weakness of varying degree in the wall of the aneurysm. Aneurysms may be intact without evidence of previous bleeding, or surrounded by fresh blood in an acute case of death from subarachnoid haemorrhage. Sometimes there is evidence of previous bleeding, consisting of a fibrous haemosiderin-laden layer surrounding the external surface of the aneurysm. Large aneurysms may be almost completely filled by lamellated mural thrombus, thus producing an angiographic appearance of a small aneurysm. Rarely, an aneurysm may become thrombosed and so is excluded from the circulation. During this process the aneurysm

may act as a source for emboli of the distal part of the circulation in the territory of the affected vessel. Large aneurysms (giant aneurysms) are especially likely to contain organised thrombus (Fig. 5.12).

Microscopic examination of an aneurysm wall shows that it differs histologically from a normal arterial wall. There is no elastic lamina or smooth muscle in the wall, which consists largely of fibrous tissue with an endothelial lining. The thin fibrous wall of the aneurysm stretches and this may account for its tendency to enlarge and rupture. Even in unruptured aneurysms, phagocytes and haemosiderin deposits are found in the wall. Not all aneurysms rupture; they are sometimes found incidentally at autopsy, or during cerebral angiography. The natural history of such unruptured aneurysms is controversial. Some neurosurgeons follow their evolution by repeated angiography, some will clip such aneurysms where feasible while others believe that the risks of this procedure outweigh any possible benefits.

Pathogenesis. Berry aneurysms are sometimes referred to as 'congenital' aneurysms but the latter is an inappropriate term since they develop in adult life, and are only very rarely found in childhood. However, both acquired and genetic factors are probably important in their pathogenesis.

A gap in the smooth muscle of the tunica media beginning abruptly at the neck of the aneurysm, at its site of origin from the bifurcation of a major vessel, has been noted in many histological studies. However, similar gaps of the muscular coat of the arterial wall are seen at these sites, even in children, without aneurysm formation, suggesting that the defective smooth muscle layer is not an inevitable precursor of aneurysm development and that additional degenerative and haemodynamic factors are important.

Similar features have been found at arterial bifurcations in the coronary, pulmonary and mesenteric arteries. The gaps in the media are said to represent the sites at which primitive mesenchysmal buds fuse to form the cerebral arterial system, and are thus probably a normal phenomenon. The intimal changes at the neck of the aneurysm, with fragmentation of the internal elastic lamina and the formation of intimal pads in some respects resemble those found in atherosclerosis, supporting the thesis that additional factors are involved. Indeed, atheromatous plaques may be found associated with aneurysms, and aneurysms occur in those cerebral vessels susceptible to atherosclerosis.

Aneurysms are not associated with hypertensive disease but *rupture* of an aneurysm is more likely to occur in hypertensive subjects, especially during sudden increases in blood pressure. Further, berry aneurysms are associated with coarctation of the aorta, a condition in which premature atherosclerosis of cerebral vessels occurs together with hypertension. Other, acquired vascular disorders, such as polyarteritis nodosa or syphilis have not been found to be associated with cerebral berry aneurysms, although autoimmune vasculitis is a rare cause of subarachnoid haemorrhage. An increased incidence of berry aneurysm has also been described in patients with polycystic kidneys, and neurofibromatosis. It has recently been suggested that one predisposing factor may be a defect of type III collagen, as occurs in one of the subtypes of Ehlers–Danlos syndrome.

Fusiform aneurysms

Atherosclerosis of the internal carotid arteries in the carotid siphon, or of the basilar artery may lead to fusiform dilatation of these vessels (Fig. 5.13). In these cases, there is usually also a history of hypertension, and atheroma is very advanced in these vessels. These fusiform aneurysms may be asymptomatic (see above), but may result in infarction in their vascular territories if complicated by embolism or thrombosis.

Complications of subarachnoid haemorrhage

The importance of cerebral infarction and its possible relationship to vasospasm is discussed above. The major late complications of subarachnoid haemorrhage are epilepsy, dementia and hydrocephalus. *Epilepsy* and *dementia* are manifestations of brain damage from the direct effects of haemorrhage into the brain from the secondary effects of brain herniation, especially of the hippocampus and temporal lobe, and from cerebral infarction.

Communicating hydrocephalus develops gradually in the days and weeks, or even several months or years after subarachnoid haemorrhage. The whole ventricular system enlarges, CSF being in free communication between the ventricles and the subarachnoid space through the aqueduct. Blood in the basal meninges, and over the convexities of the cerebral hemispheres causes a low-grade arachnoiditis so that thin fibrous adhesions develop between the pia and the arachnoid, and overlying the Virchow–Robin spaces. This causes impairment of circulation of the CSF over the hemispheres towards the sites of CSF absorp-

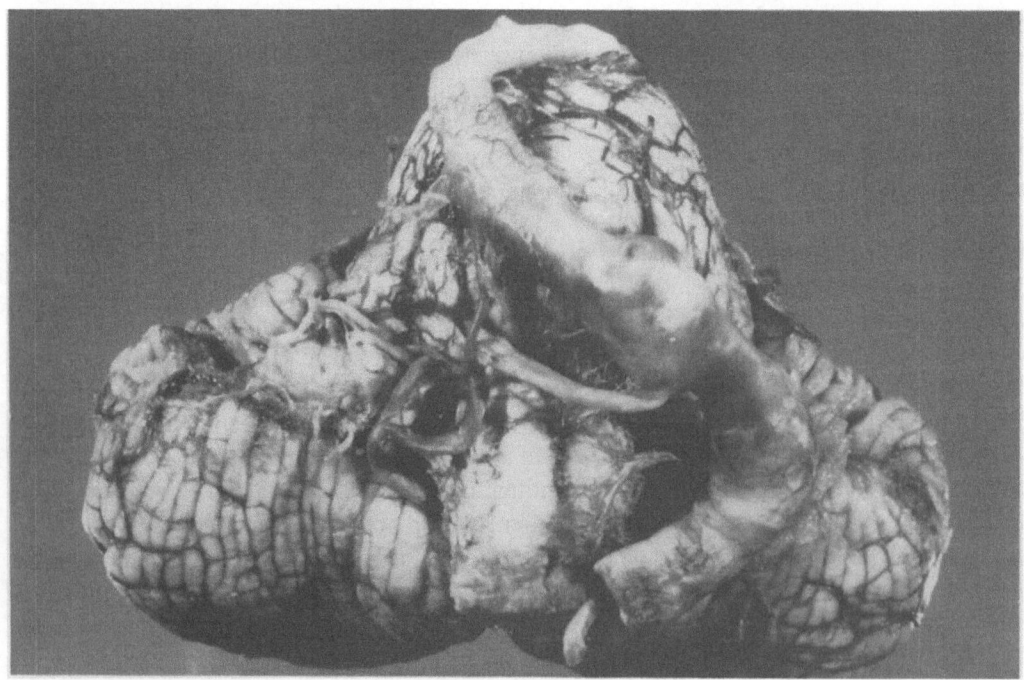

Fig. 5.13 Fusiform aneurysm. A tortuous, dilated atherosclerotic basilar artery. The left vertebral artery is dilated whereas the right vertebral artery is small.

tion in the arachnoid granulations, and impairment of absorption of CSF through the surface of the hemisphere, and so to hydrocephalus. Sometimes this hydrocephalus is accompanied by papilloedema. The hydrodynamics of the disturbance of CSF circulation and absorption can be studied by quantitative CSF hydrodynamic studies and, to some extent, by observing the diffusion of water-soluble radio-contrast material, e.g. Metrizamide, by CT scanning of the head after lumbar or cervical subarachnoid injection. Radio-isotope techniques have also been used. However, such studies are of little value in predicting the likely response to shunt operations. Monitoring the intracranial pressure is the most useful predictive test. Although hydrocephalus can be demonstrated in about a third of patients following subarachnoid haemorrhage, in only 10% does it become symptomatic. Patients may stop improving or may develop acute intracranial hypertension characterised by depressed conscious level with or without papilloedema, headache and meningism. Alternatively they may present later with features of 'normal pressure' (intermittently raised pressure) hydrocephalus characterised by gait disturbance, dementia and incontinence.

Mycotic aneurysms

Pyogenic infection of the wall of an artery, resulting from emboli in patients with septicaemia or endocarditis, but sometimes occurring from direct invasion of a vessel by a contiguous abscess or osteomyelitis, causes weakening of the vessel wall. There is a localised inflammatory response, with polymorphonuclear leukocytes, and destruction of the internal elastic lamina, and of the tunica media, and localised aneurysmal dilatation of the vessel. Rupture may occur. These aneurysms are usually small since the disease is acute. There is often infarction in the territory of the damaged vessel since the causative embolus often results in transient occlusion of the vessel, or its branches.

Dissecting aneurysms of cerebral vessels

Dissection of intracranial arteries is rare, but may occur spontaneously, in response to trauma, in syphilitic infection and in patients with congenital defects in the arterial media. It may also result from the trauma associated with arterial puncture in cerebral angiography. In spontaneously occurring cases, presenting as infarction, the middle cerebral artery is usually affected. Dissecting aneurysm is not a cause of cerebral haemorrhage.

Dissecting aneurysm of the aorta may progress to involve common carotid or brachiocephalic arteries or cause obstruction of the internal carotid artery on one or both sides thus leading to carotid territory cerebral infarction.

Vascular malformations of the brain and spinal cord

Vascular malformations are hamartomas of blood vessels in the CNS. There are three main types: arteriovenous malformations (AVM), capillary telangiectases, and cavernous angiomas. The term 'angioma' is sometimes incorrectly used in a general sense to refer to all three types. The AVM is the commonest of these three types, representing about 90% of vascular malformations causing clinical symptoms. Most, about 80%, of AVMs are supratentorial (Fig. 5.12) in location and more than half of these are situated in the central/parietal parts of a hemisphere, in the territory of the middle cerebral artery. The ratio of incidence of intracranial AVMs to cerebral aneurysms is about 1:7; occasionally these two vascular abnormalites occur together, in the same vascular territory, suggesting that they have a related congenital basis.

Arteriovenous malformations. AVMs may be small and well-localised or so large as to involve the major part of a hemisphere. Sometimes they occur as multiple, separate anomalies within the brain. The vessels forming the malformation vary in size, shape and tortuosity, but they are usually dilated, tortuous and thin-walled. Most AVMs are visible on the surface of the brain (Fig. 5.14), but extend in a wedge-shaped distribution of abnormal interconnecting arteries and veins into the subcortical white matter, and even into the deep grey nuclei. Venous drainage may occur through both deep and central veins, usually themselves dilated, and the arterial supply to the malformation is usually derived from several large, dilated branches of the middle cerebral or other major cerebral vessels. The carotid or vertebral artery in this territory is usually also enlarged and a bruit may be audible over it. The blood flow through this system of abnormal vessels may be very large and the venous drainage is sometimes arterialised and thus red in colour, indicating the extent of arterial to venous shunting within the lesion.

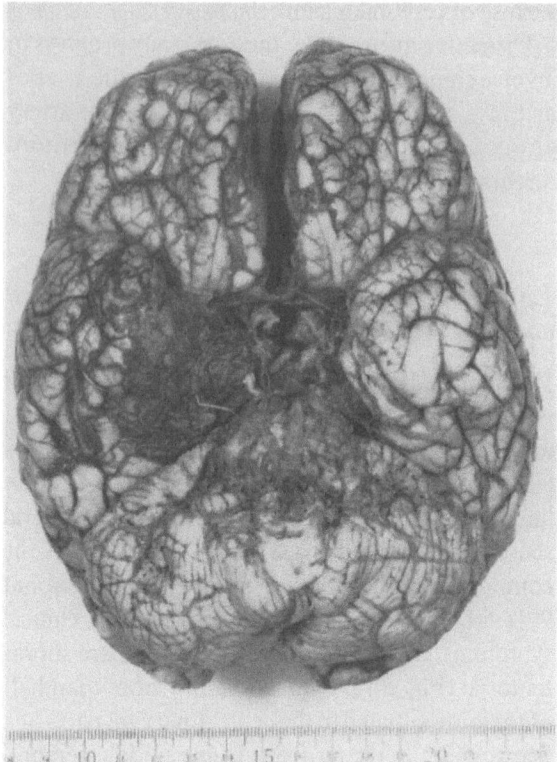

Fig. 5.14. Arteriovenous malformation. Large, tortuous vessels are prominent on the surface of the medial aspect of the left temporal lobe.

Microscopically the enlarged and abnormal vascular channels within the AVM are thin walled, with a poorly developed tunica media and elastica. The intima may be thickened, or even atheromatous and calcified. It is often difficult to distinguish arteries and veins among these abnormal vessels (Fig. 5.15). Haemosiderin is often present in and around the vessels indicating previous extravasation of small or large quantities of blood. Adjacent and intermingled cerebral tissue is usually gliotic.

Clinically, AVMs of the type discussed above produce symptoms and signs as a result of is-chaemia, gliosis, haemorrhage, mass effect or hydrocephalus. Ischaemia usually results either from the size of the arterial to venous shunt through the malformation, leading to ischaemic hypoxia of neighbouring regions of the brain, or from thrombosis within the AVM, usually leading to haemorrhagic venous infarction in the same vascular territory. Another effect of ischaemia, and of the cerebral malformation that often accompanies AVM, is focal or generalised epilepsy; this is fairly common presenting feature, especially in temporal lobe AVMs. Haemorrhage may be local and minor, leading to a slight, reversible neurological deficit

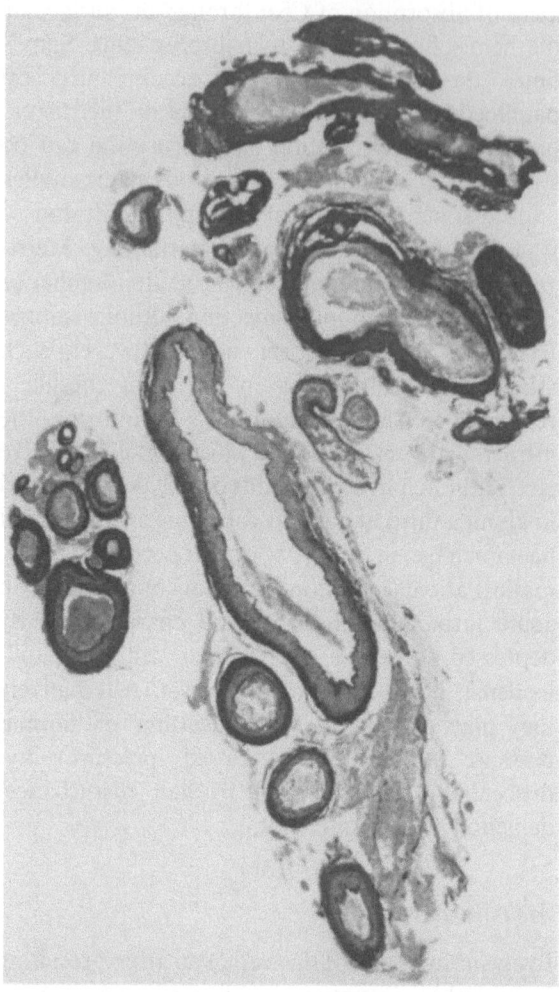

Fig. 5.15. Photomicrograph of a surgically excised arterio-venous malformation showing vessels of various sizes. Some have the structure of arteries. (Elastic van Giesen × 30)

and to headache, or large, causing a substantial haematoma. The latter may be fatal. Sometimes haemorrhage from an AVM is subarachnoid, and this does not differ from subarachnoid haemorrhage of other cause in its clinical features. Very large AVMs, together with their draining veins, may themselves cause a mass effect, leading to seizures and to a progressive neurological deficit. Cardiomegaly, with high-output cardiac failure, is an uncommon complication even in children.

Neither ligation of the arterial feeders nor embolisation leads to the long-term obliteration of an AVM. Hence, excision is required but indicated only where the AVM has bled and is accessible. Inaccessible AVMs, less than about 3.5 cm in diameter, are amenable to stereotactic radio-therapy, a promising technique not yet widely available. When epilepsy is the only symptom, surgery is not usually recommended unless the AVM is in a relatively 'silent' part of the brain in a young person. Operation in these cases is not necessarily to cure the epilepsy but to avoid the uncertain risk of bleeding in the future.

Capillary telangiectases. These lesions are silent until they burst, leading to spontaneous haemorrhage and haematoma. They may only rarely be recognised angiographically since they are very small. Many such lesions are destroyed by the haemorrhage itself, thus accounting for some cases of apparently spontaneous intracerebral or subarachnoid haemorrhage. These cryptic hamartomas are characterised by extremely thin-walled capillaries without muscle or elastic tissue layers in their walls. They are sometimes multiple.

Other forms of vascular malformation. In Sturge–Weber syndrome there is an arteriovenous malformation affecting part or all of a cerebral hemisphere composed of abnormal capillaries and arterioles, rather than large, dilated vessels, and located principally in the cortex. The lesion is often accompanied by calcification of the cerebral tissue near it, and by a trigeminal vascular naevus (port wine stain) of the face ipsilateral to the cerebral lesion. Epilepsy, hemiparesis, hemianopia, and mental retardation are characteristic clinical features, but haemorrhage does not occur.

Aneurysmal dilatation of the vein of Galen causes non-communicating hydrocephalus, usually presenting in infancy. This lesion is very rare.

In Von Hippel–Lindau disease small CNS haemangioblastomas are associated with angiomas of other tissue, especially retina, lungs, liver and kidneys. Malignant renal tumours may also occur. The disorder, one of the phakomatoses (see Chap. 11) is often familial, showing a dominant pattern of inheritance.

Spinal AVMs are usually situated on the dorsal surface of the cord but may penetrate into the substance of the cord through the dura. They resemble cerebral AVMs histologically and may present either with haemorrhage or with intermittent and remittent paraplegia in late middle life or old age, especially in men, often associated with radicular pain. Most spinal AVMs are situated in the thoracic or lumbar cord. Their draining veins, draining in a cephalad direction, are often visible at myelography. The detailed anatomy can be established by spinal angiography when surgery is contemplated. Surgical treatment is often effective not only in preventing further episodes of paraplegia but also in improving neurological function, presumably by relieving a 'shunt effect' through the AVM itself.

Cerebral tumour and cerebral haemorrhage

Cerebral haemorrhage is sometimes a presenting feature of cerebral tumours. This is particularly likely in vascular tumours, e.g. in metastases from malignant melanoma, carcinoma of the bronchus and renal carcinoma, but it also occurs with primary CNS neoplasms, particularly oligodendrogliomas and glioblastomas. In these instances the tumour may not at first be suspected.

Further reading

Anderson T W, Mackay J S (1968) A critical reappraisal of the epidemiology of cerebrovascular disease. Lancet i: 1137

Astrup J, Siesjo B K, Symon L (1981) Thresholds in cerebral ischaemia. The ischaemic penumbra. Stroke 12:723

Brierley A B, Prior P F, Calverley J, Jackson S J, Brown A W (1980) The pathogenesis of ischaemic neuronal damage along the cerebral arterial boundary zones in Papio anubis. Brain 103:929

Brierley J B, Adams J H, Graham D I, Simpson J A (1971) Neocortical death after cardiac arrest: a clinical neurophysiological and neuropathological report of two cases. Lancet ii:500

Cameron I R (1977) The chemical control of the cerebral circulation. Clin Sci Mol Med 52:549

Castaigne P, Lhermitte F, Gautier J C et al. (1973) Arterial occlusions in the vertebro-basilar system: a study of patients with post-mortem data. Brain 96:133

Crawford J V, Russell D S (1956) Cryptic arteriovenous and venous hamartomas of the brain. J Neurol Neurosurg Psychiatry 14:1

Crompton M R (1964) Cerebral infarction following the rupture of cerebral berry aneurysms. Brain 82:377

Fisher C M (1961) The pathology and pathogenesis of intracerebral haemorrhage. In: Fields W S (ed) Pathogenesis and treatment of cerebrovascular disease. Thomas, Springfield Ill, p. 562

Fisher C M (1965) Lacunes: small deep cerebral infarcts. Lancet ii:19

Freytag E (1968) Fatal hypertensive intracerebral haematomas: a survey of the pathological anatomy of 393 cases. J Neurol Neurosurg Psychiatry 31:616

Hutchinson E C, Acheson E J (1975) Strokes: Natural history, pathology and surgical treatment. Saunders, Philadelphia

Hutchinson E C, Yates P O (1961) Cerebral infarction: The role of stenosis of the extracranial cerebral arteries. Special Report Series of the Medical Research Council, No. 300. HMSO, London

Jennett B, Miller J D, Harper A M (1976) Effect of carotid artery surgery on cerebral blood flow. Excerpta Medica, Amsterdam

Kendall R E, Marshall, J (1963) Role of hypotension in the genesis of transient focal cerebral ischaemic attacks. Br Med J I:344

Lassen N A (1966) The luxury perfusion syndrome. Lancet ii:1113

Marshall J (1964) The natural history of transient ischaemic cerebrovascular attacks. Quart J Med 33:309

Marshall J (1965) The management of cerebrovascular disease. Churchill, London

McKissock W, Paine K W, Walsh L S (1960) An analysis of the results of treatment of ruptured intracranial aneurysms: report of 772 conservative cases. J Neurosurg 17:762

Pickard J D (1982) Adult communicating hydrocephalus. Br J Hosp Med 27:35

Rees J E, Bull J W D, Ross Russell W R, Marshall J, Symon L (1970) Regional cerebral blood flow in transient ischaemic attacks. Lancet ii:1240

Ross Russell W R (1968) The source of retinal emboli. Lancet ii:789

Ross Russell W R (1976) Cerebral arterial disease. Churchill Livingstone, Edinburgh

Tomlinson B E (1959) Brain changes in ruptured intracranial aneurysms. J Clin Pathol 12:391

Vander Eecken H M (1959) The anastomoses between the leptomeningeal arteries of the brain. Thomas, Springfield Ill

Wilkins R H (1980) Cerebral arterial spasm. Williams & Wilkins, Baltimore

Chapter 6

Trauma to the Nervous System

Head injuries

In the management of head injury the clinician must be aware of when and why complications occur. Although little can be done to modify the primary brain damage occurring at the time of the injury, much can be done to minimise the effects of cerebral oedema, raised intracranial pressure and brain shift which may complicate a head injury. It is not only that the life of the patient may be in danger, but disability can also be minimised by limiting the extent of damage to the brain. The role of the pathologist in the management of head injuries is to examine the clinical history and the brain of those patients who die with head injuries and to advise the clinician on the course of events and the complications which have resulted in the patient's death. It is only in this way that the clinician becomes aware of crucial aspects in the management of head injuries.

Each year 1 000 000 people in Britain receive treatment in casualty departments for mild or severe head injuries. The 100 000 patients with head injuries admitted to hospital represent about 25 % of all acute admissions; of these 5000 (5 %) receive neurosurgical care, some 1500 (1.5 %) will have residual permanent damage, or will remain in a vegetative state, and 5000 (5 %) will develop epilepsy. Up to 50 % of patients with severe head injuries will die as a direct result of their head injury; the largest group being the adolescent males (15–19 year old), a group in which head injuries cause half of all deaths. When death follows a road traffic accident, there is a 75 % chance that it will be as a direct result of a head injury; about 50 % die immediately, 15 %–20 % in neurosurgical wards and a small number in general hospital wards. Road traffic accidents cause 60 % of all head injuries resulting from deceleration/acceleration forces and the rest can be divided equally between industrial accidents and assaults.

Damage to the head depends upon the amount of force applied to it and upon the way in which the force is applied. Head injuries may be divided into (a) *blunt injuries* in which the force is applied diffusely to a large area of the head and (b) *penetrating injuries* in which the force is applied in a localised area, as in an injury causing a compound depressed fracture, or as in a missile injury. The two types of injury may coexist, especially when the energy expended upon the head is excessive. On the other hand diffuse damage to the brain may be far greater than the extent of injury to the skull would suggest, as in a high velocity penetrating missile injury.

Blunt head injuries

At the moment of impact, accelerating and decelerating forces are applied to the head. The amount of energy expended, i.e. the force of the blow, determines subsequent events. Details of the accident by eye witnesses are thus vital both at an early stage in the treatment of the patient and in retrospective assessment of the patient's progress. *Superficial structures*, including face, scalp and skull may absorb much of the energy. Patients are seen with gross superficial injuries and little neurological damage, and vice versa. Ultimately, in all cases the brain is involved and either microscopic or macroscopic mechanical damage will ensue.

Primary brain damage

This is damage that occurs at the time of impact; the resulting temporary or permanent loss of function in neural pathways depends upon the severity of the injury. There is an immediate change in the clinical condition of the patient resulting in varying degrees of alteration in function. The severity of a head injury is best indicated clinically by the extent and duration of the impairment of conscious level. Coma, where the patient is unable to obey commands, to utter recognisable words or to open his eyes, indicates extensive damage to tissue, particularly in the white matter. Although little or nothing active may be done about the primary brain damage, an early accurate assessment of the patient's clinical state is essential, as it will enable the clinician to offer some prediction of the probable complications. A record of the level of consciousness or state of coma is particularly important. Once the patient's condition has stabilised, a coma scale can be used to monitor his progress. Similarly, focal neurological deficits at or soon after the time of primary impact damage should be recorded.

At a later stage, periods of post-traumatic and retrograde amnesia may be used to predict the ultimate recovery, although both may shrink as time passes. Retrograde amnesia is rarely seen without post-traumatic amnesia, but the latter can be present on its own.

Mechanisms of primary brain damage. Mechanical trauma induced at the time of a blunt head injury induces contusion and laceration of the surface of the brain and shearing of nerve fibres and blood vessels within the white matter, particularly in the cerebral hemispheres (Fig. 6.1A). Both these types of injury are subsequently complicated by cerebral oedema, brain shift and brain distortion. The brain has a peculiar anatomical arrangement such that it is supported in cerebrospinal fluid contained within a bony box and is only held firm at the base of the skull by emerging nerve roots and by major blood vessels entering the brain. Superficially, there are relatively flimsy attachments by cortical veins to the superior sagittal sinus. Such an arrangement means that the brain moves within the skull mainly in a rotary fashion, so that those parts of the brain furthest from the axis rotate with a greater velocity and come into more violent contact with the skull. Hence, superficial damage to the cortex more commonly involves the frontal and temporal lobes, which may be grossly contused and lacerated: the so-called burst temporal lobe (Fig. 6.2) or frontal lobe. As the patient recovers from a head injury, the clinician may observe the unmistakable signs of such damage; these include apathy, loss of drive, and memory disturbances. Other parts of the brain may come into contact with irregularities within the skull, notably the falx cerebri, the lesser wings of the sphenoid and the petrous temporal ridge. Thus, laceration of the corpus callosum (Figs. 6.3, 6.4 and 6.6), superior cerebellar peduncles (Fig. 6.6) and the under surfaces of the temporal lobes may occur.

During the swirling movements of the brain within the skull (*commotio cerebri*), shearing forces are set up throughout the brain, particularly at the junction of grey and white matter, probably because of the differing consistencies of the two types of tissue. Widespread tearing and shearing of axons occur throughout the hemispheres, particularly in the white matter (Fig. 6.7a, b), which may or may not be associated with petechial haemorrhages from tearing of small blood vessels (Fig. 6.3). Such shearing forces are concentrated at the junction of mobile structures, like the cerebral hemispheres, and relatively fixed parts of the brain, such as the brain stem (Fig. 6.5). In very severe injuries avulsion of the cerebral peduncles may occur. More commonly, however, small haemorrhages and axonal shearing will be seen in the midbrain (Fig. 6.5), resulting in the familiar clinical picture of the severe head injury with fixed, dilated pupils, deep coma, and severe disturbances in motor activity on both

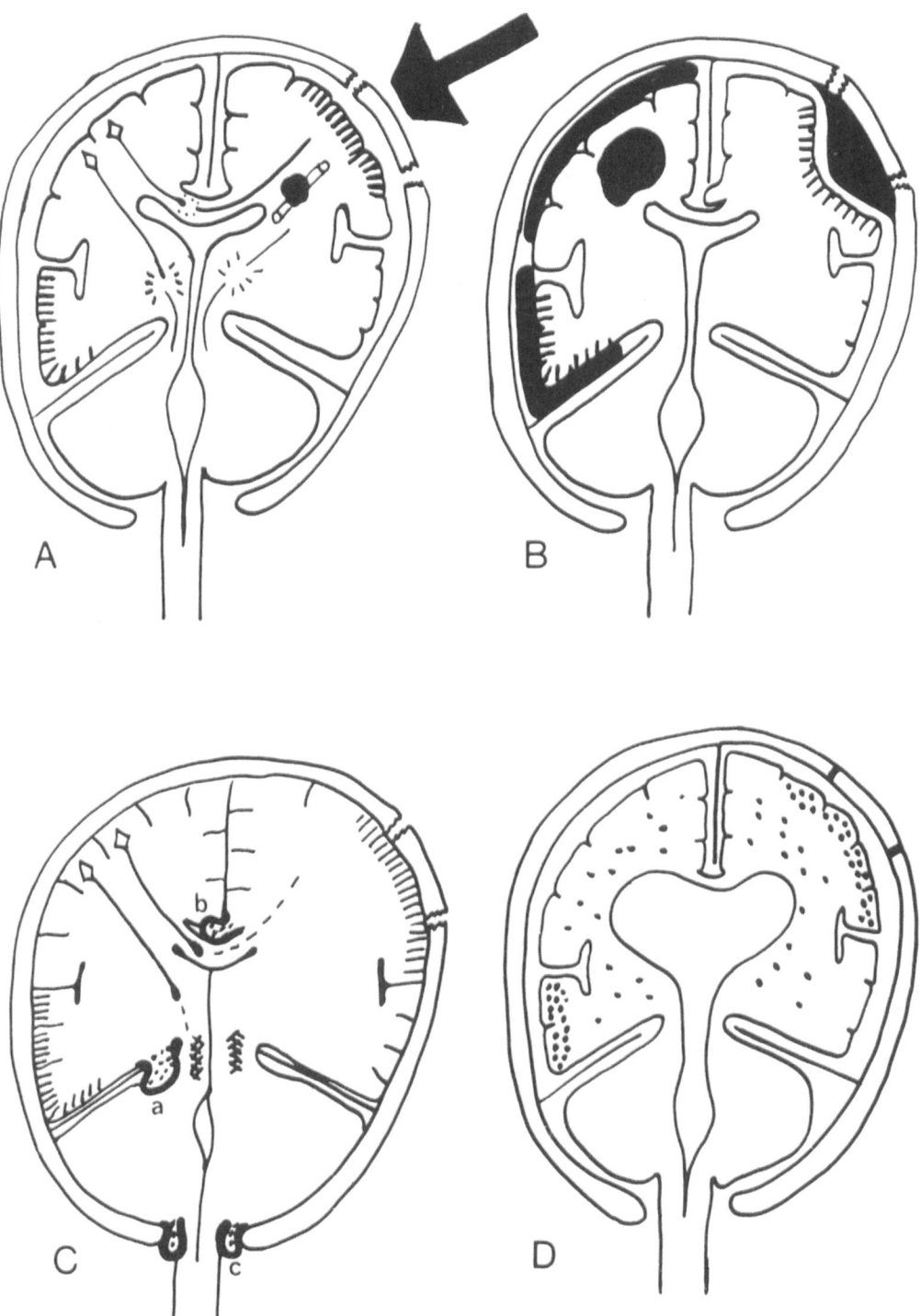

Fig. 6.1.

A *Primary brain damage.* Blunt injury (*blunt arrow*) with skull fracture, underlying brain contusion and *contre-coup* lesion (*both shaded*). Axons are severed in the white matter and small blood vessels are torn.

B *Intracranial haemorrhage associated with trauma.* Extradural haematoma underlying small fracture. Subdural haemorrhage associated with (*contre-coup*) brain contusion. Subdural haemorrhage from ruptured cortical veins. Intracerebral haemorrhage in white matter.

C *Cerebral oedema.* Swollen brain flattened against dura and skull, compressed ventricles. Herniation of parahippocampal gyrus (*a*) through the tentorial opening is associated with midbrain compression and haemorrhage. Herniation of cingulate gyrus (*b*) under the falx, and herniation of cerebellar tonsils (*c*) into the foramen magnum.

D *Late effects.* Softening and glial scarring of the surface contusions (*close stippling*). Scars resulting from shearing of nerve fibres in the white matter are represented by *widely spaced dots*. Hydrocephalus may result from fibrosis of meninges following subarachnoid haemorrhage or meningitis. Ventricular dilatation may also be due to loss of tissue from primary brain damage.

sides of the body. It is by assessing the probability of such damage that the clinician may predict the probable complications at a later stage.

Secondary brain damage

As a result of the gross lesions in the brain resulting from the primary injury, and more subtle functional effects that leave no trace, there may be profound disturbances of distant structures in the body that are under nervous control, notably the heart, the respiratory apparatus, and the airways. Disturbance of respiratory or cardiac function may occur; it may only be transitory, lasting perhaps 10 min or more, but during this time cerebral blood flow may be affected, oxygen levels may be reduced, and carbon dioxide levels in the blood may be raised, thus setting in train cerebral oedema, loss of normal autoregulatory mechanisms controlling cerebral blood flow and resulting in neuronal loss. These complications may occur soon after the head injury so that ambulance staff should be trained in the management of head injuries and they should be particularly aware of the problems which arise from airway obstruction.

Intracranial haematomas. The main effect of intracranial haematomas is that of brain displacement. Although they are relatively rare complications of head injury, haematomas constitute an important feature as they can often be removed surgically.

Extradural haematomas are commonly found in the middle cranial fossa, because a skull fracture in this region may lead to a tear in a branch of the middle meningeal artery. They usually occur in younger age groups, often with little primary brain injury, so that a lucid interval varying from a few minutes to several hours may be seen before the patient lapses into unconsciousness from the secondary effects of brain compression due to the extradural haematoma.

Acute subdural haematomas (Fig. 6.1B) occur more frequently in the elderly or in those with pre-existing cerebral atrophy. They are frequently associated with severe primary brain damage where bleeding occurs from the surface of the brain and accumulates subdurally. Although the clinical picture is that of progressive cerebral compression, a lucid interval very rarely occurs.

Chronic subdural haematomas may present days or even months after a relatively minor injury. There is confusion with fluctuating consciousness and focal neurological signs are common. The causative injury may have been forgotten and diagnosis is therefore difficult.

Intracerebral haematomas (Fig. 6.3) are usually associated with severe brain damage; they may be multiple and they may certainly contribute to the general rise in intracranial pressure and, as such, they warrant rapid diagnosis and surgical removal.

Detection and localisation of intracranial haematomas depends partly upon the clinical history and neurological signs, and partly upon confirmation by radiological techniques. X-rays may reveal pineal shift or a skull fracture in a site related to the middle meningeal artery. CT scanning may be used to localise blood clot.

Intracranial pressure following head injuries. A third major effect of diffuse blunt head injury is the change that occurs in intracranial pressure. Seventy percent of patients with severe head injuries develop raised intracranial pressure due to bleeding or oedema, but in about 10% intracranial pressure is lower than normal; in these, the clinical features are generally those of severe primary brain damage and the prognosis is usually very poor. A further 20% are found to have a relatively normal intracranial pressure and the outlook is better.

Bleeding into the brain substance or into the extradural or subdural space increases the amount of solid material within the cranial cavity. If localised and large, *haematomas* may be removed surgically. More commonly, however, the blood clot is diffusely distributed in bruised brain tissue.

Brain displacement or shift. As with other rapidly enlarging space-occupying lesions within the cerebral hemispheres, oedema occurring in association with a traumatic brain lesion may cause the cingulate gyrus to be herniated under the falx cerebri (subfalcine herniation) (Fig. 6.4). In temporal lobe lesions, the uncus and parahippocampal gyrus (Fig. 6.1C) may be displaced downwards between the midbrain and the free edge of the tentorium cerebelli (transtentorial herniation) (see Chap. 4). Side-to-side compression of the midbrain may be accompanied by multiple haemorrhages within the pons and the midbrain, by compression of the third and fourth nerves, and by compression of branches of the posterior cerebral artery with consequent infarction of the temporal and occipital lobes. Swelling of the cerebellar hemispheres may be complicated by herniation of the cerebellar tonsils through the foramen magnum (Fig. 6.1C).

Cerebral oedema inevitably accompanies severe

cerebral trauma and will produce an expansion of the intracellular and extracellular water compartment of the brain. Cerebral anoxia, either local or diffuse, is another common cause of cerebral oedema. The control of water balance in the management of cerebral oedema is perhaps the most significant problem the clinician faces in the treatment of head injured patients. The margin for error is extremely small. Volume-pressure challenge tests show that the addition of a few millilitres of fluid into the head may result in a rise of intracranial pressure above that commensurate with normal cerebral blood flow. During the stage of cerebral oedema following the injury, the volume of CSF in the head is usually reduced and the ventricles are small. On occasions, however, a CT scan may show a unilateral hydrocephalus if one foramen of Monro is blocked.

As already described, disturbance of ventilation, atelectasis from airways obstruction and pneumonia from infection all affect gas exchange within the lungs. *Hypoxia*, from whatever the cause, is a serious complication in a patient with diffuse primary brain damage from a blunt head injury. Of equal importance is the *hypercapnia* associated with these conditions and the consequent enlargement of venous and capillary components of the cerebral circulation. Airways obstruction is always associated with a rise in central venous pressure, which again results in venous congestion of the brain. Hence, good care of the airways and the use of mechanical ventilation are useful in the treatment of severe head injuries. As intracranial pressure rises cerebral blood flow decreases, leading to ischaemic brain damage, or even to death. It is estimated that failure of the cerebral circulation with ischaemic brain damage is the final cause of death in 80% of patients dying with diffuse cerebral injuries. Ischaemic brain damage may also occur when the head injury is accompanied by extensive trauma to the rest of the body with blood loss, shock and hypotension.

Late complications

When cerebral oedema has subsided in patients with widespread shearing brain lesions, and the tissue debris has been removed (Fig. 6.5), *cerebral atrophy* with large ventricles may develop. If the atrophy is severe it may be associated with a clinical picture of persistent severe neurological damage, the so-called persistent vegetative state (see Chap. 3).

Hydrocephalus may occur early after head injury due to obstruction of CSF pathways by blood and products of damaged brain. This usually improves with time and rarely requires treatment. Intermittently raised pressure (normal pressure) hydrocephalus (see Chap. 15) is an unusual late complication of head injury. It may be due to obstruction of the subarachnoid space by fibrosis following haemorrhage or meningitis complicating the primary injury. The ventricles are enlarged and the patient may present with a progressive dementia, which can be relieved by a CSF shunting procedure.

Epilepsy may occur as a complication of head injury. Seizures may occur within the first week or may begin up to 25 years after the head injury. Early seizures are not necessarily of serious prognostic significance but late onset seizures usually continue. Seizures occurring during the early days following a head injury may be associated with severe hypoxic damage to the brain.

Pathology of blunt head injuries

Minor head injuries

In patients with a minor head injury there is no skull fracture, or sign of cerebral irritation. About 40% of such patients are concussed, 30% have a depressed level of consciousness and 15% are amnesic for a few minutes following the injury. It has been suggested that precautionary admission to hospital if unnecessary if efficient use of x-ray facilities is made and adequate instructions are given to relatives for care of the patient.

Pathological studies of the brain in patients with minor head injuries are infrequent unless the patient dies soon after the accident from unrelated causes. Minor contusions on the surface of the brain and sparsely distributed foci of axonal shearing have been reported. The lesions are qualitatively similar to those seen at primary impact damage in severe blunt head injuries, but they are quantitatively much less extensive.

Severe head injuries

As stressed previously, data derived from the careful post-mortem study of the brains of patients dying with head injuries can contribute greatly to management of head injuries. The pathologist can not only judge the pattern of primary brain damage and correlate it with the sites of impact from scalp laceration and skull fracture, but in conjunction with the clinical history he can also tabulate the timing and progress of secondary complications.

The pattern of lesions seen in head injuries is summarised in Fig. 6.1.

Primary brain damage

Cortical damage occurs in the form of *contusions and lacerations*. Contusions are found both at the site of impact (*coup* lesions) and away from the site of impact (*contre-coup* lesions) (Fig. 6.1A and 6.2). They appear as surface contusions on the tops of convolutions and in the fresh state they are haemmorhagic. Contusions can usually be distinguished from recent infarction due to vascular occlusion as the contusions are seen mainly on the surface of the brain whereas infarction also involves the cortex within the depths of the sulci. In more severe contusions, damage extends into the subcortical white matter and there may be small flame-shaped haemorrhages under the surface of the brain, usually orientated at right angles to the cortical surface.

Histological studies have shown that during the first 24 h, polymorphonuclear leukocytes migrate into the areas of contusion and after some days they

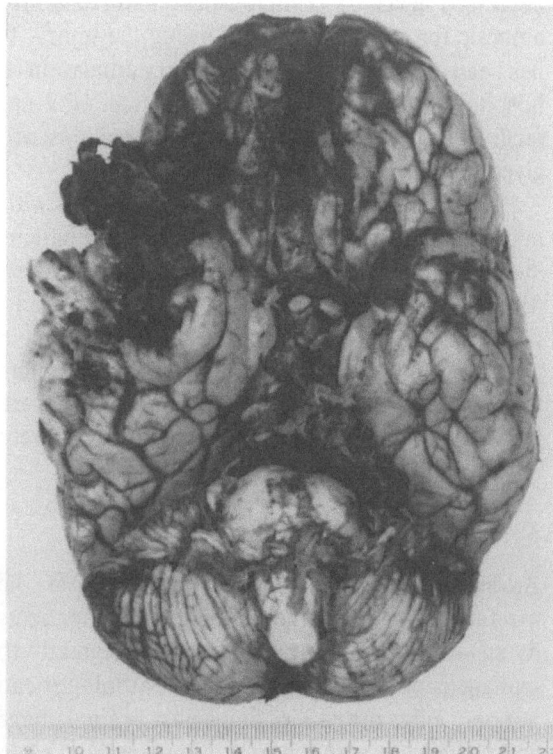

Fig. 6.2. Burst temporal lobe: basal view showing extensive contusion and disruption of the right temporal pole and inferior surface of the right frontal lobe. Less extensive contusions are seen on the left side.

are followed by macrophages. Finally the contused region becomes a soft surface lesion often discoloured orange by old blood pigment. Deep to the area of softening there is glial scarring; at this stage it is impossible to age the lesion accurately. *Contre-coup* lesions are similar histologically to the lesions directly under the point of impact. The distribution of *contre-coup* lesions is not always directly opposite the site of primary impact; the tips of the frontal lobes and temporal lobes are particularly prone to suffer these lesions.

There have been numerous explanations put forward to account for the development of contusions, particularly in relation to the *contre-coup* lesions. They probably occur in association with rotational forces as already described. The irregularity of the floor of the anterior and middle cranial fossae suggests that contusions may arise from direct contact between the brain and bone. Such contusions are not seen in infants, in whom these bony surfaces are smooth. *Contre-coup* injuries occur due to movement of the brain in a single plane resulting in impact on opposite sides of hemispheres. Such injuries are seen particularly in older people in whom there is cerebral atrophy, especially in falls in which the primary impact is occipital; serious frontal and temporal lobe damage results. Other explanations for the occurrence of contusions include the explosive release of dissolved gases in the brain tissue subjected to negative pressure as the brain lags behind the skull; this is considered to be unlikely in civilian injuries, but may be a factor in the cavitation seen in gun shot wounds of the brain.

Local brain damage also occurs during movement as the brain comes into contact with sharp features such as the falx cerebri, tentorium cerebelli and the petrous ridge.

The role of contusions in producing *coma* immediately after head injuries is unclear. The contusion index derived from the calculation of the depth and extent of contusions has shown that there is no difference in the severity of contusions between patients who lose consciousness immediately and those who have a lucid interval. It seems more probable that coma results from the damage inflicted from shearing forces applied to the white matter and more deeply in the brain at brain stem level.

Damage to *white matter* is caused by *shearing forces*. Acceleration of the cortical grey matter during impact most closely approximates to that of the skull, while the white matter lags slightly behind. Shearing forces are thus set up within the white matter; these are maximal in the frontal and occipital lobes and in long, transverse tracts such as the corpus callosum (Figs. 6.3, 6.4, 6.6). Similar forces develop in the basal ganglia, thalamus and brain stem (Fig. 6.5).

Single axons or small groups of axons which have been severed by shearing forces can be detected histologically 3–8 days after the injury as areas of oedema in myelin-stained preparations (Fig. 6.7a) or by the presence of axon balloons (Fig. 6.7b). These swellings form at the distal end of the proximal stump of the severed axon and can be seen as pale, eosinophilic, sausage-shaped or circular profiles some 50 μm in diameter in H&E-stained sections. They are more easily detected in silver-stained preparations (see Chap. 4). The distal ends of the axons degenerate and myelin breakdown products can be detected within affected tracts about 2 months after the injury, and even up to 2 years later. After this time, areas in which axonal shearing has occurred can only be detected by the

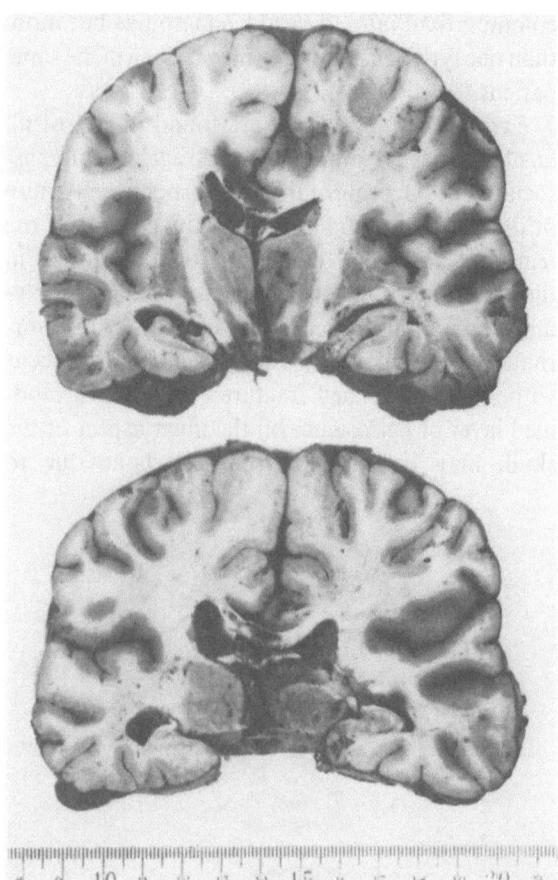

Fig. 6.4. A moderately severe head injury. The right hemisphere is oedematous and there is subfalcine herniation. There is haemorrhagic disruption of the corpus callosum.

presence of glial scars. Loss of white matter fibres produces secondary enlargement of the ventricles, atrophy of the corpus callosum and small cystic areas in the regions most affected (Fig. 6.6). Small blood vessels may be damaged at the time of primary impact so that petechial haemorrhages may occur in areas of axonal shearing.

The neurological state of the patient following the accident is probably more related to the extent of the white matter shearing damage in the brain than it is to the presence of surface contusions. Such shearing lesions may even occur without either skull fracture or surface contusions. Histological study of the brain is thus worthwhile in patients who die from head injuries even when there is little macroscopic abnormality in the brain.

Secondary brain damage

Intracranial haematomas are seen in two-thirds of all

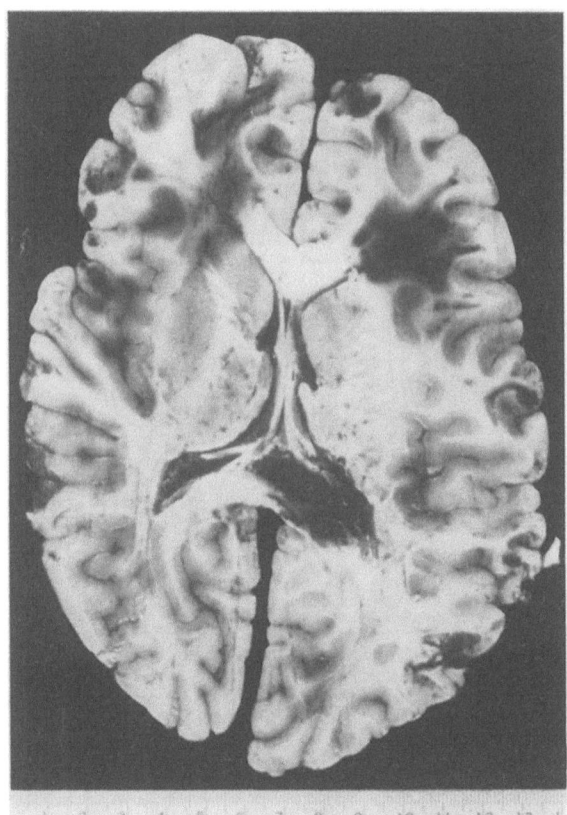

Fig. 6.3. Sagittal slice of brain following a severe head injury. There are numerous small intracerebral haematomas especially at the junction of the cortex and white matter. Larger haemorrhages are seen in the corpus callosum anteriorly and posteriorly.

autopsies of patients dying with severe head injuries. *Subdural* and *extradural* haematomas are much less common than *intracerebral* haematomas but more than one type of haematoma may be seen in the same patient.

Extradural haematomas are found in 3% of all head injuries at autopsy and are classically associated with tearing of the middle meningeal artery or its branches by fracture of the inner table of the temporal bone. Less commonly they are found in the parietal region associated with fractures involving the parietal diploic veins; extradural haemorrhage may also be seen in the frontal region or occur without an associated fracture. The dura, a modified layer of periosteum on the inner aspect of the skull, may be stripped from the bone due to

distortion at the time of impact. The resultant potential space rapidly fills with blood, which compresses the brain. Extradural haematomas are often fatal unless early recognition and evacuation of the blood clot can be achieved. Up to 70% of patients have a lucid interval between the injury and the onset of coma, as the initial impact damage is often mild. If a patient survives and the haematoma is successfully removed, the long-term prognosis is good.

A *subdural haematoma* (Fig. 6.8) accumulates in the space between the dura and the arachnoid. This space tends to be larger in older patients, in those with cerebral atrophy, in chronic alcoholics and in patients with hydrocephalus. Bleeding may occur from cortical veins, sometimes known as 'bridging veins', as they pass from the cerebral hemispheres into the superior sagittal sinus and into other sinuses, or haemorrhage may arise from severe cortical lacerations. The blood may track over the whole hemisphere and form a uniform coating layer.

A subdural haematoma may present as an acute manifestation of trauma, when the clinical picture may mimic that of an extradural haematoma. However, *acute subdural* bleeding is associated with

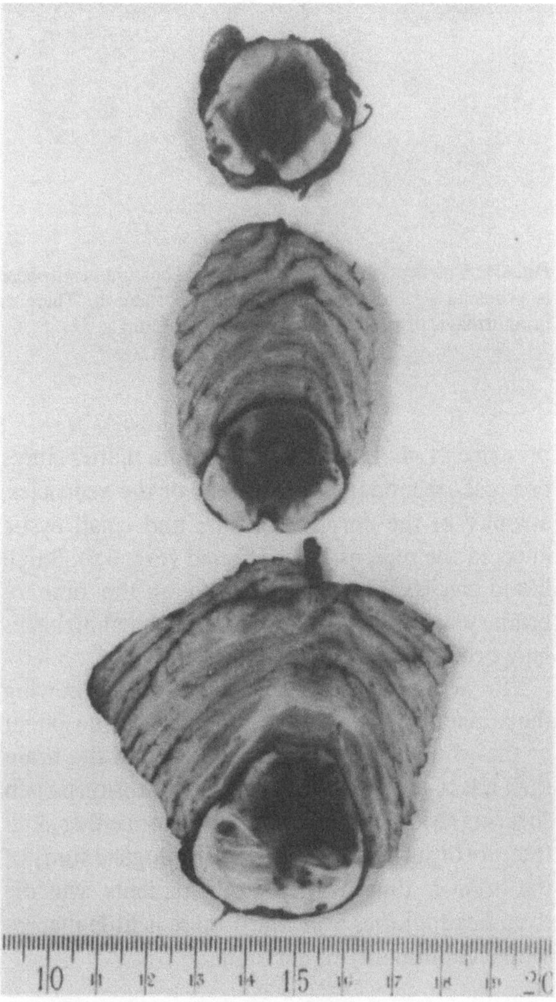

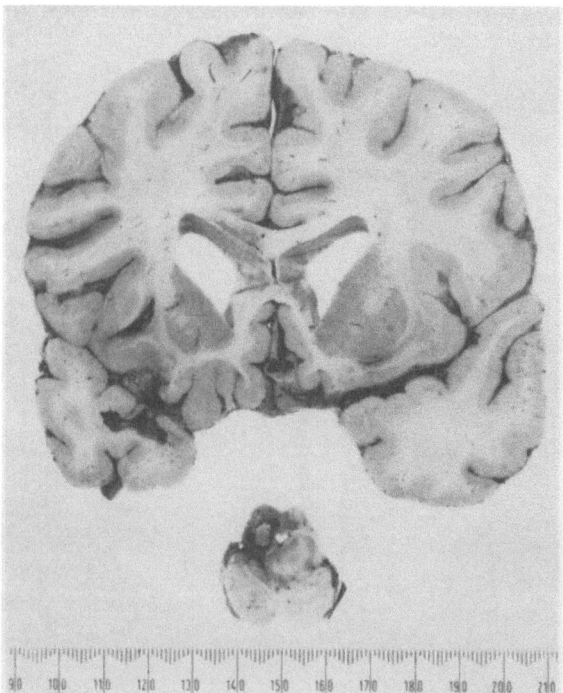

Fig. 6.5. Pons and midbrain of the same case as Fig. 6.4 showing haemorrhage into the midbrain and pons. A rim of subarachnoid blood is seen coating the anterior aspects of the pons.

Fig. 6.6. Brain from a patient surviving for 6 months in a persistent vegetative state following a head injury. There is generalised cerebral atrophy with dilatation of the ventricles. Old shearing lesions are seen in the corpus callosum and brain stem.

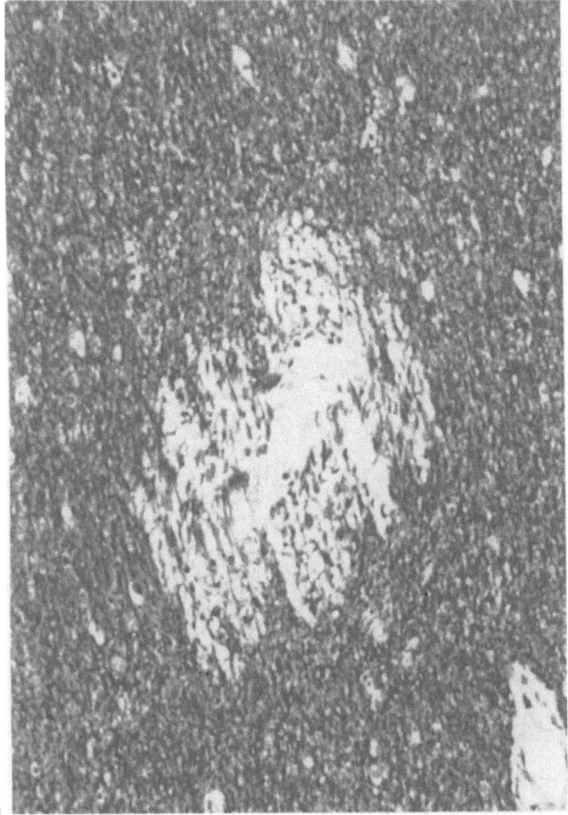

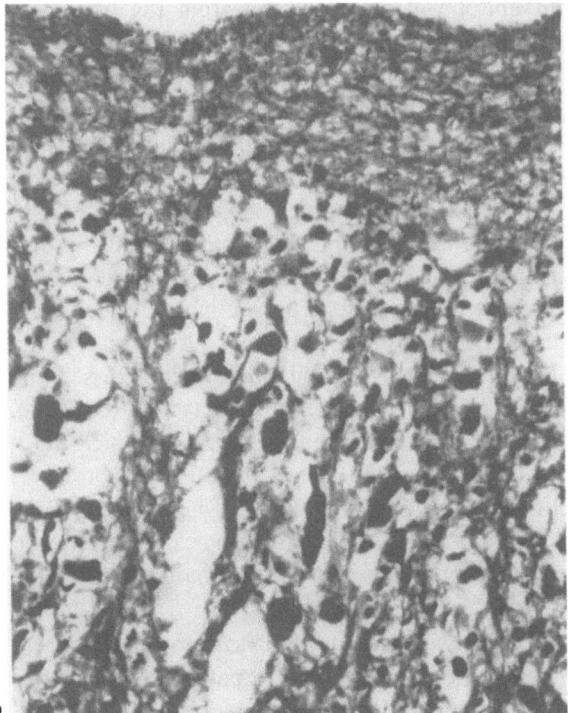

Fig. 6.7. Photomicrographs. **a** Shearing lesion around a blood vessel in the cerebral white matter of a patient dying 1 day after a head injury. (Myelin stain × 100)
b Ballooned axons in the white matter of a patient dying 6 days after cerebral trauma. (Silver stain for axons × 300)

severe primary impact damage and is usually due to cortical lacerations; a lucid interval is therefore common and the results of treatment are poor. *Chronic subdural haematomas* usually occur in association with a relatively slight initial injury and the subdural bleeding often passes unnoticed for several weeks. By this time the haematoma is largely fluid and surrounded by a 'membrane' of granulation tissue. The subdural collection increases in size because further bleeding may occur from new capillaries in the granulation tissue. A further increase in size may result from the absorption of fluid across the subdural membrane. The patient shows progressive impairment of intellectual function and fluctuating levels of consciousness. Such a slowly evolving clinical picture of chronic subdural haematoma may be difficult to recognise. Further, it must be remembered that these haematomas are frequently bilateral.

An acute subdural haematoma appears as a red gelatinous mass of fresh blood clot distributed over the surface of the hemisphere and accumulating over cortical lacerations. Later the haematoma becomes organised and macrophages invade the blood clot from the dura and to some extent from the arachnoidal surface. Granulation tissue consisting of fragile capillary loops, fibroblasts and collagen, steadily increases in thickness and maturity around the edges of the haematoma. To some extent, the age of subdural haematomas can be estimated from the thickness and maturity of the 'membrane' of granulation tissue which is usually thicker on the dural than on the arachnoidal aspect. At surgery, it may be difficult to strip the 'membranes' from the cortical surface. The contents of a subdural haematoma become fluid as the haematoma ages so that it may eventually have the consistency, and colour, of light oil.

Bleeding from blood vessels torn at the time of primary impact damage occurs, predominantly at the junction of grey and white matter (Fig. 6.3). In older patients, and in severe injury, *intracerebral haematomas* may be multiple but they vary in size. They are seen readily on CT scanning and occur in about 20% of severe head injuries; however, it is sometimes difficult to determine the clinical significance of intracerebral haematomas. Bleeding most commonly occurs in the frontal and temporal lobes, and may be in continuity with subdural haemorrhage or associated with considerable brain laceration—a burst lobe (Fig. 6.2).

Cerebral oedema commonly occurs as a reaction to brain injury. After primary impact damage to the

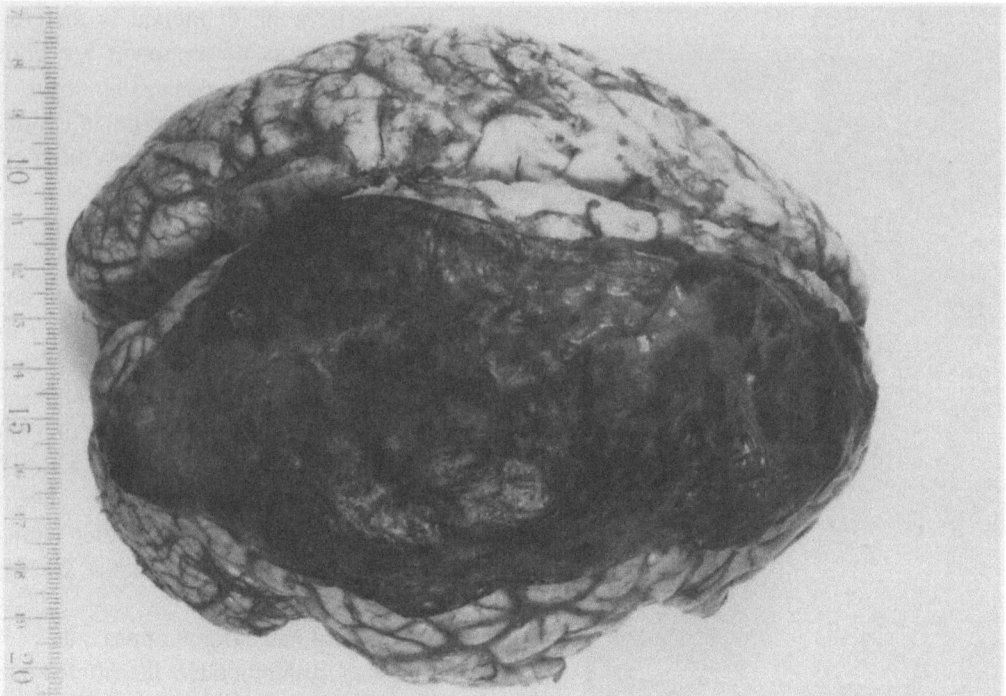

Fig. 6.8. A large subdural haematoma extending over the convexity of the right hemisphere. The dura has been removed.

brain, fluid starts to accumulate very quickly, becoming clinically important within the next 24–48 h. Further brain tissue damage due to hypoxia, ischaemia and brain shift may induce the accumulation of even more oedema fluid.

Localised oedema occurs at the sites of injury where fluid accumulates in damaged cells—*cytotoxic* oedema. Generalised cerebral oedema of the *vasogenic* type, however, is a much more important complication of head injuries. The blood–brain barrier is broken down and protein and water enters the extracellular space, particularly in the white matter, and may spread from the initial area of damage to involve much of the hemisphere.

At autopsy, the oedematous brain is heavier than normal and shows flattening of the gyri and narrowing of the sulci, particularly over the vertices. The ventricles are usually compressed and there is herniation of the parahippocampal gyrus through the tentorial opening, causing midbrain compression, and, less frequently, cerebellar tonsillar herniation. The consequences of such brain shift are discussed below. When the brain is cut, the oedematous areas are softer than normal brain and the extracelluar space in the white matter, normally about 15 % of brain volume, is greatly increased. Zones of cerebral oedema can usually be detected on myelin stains because the oedematous white matter appears pale when compared with normal tissue.

High molecular weight diuretic agents such as mannitol will remove water from the brain and reduce intracranial pressure. They probably act upon normal parts of the brain with an intact blood–brain barrier. If given early during the phase of development of cerebral oedema, they may increase oedema due to the large molecules of the drug entering the brain as oedema develops. High-dose glucocorticoid therapy, such as dexamethasone, is thought to reduce the extent of cerebral oedema and may also be useful in preventing its development.

When the pressure in the intracranial cavity becomes very high, capillaries are compressed and there is further ischaemic damage to the brain, particularly in the damaged area, in which autoregulation may be lost. Ultimately cerebral perfusion becomes inadequate and death occurs. This stage can be identified radiologically because no angiographic contrast can be made to enter the head.

Brain shift and displacement can result from localised or asymmetrical expansion of the intracranial components, either because of cerebral oedema or intracranial haemorrhage. This change in volume may be accommodated initially by compression of the ventricular system as CSF is driven from the skull. In unilateral lesions, the ipsilateral ventricle collapses first but this is not always followed by collapse of the contralateral ventricle. As one cerebral hemisphere expands, the cingulate gyrus is forced under the falx cerebri. Such subfalcine herniation can be detected radiologically either by CT scanning or by angiography. Occasionally, shift of the brain across the midline can obstruct the opposite foramen of Monro so that the contralateral ventricle dilates, thus fixing the injured hemisphere and preventing further displacement.

Expansion of the brain in the *supratentorial* compartment, whether unilateral or bilateral, results in the downward displacement of the brain through the tentorial opening. The oculomotor nerve and branches of the posterior cerebral artery may be compressed by the herniated parahippocampal gyrus, leading to the signs of a third nerve palsy with a fixed dilated pupil, and to hemianopia from infarction of the calcarine (visual) cortex in the territory of the posterior cerebral artery. The parahippocampal cortex may itself undergo necrosis due to pressure from the free edge of the tentorium cerebelli. One of the most important complications of transtentorial herniation is compression of the midbrain with the induction of central flame-shaped haemorrhages (Duret haemorrhages) in the substance of the midbrain; these haemorrhages are probably venous in origin. This is a frequent finding in patients dying with uncontrolled raised intracranial pressure. A less severe form of damage may occur in the compressed midbrain when the contralateral cerebral peduncle is caught against the free edge of the tentorium; nerve fibres and blood vessels are damaged within a haemorrhagic patch on the peduncle (*Kernohan's notch*).

Further caudal brain displacement, particularly when there is associated brain swelling in the posterior fossa, results in collapse of the fourth ventricle and ultimately death from brain stem compression associated with cerebellar tonsillar herniation through the foramen magnum.

The possibility that *ischaemic or hypoxic damage* to the brain following a head injury can be prevented by correct management makes it very important that the pathologist is aware that these complications can follow a head injury. It is also important for clinicopathological correlation to be made in relation to damage to organs other than the brain since this also affects the outcome.

Cerebral ischaemia and hypoxia can result from several factors which often coexist. These include: (a) direct damage to cardiovascular and respiratory central control mechanisms; (b) associated damage to heart and lungs; (c) respiratory and cardiac malfunction due to the onset of shock, airways obstruction and epilepsy; (d) effects of a progressive rise in intracranial pressure with failure of compensatory mechanisms and a decrease in cerebral perfusion; and (e) spasm or constriction of major blood vessels as a direct response to injury or from compression in relation to haematoma formation or brain herniation.

Certain neuronal groups are more vulnerable to hypoxia than others. These include the pyramidal cells in the hippocampus, the basal ganglia and the cortex. Purkinje cells in the cerebellum are also selectively damaged by hypoxia.

Boundary zone infarcts (see Chap. 5) may occur in those regions of the brain in which the middle, anterior and posterior cerebral artery territories abut. Such ischaemic lesions occur particularly when there are periods of hypotension or vessel spasm induced by blood in the subarachnoid space.

Meningitis may follow head injury when fractures involving the air sinuses, the ethmoid bone and the middle ear occur. Such fractures allow CSF to leak from the intracranial cavity and may thus open a route for infection to the CNS. *Streptococcus pneumoniae* is the commonest such infection, and penicillin and sulphonamides are often used prophylatically when there is a sinus fracture involving the skull.

Pathology of the brain in old head injuries. It may not be possible to estimate accurately the age of lesions in a brain when injury has occurred some months or years previously, but an assessment of the distribution of the lesions is feasible.

Old surface contusions appear as sunken, soft patches with orange discoloration and they are usually found in the frontal lobes, particularly on the under surface and near the poles, or at similar sites in the temporal lobes. Macroscopic or microscopic cystic lesions may be seen in the white matter in areas where nerve fibres have previously been damaged or blood vessels have been torn (Fig. 6.6); macrophages and reactive astrocytes may be seen for many months after the initial injury. The corpus callosum is often thin. The ventricles may be dilated through loss of white matter. Hydrocephalus may occur due to blockage of the CSF drainage pathways by fibrosis of the meninges following subarachnoid haemorrhage or meningitis. The effects of previous ischaemia can be detected especially when cortical damage extends into the depths of the sulci rather than just involving the gyral apices as in contusional damage.

All these features may be found some years after the accident, so that adequate correlation with the clinical data can be made.

Penetrating head injuries

Such injuries are less common than blunt head injuries and only account for some 15 % of the total. The most serious penetrating injuries are caused by high-velocity missiles. Bullets may pass into the skull and take bone fragments and infected material deep into the brain tissue. As a bullet passes through the brain it leaves a localised track with a much wider sleeve of necrotic haemorrhagic tissue surrounding it (Fig. 6.9). The more extensive area of

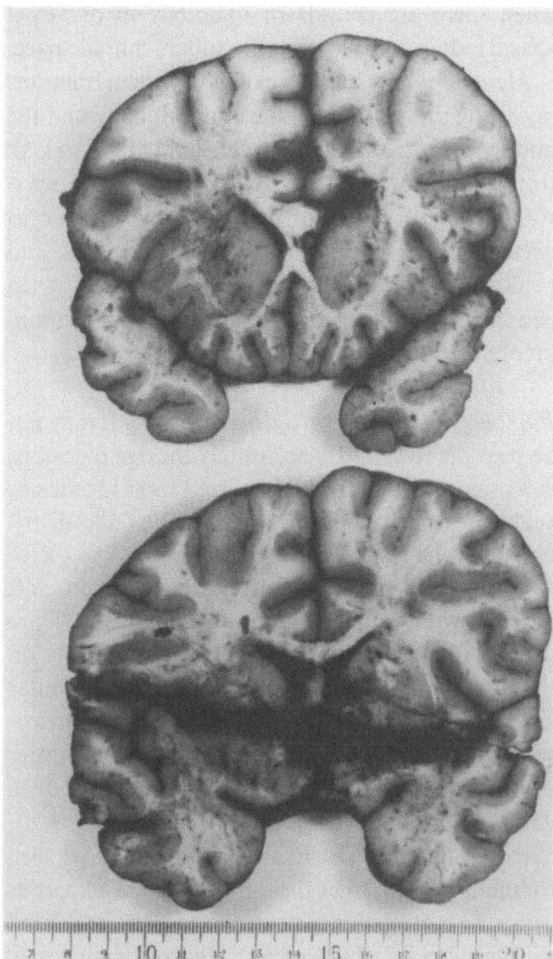

Fig. 6.9. A penetrating injury caused by a bullet. The bullet track is filled with blood and the surrounding brain is swollen and shows petechial haemorrhages.

damage is probably caused from shock waves generated by the missile. Low-velocity missiles may cause widespread damage within the brain as they lack the energy to leave the skull and thus ricochet off the inside of the calvarium and re-enter the brain.

Post-traumatic *epilepsy* occurs in up to 60 % of patients who survive penetrating injuries and is the principal complication of this type of trauma.

Spinal cord trauma

The problems of management of spinal cord trauma bear some similarities to those encountered in the management of head injuries. Primary damage to the cord may result in a complete transection at the time of injury or, as happens in many cases, some neurological function is preserved immediately after the injury but tissue damage then becomes more extensive and neurological function deteriorates. As with head injuries, it is important that the accounts of those observing the patient soon after the accident should be noted as part of the clinical history.

Pathological studies are important for correlation of the clinical course and the degree of injury that the cord sustained. However, since many patients with spinal cord injuries survive, experimental studies have proved essential for the elucidation of mechanisms of trauma and, in particular, the characterisation of processes involved in the extension of damage following trauma.

Traumatic lesions to the spinal cord are the cause of admission for over half the cases in large hospitals for paraplegic and tetraplegic patients. In a civilian population, 80 %–90 % of all new cases are due to road traffic accidents and 5 % to missile injuries with an incidence of 19 new patients per million population per year. Seventy percent of these patients are under 40 and nearly 90 % are men. Most road traffic accidents and swimming injuries involve the cervical and thoracic spine, whereas the crush injuries seen in mining accidents more commonly damage the lumbar spine. Missile injuries involve both thoracic and cervical cord equally.

Complete spinal cord transection following trauma is most commonly seen in the lower thoracic region; motor and sphincter function, and sensation below the level of the lesion are lost from the time of injury. *Incomplete* lesions involve the cervical cord and the cauda equina with an almost equal distribution. Early mortality among patients with spinal cord lesions is related to the site of the injury and the extent of the associated pathology. Patients surviving complete high cervical lesions have an early mortality (5%–15%) while partial cauda equina lesions are often compatible with an almost normal life expectancy. Modern methods of management have resulted in prolonged survival with a reasonable quality of life even for the patient with a cervical lesion; many live at home and are in full employment.

Primary damage to the spinal cord

Mechanisms of injury. Most injuries to the spinal cord result from a combination of flexion, rotation, extension and compression. It is only by considering the force and position of the body in relation to the injury that the major components can be identified.

In *extension* injuries of the cervical spine, or more correctly, retroflexion injuries, hyperextension forces the spinous and articular processes of the midcervical vertebrae together; they then act as a fulcrum for the separation of vertebral bodies and their adjacent intervertebral discs, thus causing dislocation between the vertebrae. Macroscopic examination of the spine following such an injury may only reveal excessive mobility and local haemorrhages under the longitudinal ligaments. With gross violence to the neck, the anterior longitudinal ligaments are torn and the posterior longitudinal ligaments are squeezed against the cord. Patients with cervical spondylosis or ankylosing spondylitis may suffer severe cord damage from what appears externally to be only minor trauma, e.g. head positioning under general anaesthesia. Spinal cord damage in these cases is probably caused by a combination of stretching and crushing the cord and from ischaemia following damage to the spinal arteries.

Excessive *flexion* of the cervical spine causes compression of the vertebral bodies; the bone fractures and fragments are displaced posteriorly causing damage to the spinal cord. If a *rotational* component is present, there may be unilateral or bilateral fractures, with dislocation and temporary narrowing of the spinal canal and consequent damage to the cord (Figs. 6.10, 6.11).

Compressive fractures are usually seen in the lumbar vertebrae. Fragments of bone may be displaced backwards into the spinal canal or, if the spinal column is acutely angulated, stretching and compression of the theca may occur.

The exact *mechanism* by which primary damage to the cord has been produced is often not clearly understood in cases of closed spinal injuries. At first sight the damage would appear to be due to mechanical distortion of the neural canal and to direct contusion and laceration of the cord itself. This, however, does not explain the occasional serious cord lesion where there is no macroscopic damage to the spine or cord itself and no external signs of trauma despite the presence of a neurological lesion indicating a complete cord transection.

Secondary damage to the spinal cord

As with head injuries, there is little that can be done to affect the primary damage to neurological tissue which occurs at the time of injury. Axons may be sheared and tracts disrupted or the cord completely transected. But clinical observations have shown that patients may deteriorate following spinal cord trauma and their neurological deficit may increase.

Experimental studies have been the main source of information regarding the secondary changes which take place in the cord following trauma. Using animal models such as rabbits and dogs, and employing systems of controlled contusion of the cord, it has been shown that a primary area of haemorrhage and necrosis is induced in the centre of the cord at the time of injury. Extension of the lesion coincides with the onset of oedema within the cord and disruption of the microcirculation, often with thrombotic occlusion of small vessels within the cord. The mechanism of microcirculatory disturbance within the cord is not fully known but it has been suggested that the release of biogenic amines may be one factor inducing vascular damage. The results, however, are clear; extensive ischaemic damage to the cord around the area of primary injury occurs. In this way the area of damage may extend both up and down from the site of injury and radially from the original central area of necrosis.

Open injuries to the cord

Injuries from *missiles* or *stab wounds* may cause direct trauma to the cord with complete or partial transection of the cord and its roots. Bullets, for example, may lodge in the cord or in extramedullary tissue, or bony fragments from shattered vertebrae may cause secondary damage to the cord by disrupting blood vessels and by introducing infected material into the wound.

High-velocity missile tracts passing near the cord may cause severe tissue pressure changes from shock wave injury so that complete loss of spinal cord function may be seen with little obvious macroscopic damage.

Stab wounds more commonly result in incomplete spinal cord lesions as the spinal laminae usually prevent the knife entering from behind. The damage may be discrete with little bleeding, though subsequent infection can occur.

Pathology of spinal cord injuries

Bony lesions

The accessibility of the spine to radiological study frequently allows an accurate assessment of the bony lesions in spinal trauma to be assessed during life. Such radiological investigations are often a valuable guide to the pathologist in localising the lesion for careful dissection. In many cases it may be advisable to remove the injured portion of spine complete, fix it, and then either dissect the column and cord or section it in the sagittal plane with a band saw (Fig. 6.10). In this way fracture–dislocations, crush fractures, ligamentous damage and disc protrusions can all be observed.

Extradural haematomas

Although uncommon, extradural haematomas may accumulate following relatively minor spinal trauma. They occur particularly in the elderly and if large they may cause spinal cord compression and infarction.

Traumatic lesions of the spinal cord

When the damage to the cord is very mild, a period of concussion may ensue with disturbance of neurological function lasting only a few days. Little is known in man about the effects of such mild trauma upon the tissue but, by analogy with other parts of the nervous system, when temporary functional disturbances occur following trauma there is little permanent damage to axons, although some demyelination may take place.

The appearances of the spinal cord following *severe trauma* vary depending upon the interval between trauma and autopsy. In the first 24 h, a severely injured cord with complete transection may show haemorrhage and softening at the site of trauma (Fig. 6.10). In less severe trauma, the external surface of the cord may show little evidence

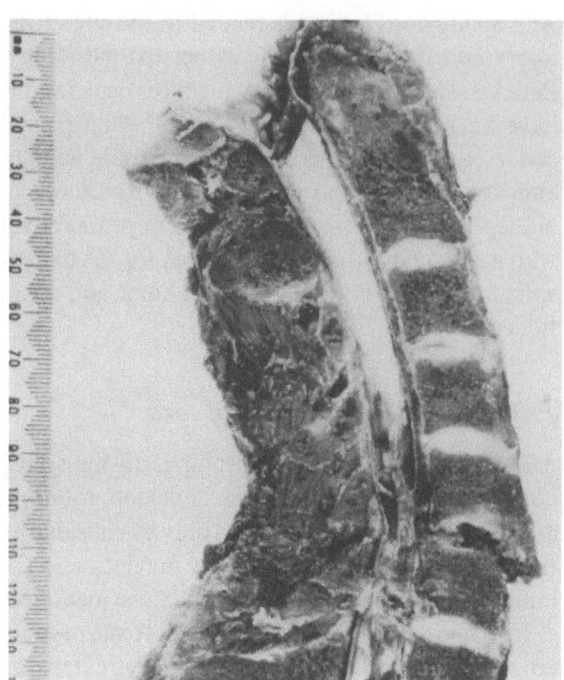

Fig. 6.10. Spinal cord injury following a fracture dislocation of C5 on C6. Extensive contusion of the spinal cord is seen at this level.

of direct injury and may only show venous stasis. Sectioning of the cord either in the sagittal plane or horizontally, reveals an area of fresh haemorrhage and necrosis in the centre of the cord which may extend for several segments above and below the point of injury. Even during the first hour, and certainly at the end of 24 h, more peripheral parts of the cord become oedematous and infarction may be seen due to disturbance of the microcirculation. Microscopically, petechial haemorrhages are seen in the ischaemic regions and, macroscopically, neurons and glial elements show ischaemic changes.

In *older lesions*, from a few days to several months, softening and cystic change will be seen in the damaged area (Fig. 6.11). Histologically, the early inflammatory exudate of polymorphs in the acute stage is supplanted by macrophage invasion and destruction of tissue debris by lipid-filled phagocytes. Iron pigment seen in macrophages within the lesion reflects the haemorrhagic nature of the primary damage.

Transection of *ascending* and *descending tracts* may be detected locally near the trauma by the presence of axon balloons; these are the swollen distal ends of the proximal axons and are similar to those seen in shearing lesions in cerebral trauma. The axon balloons soon disappear as no effective

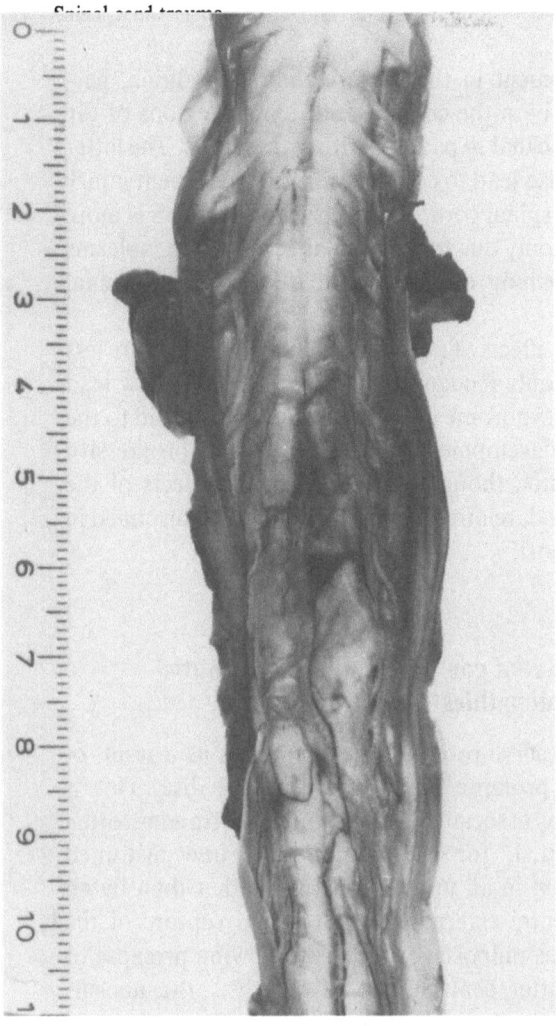

Fig. 6.11. Spinal cord injury showing necrosis and cavitation of the cord. In this case *compression* of the cord occurred without an associated fracture.

through alternative pathways and local redistribution of synaptic connections.

Late complications

Bacterial infection from foreign bodies introduced into the subarachnoid space at the time of injury, via a CSF leak or from infection in the bone surrounding the cord, may cause *meningitis* following spinal cord trauma. Other complications occurring several years after the injury may be due to the effect of a narrowed spinal canal upon the cord, to secondary arachnoid lesions or to persistent vascular insufficiency. Intramedullary cavities which form following the removal of the necrotic material after the injury may track downwards and occasionally upwards to the medulla in a similar way to syringomyelia. Such cavities are surrounded by gliomesodermal scar tissue and tend to extend into the dorsolateral quadrants of the cord. The fluid within a *post-traumatic syringomyelia* cavity has a high protein content but the syrinx rarely causes neurological complications.

Delayed myelopathy involving the posterior and lateral columns occurs in the craniocervical region and probably results from compression of the cord and associated vascular insufficiency and is similar to that seen in cervical spondylosis (Fig. 6.12). Histological examination of these lesions shows diffuse loss of myelin staining and gliosis. Unstable fractures in the spine are rarely a cause for concern as most bony injuries are stabilised after 4 months except when another disease process delays healing. This particularly occurs when there are collapsed vertebrae due to the presence of metastatic tumour.

Prospectus

Apart from stabilising fractures and dislocations of the spine, the results of clinical treatment of the spinal injuries have been disappointing. Whatever treatment is instituted, it seems that 60 % of patients show some improvement and a variable restoration of neurological function. It is clear that despite some careful studies of the pathology of spinal cord trauma, the mechanisms of primary and secondary damage are not fully understood. It is only through a full appreciation of the factors involved, particularly in the progression of neurological deficit following spinal cord trauma, that satisfactory management can be instituted to minimise the long-term neurological defects.

regeneration of severed axons occurs in the cord. More distal to the site of injury, axonal degeneration can be detected by staining for myelin breakdown products with Marchi or Oil-Red-O techniques.

As the debris is progressively removed, the cord may become shrunken, cystic and gliosed. Fibrosis may also occur in the cord and if the injury has involved root entry zones, Schwann cells may invade the cord and even form myelin sheaths. Although there is little or no evidence for effective axonal regeneration in the long tracts severed by spinal cord trauma, some recovery of the patient's neurological function may be observed. Such recovery is thought to be due to 'plasticity', a term which is used to define the way in which the damaged nervous system may continue to function

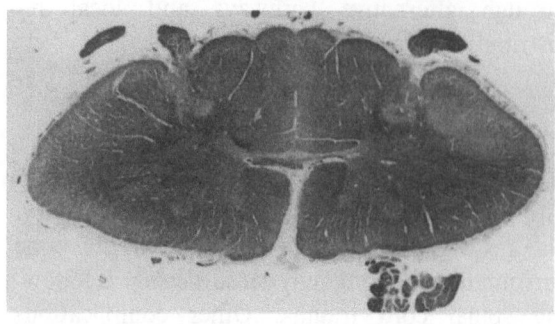

Fig. 6.12. Histological section of the cervical cord in a patient with severe cervical spondylosis. Pallor of staining in the right lateral corticospinal tract and in the gracile tracts of the dorsal columns indicates that there has been damage to the axons in these long tracts. (Myelin stain × 12)

Chronic and recurrent trauma to the nervous system

Recurrent minor trauma to the *peripheral nervous system* can lead to progressive and permanent defects (Table 6.1), as in the peripheral nerve palsies associated with *compression* of the median nerve at the wrist and with *recurrent trauma* to the relatively vulnerable ulnar and common peroneal nerves at the elbow and at the head of the fibula respectively. These peripheral nerve lesions are discussed in Chap. 16.

The *spinal roots* are vulnerable to damage from compression by prolapsed disc material, or from

Table 6.1. Syndromes of recurrent trauma to the nervous system

Peripheral nerves	Peripheral nerve entrapment and compression syndromes (see Chap. 16)
Nerve roots	Disc prolapse: cervical, thoracic and lumbosacral spondylosis
Cord	Cervical spondylosis with myelopathy syndrome of the narrow spinal canal claudication of the cauda equina achondroplasia
Brain	Dementia pugilistica (boxer's encephalopathy) (see Chap. 15)

entrapment in their intervertebral foramina, particularly in the cervical and lumbar regions of the spinal canal in patients with spondylosis. The latter may also lead to compression or to recurrent injury of the spinal cord. *Spinal cord* compression is more commonly due to primary or secondary neoplasms encroaching on the available space in the spinal canal.

The effects of repeated trauma to the *head* are less commonly recognised. Boxing, however, may lead to the syndrome of 'punch-drunkenness' and to the later development of an insidiously progressive dementia, thought to be due to the effects of the repeated, relatively minor head injuries sustained in this sport.

Nerve root compression, and traumatic radiculopathies

Acute nerve root compression arises as a result of acute prolapse of an intervertebral disc. This is usually associated with significant trauma, often sustained, for example, during unaccustomed exertion in an unusual posture, rather than by an accidental external force. There is rupture of the annulus pulposus of the disc, allowing prolapse of the softer central part of the disc, the nucleus pulposus, into the spinal canal. Disc prolapse occurs most commonly at C5/6 and L5/S1 levels, causing radicular pain, local pain in the spine and paraspinal region and sometimes weakness and sensory loss in the appropriate segmental distribution. Most disc prolapses are laterally situated so that only the nerve root is at risk. However, in the cervical and thoracic regions the cord is also at risk, particularly if the disc prolapse is central rather than lateral, and an acute paraplegia may then develop, requiring urgent surgical decompression. In severe injuries, especially road traffic accidents, root avulsion may occur.

Pathology

The compressed nerve root often appears thickened, indicating that there has been sufficient time for endoneurial fibrosis to develop. There may be severe axonal damage with wallerian degeneration distal to the site of injury. Neurogenic atrophy may be seen in muscles innervated by the affected nerve roots. Spinal cord compression and nerve root compression are more likely to occur if the spinal canal is congenitally narrow, a relatively common anomaly, and in achondroplastic subjects.

Root and cord lesions in spondylosis

With increasing age the spinal column shows changes due to degenerative osteoarthritis leading to restriction of movement, local pain and sometimes to root entrapment and cord compression. These changes are most marked in the cervical and lumbar regions, the parts of the spine in which most movement takes place. Calcification occurs at the margins of vertebral bodies, often in relation to small and otherwise insignificant bulges of the annulus fibrosus of the intervertebral disc. Calcified *osteophytes* form which may encroach sufficiently on the lateral recess of the spinal canal or on the intervertebral foramen itself to compress the nerve root during certain postures or movements, thus inducing radicular pain, or even weakness and sensory loss in the root distribution. The affected nerve roots are thickened and their 'root sleeve' region can no longer be demonstrated by myelography. Severe encroachment on the intervertebral foramen may interfere with the blood supply of the root entry zone, or even of the spinal cord itself, because the circulation in the radicular artery accompanying the nerve root may be compromised.

There is a risk of cord compression when the cervical spinal canal is congenitally narrow, an anomaly due to unusual shortness of the vertebral laminae so that the lateral recesses of the spinal canal are flattened and its largest sagittal diameter is decreased to less than about 14 mm. Cord compression is most likely not in the neutral, head erect position, but in neck extension, when the slight buckling of the posterior spinal ligament is enough to indent the cord against the bulging intervertebral discs. This can be seen both at autopsy and at laminectomy. The paraplegia found in cervical spondylosis due to *cervical spondylotic myelopathy* thus results from recurrent minor compressive injury associated with head and neck movement, and perhaps from compromise of the cervical cord circulation due both to the cord compression and to the effects of compression of the radicular feeding vessels.

When the cauda equina is affected by spondylotic compression, a characteristic syndrome may result. This syndrome of *claudication of the cauda equina* consists of pain, weakness and dysaesthesiae occurring in a lumbosacral distribution during exercise, and relieved by rest. There is usually a history of sciatica, or back injury, and of ischaemic or hypertensive vascular disease. Investigation reveals spondylotic changes with compression of the cauda equina by intervertebral disc protrusion, and there is usually a congenitally narrow spinal canal.

Pathology

The commonest sites of cord compression associated with spondylosis are C4/5, C5/6, C6/7 and C3/4. The cord is indented and flattened anteriorly by osteophytes and protruded disc material and posteriorly by the ligamentum flavum. Above the zone of cord compression there is atrophy and loss of myelin staining of ascending tracts, especially of posterior columns and spinothalamic tracts, and below this zone there is similar atrophy of descending fibre systems, especially of the corticospinal tracts. These changes are frequently asymmetrical. The anterior horns show atrophy, loss of anterior horn cells and gliosis, which may extend below the levels of the midcervical compression to the upper two or three thoracic segments, presumably as a result of secondary vascular factors, especially venous congestion resulting from chronic cord compression. The arachnoid in the region of cord compression is often slightly thickened, and the spinal roots in this region are invariably somewhat atrophic, although their perineurial tissue may be thickened.

Spinal cord and nerve root compression by tumour or infection

Tumours frequently cause compression of the spinal cord and of the nerve roots. Metastatic tumour is the most frequent cause but primary tumours, such as meningiomas and schwannomas, arising within the spinal canal, may also present with cord and root compression. The prognosis is largely determined by the speed of onset and severity of the neurological signs. In patients in whom complete paraplegia and sensory loss with loss of sphincter function has occurred as a result of cord compression by metastatic tumour, it is unlikely that any useful recovery will result from surgical decompression, presumably because the cord has been irreversibly damaged. In these patients the onset of neurological disability is often abrupt or subacute during a few days, suggesting that vascular factors, presumably due to thrombosis or compression of the blood supply to the cord, are responsible. In patients with slowly growing lesions within the spinal canal, on the other hand, even virtually complete paraplegia may improve dramatically in the weeks and months following successful removal of the neoplasm, and decompression of the cord. This difference in prognosis and in pathogenesis of the cord lesion is probably due, in large part, to the vascular changes that occur in the cord when metastatic tumour invades a vertebral body, often causing its collapse, or infiltrates an intervertebral foramen and surrounds the cord as a tight, oedematous or even necrotic cuff, even though this lesion is extradural in location.

Infection may also cause cord compression. Unlike metastatic tumours, infections causing cord compression usually begin in the intervertebral discs, or in the subdural space. *Tuberculosis* of the spine, leading to Pott's paraplegia, almost always begins in a disc space. It secondarily invades the adjacent vertebral bodies, the paravertebral space, the subdural space and even the subarachnoid space, thus causing spinal tuberculous meningitis and radiculitis. *Pyogenic* infections may begin in a similar location, in the vertebral bodies, or in the subdural space (spinal subdural empyema). Infections that invade the subdural space often cause paraplegia not by their mass effect, but by leading to cord infarction from pyogenic thrombosis of the venous drainage of the cord, or by invasion of the spinal arterial system.

Radiation myelopathy and encephalopathy

Although the CNS is relatively resistant to injury by ionizing radiation, doses used in radiation therapy for cancer are in the range at which radiation damage to the CNS can occur. For this reason, neoplasms in the nervous system are usually treated by a carefully fractionated regime utilising multiple planes of irradiation to avoid exposing the normal brain or spinal cord to more than small doses. Doses in excess of 3500 rads may lead to spinal cord damage as a late complication, but similar doses applied to the brain seem rather less likely to produce clinically discernible effects although pathological changes may be demonstrable.

After excessive spinal cord irradiation a progressive myelopathy develops gradually 3 months to 3 years after exposure. An acute reaction consisting of Lhermitte's phenomenon may occur in the first 6 weeks to 3 months after irradiation but this is benign and does not presage the development of a chronic progressive myelopathy. It is probably due to partial demyelination in the posterior columns. The clinical picture of progressive radiation myelopathy consists of dysaesthesiae, progressive paraparesis with sensory impairment below the level of irradiation, and sphincter involvement. Amyotrophy from anterior horn cell damage occurs at the level of lesion. Rarely the cord lesions may progress abruptly.

Pathology

The cord is shrunken in the irradiated zone. Histologically there is neuronal loss in the anterior horns and in the posterior root ganglia. The white matter shows diffuse spongy degeneration with marked loss of axons. In many cases there are areas of infarction in the cord. The blood vessels show marked intimal and medial thickening, with evidence of thrombosis and recanalisation, but this arterial and capillary abnormality is not accompanied by fibrinoid necrosis or inflammatory cell infiltration of the vessel walls. Degeneration of ascending or descending tracts is found above and below the level of the irradiation damage itself.

The changes found in the brain associated with 'radiation' necrosis are similar to those found in the cord.

The nerve roots and peripheral nerves are less vulnerable to radiation injury than the CNS, but a progressive disability sometimes occurs after irradiation of the brachial plexus region. In most cases, however, this is due not to radiation injury but to malignant infiltration of the plexus.

Further reading

Adams J H, Graham D I, Scott G, Parker L S, Doyle D (1980) Brain damage in fatal non-missile head injury. J Clin Pathol 33: 1132

Freytag E (1963) Autopsy findings in head injuries from blunt forces: statistical evaluation of 1367 cases. Arch Pathol 75: 402

Freytag E (1963) Autopsy findings in head injuries from firearms: statistical evaluation of 254 cases. Arch Pathol 76: 215

Graham D I, Adams J H (1971) Ischaemic brain damage in fatal head injuries. Lancet i: 265

Guttmann L (1973) Spinal cord injuries. Oxford University Press, Oxford

Holbourn A H S (1945) The mechanics of brain injuries. Br Med Bull 3: 147

Jennett B (1962) Epilepsy after blunt head injuries. Heinemann, London

Jennett B, Bond M (1975) Assessment of outcome after severe brain damage: a practical scale. Lancet i: 480

Jennett B, Teasdale G, Braakman R et al. (1979) Prognosis of patients with severe head injury. J Neurosurg 4:283

Klatzo I (1967) Neuropathological aspects of brain oedema. J Neuropathol Exp Neurol 26: 1

Plum F, Posner J B (1972) The diagnosis of stupor and coma, 2nd edn. Davis, Philadelphia

Strich S J (1961) Shearing of nerve fibres as a cause of brain damage due to head injury: a study of 20 cases. Lancet ii: 433

Strich S J (1976) Cerebral trauma. In: Blackwood W, Corsellis J A N (eds) Greenfield's neuropathology. Arnold, London, p 327

Chapter 7

Intracranial and Spinal Tumours

Classification

Diagnosis and treatment of intracranial and spinal tumours form an important part of the workload of neurosurgical, neuroradiological and neuropathological services. Therapy for many of the malignant brain tumours is still far from satisfactory but accurate diagnosis, and especially the detection of meningiomas and other benign tumours is an essential part of good clinical management.

For the purposes of classification, intracranial and spinal tumours may be divided into primary tumours and metastatic tumours. In the latter group, lung, breast, kidney and malignant melanoma are the most common primary sites.

Although ultimately classified according to the cell of origin (Table 7.1) primary intracranial and spinal tumours can be broadly subdivided into two major groups; *firstly* neuroectodermal (neuroepithelial) tumours (gliomas and medulloblastomas) arising from brain or spinal cord neural tissue and, *secondly* those tumours derived from other structures within the cranial cavity or spinal canal.

Tumours in the second group include meningiomas, schwannomas, pituitary adenomas, craniopharyngiomas and tumours and malformations arising from vascular elements. Most of the tumours in this group are benign and in many cases the patients may be cured by surgical removal of the tumour. On the other hand, it is usually not possible to remove neuroectodermal tumours completely except in a few instances, such as colloid cysts of the third ventricle, choroid plexus papillomas, or the occasional well-circumscribed oligodendroglioma or cerebellar astrocytoma. Furthermore, only a few neuroectodermal tumours, e.g. medulloblastomas, are sensitive to irradiation or chemotherapy.

Benign and malignant brain tumours

When compared with tumours arising from other tissues, the concept of benign and malignant is rather different when applied to neuroectodermal tumours. *Well-differentiated* neuroectodermal tumours e.g. astrocytomas, oligodendrogliomas and ependymomas are rarely encapsulated and, in most cases, they diffusely infiltrate the surrounding tissue. Despite their low growth rate, they may eventually kill the patient especially if they are growing in the medulla, pons, midbrain, or deep in the hemisphere since in these sites they are inoperable. In addition, well-differentiated tumours, particularly astrocytomas, may become 'malignant', poorly differentiated tumours after a number of years.

The definition of *malignancy* when applied to neuroectodermal tumours is also different from that applied to tumours elsewhere in the body. *Poorly differentiated*, or malignant, neuroectodermal tumours do not, except on very rare occasions, metastasize outside the CNS. They do, however, spread within the brain and spinal cord, both by direct infiltration through brain tissue and by spread through the CSF. The major deleterious effects of neuroectodermal tumours are due to destruction of neural tissue, to their mass effect and, in some cases, due to obstruction of CSF flow which results in hydrocephalus.

Lack of clear criteria for distinguishing benign from malignant tumours within the CNS, and the almost continuous range of variation from well-differentiated to anaplastic forms of tumour arising from the different cell types, has led to the adoption of a simplified grading system. In 1949, Kernohan introduced a grading system on a scale 1–4; this facilitated communication between pathologists and clinicians, but it does have defects which, if not recognised, may lead to confusion. Most of the data regarding the grading system for neuroectodermal tumours were originally derived from the study of post-mortem brains. The role of histology in the diagnosis of neuroectodermal tumours has now shifted in emphasis to the study of biopsy material, in which only small fragments of the tumour may be available for examination. Heterogeneity of histological patterns in many neuroectodermal tumours, therefore, presents problems for the use of a rigid grading system when applied to biopsy material. This is particularly apparent when a well-differentiated area of an otherwise poorly differentiated tumour is all that is available in a biopsy. Thus, assessment of the degree of malignancy of the tumour must be based upon an appreciation of the clinical presentation and course, together with the histological picture in the biopsy. Despite the disadvantages of the grading system, it is still widely used and can be summarised as follows: grade 1 and 2 tumours are well differentiated; grade 3 tumours are poorly differentiated and grade 4 tumours are anaplastic.

Table 7.1. Classification and incidence of intracranial and spinal tumours

PRIMARY INTRACRANIAL TUMOURS (adapted from WHO classification 1979)	Percentage of total	
	All ages	Children
Tumours of neuroectodermal (neuro–epithelial) tissue		
Astrocytic tumours	10%	50%
Astrocytoma		
Glioblastoma multiforme and anaplastic astrocytoma	30%	
Oligodendroglial tumours	3%	
Oligodendroglioma		
Mixed oligo-astrocytoma		
Anaplastic (malignant) oligodendroglioma		
Ependymal tumours	3%	14%
Ependymoma		
Anaplastic (malignant) ependymoma		
Embryonal tumours..	3%	35%
Medulloblastoma		
Choroid plexus tumours..	1%	
Choroid plexus papilloma		
Anaplastic (malignant) choroid plexus papilloma		
Malformative lesions...	1%	
Colloid cyst of the third ventricle		
Tumours of nerve sheath cells	10%	
Schwannoma (neurilemmoma)		
Neurofibroma		
Tumours of meningeal tissue	15%	
Meningioma		
Meningeal sarcoma		
Primary malignant lymphomas of brain	< 1%	
(original name: microglioma-reticulum cell sarcoma)		
Tumours and hamartomas of blood vessel origin	10%	
Haemangioblastoma		
Cavernous haemangioma		
Capillary telangiectasis		
Arteriovenous malformations		
Tumours of pituitary origin		
Adenomas of anterior pituitary	7%	
Craniopharyngiomas and supracellar cysts...................................	3%	
Tumours of the pineal	1%	

METASTATIC INTRACRANIAL TUMOURS	Percentage of total
Carcinoma—bronchus and lung	~2%[a]
—breast	of all
—kidney	intracranial
Malignant melanoma	tumours
Leukaemias and lymphomas	

SPINAL TUMOURS	Percentage of total
Tumours of neuroepithelial tissue	25%
Ependymoma (60%)	
Astrocytoma (25%)	
Glioblastoma (15%)	
Non-glial tumours	75%
Meningioma	
Schwannomas	
Metastases	

[a]This figure is difficult to estimate; see text

Incidence of intracranial and spinal tumours

In 1975 there were 123782 deaths from malignant neoplasms in England and Wales which represents 21 % of the 582825 deaths from all causes. Twenty-three percent of all male deaths were from malignant neoplasms as were 20 % of all female deaths. The most common cancer causing death in women was breast cancer (22 %), whereas lung cancer was the most common tumour in men and represented 38 % of all cancer deaths in males. *CNS* tumours are the second most numerous form of cancer in children and the sixth most common form in adults. Some 2 % of all tumours in adults are in the brain and about 0.7 % are neuroectodermal in origin. In children, most brain tumours occur in the posterior fossa in the midline, either in the cerebellum or brain stem whereas in adults most of the tumours are above the tentorium in one or other cerebral hemisphere.

Estimates of the incidence of the various types of tumour within the brain vary depending upon whether the surveys are taken from post-mortem records or from biopsy surveys. The various figures available therefore give an approximate picture of the incidence of these tumours.

In the Wessex Region of Southern England, the annual incidence of gliomas (i.e. neuroectodermal tumours excluding medulloblastoma) in the adult population is 3.94 per 100000. Poorly differentiated cerebral gliomas (glioblastoma) have the highest incidence with a peak annual incidence of 7.3 per 100000 in the sixth decade. Glioblastoma (malignant glioma) is more common in males whereas meningiomas tend to occur more commonly in females.

Just as the true incidence of intracranial tumours is difficult to obtain, so are accurate data on the age-related incidence of neuroectodermal tumours. Figure 7.1 illustrates the pattern of incidence of neuroectodermal tumours related to age of the patient. Well-differentiated astrocytomas and medulloblastomas are the most common neuroectodermal tumours of childhood but ependymomas, usually in the posterior fossa, also occur in this age group. Cerebral astrocytomas are found in younger

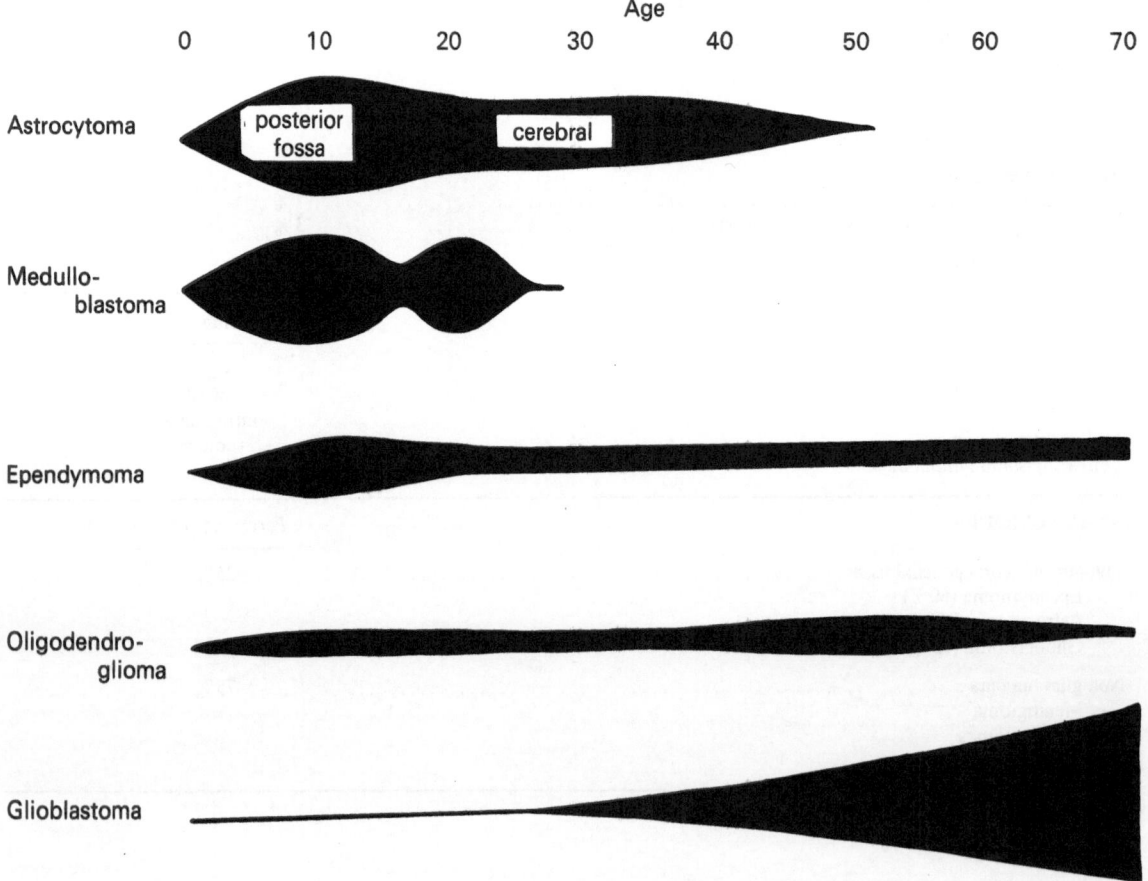

Fig. 7.1. Diagram to show the pattern of incidence of neuro-epithelial tumours (gliomas and medulloblastomas) related to age.

adults but in older age groups they either become less well differentiated (malignant) or arise de novo as glioblastomas. Oligodendrogliomas are uncommon in the posterior fossa and in younger children; they do occur in the cerebral hemispheres, however, in all age groups but, in older people, they tend to be more aggressive and may behave in a similar way to glioblastomas.

Site

In addition to the variation in incidence of different types of tumour with age, most intracranial and spinal tumours show a distinct predilection for site

(Fig. 7.2). Cerebral astrocytomas and glioblastomas occur more commonly in the frontal and temporal lobes, and although they do occur in the parietal lobes they are uncommon in the occipital lobes. Both these tumours may be located in the central, thalamic, regions of the brain. Oligodendrogliomas have similar sites of predilection. Ependymomas and choroid plexus papillomas most commonly involve the ventricular system although ependymomas arising in the spinal cord often spread throughout the neuraxis. Astrocytomas in the cerebellum and brain stem are one of the commonest tumours in childhood along with medulloblastomas, which most frequently arise in

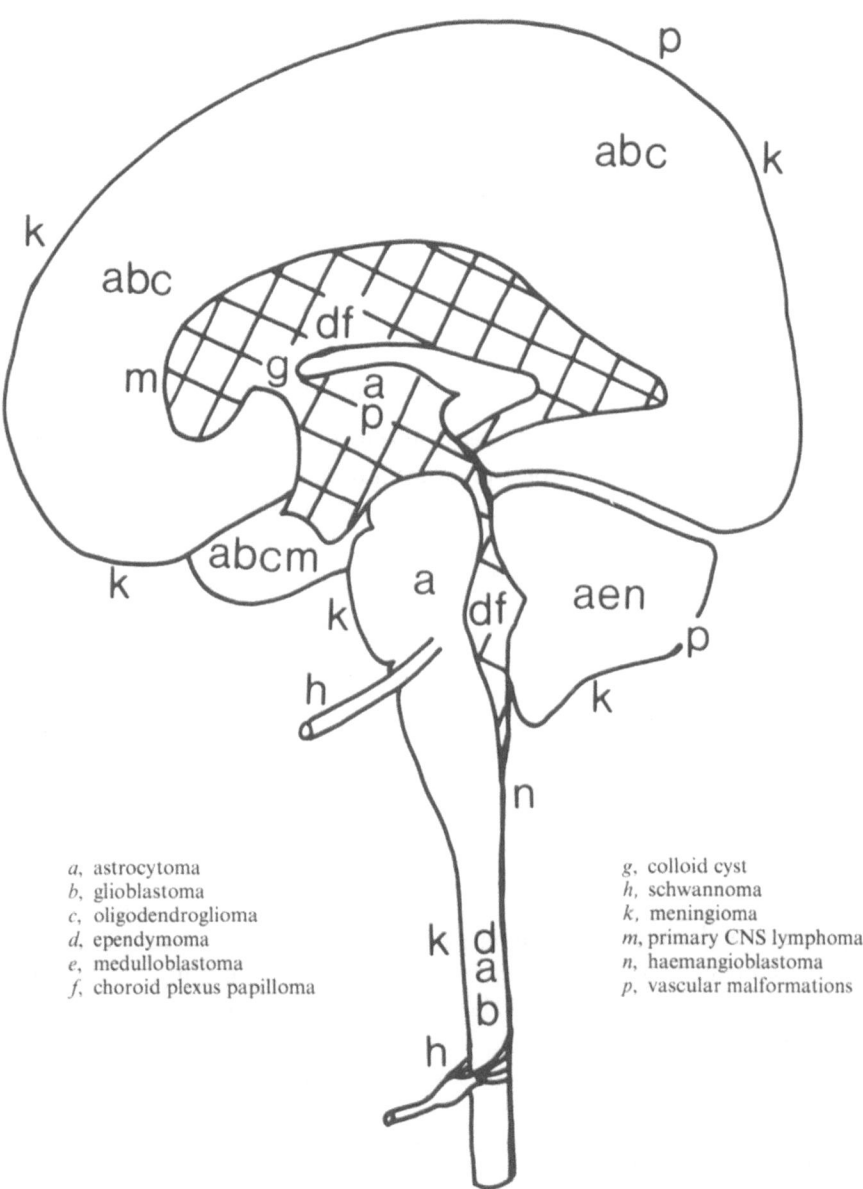

a, astrocytoma
b, glioblastoma
c, oligodendroglioma
d, ependymoma
e, medulloblastoma
f, choroid plexus papilloma

g, colloid cyst
h, schwannoma
k, meningioma
m, primary CNS lymphoma
n, haemangioblastoma
p, vascular malformations

Fig. 7.2. Diagram to show main sites of intracranial and spinal tumours.

the midline of the cerebellum. Colloid cysts may block CSF flow from the lateral ventricles due to their unique site in the third ventricle near the foramina of Monro. Meningiomas may be found at any site over the surface of the brain and cord. They arise from the arachnoid and are usually attached to the dura. Occasionally, meningiomas grow within the brain or the ventricular system. Although most commonly associated with the eighth nerve, schwannomas (acoustic neuromas) may also arise from the fifth nerve and from other cranial and spinal nerve roots. Arteriovenous malformations may be sited deep within the cerebral hemispheres or cerebellum, but are often found on the surface of the brain. Although the cerebellum is the most common site for haemangioblastomas, these tumours also occur on the surface of the spinal cord and medulla. Primary lymphomas of the CNS usually involve the cerebral hemispheres and have a predilection for the periventricular regions and the frontal and temporal lobes. Metastatic carcinoma and malignant melanoma, on the other hand, may be widely distributed throughout the brain and may even form a diffuse meningeal infiltration (carcinomatous meningitis).

Clinical presentation of intracranial tumours

The clinical presentation of intracranial and spinal tumours was considered briefly in Chap. 3 and is reviewed in detail by Northfield (1973). The rate at which symptoms develop depends upon the nature of the tumour, its situation and the age of the patient. Presenting symptoms are due to focal destruction of neural tissue, to oedema, to distortion of the intracranial contents or to raised intracranial pressure.

Focal deficit and silent areas

When progressive focal clinical deficit occurs, the diagnosis is relatively easy because the pattern of symptoms and signs allows accurate localisation of the area of the brain involved. By contrast, there are certain sites in the brain at which tumours may arise without producing a focal clinical abnormality. Such 'silent areas' are the non-dominant temporal lobe, the corpus callosum, the frontal lobe and the thalamus. Tumours of the temporal lobe may produce their first symptom by causing transtentorial herniation and compression of the brain stem

(see Chap. 4); some thalamic tumours can obstruct the third ventricle and upper aqueduct and cause hydrocephalus. Other sites are silent in the sense that small tumours can obstruct the passage of CSF and present by raising intracranial pressure. Lesions in the region of the pineal gland and pineal recess, the vermis of the cerebellum and the third ventricle characteristically present in this way. It is often impossible to distinguish clinically between the presence of multiple lesions in the brain and the combination of a single lesion with raised intracranial pressure.

Tumours of the frontal lobes may cause progressive dementia without other focal signs, with drowsiness appearing for the first time only as intracranial pressure rises in the late stages of the disease. Features suggesting parkinsonism may further complicate the clinical picture, although these effects are not usually due to infiltration of the basal ganglia but probably due to the combined effects of tissue destruction in the frontal lobes and distortion of the premotor cortex and its connections with the basal ganglia. Such tumours are clearly not silent but their effects may be misdiagnosed as being due to degenerative disease, especially in the elderly.

Raised intracranial pressure

It is least difficult to diagnose raised intracranial pressure when it occurs suddenly, producing headache, nausea, decline in the level of consciousness and visual failure. Chronically raised pressure of insidious onset may produce visual failure without other signs and this may go unrecognised by the patient and undetected by the clinician unless specifically sought. Enlarged physiological blind spots with or without reduced visual acuity are a much more reliable sign of raised intracranial pressure than papilloedema. Neither the site of the lesion nor its duration can be inferred from the presence or absence of papilloedema. It is a helpful diagnostic sign when present, but papilloedema is absent in two thirds of patients with intracerebral tumours at the time of surgery. Contrary to popular belief, headache is an unhelpful symptom. The most reliable feature in patients with tumours is that the headache is a new symptom for that patient; otherwise it is of poor diagnostic or localising value.

The effects of an expanding lesion upon intracranial pressure may vary with the age of the patient. Some degree of decompression may occur in infants and young children and even in older children due to separation of the skull sutures or to a change in the shape of the skull; in particular the temporal fossae may be modified by long-standing raised intracranial pressure. In the elderly, the volume of cerebral tissue within the skull is reduced by degenerative changes, thereby providing more room for a lesion to expand before it causes the intracranial pressure to rise.

Epilepsy

Epilepsy occurs in one-third of patients with brain tumours. Clinically, the seizures may be focal or generalised in nature although a focus can usually be detected on the electroencephalogram when the epilepsy is due to a tumour in the cerebral hemisphere. When epilepsy does occur, it tends to do so early in the growth of the tumour. Thus epilepsy is the presenting symptom in approximately 50% of those parietal tumours which cause epilepsy, 80% of those frontal tumours and 90% of those temporal tumours which cause epilepsy. Overall, epilepsy occurs four times more frequently in slowly growing tumours such as oligodendrogliomas (81% of cases) than in rapidly growing tumours such as metastases (19% of cases).

Diagnosis of intracranial tumours

Radiology—x-rays, isotope and CT scans

Diagnosis based upon the clinical criteria above is greatly assisted by radiological investigation and particularly by computerised axial tomography (CT). As a first step in the investigation of a patient with a possible tumour, plain x-rays of the skull may reveal evidence of raised intracranial pressure, pathological bone erosion or calcification, or lateral shift of the calcified pineal gland. A chest x-ray showing evidence of malignant disease may suggest the diagnosis of cerebral metastatic carcinoma without incurring the expense of a CT scan.

In the absence of adequate CT scanning facilities, *radio-isotope scans* are widely used, but they often give false negative results with relatively avascular tumours. A radioactive isotope (Technetium[99]) is injected intravenously and, due to a defective blood–brain barrier, it enters tumour tissue at a higher rate than normal brain, producing a 'hot spot' in a scan of the affected area. Resolution is poor near the skull base and in the posterior fossa because the mucous membranes and salivary glands also take up isotope in greater concentration than

normal brain and therefore obscure the evidence of tumour in these areas. Tumours and infarcts may both give a positive uptake but a second scan 8 weeks later will have returned to normal in most cases of infarction.

The various structures within the skull have different radiological densities that are all much less than the density of bone, so that conventional skull x-rays can detect changes in the configuration only of bone, or of materials of similar density, such as calcium. In *CT scanning*, a narrow x-ray beam is passed through the head while its source and a crystal detector rotate around the head through 180°. As the path of the x-ray beam rotates, the absorption of the beam changes. The signals from the x-ray detector are computed to reconstruct a picture of the areas of different radiological density within the skull. The signals are recorded on a disc and the radiologist can subsequently use the computer to manipulate the data in order to achieve optimum visual contrast or to establish the precise radiological density in the area of tissue under study.

Bone, calcium and fresh blood are radiologically dense; tumour tissue may appear more or less dense than normal brain and oedema appears as a surrounding area of decreased density (Fig. 7.5a). CT scanning not only shows the location of the lesion or lesions, but provides evidence of the extent of surrounding oedema, the degree of shift of the intracranial contents and the size of the ventricles. Radiological *contrast medium* injected intravenously enters the abnormal tissue where the blood–brain barrier is defective and thus alters its radiological density and provides further evidence of the nature of the lesion. After injection of the contrast medium, areas of the tumour which previously had a reduced or normal radiological density may become abnormally dense but the appearances of oedema are unchanged (Fig. 7.5b). CT radiographs are conventionally displayed as horizontal 'slices' parallel to the skull base but precise localisation of the lesion may require computerised conversion of the image to the sagittal or coronal plane. Angiography is necessary only to exclude aneurysms and vascular malformations and to delineate the blood supply of a tumour when the surgeon particularly requires this information.

Despite the immense advance of CT scanning, it does not provide a histological diagnosis and even the general nature of a space-occupying lesion in some cases remains in doubt. The surgeon may still have to plan an operative approach that would be appropriate for both a tumour and an abscess, or for both a tumour and an infarct; the *diagnosis* of the lesion may be confirmed only at the time of surgery or by histological examination of a biopsy.

Biopsy of brain tumours

One of the most difficult decisions in the management of a patient with a single cerebral tumour is whether or not it should be biopsied. Despite the advance of CT scanning, histological examination remains the only certain method of diagnosis and only in exceptional circumstances should biopsy *not* be performed. The clinical management of a patient with radiological evidence of metastases is particularly difficult. If the patient has a histologically proven primary tumour in a site known to metastasize commonly to the brain, then it is reasonable to assume that the cerebral lesions are metastases provided the clinical and radiological evidence is convincing. Mistakes, however, do occur and patients may die from potentially *treatable* conditions such as *meningioma* or *abscess*, when the diagnosis is accepted without histological verification or when the only histological evidence has been obtained from a primary site that rarely metastasizes to the brain. Most tumours of the gastrointestinal tract fall into this category. It is particularly important to exclude tumours susceptible to parenteral treatment, such as certain breast carcinomas, before committing the patient to symptomatic treatment only. The prognosis of individual tumours is considered with their histopathological features later in this chapter.

Cerebral biopsy: burr-hole or craniotomy?

Needle biopsy via a burr-hole has a number of advantages. It is a rapid procedure which requires a minimum of anaesthesia and is particularly suitable for patients who are suffering a severe neurological deficit and whose prognosis appears poor irrespective of the histological diagnosis. If the mass could be an abscess, or is cystic, aspiration via a burr-hole may be the treatment of choice as well as providing a histological diagnosis.

The disadvantages of burr-hole biopsy are that only small fragments of tissue are obtained and that the target may be missed by the needle. Furthermore, the needle may provoke a haemorrhage that causes damage in the absence of the decompressive effects of a craniotomy.

Obtaining a biopsy, either through a burr-hole or

craniotomy flap, increases the immediate risk to the patient due to haemorrhage, oedema or disturbance of brain tissue during the operation. A clinical decision may therefore be required as to how vigorously to treat such complications or further deterioration in the patient's condition; such decisions are made in the light of the histological evidence, even when it is only on the provisional interpretation of a *tissue smear* or *cryostat* (frozen) *section*. Until malignancy has been positively identified, neurosurgeons will, on the whole, continue to intervene surgically in order to preserve the patient's prospects.

The rigour with which a firm histological diagnosis of a tumour is pursued depends also upon local policy concerning the use of palliative chemotherapy and radiotherapy for the underlying condition. In the present state of knowledge, chemotherapy can rarely be justified for an individual patient on clinical and histological grounds alone, since the results of treatment to date differ so little from the outcome in untreated cases. However, advances in the treatment of gliomas can be made only by careful evaluation and comparison of the different therapies as they develop and a neurosurgeon involved in such work is likely to biopsy more extensively than one whose management is dictated by individual clinical considerations alone.

Intracranial tumours of neuro-epithelial origin

Approximately 50% of intracranial tumours arise from neuro-epithelial tissue (Table 7.1), and the rest arise from structures outside the brain or from vascular or connective tissue elements within the brain itself. Most of the neuro-epithelial tumours, especially in adults, arise from different types of glial cells within the brain and therefore form the group of tumours called *gliomas*; the only neuro-epithelial tumours excluded from this group are those which are thought to arise from neurons, i.e. medulloblastoma and neuroblastoma.

Astrocytomas

Clinical features

Astrocytomas are well-differentiated tumours arising from astrocytes; they occur mainly in the brain stem and cerebellum in the posterior fossa of children or in the cerebral hemispheres of young adults. Thalamic subependymal astrocytomas may occur in association with tuberous sclerosis. Depending upon the site, astrocytomas usually present with slowly progressive neurological signs. In children with *brain stem tumours*, the pyramidal tracts may be affected, producing spastic hemiplegia or quadriplegia. If the tumour spreads into the floor of the fourth ventricle, cranial nerve nuclei may be damaged and cranial nerve palsies may ensue. Astrocytomas in the cerebellum are frequently cystic and may present with cerebellar ataxia or cause raised intracranial pressure with or without hydrocephalus.

Cerebral astrocytomas in children or young adults may present with a long history of focal or temporal lobe epilepsy, focal weakness or signs of raised intracranial pressure.

Skull x-ray may reveal the calcification which frequently occurs in cerebral astrocytomas. CT scanning usually reveals the tumour mass which may or may not enhance following contrast injection, depending upon how significantly the blood–brain barrier within the tumour is altered. Astrocytomas encroaching upon the ventricles may also be defined by CT scanning but in rare instances where the tumour has the same radiological density as normal brain, air encephalography may still be required to locate the abnormal region.

The *prognosis* and *complications* of astrocytomas depend upon the site and speed of growth of the tumour. Those arising in the *cerebellar hemispheres* may be completely excised, and with surgery alone or with surgery and irradiation the 15-year survival rate is nearly 80%. *Brain stem* astrocytomas represent some 12% of childhood tumours but they have a less favourable prognosis as they are usually inoperable; the 3-year survival rate is about 19% following irradiation. Usually the patient dies as the tumour expands and infiltrates into long tracts and vital centres in the brain stem.

Cerebral astrocytomas may be accessible to surgical excision but this is often incomplete and the tumour may undergo *malignant (anaplastic) change* after 5 or 10 years and behave ultimately in a similar way to a glioblastoma. The treatment of choice in astrocytomas appears to be surgical excision and irradiation.

Pathology

The *macroscopic* appearances of an astrocytoma in the brain at surgery or post-mortem are usually quite characteristic. *Cerebellar* astrocytomas are often cystic with proteinaceous fluid within the cyst and a small nodule of firm or gelatinous, creamy-white tumour tissue in the wall of the cyst. *Pontine* and other *brain stem* gliomas show diffuse enlargement of the region which often more or less maintains its original shape, although enlarged in size. Similarly, *cerebral* astrocytomas may appear as swelling of the hemisphere. Some astrocytomas are soft and gelatinous whereas others are tough and fibrous; in most cases it is difficult, if not impossible, to define the border of an astrocytoma as it diffusely infiltrates the surrounding tissue (Fig. 7.3). Occasionally the tumour spreads through the subarachnoid space or ventricles and forms a gelatinous coating to the brain surfaces.

Fatal *complications* from astrocytomas vary in their nature. The tumour tissue may replace vital centres in the brain stem. Alternatively there may be sudden haemorrhage into a cerebral astrocytoma causing a rise in intracranial pressure and brain stem compression due to transtentorial herniation (see Chap. 4). Herniation of the cerebellar tonsils through the foramen magnum may occur with cerebellar tumours or acute hydrocephalus may result from blockage of the ventricular system by tumour or from displacement of the brain stem by a tumour mass.

Histology

Histologically there is some variation in the appearance of astrocytomas. *Protoplasmic* astrocytomas often have a soft, gelatinous consistency and are composed of cells which extend a few delicate processes to form a cobweb-like structure between the cell bodies (Fig. 7.4). Few, if any, intracytoplasmic glial fibrils are present in the processes and the cells are often separated by microcystic cavities. There is some variation in nuclear shape and size but usually the cells have moderately regular, round nuclei. *Fibrillary* astrocytomas may also be soft in consistency and similar to protoplasmic astrocytomas but their processes contain more glial fibrils. Some tumours are firm and rubbery and composed of tightly packed spindle-shaped astrocytic cells containing large numbers of intracellular glial fibrils. Such tumours are often called *pilocytic* astrocytomas and may contain thickened, brightly eosinophilic processes (Rosenthal fibres). In some astrocytomas, the tumour cells are plump with abundant eosinophilic cytoplasm and eccentric nuclei; they superficially

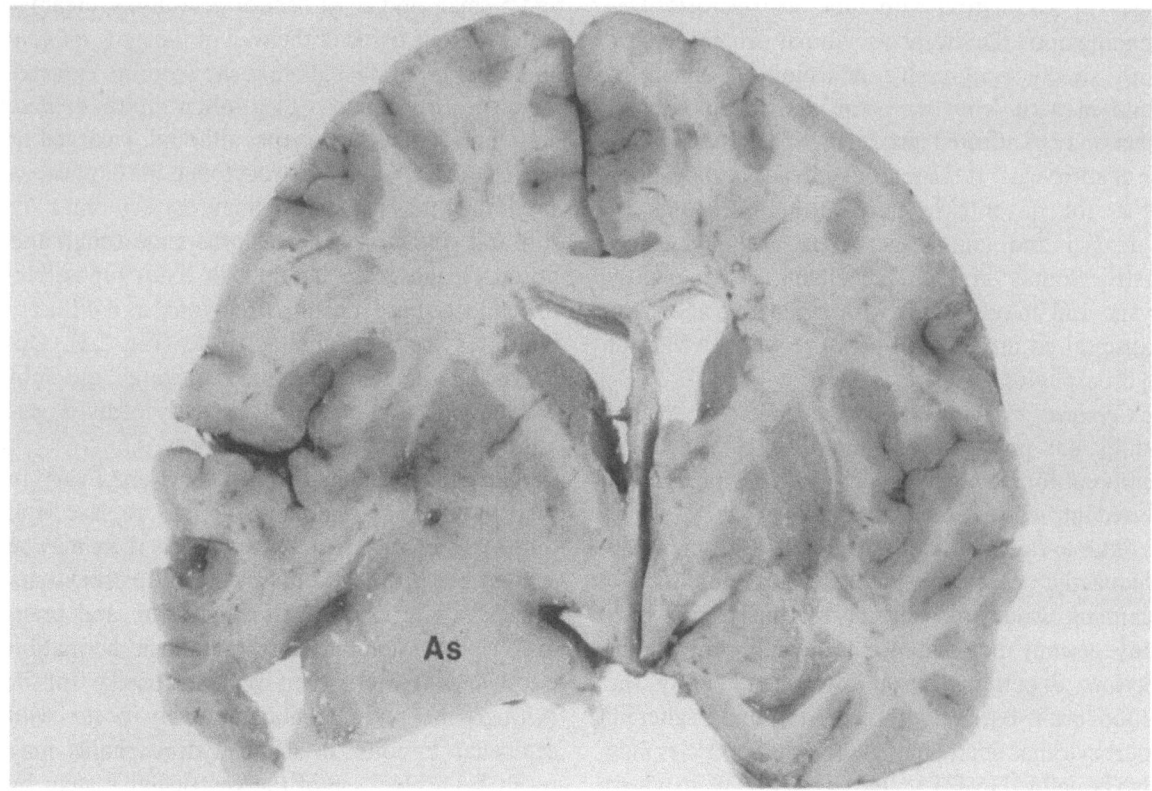

Fig. 7.3. Cerebral astrocytoma (*As*).

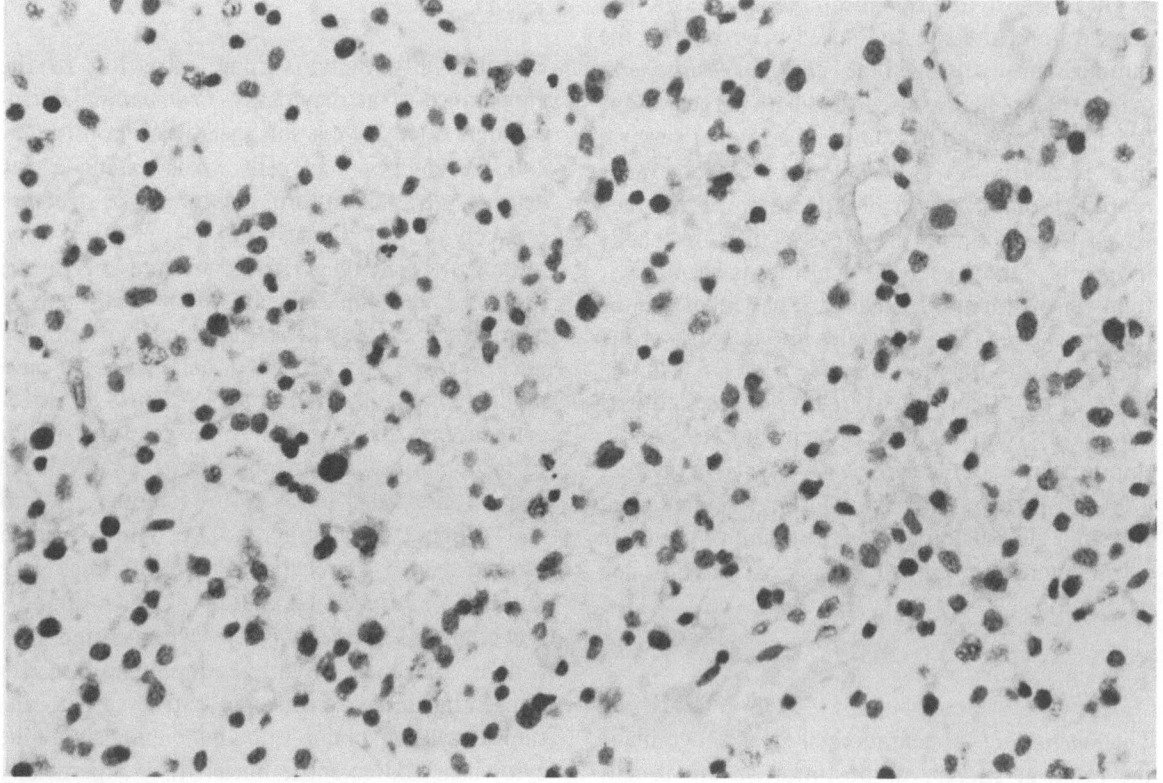

Fig. 7.4. Protoplasmic astrocytoma. (H & E ×400)

resemble hypertrophic reactive astrocytes seen in areas of brain damage. Such *gemistocytic* cells form the majority of the tumour in gemistocytic astrocytomas and they are seen to a greater or lesser extent in other astrocytic tumours.

Astrocytomas infiltrate the surrounding tissue to varying degrees and their stage of differentiation is partly judged on nuclear form. In well-differentiated astrocytomas, the nuclei are round or elongated but are equal in size and show little variation in shape or density of staining. Poorly differentiated tumours may contain cells in mitosis and show nuclear pleomorphism with an increase in the density of staining of the nuclei (hyperchromasia) and focal anaplasia.

Surgical pathology

Rapid diagnosis of astrocytomas may be made on a smear or cryostat section. The monomorphic nature of the cellular content in a smear may suggest the presence of tumour, particularly if the cells show a delicate network of processes. When the astrocytes resemble reactive astrocytes it may be difficult to distinguish a tumour from reactive gliosis, although the absence of macrophages and inflammatory cells in the smear may suggest a tumour rather than the damaged tissue around an infarct or abscess. Cryostat sections are valuable when the tissue is too tough to smear. In such cases the cryostat sections are usually of better quality than sections from soft tumours and may be more suitable for histological identification of the tumour. The use of Holzer or other techniques for astrocytes, e.g. basic fuchsin, amido black, naphthol yellow (FAN) method (Miquel et al. 1968) on cryostat sections may be useful in the identification of astrocytomas.

The characterisation of a tumour in paraffin sections is usually straightforward when the tissue supplied by the surgeon is sufficient. With smaller fragments of tumours it may be useful to characterise the cells by immunoperoxidase staining for GFAP or by electron microscopy through the presence of glial fibrils within the cytoplasm.

Glioblastomas and anaplastic astrocytomas

Clinical features

The majority of glioblastomas occur in patients over the age of 40 and they usually arise in the cerebral hemispheres (Figs. 7.1, 7.2). Depending upon the site, the patient may present with a few months' history of progressive personality change, intellectual deterioration, focal neurological signs or epilepsy. In some cases, the first indication of the presence of a tumour may be the headache, alteration in consciousness, and papilloedema of raised intracranial pressure. When the tumour has arisen first as a well-differentiated astrocytoma, the patient may present with a long history but as foci of anaplastic change develop and the tumour becomes an anaplastic astrocytoma recent rapid deterioration occurs as outlined above.

Radiographic investigation may reveal shift of the pineal on straight skull x-ray; evidence of bony erosion within the skull or thinning of the calvarium may be observed if the tumour has originated in a more benign, slowly growing form. The site of the tumour is often evident on a Technetium[99] isotope scan and a glioblastoma is usually obvious on a CT scan in which the viable tumour with its deficient blood–brain barrier is outlined by Conray enhancement (Fig. 7.5b). An area of cerebral oedema which usually surrounds a glioblastoma can be seen on the CT scan as an area of decreased attenuation (black on the scan) (Fig. 7.5a).

Although symptomatic improvement in patients with glioblastoma may follow *treatment* of the peritumoral oedema with dexamethasone, or decompression of the tumour by removal of cystic fluid, the overall prognosis is poor especially for patients with the more anaplastic gliomas. Even with surgical excision of the tumour mass and postoperative irradiation, less than 5 % of patients survive for 12 months. Although chemotherapy with BCNU and with methotrexate have been tried, there is a barely significant increase in survival times following these treatments. Currently, much emphasis is placed upon the quality of survival in addition to the length of survival; if the treatment of the tumour deprives the patient of a reasonable life then many would consider the treatment unjustifiable.

Pathology

The *gross pathology* of glioblastoma is most clearly seen in post-mortem brains. About 73 % of glioblastomas occur equally distributed between the frontal and temporal lobes. A further 20 % occur in the parietal region whereas the occipital region and the posterior fossa are uncommon sites for this tumour. Figure 7.6 shows a cystic glioblastoma in the frontal lobe corresponding to the CT scan seen in Fig. 7.5;

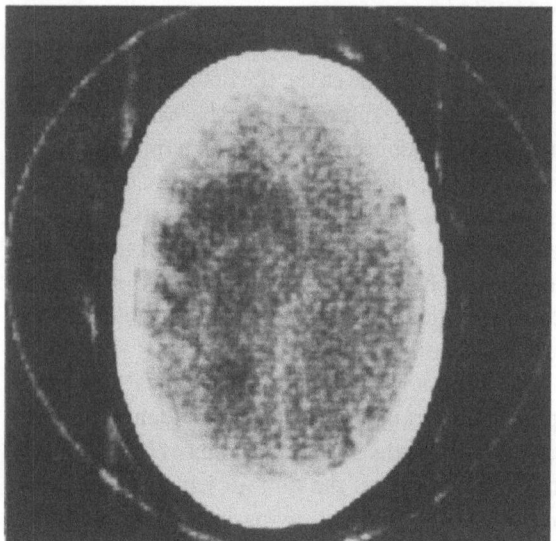

Fig. 7.5a Unenhanced CT scan showing an area of *oedema* (*black*) in the left hemisphere.

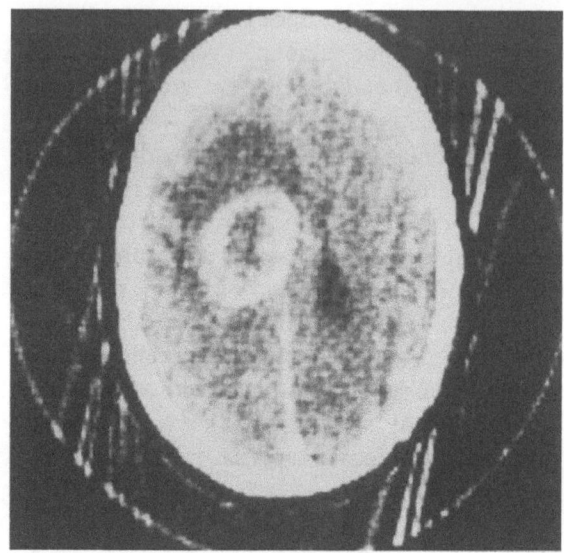

b CT scan enhanced with Conray. The plane is similar to that in Fig. 7.5a but the cystic glioblastoma is outlined in *white*.

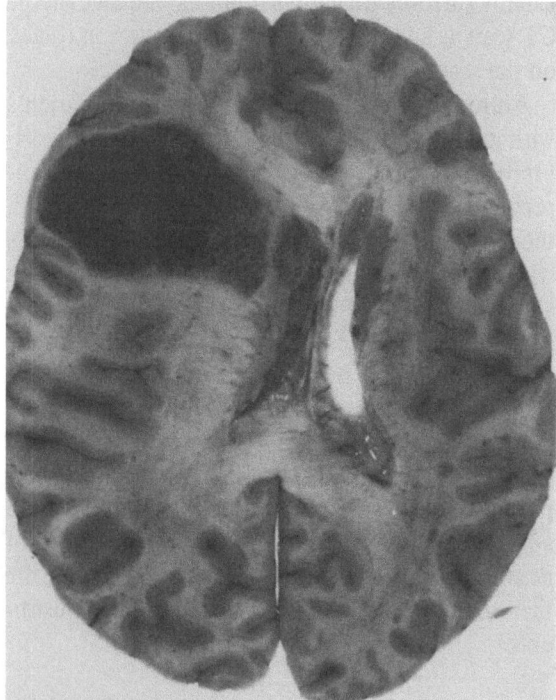

Fig. 7.6. Cystic glioblastoma similar to that in Fig. 7.5, with shift of the midline to the right.

it has a cystic centre and viable tumour is seen around its periphery. Enlargement of the hemisphere due to tumour and surrounding oedema has displaced the midline towards the right. Despite the apparent circumscribed margin of the tumour, glioblastoma cells infiltrate the surrounding brain.

Some tumours are very large and may follow white matter tracts such as the fornix and corpus callosum (Fig. 7.7), spreading from one hemisphere into the other. Necrosis is commonly seen and haemorrhage may occur during the course of the illness or as a terminal event. The major complications of gliomas which eventually kill the patient are either replacement of vital neurological tissue, or the displacement effects of the tumour mass and its surrounding oedema with transtentorial herniation of the parahippocampal gyrus, brain stem compression and consequent haemorrhage. Spread throughout the ventricular system and in the subarachnoid space may occur in glioblastoma. Satellite nodules of tumour, distant from the primary site, may cause confusion on CT scanning, as the multiple lesions may be interpreted as metastatic tumour from a non-neural primary.

Histology

The histology of glioblastomas varies not only from tumour to tumour but also within the same tumour; a feature which justifies the name of *glioblastoma multiforme*. In the centre of the tumour there is usually an area of necrosis surrounded by viable but degenerate tumour showing extensive nuclear and cytoplasmic *pleomorphism*, multinucleate cells, and hyperchromasia (Fig. 7.8). Abnormal mitoses may also be seen in such degenerate areas. Studies with isotope-labelled thymidine suggest that there is little cell replication in the central degenerate areas. In

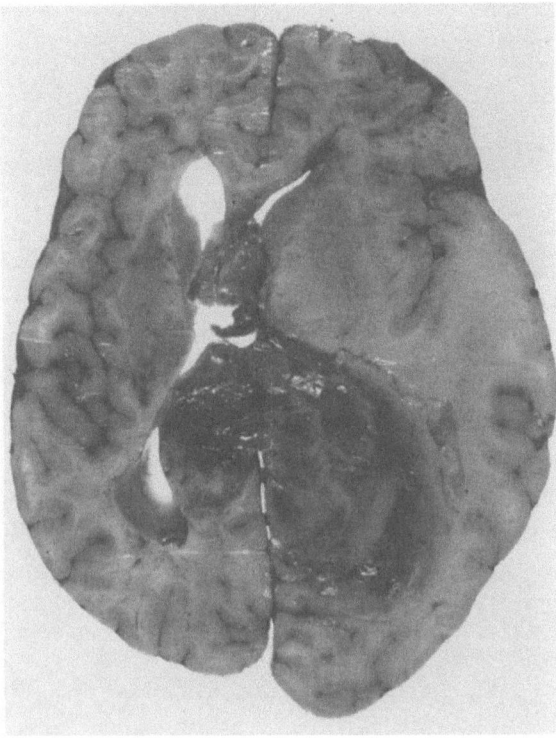

Fig. 7.7. A 'butterfly' glioblastoma involving both hemispheres via the corpus callosum.

the main body of the tumour, away from the degenerate areas, there may be considerable variation in the cytology of the tumour cells. Figure 7.9 shows a common pattern of spindle-shaped hyperchromatic nuclei which vary in shape and size and form *pseudo-palisades* around small areas of necrosis; this is a typical feature of glioblastomas. At the growing edge of the tumour (Fig. 7.10) glioblastoma cells, often with small hyperchromatic elongated nuclei and few processes, insinuate themselves between the neurons and glial cells of the normal brain. Such invasion is not as diffuse as in better differentiated astrocytomas but it is still difficult to identify a true border between tumour and normal brain. There is only rarely an astrocytic reaction to the invasion of a glioma but perivascular lymphocyte accumulation is commonly seen in this infiltrating zone.

In addition to the poorly differentiated and pleomorphic nature of the cells and the presence of necrosis within the tumour, blood vessel changes with *capillary endothelial proliferation* are a major feature which distinguishes a glioblastoma from a well-differentiated cerebral astrocytoma. The abnormal proliferation of small capillary vascular channels and their surrounding pericytes can be

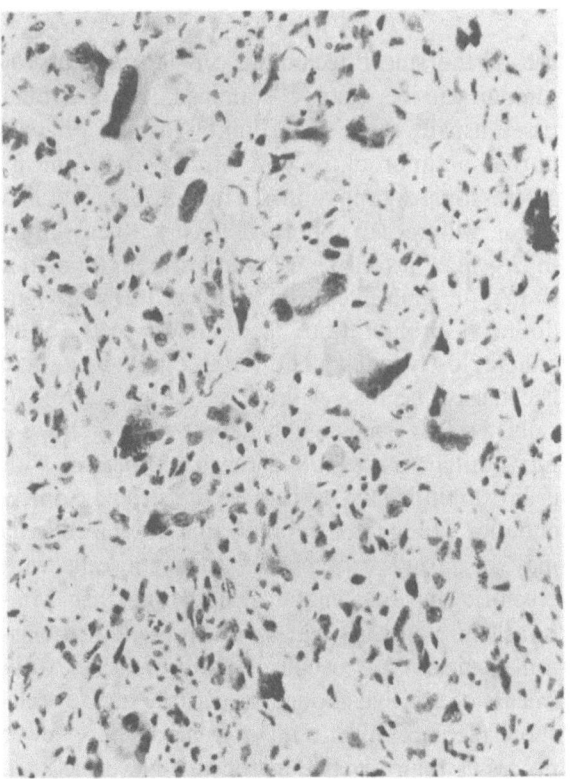

Fig. 7.8. Central area of glioblastoma showing bizarre cells with hyperchromatic nuclei. (H & E × 180)

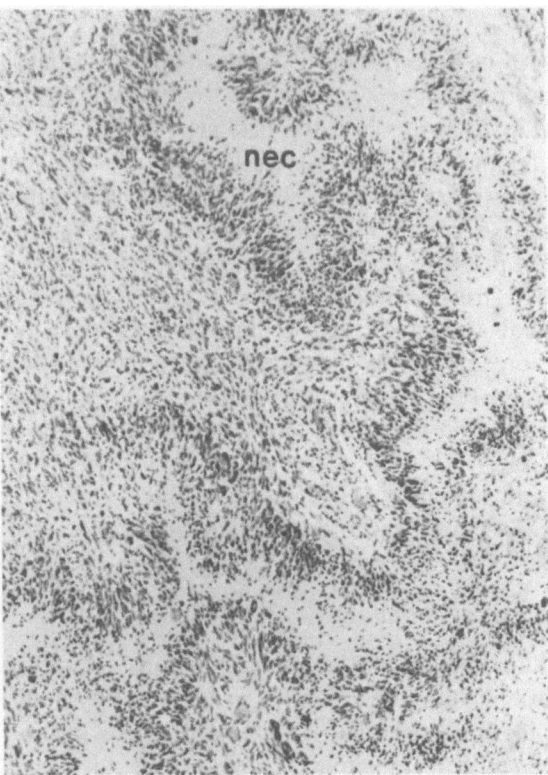

Fig. 7.9. Pseudo-palisading of tumour cells around an area of necrosis (*nec*) in a glioblastoma. (H & E × 75)

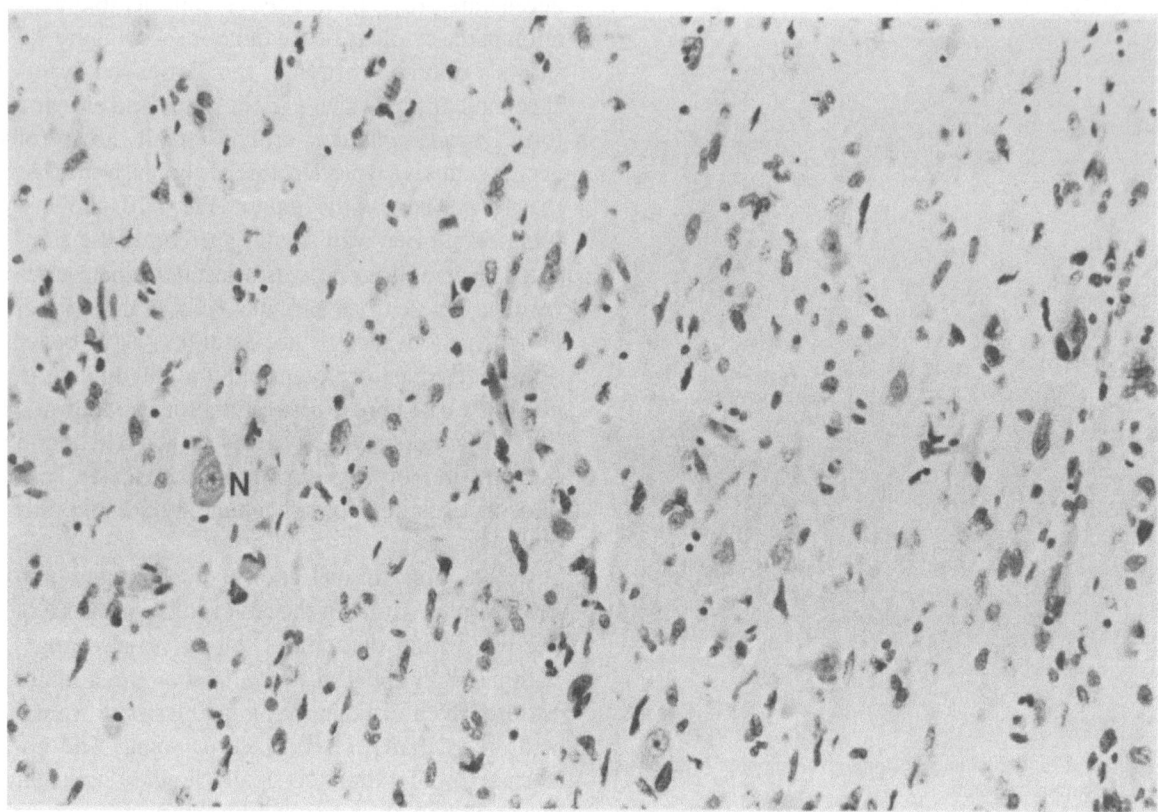

Fig. 7.10. Infiltrating edge of glioblastoma showing numerous small hyperchromatic tumour cell nuclei but neurons (*N*) are still preserved. (H & E × 250)

seen in H & E-stained sections (Fig. 7.11) but is more prominently displayed by reticulin stains (Fig. 7.12) in which the basement membranes of endothelial cells and pericytes are well demonstrated. An increase in the number of capillaries is seen in the infiltrating zone of the tumour but prominent capillary endothelial proliferation is only usually observed towards the centre of the glioblastoma. The blood–brain barrier is probably more intact in the infiltrating zone at the periphery of the tumour than in the central region; this may mean that the growing edge of the tumour is less accessible to blood-borne chemotherapeutic agents.

In a minority of glioblastomas, there is extensive connective tissue formation (gliosarcoma).

Surgical pathology

Rapid diagnosis of a glioblastoma may entail the examination of cores of tissue extracted by needle biopsy through a burr-hole, or larger pieces of tissue removed at craniotomy. Tumour tissue can usually be distinguished from the surrounding normal brain by its dark brown or dark grey colour. By the use of the smear technique, small fragments of tumour can be quickly examined. Glioblastoma tissue usually smears in a lumpy fashion whereas normal brain produces a uniformly smooth smear. Microscopic examination of a toluidine blue stained smear will reveal abnormal vessels where large, thick-walled arteries have short, stumpy branches ending in club-like formations of capillary endothelial proliferation. The tumour cells often adhere closely to the blood vessels especially if there is extensive necrosis within the tumour. Cytologically, a smear from a glioblastoma usually shows a fine fibrillary background of glial processes with cells exhibiting various degrees of astrocytic differentiation. Elongated bipolar spindle-shaped cells may be mixed with plump astrocytic cells with eccentric hyperchromatic nuclei (Fig. 7.13). Multinucleate giant cells may also be present. Glioblastoma smears can usually be distinguished from smears of reactive gliotic tissue as the tumour cells show pleomorphism and, in general, have fewer processes than reactive astrocytes. Nevertheless a continuous range of cytological features extending from non-neoplastic astrocytes to unrecognisable

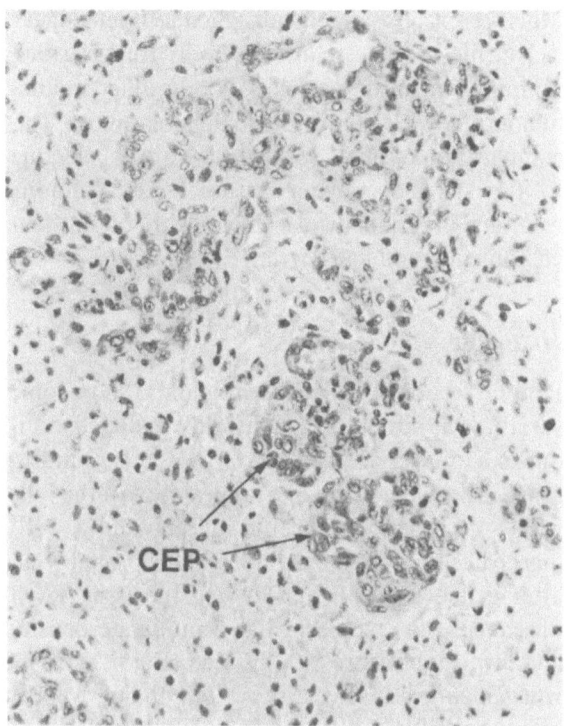

Fig. 7.11. Glioblastoma showing capillary endothelial proliferation (*CEP*). (H & E × 180)

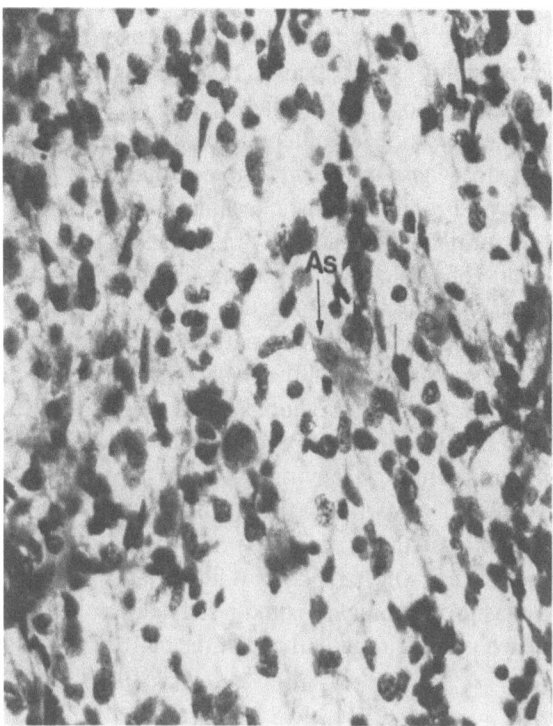

Fig. 7.13. Smear of glioblastoma showing nuclear pleomorphism. Some cells (*As*) have astrocytic features. (Toluidine blue stain × 36)

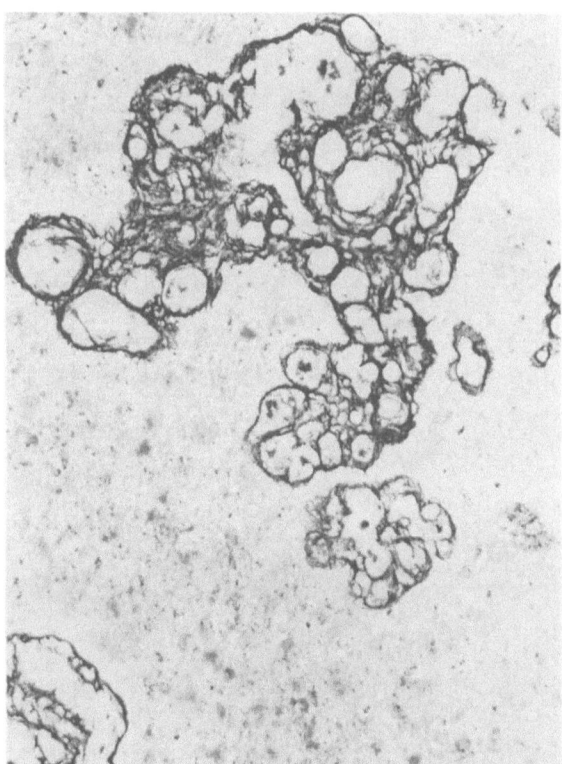

Fig. 7.12. Glioblastoma: same field as in Fig. 7.11. Basement membranes of endothelial cells and pericytes are outlined in *black*. (Reticulin stain × 180)

anaplastic tumour cells may make the categorisation of individual cells impossible.

The presence of extensive connective tissue within a glioblastoma may make it difficult to smear. Cryostat sections of such tough tumours are often more useful than the smears.

Although the majority of glioblastomas show astrocytic features, some tumours are so *anaplastic* that the origin of the cells cannot be determined histologically. In addition, some glioblastomas contain areas which have some of the features of oligodendrogliomas. It is probable that glioblastoma is the anaplastic form not only of astrocytoma, but also of oligodendroglioma and ependymoma.

A number of investigations may be carried out on glioblastomas to characterise their astrocytic components. PTAH and Holzer techniques applied to paraffin sections will stain astrocyte processes. Similarly, glial fibrillary acidic protein (GFAP) can be identified by immunoperoxidase or immunofluorescence staining in glioblastomas; in general the better differentiated cells contain more GFAP. Electron microscopy can also be used to define the 9-nm glial fibrils composed of GFAP within the tumour cells. In addition to the production of glial fibrils, many astrocytic cells in glioblastomas retain the capacity of normal astrocytes to take up protein by pinocytosis from the surrounding extracellular fluid; this capacity is only lost in the most poorly differentiated cells.

The detection of different isoenzymes of lactic dehydrogenase by electrophoresis has also been used as a rapid diagnostic technique to distinguish tumour tissue from normal brain tissue as the LDH profile of isoenzymes in gliomas is similar to fetal brain. Furthermore, metastatic non-glial tumours have a different isoenzyme pattern from gliomas.

Tissue culture techniques have been employed in the investigation of gliomas, particularly to test susceptibility to chemotherapeutic agents. Well-differentiated astrocytomas show a distinctive pattern of growth in tissue culture with highly branched stellate cells which move only slowly in the culture, whereas poorly differentiated glioblastomas grow mainly as spindle-shaped bipolar cells which migrate rapidly through the culture.

Oligodendrogliomas

Clinical features

Oligodendrogliomas usually occur in the cerebral hemispheres and are rarely seen in the posterior fossa. They may occur at any age but are most common in the frontal, temporal and parietal lobes of adults. In younger patients, oligodendrogliomas may present with temporal lobe epilepsy or with a history of slowly progressive focal neurological signs or raised intracranial pressure. In older patients, the tumours may be more aggressive and the history may resemble that of a glioblastoma.

Calcification within the tumour may be visible on a straight skull x-ray or on an unenhanced CT scan. Well-differentiated oligodendrogliomas may show little enhancement on CT scanning and minimal oedema; poorly differentiated oligodendrogliomas, on the other hand, may enhance in a similar way to glioblastomas and may be accompanied by oedema of the surrounding tissue. The prognosis in well-differentiated oligodendrogliomas is favourable and patients may survive for many years. Those tumours which are accessible to surgery can be treated by excision, especially as a proportion of the tumours are well circumscribed and localised. Although of doubtful benefit, radiotherapy may be used together with steroids to treat oligodendrogliomas in surgically inaccessible sites.

Pathology

Macroscopically, oligodendrogliomas often appear as purple-brown, relatively well-circumscribed tumours with little necrosis. Poorly differentiated tumours, however, may resemble glioblastomas. The complications seen at post-mortem are usually due to the space-occupying nature of the tumour resulting in brain displacement with brain stem compression and haemorrhage.

Histology

Paraffin sections of oligodendrogliomas show some variation in structure. In well-differentiated tumours, the nuclei are uniform in size and round in shape. The classic 'box-like' appearance of the cells with a clear halo round the nucleus and a well-marked cell border may be seen but is probably an artefact due to poor fixation. When the tissue is well preserved, the cytoplasm has a moderate density and few cell processes can be seen (Fig. 7.14). The *vascular pattern* is often distinctive with thin-walled, highly branched vessels (Fig. 7.14) which are particularly characteristic in sections stained for

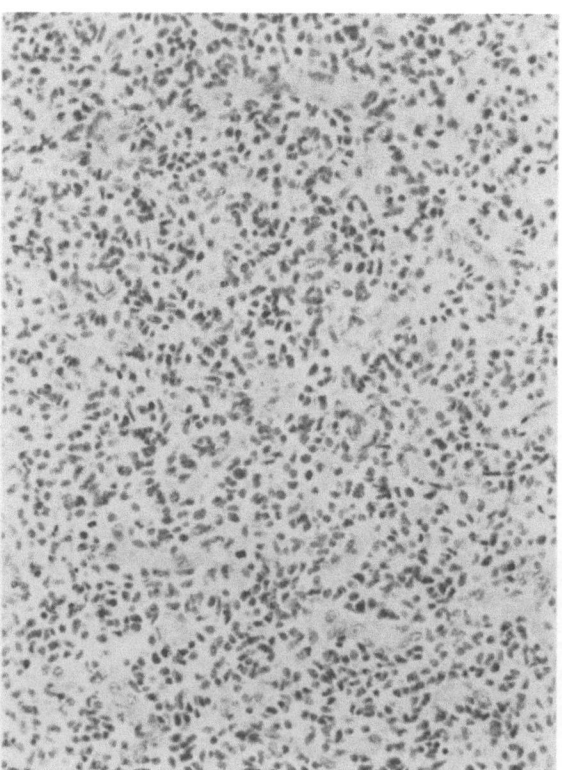

Fig. 7.14. Oligodendroglioma with numerous branched blood vessels. (H & E × 175)

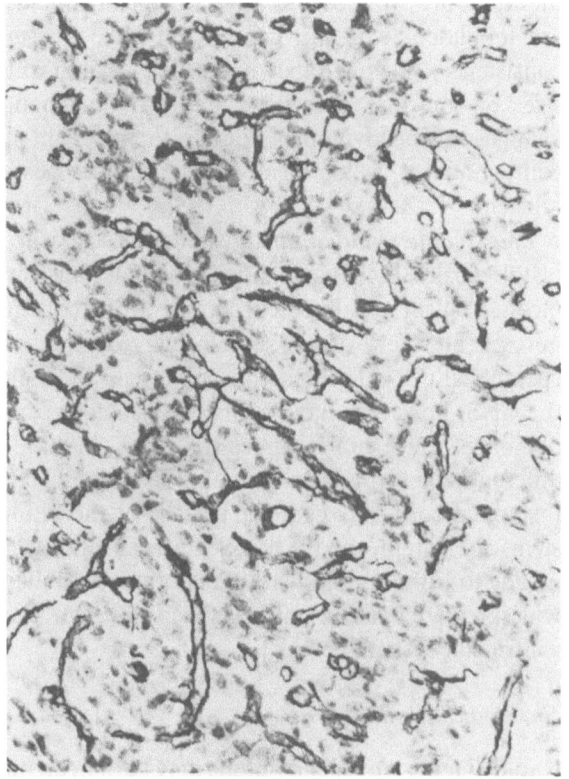

Fig. 7.15. Same oligodendroglioma as in Fig. 7.14, showing thin-walled branched blood vessels. (Reticulin stain × 175)

reticulin (Fig. 7.15). Some oligodendrogliomas are very well circumscribed histologically but the majority show a diffuse spread of tumour cells into the surrounding white matter and cortex. In many cases, the tumour oligodendrocytes accumulate in the surface layers of the cortex and may seed into the subarachnoid CSF. In the less well-differentiated oligodendrogliomas, there are moderate numbers of mitoses and increased variation in nuclear shape and size. Endothelial cells associated with the vessels may become plump and a diffuse endothelial proliferation may be seen; the complex capillary budding seen in glioblastomas is not usually present in pure oligodendrogliomas. Necrosis is rarely a feature of oligodendrogliomas except when they have become poorly differentiated or anaplastic and are, in effect, glioblastomas.

Pure oligodendrogliomas are comparatively rare, as a high proportion of oligodendrogliomas contain astrocytic tumour cells. It is possible that the astrocytic element in these tumours may also become anaplastic and the tumour progress to glioblastoma.

Surgical pathology

Rapid diagnosis of oligodendrogliomas from biopsy material can be made on smears or cryostat sections. Often the cells have a monomorphic appearance with small round nuclei and a small number of fine cytoplasmic processes. The long, thin, branched vessels seen in smears of oligodendrogliomas may be a clue to the origin and diagnosis of the tumour. Oligodendrocytes and oligodendrogliomas do not contain GFAP although they may exhibit oligodendrocyte surface markers such as galactocerebroside, especially in tissue culture. The presence of calcospherites may be useful in determining the origin of a tumour both in smears and in sections. Electron microscopically oligodendrogliomas may exhibit whorl-like structures resembling uncompacted myelin within their processes.

Oligodendrogliomas in tissue culture grow as small rounded cells with few processes.

Ependymomas

Clinical features

Ependymomas occur at all ages; they arise from the ventricular lining and may originate in the cerebral hemispheres or in the posterior fossa. Ependymomas commonly involve the spinal cord either primarily or through seeding in the CSF. They may present with raised intracranial pressure due to hydrocephalus from blockage of the ventricular system or with signs of brain stem or hemisphere invasion. If an ependymoma involves the spinal cord, the patient may complain of backache or symptoms referable to specific spinal roots. In some cases the cranial nerves may be involved. The tumour may be located on a CT scan or the presence of tumour within the spinal cord may be detected by myelography. Ependymoma cells free within the subarachnoid space or within the ventricles may be detected by examination of cytospin deposits from fresh CSF.

Treatment involves relief of hydrocephalus and surgical excision of ependymoma from the fourth ventricle or from cerebral ventricles, although the propensity of ependymoma to seed throughout the CSF means that local excision is usually ineffective. Irradiation of the neuraxis is the treatment of choice and the 5-year survival rate for ependymoma is 30%–40%.

Pathology

At post-mortem, friable, light-brown tissue may be found filling the ventricular system and coating the spinal cord. It often surrounds the spinal and cranial nerve roots. Ependymomas may also infiltrate the brain tissue and death may occur due to involvement of the brain stem or due to hydrocephalus.

Histology

Histologically *well-differentiated* ependymomas are composed of cells with regular round nuclei and a cell shape which sometimes resembles the square or cuboidal configuration of an ependymal cell. *Rosettes* may be seen within the tumour with cuboidal cells surrounding the central lumen. *Pseudo-rosettes* are rather more common (Fig. 7.16); the cells are arranged around blood vessels giving a characteristic pink fibrillary halo around vessels in an H & E section. Varying amounts of glial fibrillary material may be produced by the tumour cells and this is stainable by PTAH or Holtzer techniques. In *subependymomas*, there is a very large amount of glial fibrillary material and the cell nuclei are usually grouped in small islands within the tumour. Macroscopically, subependymomas are lobulated, white in colour and have a firm consistency. Although they may reach a significant size, or, on rare occasions, undergo malignant change, subependymomas may be found as small white nodules as an incidental finding at post-mortem.

Poorly differentiated ependymomas also occur; histologically they may show moderate nuclear pleomorphism and hyperchromasia with frequent mitoses and few of the cytological features of ependymal cells. Their method of spread through the CNS, however, may be characteristic of ependymomas but more aggressive than in well-differentiated forms. Such tumours spreading from the spinal cord may coat the surface of the brain stem, cerebellum, and the base of the brain and even invade to form nodules within the brain. A similar widespread extension may be seen through the ventricular system.

Surgical pathology

Rapid diagnosis of ependymoma may be difficult on a smear alone as the tumour may resemble an

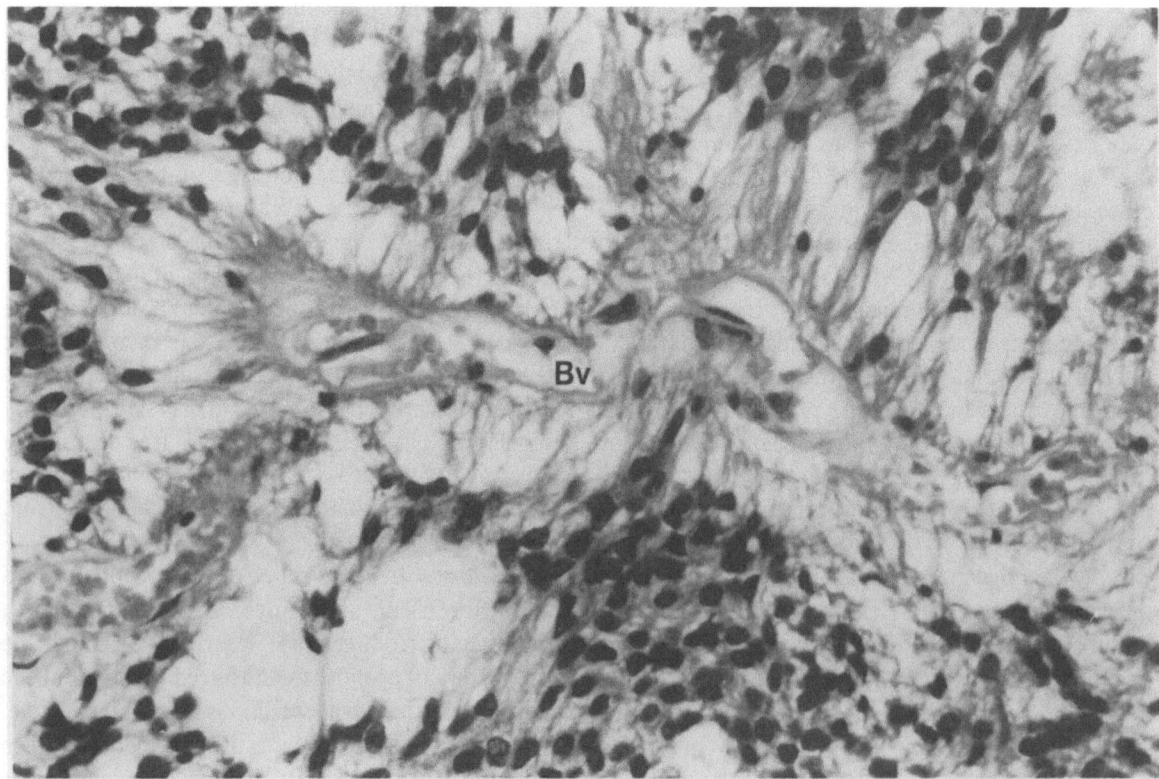

Fig. 7.16. Ependymoma. Tumour cells have formed a pseudo-rosette with long fibrillary processes extending to a blood vessel (*Bv*). (H & E × 460)

astrocytoma. Cryostat sections are often helpful as they may depict rosettes and pseudo-rosettes within the tumour tissue. The ependymal origin of the cells in the tumour may be confirmed in paraffin sections by the identification of blepharoplasts in PTAH stained sections (see Chap. 2, Fig. 2.12). These bodies are, in effect, the basal bodies of cilia; it is often easier to look for the cilia on the cells in electron microscope preparations when there is difficulty with the histological diagnosis.

Medulloblastomas

Clinical features

Medulloblastoma is one of the commonest tumours of childhood; it also occurs in adults, but less frequently. In children, these tumours arise almost exclusively in the vermis in the *midline of the cerebellum* in the posterior fossa; in adults they may occur more laterally in the cerebellar hemisphere. Clinically, medulloblastomas may present with cerebellar ataxia or brain stem signs of cranial nerve palsy or long tract signs due to invasion of the pons and medulla. Alternatively, hydrocephalus may be a presenting symptom due to occlusion of the fourth ventricle by tumour so that the child either presents with an enlarging head or with raised intracranial pressure. The tumour can be localised by CT scanning which may also show enlargement of the lateral ventricles; confirmation of the nature of the tumour may require a posterior fossa craniectomy but medulloblastoma cells may also be found in lumbar CSF. Complete surgical removal of the tumour from the posterior fossa is usually not possible as it infiltrates the cerebellum and brain stem. Furthermore, medulloblastoma seeds readily throughout the CSF so that adequate treatment entails surgical removal of the bulk of the tumour from the posterior fossa and x-irradiation to the posterior fossa and the spinal cord. Surgery and radiotherapy have given a 5-year survival rate of 40% but there may be recurrence of the tumour even after 5 years.

Pathology

Medulloblastoma may spread from the posterior fossa in the CSF to coat the brain and cord with a soft, opalescent, gelatinous tissue reminiscent of sugar icing in appearance. In addition, the tumour invades the surface of the brain from the sub-arachnoid space.

Histology

Medulloblastomas are composed of small cells with densely staining ovoid nuclei and little cytoplasm drawn out into the few fine fibrillary processes. Mitotic figures are common and there may be rosette formation in which the nuclei are arranged in a circle with their fibrillary processes extending into the centre. Very occasionally other elements resembling oligodendroglial cells or striated and smooth muscle cells may be seen within the tumour. The pattern of invasion of medulloblastoma is usually quite characteristic; in sections of the cerebellum groups and nodules of tumour cells extend into the cerebellar tissue from the surface (Fig. 7.17). When the tumour has invaded the subarachnoid space, there may be proliferation of connective tissue, and in some tumours, the *desmoplastic* variety, the tissue is firm and contains an extensive connective tissue component.

The resemblance between medulloblastoma cells and the germinal external granular layer of the cerebellum, present in the first year of life (see Chap. 11), suggests that medulloblastomas are derived from immature neuronal elements.

Surgical pathology

Smear preparations used in the rapid diagnosis of medulloblastomas give a characteristically uniform smear with a monomorphic cellular pattern consisting of small cells with densely staining nuclei; mitoses may be seen in the smears. Cryostat sections are useful for examination of the tough desmoplastic variety of medulloblastoma and in identifying the characteristic pattern of invasion into the cerebellum.

Neuronal tumours other than medulloblastomas do occasionally occur in the cerebral hemispheres. These are chiefly neuroblastomas, poorly differentiated neuronal tumours, or the more mature ganglioneuromas. Mixed gangliogliomas consisting of neurons and astrocytic cells also occasionally occur in the cerebral hemispheres.

Choroid plexus papillomas

Clinical features

Papillomas of the choroid plexus are uncommon tumours which occur in the lateral, third and fourth ventricles, usually in adults. They frequently present with headache, papilloedema and hydrocephalus

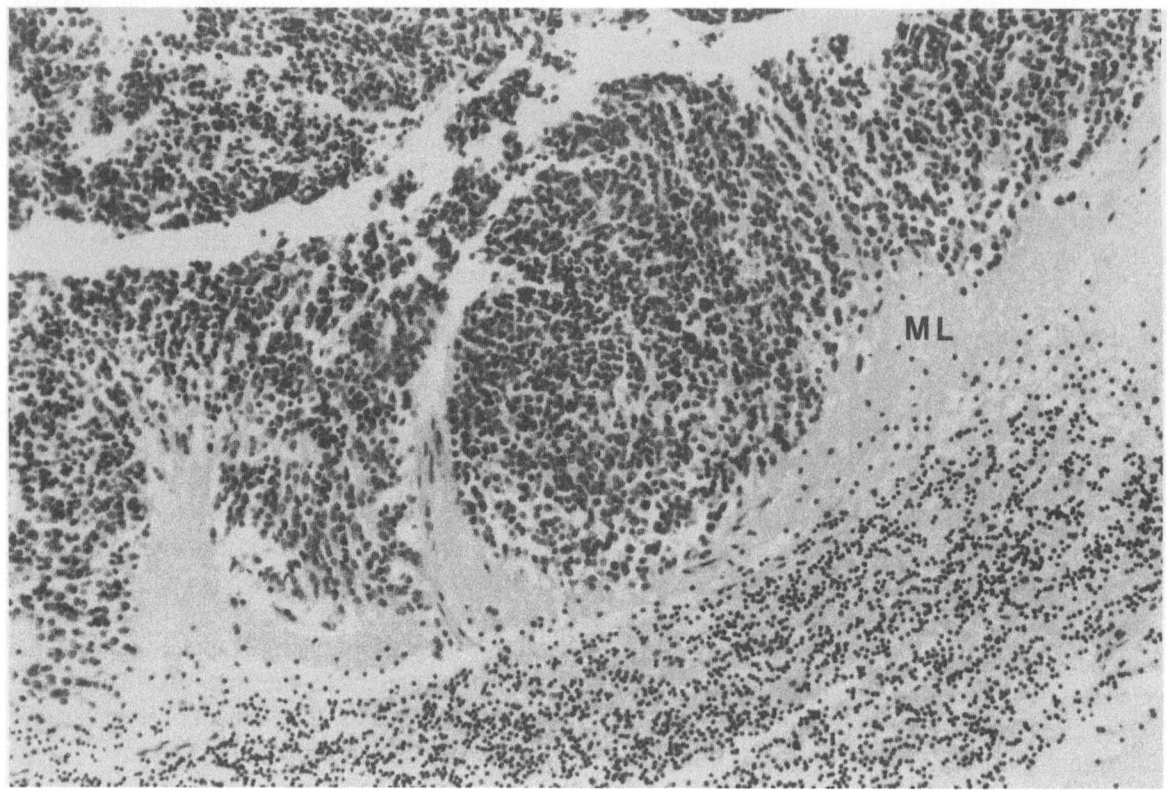

Fig. 7.17. Medulloblastoma. Tumour cells have invaded the molecular layer (*ML*) of the cerebellum. (H & E ×210)

due to blockage of the CSF drainage pathways from the ventricles. Occasionally the hydrocephalus is thought to be due to over-secretion of the CSF. CT scans reveal a highly enhancing lesion in the ventricles; air encephalography or cerebral angiography may also be used to demonstrate choroid plexus papillomas. Complete surgical excision of the tumour often leads to a cure but, in some cases, the tumour is too large to remove, or it fragments and may seed within the ventricular system. Treatment of the hydrocephalus by shunting may also be necessary.

Pathology and surgical histology

Cysts and nodules of calcification or small calco-spherites are not uncommon in the choroid plexus, which itself has a fine papillomatous surface appearance. On macroscopic inspection, choroid plexus tumours are papillomatous enlargements of the choroid plexus. Histologically they reveal a vascular stroma covered by cuboidal or columnar cells which are often larger than the low cuboidal cells of the normal choroid plexus. In some cases,

the epithelium of the papilloma shows nuclear pleomorphism and irregularity of cell shape; malignant forms of choroid plexus papilloma occur and may spread throughout the CSF.

Confusion may occur between choroid plexus papillomas and well-differentiated adenocarcinomas, particularly from the lung. The connection of the papilloma with the choroid plexus and the exclusion of a primary carcinoma may facilitate the correct diagnosis.

Choroid plexus papillomas are usually recognised at surgery by their site and papillomatous appearance. However, histological confirmation may be obtained by recognising the papillomatous character of the tumour in smears and cryostat sections.

Colloid cysts of the third ventricle

Although colloid cysts usually present in adults, they are probably maldevelopmental in origin. They develop as thin-walled cysts filled with proteinaceous fluid and lined on the inner aspect by low cuboidal or columnar epithelium which resembles ependyma; in many cases the epithelium is ciliated. Colloid cysts develop at the anterior end of the third ventricle near the foramina of Monro, and thus usually present with signs of raised intracranial pressure and hydrocephalus which may be intermittent. The presence of a cyst can be detected by CT scanning, where it enhances strongly, or by air encephalography, where it deforms the ventricular outline. Surgical excision of a colloid cyst usually cures the patient, but if the cyst remains undiagnosed, the patient may die with acute hydrocephalus. In some cases the cyst may be large and have a thick fibrous wall containing blood pigment and cholesterol clefts, suggesting recurrent haemorrhage. Absence of an intact epithelial lining in the cyst may make a firm diagnosis of colloid cyst difficult.

Tumours of nerve sheath cells

Benign tumours of nerve sheaths are divided into two major groups, schwannomas and neurofibromas. *Malignant tumours of nerve sheath* are uncommon and are either malignant schwannomas, malignant neurofibromas associated with von Recklinghausen's disease, or fibrosarcomas of nerve sheath. The significance of the difference between schwannomas and neurofibromas is often not fully appreciated. Schwannomas are tumours of Schwann cells which are usually solitary, seldom recur following complete surgical removal and very rarely undergo malignant change. Neurofibromas, on the other hand, are tumours composed of Schwann cells and other cellular elements; they are frequently multiple and regrowth and malignant change may occur.

Schwannomas

Schwannomas are benign tumours of Schwann cells, which are the myelin-forming satellite cells surrounding axons in peripheral nerves. A number of synonyms exist for schwannomas, e.g. neurilemmoma (from neurilemma, an outdated term for Schwann cell and other structures that ensheath individual axons) and neurinoma (tumour of nerve). Acoustic neuroma is a schwannoma (of the eighth cranial nerve) but use of the term neuroma is otherwise usually reserved for non-neoplastic swellings of nerve, e.g. amputation neuroma (Weller and Cervós-Navarro, 1977).

Although schwannomas may occur at any age, they most commonly present in adults and are more frequently found in females than in males. Schwannomas occur in every part of the peripheral nervous system but are most commonly found on the sensory cranial nerves and the sensory posterior spinal roots. The acoustic nerve is the site of origin of more than 60% of all schwannomas, although they may also occur on the fifth nerve. Schwannomas may reach a considerable size in the abdomen or posterior mediastinum, where it may be difficult to detect the nerve of origin.

Clinical features

Clinically, schwannomas arising on the *eighth nerve* (acoustic neuromas) present with deafness and tinnitus although vestibular signs and symptoms may also occur. When they are large, 3–4 cm in diameter, acoustic neuromas may be associated with hydrocephalus probably due to displacement of the brain stem and interference with CSF flow. Such an occurrence is marked by the onset of raised intracranial pressure and unless the hydrocephalus is treated, the patient may die. The presence of an acoustic schwannoma may be suspected on skull x-ray and confirmed by tomography of the internal auditory meatus because the tumour usually causes enlargement of the internal auditory meatus by eroding bone. Strong enhancement of acoustic schwannomas is seen on CT scans, in which the tumour can be observed in the cerebellopontine angle, its size estimated and any consequent hydrocephalus assessed.

Schwannomas arising from *spinal nerve roots* may present with pain radiating along the course of the nerve. Symptoms may also be caused by compression of motor roots with lower motor neuron weakness at the segmental level of the tumour. Spasticity at lower levels may also be present due to spinal cord compression. Tumours on nerve trunks may cause problems from compression of the involved nerve; tumours elsewhere may cause problems due to their mass effect.

Treatment of schwannomas is by surgical excision and the tumour rarely recurs. The nerve from which a schwannoma arises, however, may be damaged during the operation as the nerve fibres may be stretched over the surface of the schwannoma capsule and be macroscopically unidentifiable at surgery. The nearby facial nerve may also be damaged during surgical excision of acoustic schwannomas.

Pathology

Macroscopically, schwannomas usually have a smooth encapsulated surface; their attachment to a specific nerve may or may not be apparent and in some cases those arising from nerve roots have a dumb-bell shape as they have grown on each side of an intravertebral foramen.

Histology

Although schwannomas show some variation in their microscopical structure, *two* main histological patterns are usually seen intermingled within each tumour. Sheets of spindle cells with elongated nuclei form the *Antoni type A* areas; frequently the parallel nuclei are ranged in rows producing palisading. Electron microscopically, the Antoni type A areas are composed of Schwann cells with prominent basement membranes; the edges of the cells can be delineated in the light microscope by staining the basement membrane with reticulin techniques. *Antoni type B* areas are more loosely packed regions of the tumour composed of cells with small nuclei and spaces between the cells. Elements other than Schwann cells, e.g. mast cells, are usually present within the Antoni type B areas but not in the Antoni type A region. In large schwannomas, particularly those arising from the acoustic nerve, there may be areas of fibrosis which are probably due to past infarction within the tumour. Tumour cell nuclei may show some pleomorphism and hyperchromasia but the absence of mitoses in these tumours is usually sufficient to exclude any suggestion of malignancy. Nerve fibres may be seen within the capsule of schwannomas but are not usually seen within the tumour itself.

Surgical pathology

Rapid histological diagnosis is usually required only when there is some doubt about the exact identity of a cerebellopontine angle tumour at surgery. In these cases schwannomas can be differentiated from gliomas, meningiomas, and haemangioblastomas on cryostat section by the spindle-shaped nature of the cells with their closely applied reticulin sheaths, and by the absence of the whorl-like structures seen in meningiomas. Smears are usually not possible as schwannomas are generally very tough.

Neurofibromas

Clinical features

Neurofibromas may not develop fully until adult life although they may be found at any age. They occur at many sites throughout the body but are typically found on skin, along deep nerves and associated with gut or retroperitoneal tissue. Clinically, neurofibromas may present as a mass or due to their interference with neural function.

Pathology

Single neurofibromas appear to be uncommon; most are multiple and may, in many cases, be related to von Recklinghausen's phakomatosis (multiple neurofibromatosis) (see Chap. 11). In the skin, neurofibromas may be multiple, pedunculated, soft rubbery nodules, but when they occur in association with major nerves, they may have a plexiform appearance where the nerve enters and becomes enmeshed within a poorly encapsulated mass of neurofibroma. Such a lack of ill-defined capsule is typical of neurofibroma and helps distinguish it from a schwannoma. Occasionally, aggressive neurofibromas may erode bone or may undergo *malignant* change.

Surgical histology

Histologically, neurofibromas are an ill-defined mixture of cells and neural tissue. Nerve fibres, often retaining their myelin sheaths, traverse the tangled mass of Schwann cells, fibroblasts and other connective tissue elements such as mast cells. Rarely are there well-defined areas of Antoni type A tissue in neurofibromas.

Other tumours may be associated with von Recklinghausen's disease such as gliomas, meningiomas, and especially bilateral acoustic schwannomas. There may be an associated overgrowth of the soft tissue surrounding nerves that are enlarged by neurofibromas; in severe forms, the skin and soft tissue in the involved areas hangs in thick, loose folds (elephantiasis nervosa). Occasionally there is localised hypertrophy of a finger or appendix in patients with neurofibromatosis.

Meningiomas

Meningiomas may present at any age but they are

more commonly seen in the older age groups, particularly in women. The tumours probably arise from arachnoid cells and are mostly attached to the dura from which they extend into the subdural space. Meningiomas are most commonly seen attached to the dura on the base of the skull or on the inner side of the calvarium; they also occur in the spinal canal and less frequently within the cerebral ventricles or even within the cerebral tissue itself. Occasionally, meningiomas are found in the orbit.

Clinical features

The clinical presentation depends upon the site of the tumour and its rapidity of growth. Large tumours frequently present as space-occupying lesions with raised intracranial pressure and may be confused clinically with gliomas. Others may present with compression of the optic nerve or with cranial nerve or spinal cord compression. Examination of the patient may reveal an *exostosis* on the outer aspect of the skull over the site of a calvarial meningioma; such an exostosis may have been present for many years. Skull x-rays may show destruction or thickening of adjacent bone, calcification within the tumour, or shift of the pineal, and angiography will often demonstrate the highly vascular nature of many meningiomas. A Technetium[99] isotope scan is always abnormal unless the tumour is very small or located in the masked areas at the base of the skull or posterior fossa. An enhanced CT scan will show the position of a meningioma as the tumour lacks the blood–brain barrier of normal neural tissue and thus allows entry of radio-opaque contrast medium. The tumour thus has a typical radiological appearance, often allowing the diagnosis to be established with reasonable certainty before biopsy or removal is attempted.

A *spinal* meningioma may be suspected when erosion of the vertebral pedicles is seen on plain radiographs; the tumour may be further delineated by myelography.

Treatment of meningiomas is by surgical excision but this may be difficult if the tumour is large or inaccessible. Further complication may occur if the tumour arises from the falx cerebri when removal may endanger the superior sagittal sinus and thus jeopardise cerebral venous drainage. Recurrence

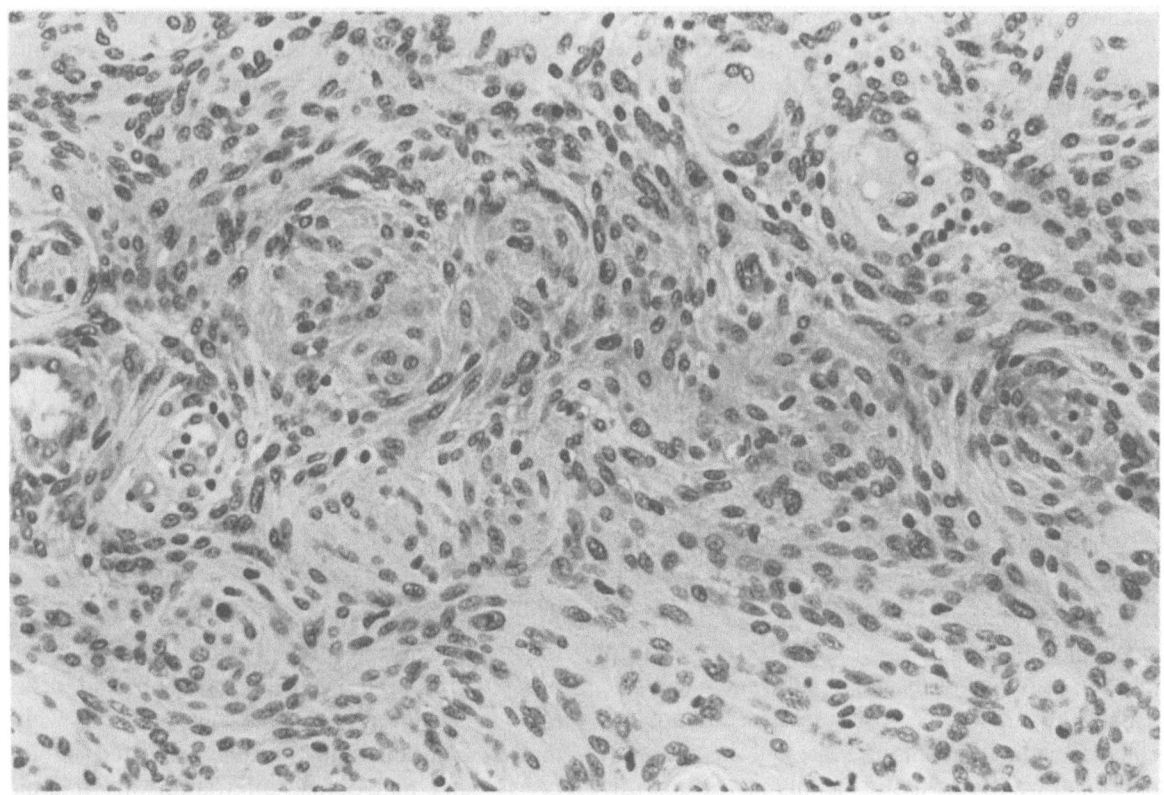

Fig. 7.18. Meningioma showing meningotheliomatous pattern with some whorl formation. (H & E × 270)

may follow a difficult or incomplete excision due to regrowth of residual tumour tissue. Elderly patients with little clinical deficit may be best served by leaving the tumour in place.

The effects of meningiomas upon the adjacent brain tissue vary. In many cases, the tumour is easily separated from underlying compressed and atrophic brain but other tumours are very adherent to the underlying neural tissue and may be associated with extensive oedema of the underlying brain. Complications, therefore, occur due to the mass effect of the tumour and any accompanying oedema.

Histopathology

Microscopically, there is a wide variation in histological pattern within meningiomas. In general, the cells have nuclei which are uniform in size and often have one or two small nucleoli and pale centres. Sheets of cells with indistinct cytoplasmic margins may be seen in the *meningotheliomatous* type where cellular whorls are often poorly formed (Fig. 7.18). Spindle-shaped cells are a feature of the *transitional* and *fibroblastic* types of meningioma where whorls are often more prominent. Small calcospherites or *psammoma bodies* may be seen in meningiomas especially in spinal tumours. Less common types of meningioma include the *angioblastic* variety where there may be little resemblance between the stromal cells and other meningioma cells and the major feature is the plethora of thin-walled blood vessels; some of these tumours resemble haemangiopericytomas seen elsewhere in the body.

Malignant meningiomas are uncommon but in some cases poorly differentiated meningiomas actively invade adjacent brain tissue. *Fibrosarcomas* and *malignant fibrous histiocytomas* also arise from the meninges and metastasize to organs other than the brain.

Surgical pathology

Rapid diagnosis of meningiomas may be an important way of distinguishing between an operable meningioma and an inoperable glioma. In many cases, the meningioma tissue is too tough to smear and the histology of meningioma in these cases is usually apparent in cryostat sections. Bands of collagen within the tumour tissue and the presence of cellular whorls are useful identifying features for meningioma. Some tumours are very soft and smear

easily; in these cases the uniformity of the oval, pale nuclei with their elongated fibrillary cytoplasm are helpful features in distinguishing the tumour from a glioma. The presence of meningioma whorls can also be seen in smears and the abundance of mast cells in some tumours may be a useful pointer.

Meningioma whorls even form in cultures of some tumours, but mostly the cells are elongated and can be distinguished from glial cells on their nuclear and cytoplasmic morphology. Electron microscopy reveals complex interdigitation of cellular processes in many meningiomas and the presence of desmosomes and intracellular fibrils; these features, however, are inconstant and are not found in every type of meningioma.

Primary malignant lymphomas of the brain

Clinical features

Primary brain lymphomas usually present in adults and involve the deep structures of the cerebral hemispheres. Often, the clinical history and presentation are similar to that of a glioblastoma. Other cases present with diffuse tumour and progressive dementia. The introduction of organ transplantation and long-term treatment of lymphomas, especially Hodgkin's disease, with chemotherapeutic and immunosuppressive agents has been accompanied by an associated rise in the incidence of primary lymphomas in the brain although the exact mechanism is not clear.

The diagnosis may be suspected from the history and CT scans may occasionally reveal a localised mass; more commonly the tumour is diffuse and involves particularly the periventricular white matter. Confirmation of the diagnosis is made on biopsy and the tumour is treated by radiotherapy. However, the patient usually dies with cerebral oedema and the spread of the lymphoma throughout the brain.

Histopathology

Macroscopically it may be difficult to define exactly the region involved by the primary lymphoma but often the affected hemisphere is soft and oedematous. Histologically, the subependymal white matter is usually most heavily involved by the perivascular and diffuse infiltration of lymphoid cells which show some nuclear pleomorphism and sometimes giant cell formation. There is often an accompanying proliferation of microglial cells whose identification within the lymphoma by early workers in the field led to the categorisation of this tumour as a *microglioma*. Recent immunoperoxidase studies suggest, however, that at least some of the tumours are B-cell lymphomas although others may be of histiocytic origin. Despite their presentation with mainly cerebral symptoms, primary brain lymphomas are often widespread throughout the cerebellum and brain stem.

Surgical pathology

Rapid diagnosis of lymphomas from brain biopsy may be made on a smear where large numbers of lymphoid cells may be seen diffusely infiltrating brain tissue and accumulating around blood vessels. In cryostat sections, the proliferation of reticulin around the blood vessels in association with perivascular lymphoma accumulation, together with the diffuse spread of the lymphoma cells throughout the surrounding brain tissue, may be sufficient to establish the diagnosis. Perivascular reticulin proliferation also occurs in inflammatory lesions whenever there is accumulation of inflammatory cells around the vessels, and diffuse invasion of brain by non-neural tumour cells usually only occurs in primary cerebral lymphomas, occasionally with metastatic malignant melanomas and rarely with metastatic carcinoma.

Tumours and malformations of blood vessel origin

Haemangioblastomas ·

These tumours are usually found in adults and occur most commonly in the cerebellum, either in the midline or in one hemisphere. They may, however, occur at the lower border of the medulla or in association with the spinal cord, usually arising from the pial surface. Some are found in the filum terminale at the lower end of the cord. Haemangioblastomas are very rare in the supratentorial region. Although usually single, haemangioblastomas may be multiple and may be associated with the von Hippel–Lindau syndrome. Often familial, this syndrome may have one or more forms of expression which include haemangioblastomas of the retina, cerebellum and spinal cord together with a high incidence of renal carcinoma.

Clinical features

Patients with haemangioblastomas may present with cerebellar ataxia and nystagmus or they may develop raised intracranial pressure with vomiting, headache, papilloedema and alteration in their level of consciousness. A proportion of the patients with this tumour have polycythaemia which usually resolves following removal of the haemangioblastoma. Spinal tumours present with root or cord compression.

Pre-operative localisation and diagnosis of haemangioblastomas in the cerebellum may be made on vertebral angiograms, which demonstrate the high vascularity of the tumours. Haemangioblastomas enhance on CT scans, which may also show an associated cyst within the cerebellum. *Treatment* is by surgical excision and complete removal offers a good prognosis.

Pathology

Macroscopically, haemangioblastomas often grow as a mural nodule within a cerebellar cyst. Haemorrhage from the tumour may give the gliotic wall of the cyst a rusty appearance but usually the majority of the cyst wall is free of tumour. A characteristic yellow or brown fleshy appearance is seen when the tumour is cut across.

Histology

Haemangioblastomas are composed of a myriad of thin-walled blood vessels with interposed packets of foamy, lipid-containing cells with small round nuclei. Reticulin stains outline the blood vessels and show the fine packing of the stromal cells. The margins of the tumour are usually poorly defined and fade gradually into the surrounding gliotic cerebellar tissue. The origin of the stromal cells is difficult to establish; they may be derived from meningeal cells or possibly from vascular elements but they do not exhibit the *factor VIII-related antigen* marker of normal endothelial cells when stained for this protein by immunoperoxidase. Electron microscopy has not elucidated the origin of the stromal cells.

Surgical pathology

Rapid diagnosis of the tumour is most satisfactorily made when cryostat sections of the yellow-brown, fleshy tumour tissue are stained by H&E and Oil-red-O to demonstrate the lipid-rich stromal cells. Reticulin stains are useful for demonstrating the thin-walled vessels and packaging of the stromal cells.

Capillary telangiectases

These lesions consist of collections of dilated capillaries which are usually seen as incidental findings at post-mortem. They are most commonly found in the pons, the cerebral cortex, or in the subcortical white matter where they may resemble petechial haemorrhages on gross inspection. If a large area of the pons is involved, the patient may develop slowly progressive long tract signs and cranial nerve palsies. Occasionally there is fatal haemorrhage associated with such a lesion. *Histologically*, capillary telangiectases are seen as groups of thin-walled capillary vessels separated by normal brain tissue. There is rarely evidence of haemorrhage or gliosis.

Cavernous angiomas

As vascular malformations rather than true tumours, cavernous angiomas consist of closely packed, thin-walled vascular spaces with no intervening brain tissue. *Clinically*, the patient may present with focal epilepsy, or hydrocephalus if the malformation is in the ventricles, or with subarachnoid haemorrhage. In one-third of cases cavernous angiomas are multiple. They are most commonly seen in the cerebral hemispheres but also occur in the pons, spinal cord, and cerebellum. Although they enhance on CT scan, they may not be visible on angiography.

Where possible, the lesions are excised surgically if they are producing neurological signs and symptoms. Cavernous angiomas may vary in size from a few millimetres to several centimetres in diameter and appear grossly as a mass of small vascular channels. *Histologically* the dilated abnormal vessels are crowded together and not separated by brain tissue.

Arteriovenous malformations (see Chap. 5)

Structurally, arteriovenous malformations are an intimate admixture of arteries and veins which occur more frequently in males than females. They may present at birth as large malformations associated with gross brain destruction and sometimes with cardiac failure. More commonly, arterio-

venous malformations present during the second decade with focal neurological signs, with epilepsy, or with the signs of a subarachnoid haemorrhage. The cerebral hemispheres are a common site of origin especially in the region of supply of the middle cerebral artery, where the malformations may involve the leptomeninges or be located deep within the hemisphere. In a proportion of cases, A–V malformations are associated with berry aneurysms in other parts of the cerebral circulation. Repeated bleeds from a vascular malformation may occur with increasing destruction of the surrounding neural tissue; in some cases fatal haemorrhage may ensue.

The exact extent and the course of the vessels supplying the malformation may be determined by cerebral angiography. Depending upon the site, the malformations may be accessible to surgical excision.

When viewed *microscopically*, arteriovenous malformations are seen as a tangle of vessels, of which a proportion exhibit the histological features of arteries with a well-formed media and internal elastic lamina. Some vessels resemble veins, but many of the dilated vascular spaces are surrounded only by a fibrous wall. Evidence of previous haemorrhage is often seen around the lesion with gliosis of the surrounding brain. In cases where there is a cerebral or cerebellar haemorrhage at an odd site or at an inappropriate age, an arteriovenous malformation may be found in association with the haemorrhage, that is, if the malformation is not itself destroyed by the bleed.

Arteriovenous malformations also occur in the spinal meninges and may be associated with gross dilation of spinal cord veins and damage to the cord.

Tumours of the pituitary

Pituitary tumours are discussed in Chap. 8.

Tumours of the pineal

The pineal gland, or epiphysis, develops from the dorsal region of the forebrain. It is an uncommon site for tumours but four main types do occur. *Teratomas*, including germinomas, are almost completely restricted to males and usually occur under the age of 20 years. Histologically, they present a wide range of appearances reflecting the potential of the constituent cells.

Pinealomas are less common and arise from pineal parenchymal cells. *Glial* tumours also may arise from the pineal and are sometimes cystic. *Dermoid cysts* may also be found in the region of the pineal.

Metastatic intracranial tumours

Clinical features

The true incidence of metastatic tumour involvement of the CNS is difficult to obtain as the clinical signs of cerebral metastases, or their presence at post-mortem, may be overshadowed by complications at the site of primary tumour growth. Metastatic disease in the brain usually occurs in older patients in line with the occurrence of most tumours. No site is necessarily exempt but the cerebral hemispheres and cerebellum are both commonly the sites of metastatic carcinoma. Patients may present clinically with raised intracranial pressure due to the mass of metastasis and the accompanying oedema. Alternatively, epilepsy or focal neurological signs may be the presenting features. Technetium^{99m} isotope scans or CT scans may

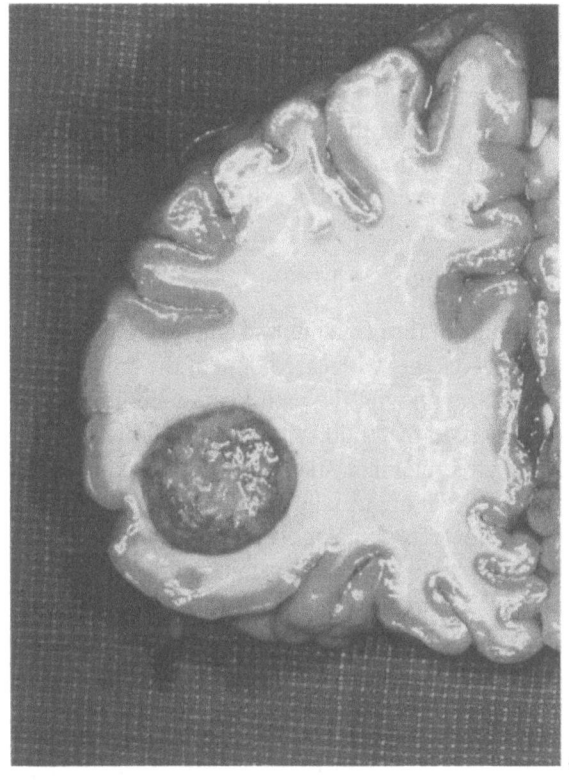

a

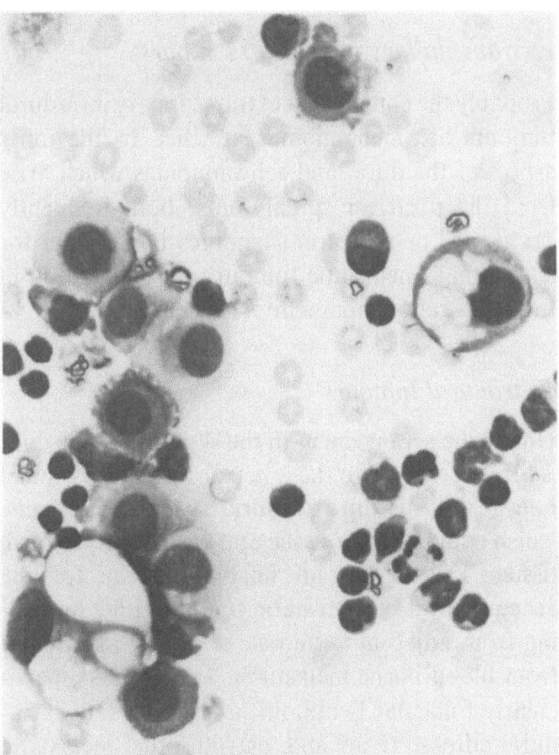

Fig. 7.19. Metastatic carcinoma cells in the CSF of a patient with carcinomatous meningitis. Vacuolated cells contain mucus. Cytospin preparation stained with Diffquick. (× 580)

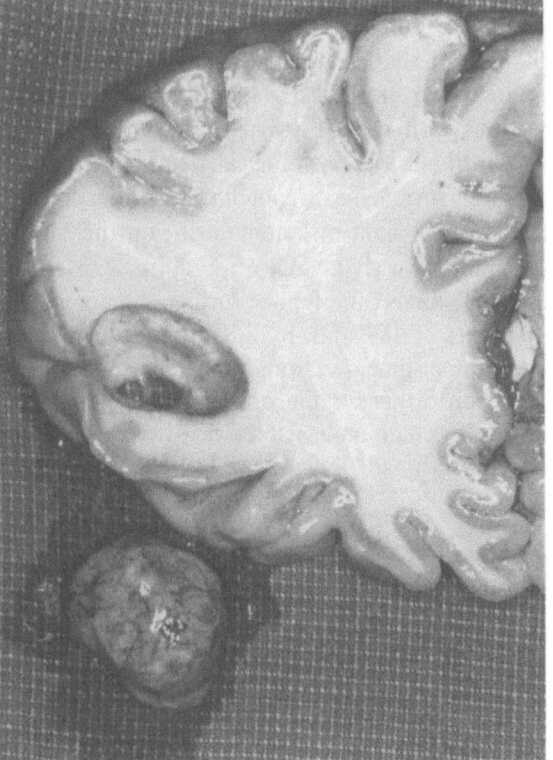

b

Fig. 7.20a Coronal slice of unfixed brain showing a single well-circumscribed metastasis.
b Handling the brain slice has caused the metastasis to fall out, revealing a smooth plane of separation.

reveal multiple spherical enhancing lesions surrounded by oedema. Isolated cerebral or cerebellar metastases may be treated by surgical excision, particularly as the lesions often shell out from the surrounding brain tissue; the ultimate prognosis may depend upon the complications arising from the primary tumour, or from metastases elsewhere in the body.

Histopathology

Carcinoma of the bronchus and adenocarcinoma of the lung, together with carcinoma of the breast and kidney are among the commonest tumours to metastasise to the brain. Malignant melanoma also has a high rate of metastasis to the brain, where the secondary foci are usually multiple and may cause fatal intracerebral haemorrhage. In addition to *localised focal metastases*, carcinomas and malignant melanoma may spread diffusely within the subarachnoid space (*carcinomatous meningitis*), invade nerve roots and may present with cranial nerve palsies. Histological diagnosis may be achieved by examination of a centrifuged (cytospin) deposit from fresh CSF (Fig. 7.19). Leukaemias also frequently involve the meninges of the CNS.

The gross appearance of a cerebral metastasis is usually very different from that of a glioma. Often spherical in shape, most metastases are sharply demarcated from the surrounding brain and may shell out with ease (Fig. 7.20). A similar sharp demarcation is seen histologically since carcinoma cells rarely invade the surrounding brain in a diffuse manner. Malignant melanoma cells, on the other hand, may diffusely involve cerebral tissue. Metastatic carcinomas can often be further characterised by mucus stains and by identifying organoid patterns. On some occasions it may be necessary to suggest an origin for the primary tumour, which may itself remain undetected even after presenting as a metastasis.

Surgical pathology

Rapid histological diagnosis of metastatic tumour may be made on smears from a burr-hole biopsy or from tissue taken at craniotomy. Groups of epithelial cells or cells with a morphology very different from that of glial cells may be readily identified among the fibrillary glial tissue of the surrounding brain. Cryostat sections stained with PAS for mucus are often helpful in characterising the origin of the metastasis.

Spinal tumours

Although gliomas (astrocytoma and ependymoma) of the spinal cord and cauda equina lipomas associated with spina bifida occur in children, the majority of tumours in the spinal column present in adults. It is difficult to obtain exact figures of their incidence, but in neurological and neuropathological practice, tumours affecting the spinal cord are much less common than those affecting the brain. Tumours in the spine can be broadly classified according to their relationship to the spinal cord.

Classification

Intramedullary tumours

Tumours which arise and expand within the spinal cord itself are usually gliomas. Well-differentiated astrocytomas and ependymomas present in children but ependymomas also occur in adults as do the less common glioblastomas. Cavernous angiomas or arteriovenous malformations may also be found in the spinal cord and metastatic tumours occasionally occur in this site.

Extramedullary intradural tumours

Probably the commonest extramedullary intradural tumours are meningiomas attached to the inner aspect of the dura, and schwannomas which arise from the posterior spinal roots; both frequently cause cord or nerve root compression. Except for leukaemias, metastatic tumours are uncommon in the subdural or subarachnoid space.

Extradural tumours

Unlike the arrangement in the skull where the dura is firmly attached to the inner surface of the cranial bones, there is an extradural space in the spine which contains fatty tissue and vascular connective tissue. This is not an uncommon site for the accumulation of metastatic tumour either spreading from adjacent vertebrae or arising apparently from blood-borne metastases. Lymphomas, particularly follicular lymphomas, also infiltrate extradural adipose tissue and, as with other metastatic tumours, they may form a space-occupying mass which results in spinal cord compression (see Chap. 6).

Tumours of the vertebrae

Metastatic tumours, commonly from lung, breast, thryoid and prostate, are more frequently found in the vertebral column than are primary tumours of bone. Hodgkin's disease and myeloma may also involve the vertebrae. Primary tumours of the vertebrae include cavernous haemangiomas, osteoblastoma, giant cell tumour of bone, and chordoma; the latter usually arises in the sacral region or in the clivus of the skull. The main effects of vertebral tumours are due either to expansion of the tumour tissue into the spinal canal causing cord compression, or to collapse of the affected vertebrae with subsequent damage to the spinal cord or to nerve roots.

Clinical presentation, investigation and treatment

Neurological disability due to tumours affecting the spinal cord arises either from direct pressure on the cord, which may damage long tracts, or from compression of veins causing congestion and oedema of the cord below or above the lesion. Damage to the arterial supply of the cord may result in spinal cord infarction. The exact clinical picture depends upon the site and the rate of progression of the lesion involving the cord. In general, slow compression of the cord results in spastic weakness of the limbs below the lesion due to involvement of the corticospinal tracts, followed by sensory loss as evidence of posterior column damage. Lastly the spinothalamic tracts, which carry pain and temperature sensation, may be affected. Sphincter disturbances and urinary problems usually occur at a late stage but are a particularly prominent early feature in cauda equina and conus medullaris tumours. Involvement of anterior roots produces local segmental weakness and muscle wasting with fasciculation, whereas posterior root compression often presents with a burning sensation and soreness of the skin aggravated by coughing and referable to the area supplied by that root. Backache is often an early symptom of involvement of the cord and roots by tumour.

X-rays of the spinal column may reveal collapse or bony erosion due to metastatic tumour or characteristic changes due to primary bone tumours. Bony erosion from the presence of a long-standing schwannoma or meningioma may be seen radiographically. Myelography may outline expanded regions of the spinal cord involved by intra-medullary tumour or identify levels at which the cord is compressed by extramedullary tumour tissue. If there is a block in CSF flow within the spinal column, the CSF below the lesion is usually xanthochromic and has a raised protein level.

Whole body CT scans produce clear, horizontal or transverse sectional views of the spinal cord, surrounding spaces and vertebral bodies, and may give a clear indication of the nature of the spinal cord compression.

Treatment of spinal cord lesions resulting from tumours depends upon decompression of the spinal canal either by laminectomy or by removal of benign tumours such as meningiomas and schwannomas. Acute compression can often be relieved by the removal of extradural masses of metastatic tumour. Compression by radiosensitive tumours such as myeloma may be relieved more effectively by radiotherapy than by laminectomy, perhaps because the blood supply to the ischaemic cord is less traumatised in the process. A diagnosis of myeloma may occasionally be accepted without recourse to biopsy if an M-band globulin is present in the blood, Bence-Jones protein is found in the urine, and there is radiological evidence of cord compression by a lesion having the characteristic appearances of myeloma. In these circumstances the decision to biopsy may depend upon whether compression is occurring sufficiently slowly for a trial of radiotherapy to be safe. The long-term prognosis is often good in benign tumours but poor when malignant neoplasms are involved, especially as the rapidity with which the cord has been compressed has a profound effect upon the outcome of decompression. In general, the faster the compression the worse the prognosis. Once all motor and sensory function below the lesion has been lost, even for as short a time as half-an-hour, useful function is unlikely to be restored by surgical decompression. Any recovery of neurological function that occurs following decompression is probably due to the resolution of oedema, as effective regeneration of axons within the cord does not occur.

Pathology

The approximate incidence of different types of tumour involving the spinal cord is shown in Table 7.1, p. 106. Well-differentiated *astrocytomas* and *ependymomas* appear grossly as featureless expansions of the cord with or without extension into the subarachnoid space. *Glioblastoma*, on the other hand, may be recognisable within the cord as an area of necrosis and tumour tissue which can be distinguished from surrounding normal cord; *metastases* can be similarly recognised. The histology of these lesions resembles that of metastases in the brain.

Meningiomas are usually attached to the dura or arachnoid within the spinal subdural space. They are usually lobulated and often gritty due to the presence of large numbers of psammoma bodies. *Schwannomas* most commonly present as smooth, encapsulated nodules which may extend in a dumbbell fashion through an intervertebral foramen along with the affected spinal root. Both meningiomas and schwannomas have a similar histology to their intracranial counterparts.

Most metastatic tumours, including lymphomas, are seen in the extradural space or in the surrounding vertebral bones.

Rapid diagnosis of intraspinal tumours may be made on smears, if the tumour is soft, or cryostat sections if the tumour tissue is very firm. Imprint preparations may be useful in defining lymphomas in extradural space and are made by dabbing fresh tissue on to a slide and staining the imprints with Leishman's or other suitable haematological stain. Difficulty may arise in the diagnosis of intramedullary tumours, as the amount of tissue removed may be small in order to prevent too much neurological damage. Under these circumstances it may be better to fix the tissue immediately and examine it either in paraffin section or in resin sections, instead of attempting to make a diagnosis on a smear or cryostat section.

Further reading

Adams J H, Graham D I, Doyle D (1981) Brain biopsy. The smear technique for neurosurgical biopsies. Chapman & Hall, London

Barker D J P, Weller R O, Garfield J S (1976) Epidemiology of primary tumours of the brain and spinal cord: a regional survey in Southern England. J Neurol Neurosurg Psychiatry 39:290

Harkin J C, Reed R J (1969) Tumours of the peripheral nervous system. 2nd series, Fascicle 3. Armed Forces Institute of Pathology, Washington DC

Hoshino T, Townsend J J, Muraoka I, Wilson C B (1980) An autoradiographic study of human gliomas: Growth kinetics of anaplastic astrocytoma and glioblastoma multiforme. Brain 103:967

McCormick D, Allen I V (1976) The value of LDH isoenzymes in the rapid diagnosis of brain tumours. Neuropathol Appl Neurobiol 2:269

Miquel J, Calco W, Rubinstein L J (1968) A simple and rapid stain for the biopsy diagnosis of brain tumors. J Neuropathol Exp Neurol 27:517

Northfield D W C (1973) Surgery of the central nervous system. Blackwell Scientific, Oxford

Russell D S, Rubinstein L J (1977) Pathology of tumours of the nervous system, 4th edn. Arnold, London

Thomas D G T, Graham D I (eds) (1980) Brain tumours: Scientific basis, clinical investigation and current therapy. Butterworths, London

Walton J N (1977) Brain's diseases of the nervous system, 8th edn. Oxford University Press, Oxford

Weller R O, Cervós-Navarro J (1977) Pathology of peripheral nerves. Butterworths, London, Boston, p 145

Zulch K J (ed) (1979) Histological typing of tumours of the central nervous system—International histological classification of tumours. World Health Organization, Geneva

Chapter 8

Pituitary Tumours

Three major types of tumour arise within, or in relation to, the pituitary fossa, viz: *pituitary adenomas* from the anterior pituitary, *craniopharyngiomas* or *suprasellar cysts* from epithelial elements related to the pituitary, and *gliomas* of the posterior pituitary which are usually well-differentiated astrocytomas. The latter are rare tumours and behave in a similar way to hypothalamic or cerebral astrocytomas.

Pituitary tumours may cause complications due to their expansion, with compression of the optic chiasm resulting in visual symptoms and eventually blindness. Tumours may expand to involve other parasellar structures such as the oculomotor nerve, cavernous sinus and hypothalamus. Endocrine problems arise either due to hypersecretion of hormones from pituitary adenomas or due to hypopituitarism resulting from the destruction of normal pituitary tissue.

Pituitary adenomas

Clinical aspects

The diagnosis and management of pituitary adenomas has altered radically in the last decade. In particular, the advent of radioimmunoassays for prolactin, adrenocorticotrophic hormone (ACTH) and growth hormone has led to early diagnosis and to the recognition of excessive hormone secretion by tumours which were formerly thought to be endocrinologically inactive. These advances have,

in turn, prompted the revival of a surgical approach to pituitary adenomas via the trans-sphenoidal or transethmoidal routes. Such techniques allow the selective microsurgical removal of small but endocrinologically active tumours. Thus, the removal of an adenoma may be indicated on endocrine grounds and surgical treatment is no longer confined to transfrontal operations with the purpose of removing a mass lesion causing visual failure by chiasmal compression. A further factor in changing management has been the introduction of drugs, the primary effect of which is to control excessive hormone secretion.

In parallel with these changes in clinical management has come a reappraisal of the histological diagnosis and pathological classification of pituitary adenomas. This chapter, therefore, includes brief descriptions of the major advances in the clinical management and pathological evaluation of pituitary adenomas.

Radioimmunoassay (RIA) of hormones in plasma

The introduction of *growth hormone* RIA in plasma has led to earlier diagnosis of acromegaly and to the realisation that burnt-out cases are extremely rare, if indeed they occur at all. The relationship between growth hormone (GH) levels and disease activity is not linear, perhaps because of a discrepancy between biologically active and immunoreactive hormones. Nevertheless, GH assay remains the best biochemical parameter for diagnosis and for judging the effect of treatment. As with many anterior pituitary hormones, the secretion of GH is pulsatile and the assessment of secretion rates demands dynamic endocrine investigation rather than reliance upon a single plasma level. The failure of a glucose load to suppress GH secretion in acromegaly is the most widely used and reliable diagnostic manoeuvre.

The increasingly widespread availability of *prolactin* RIA has added several dimensions to the management of pituitary adenomas. *First*, it is now known that approximately 60% of tumours formerly classified as chromophobe adenomas are, in fact, prolactinomas capable of secreting large quantities of prolactin both in vivo and in vitro. *Second*, the presence of hyperprolactinaemia is now recognised to be the cause of amenorrhoea and infertility as well as impotence and galactorrhoea in many patients with pituitary adenomas. This association has profoundly altered the supposition that loss of gonadal function in patients with pituitary adenomas is due to hypopituitarism as a result of destruction of the normal tissue secreting gonadotrophic hormones. Indeed, there is now ample evidence that the correction of hyperprolactinaemia alone can restore gonadal activity in a proportion of cases. *Third*, prolactin RIA has led to early diagnosis of small tumours including microadenomas a few millimetres in diameter. It is now commonplace for small prolactinomas to be diagnosed in patients attending infertility clinics on the basis of hyperprolactinaemia and on radiological changes which may only be evident on tomograms of the pituitary fossa.

A changing view of the aetiology and management of Cushing's syndrome has likewise followed the use of RIA of *adrenocorticotrophin (ACTH)*. Whereas Cushing's syndrome was long thought to be due most commonly to primary hypertrophy of the adrenals, it is now realised that the majority of patients harbour an ACTH-secreting tumour of the pituitary. Adrenalectomy for Cushing's syndrome may, therefore, lead to Nelson's syndrome in which an ACTH-secreting tumour is associated with progressive pigmentation of the skin.

Trans-sphenoidal surgery

A surgical approach to the pituitary via the sphenoidal sinus was originally used by Cushing but subsequently abandoned by him because of the risk of CSF leakage and meningitis postoperatively and because large tumours with suprasellar extension

could not be adequately excised. In recent years the operation has found favour again since small intrasellar tumours are accessible by this route without the attendant risks of transfrontal craniotomy, which involves retraction of the frontal lobes and exploration of the pituitary from above the optic chiasm. A further advantage of trans-sphenoidal surgery is that selective removal of a tumour may be possible and enough normal pituitary may be left behind so that postoperative replacement hormone therapy can be avoided in a significant number of patients. In large series of tumours treated by trans-sphenoidal surgery, the operative mortality has been very low and the morbidity confined to the occasional patient with postoperative CSF rhinorrhoea; this may cease spontaneously or following the insertion of a muscle plug. Although it remains true that large suprasellar tumours cannot be removed trans-sphenoidally, there is an increasing tendency for surgeons to favour the trans-sphenoidal approach in patients with limited suprasellar extension.

Drug treatment

The introduction of drugs which suppress excessive hormone secretion by pituitary tumours stems from advances in our understanding of the physiological control exerted by the hypothalamus over the normal pituitary. Secretion of each anterior pituitary hormone is regulated by releasing or inhibiting factors synthesised in the hypothalamus and secreted into the hypophyseal portal system. The first of these factors to be isolated and synthesised was the thyrotrophin-releasing hormone which proved to be a small peptide; since then a number of other small peptides including the releasing hormone for luteinizing hormone have been similarly identified. More recently it has become clear that classic neurotransmitters including dopamine and 5-hydroxytryptamine are also involved in the servo-system operating between the hypothalamus and the pituitary. It is now widely accepted that the most important regulatory factor for prolactin secretion is dopamine, which acts as a prolactin inhibiting factor (PIF). The experimental evidence for this view has now been amply confirmed by clinical experience showing that prolactin secretion in both normal subjects and in patients with prolactinomas can be suppressed by dopamine agonist drugs. *Bromocriptine* has proved to be the most useful dopamine agonist; in relatively small doses, it is almost universally effective in lowering prolactin levels to normal in patients with pro-lactinomas. At the same time, treatment with bromocriptine frequently restores fertility and abolishes galactorrhoea.

Dopamine is also involved in the regulation of growth hormone secretion and in normal subjects dopamine agonists such as L-dopa stimulate growth hormone secretion. Paradoxically, in patients with acromegaly, the effect of dopamine agonists is to suppress growth hormone secretion. The mechanism for this paradoxical response in acromegaly is not yet clearly understood but the empirical observation has led to the use of *bromocriptine* in the treatment of patients with the disease. Although there is no doubt that bromocriptine has a place in the management of acromegaly, the drug is less effective in controlling excessive growth hormone secretion than in controlling excessive prolactin secretion.

Cushing's syndrome may also be controlled by drug therapy in a proportion of cases. The drug concerned is *cyproheptadine* and it is thought to inhibit ACTH secretion in Cushing's syndrome by its action as a 5-hydroxytryptamine antagonist. In some patients the effect of cyproheptadine is striking, and in cases of Nelson's syndrome pigmentation may be controlled, but the drug is by no means universally effective.

Management

Endocrinologically silent tumours. Although the majority of tumours which were formerly classified as chromophobe adenomas are now recognised to be prolactinomas, there remains a substantial minority with endocrine effects that are confined to hypopituitarism. Since such tumours do not secrete excessive amounts of any known hormone, diagnosis is often delayed and endocrinologically silent tumours therefore tend to present with large suprasellar extensions causing chiasmal compression. In these patients the purpose of treatment is to remove or destroy a space-occupying lesion in order to preserve vision. Endocrine considerations play only a small part in the management and are confined largely to post-operative replacement therapy. Transfrontal hypophysectomy followed by a course of radiotherapy which further reduces the risk of recurrence therefore remains the conventional treatment of large tumours. Although it is becoming rarer for prolactinomas or growth-hormone-secreting tumours to present as space-occupying lesions, such cases do occur and in these

circumstances the preservation of vision will be the over-riding consideration in deciding management.

Acromegaly. The classic appearance of the acromegalic patient is easily recognised, though not usually by the patient himself because of the insidious onset of the disease. Most patients do not, in fact, present with symptoms referable to acromegaly but are recognised to have the condition in the course of treatment for an unrelated disease. Only then is the typical history of chronic headaches, acroparaesthesiae and excessive sweating obtained. The fact that acromegaly is a chronic condition which does not present per se does not, however, imply that it is a benign condition. Patients with untreated acromegaly have an increased mortality rate due to a combination of the diabetes mellitus, hypertension, and respiratory disorders which accompany the excessive secretion of growth hormone. The lowering of growth hormone secretion in acromegaly is thus of considerable importance and the variety of treatments used is an indication that no one method is entirely successful in all patients.

Prior to the revival of trans-sphenoidal hypophysectomy, conventional external *radiotherapy* was the most widely used treatment for acromegaly. In terms of risk, radiotherapy has a clear advantage over transfrontal surgery and with improvements in radiotherapeutic techniques such serious complications as necrosis of adjoining brain structures have become comparatively rare. One disadvantage of radiotherapy is that suppression of growth hormone levels is frequently inadequate in the immediate post-treatment period, although up to 75% of patients may have a satisfactory response 5 years after radiotherapy has been given. A greater immediate effect has been achieved in the United States using proton beam therapy but this only at the expense of a higher rate of complications from the treatment.

Bromocriptine has not proved to be adequate for the control of excessive growth hormone secretion. Although clinical symptoms are frequently abolished with this drug, growth hormone levels are satisfactorily lowered in only about 50% of cases and a significant number of patients cannot tolerate the drug because of nausea and vomiting. It is also important to bear in mind that dopamine agonist drugs probably have little effect upon the size of the pituitary adenoma which may, therefore, remain a potential threat to vision. For these reasons it is generally held that bromocriptine is a useful adjunct in the treatment of acromegaly, to be employed either to suppress residual growth hormone secretion after a partial hypophysectomy, or to control growth hormone secretion when radiotherapy is only partially successful.

Because of the limitations of external radiotherapy and medical treatment, an increasing number of centres in Britain and the United States now advocate *trans-sphenoidal hypophysectomy* as the primary treatment for a patient with acromegaly. A satisfactory fall in growth hormone levels occurs in approximately two-thirds of patients immediately after operation, leaving radiotherapy or bromocriptine as adjuncts to treatment in those patients with persistently high levels. In comparing radiotherapy and surgery as first-line treatments, it is important to remember that surgical removal of a tumour following a course of radiotherapy is technically very much more difficult because of the fibrosis affecting the tumour and surrounding tissues.

Clearly one of the major factors affecting the management of acromegaly will be the facilities and expertise available in a particular centre. At the present time it would appear that where the surgical skill is available, trans-sphenoidal surgery offers advantages over other forms of treatment.

Prolactinomas. As in acromegaly, the treatment of small prolactinomas with a view to correcting an endocrine disorder remains controversial. In many patients whose infertility is due to hyperprolactinaemia, pregnancy may occur following suppression of high prolactin levels with bromocriptine. The argument against bromocriptine alone centres on the theoretical risk of rapid enlargement of a small pituitary tumour during pregnancy. Although there is no doubt that this sequence of events can occur, the degree of risk is not yet clear. Nevertheless, there are those who advocate treatment of the primary lesion before proceeding to a pregnancy and both trans-sphenoidal surgery and prophylactic radiotherapy have been used. At present it would appear that at least in those patients with larger prolactinomas, trans-sphenoidal removal of the tumour offers the more certain safeguard against rapid expansion of the tumour and chiasmal compression during pregnancy.

There is an increasing number of patients in whom the diagnosis of a prolactinoma can be made on the basis of hyperprolactinaemia and often minor radiological change in the pituitary fossa. The diagnosis may, for example, follow a routine skull x-ray taken after a minor head injury. In such cases, in which there is no endocrine indication for treatment and when visual pathways are not threatened by a small tumour, management may be confined to a clinical review and a repeat skull x-ray at a later date. Although large prolactinomas were clearly small prolactinomas originally, it is likely that many small tumours never reach sufficient size to act as a space-occupying lesion.

Cushing's syndrome. The recognition that most patients with Cushing's syndrome have hypersecretion of ACTH has led to attempts to treat these at pituitary level rather than by adrenalectomy. External radiotherapy to the pituitary has not proved satisfactory in many patients whose Cushing's syndrome has ultimately required bilateral adrenalectomy but the results of trans-sphenoidal surgery in those patients with a demonstrable pituitary tumour are more encouraging. The role of cyproheptadine remains as an adjunct to other forms of treatment rather than as first-line therapy.

Histopathology

Normal pituitary

The normal anterior pituitary is a very vascular tissue with many thin-walled blood vessels separating groups of cuboidal or polygonal cells. When stained with H & E (Fig. 8.1), three major types of cell may be distinguished. Some 40 % of the cells are acidophil (eosinophil) with bright pink cytoplasm, and 10 % stain blue (basophil). Approximately half the cells in the pituitary have little or no staining in their cytoplasm (*chromophobe* cells). When the tissue is stained with a PAS orange G method, the eosinophils stain yellow and the basophils stain as PAS-positive cells. Again the chromophobes are unstained. The different types of cell are often grouped together and not evenly distributed throughout the anterior pituitary. *Eosinophil* cells are the source of prolactin and growth hormone whereas follicle stimulating hormone (FSH), luteinizing hormone (LH), thyroid stimulating hormone (TSH) and adrenocorticotrophic hormone (ACTH) are secreted by *basophils*. Some of the chromophobe cells probably also secrete ACTH.

Electron microscopically, cells within the anterior pituitary are seen to contain dense intracellular granules 200–800 nm in diameter. Cells secreting prolactin contain the largest granules.

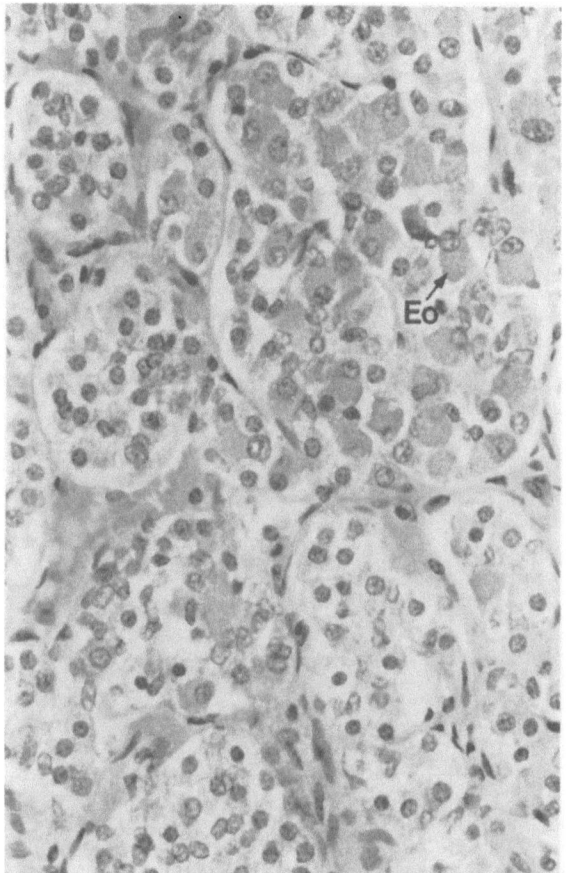

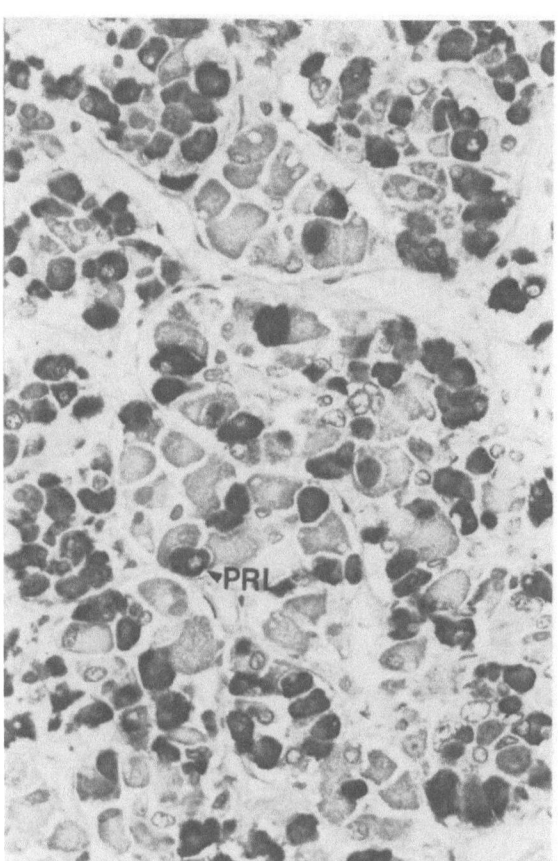

Fig. 8.1. Normal pituitary showing eosinophils (*Eo*) with stained cytoplasm and unstained chromophobe cells. (H & E × 350)

Fig. 8.2. Normal pituitary stained for prolactin (*PRL*). (PAP technique × 350)

Although the chemical differences between the pituitary hormones allow some degree of localisation of cells secreting particular hormones, standard histological techniques are very imprecise. Similarly, the classification of secretory activity in individual cells by electron microscopy is both laborious and of doubtful reliability. *Immunoperoxidase* techniques, on the other hand, have proved to be highly specific in their localisation of hormone secretion to individual cells and to intracellular granules. The use of immunocytochemistry allows much better correlation between the histopathology and the clinical behaviour of pituitary adenomas than was possible with the older routine techniques. Figure 8.2 shows the pattern obtained when anterior pituitary is stained for a specific hormone, prolactin.

The neural origin of the *posterior pituitary* is reflected in its histological structure. Pituicytes in this region are elongated and have long fibrillary processes resembling glia.

Adenomas

Depending upon the techniques employed for their study, pituitary adenomas may be classified in one or several ways.

Histology. Various histological patterns can be recognised in tumours of the anterior pituitary. There may be a diffuse pattern of polygonal cells with regular, round nuclei often containing a small nucleolus (Fig. 8.3). Alternatively, the tumour may show a sinusoidal pattern with either small cells gathered around vascular tufts or elongated columnar cells arranged around blood vessels (Fig. 8.4). None of the histological types accurately reflect the hormonal activity of the tumour but they do allow distinction between the tumour and normal pituitary.

Immunocytochemistry. A number of combined clinical and immunocytochemical studies of pitu-

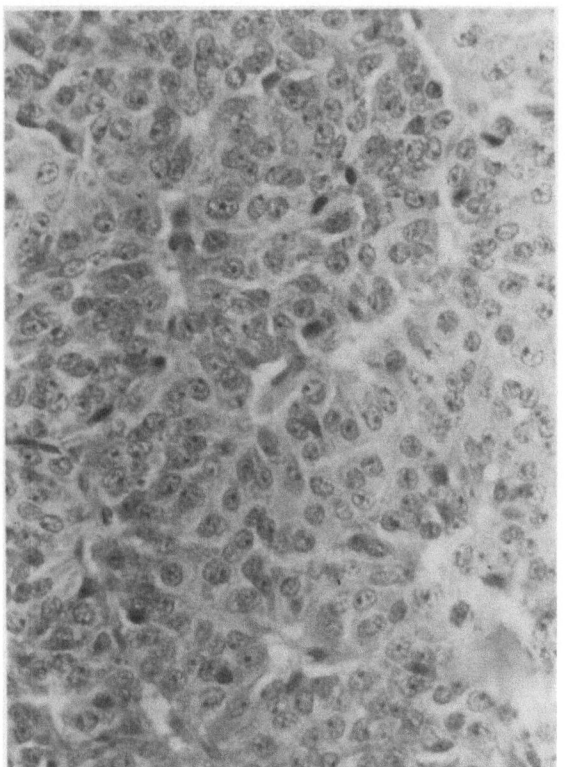

Fig. 8.3. Pituitary adenoma: diffuse pattern. (H & E × 300)

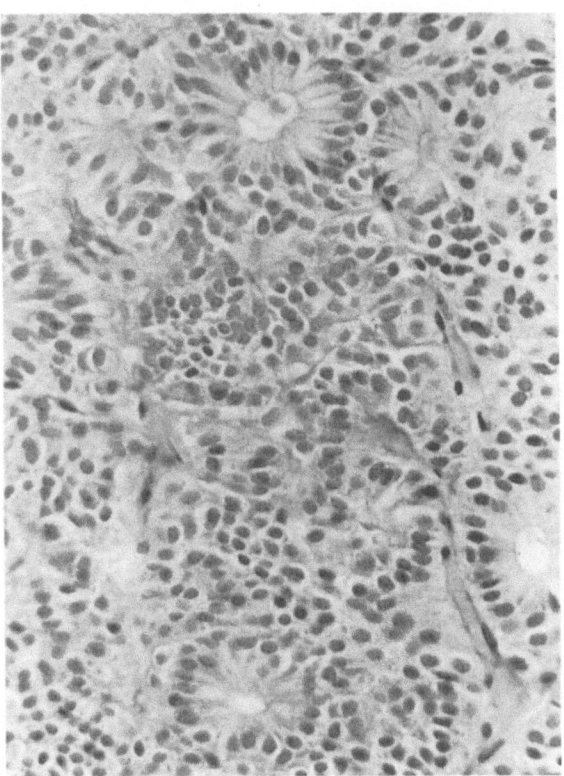

Fig. 8.4. Pituitary adenoma: sinusoidal pattern. (H & E × 300)

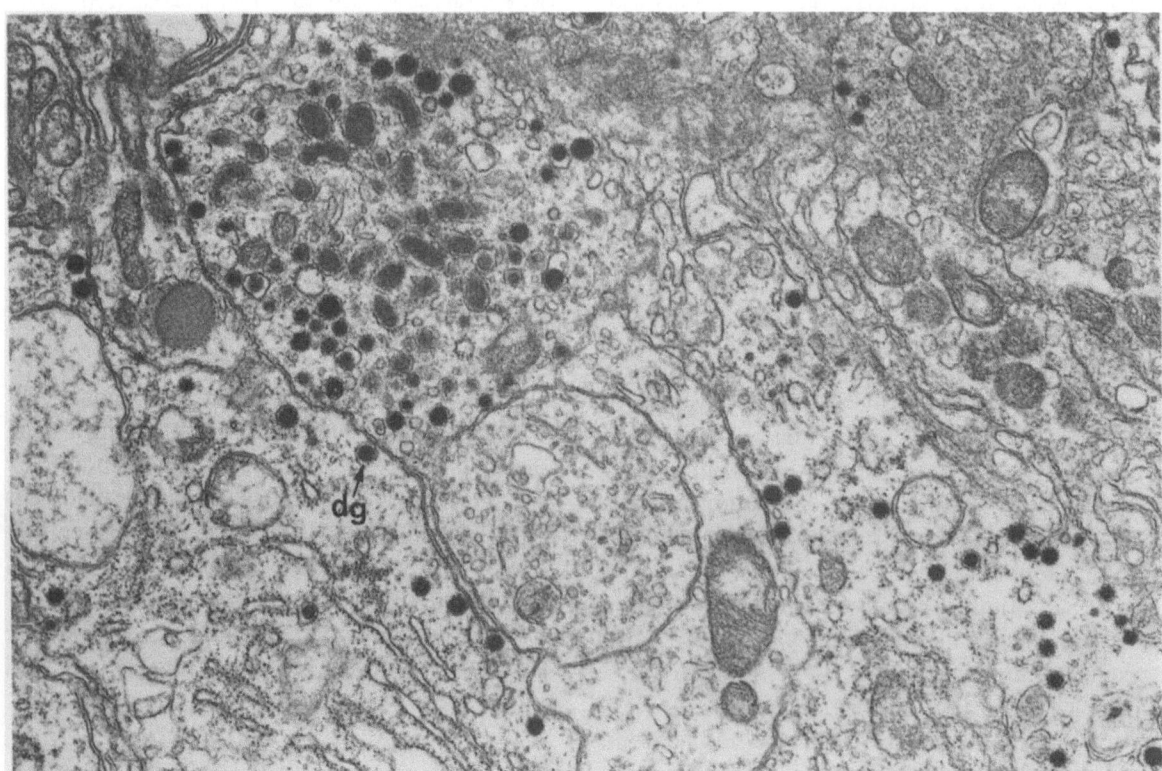

Fig. 8.5. Non-secreting pituitary adenoma. Dense 120–170 nm granules (*dg*) are present in the cytoplasm. (EM × 17500)

itary adenomas have shown a close correlation between raised serum hormone levels and the detection of hormones within the cells of the pituitary adenomas. There is some variation in the proportions of each tumour type in the different series. In 50 patients examined by Martinez et al. (1980), 47 tumours were removed by the trans-sphenoidal route and 3 by transfrontal hypophysectomy. These authors found by immunoperoxidase and ultrastructural characteristics that 25 tumours (50%) were prolactin cell adenomas, 4 (8%) contained growth hormone secreting cells, 1 (2%) was a mixed growth hormone–prolactin cell tumour and 3 (6%) were adrenocorticotrophic cell tumours. The remaining 17 tumours (34%) were undifferentiated cell adenomas and showed no secretion of growth hormone, prolactin or ACTH.

Electron microscopy. Pituitary adenoma cells may be densely or sparsely granulated on electron microscopy and in many cases the size of the granules reflects the type of hormone secretion. However, electron microscopic evaluation is not as reliable as immunoperoxidase characterisation of the cells. In those tumours which show no immunoreactivity for pituitary hormones, the tumour cells may still contain sparse 120–200 nm diameter dense granules within the cytoplasm (Fig. 8.5).

Old classification. Before the introduction of RIA for the clinical measurement of pituitary hormones in the plasma and before the widespread use of immunocytochemistry for the specific localisation of pituitary hormones within tumour cells, the classification of pituitary adenomas was based upon the staining characteristics of the cells in techniques such as H & E and PAS Orange G. Adenomas were separated into chromophobe adenomas (79%), eosinophil adenomas (15%), basophil adenomas (6%). Although in some cases eosinophil adenomas are found in patients with acromegaly, and basophil adenomas in Cushing's disease, the clinicopathological correlation is poor. This classification can now only be used in a descriptive manner and not as an accurate indication of the hormonal activity of the tumour.

Surgical pathology. The introduction of microsurgical trans-sphenoidal techniques for the treatment of pituitary adenomas allows the selective removal of tumour, and in many cases the retention of functioning normal pituitary tissue. Histological identification of tumour may be required during the

operation so that selective removal may be accomplished. In these cases, rapid assessment of the tissue can be made by preparing toluidine blue–stained smears of small fragments of tissue. Smears of adenomas appear, in general, as monomorphic sheets of cells which can be distinguished from the more polymorphic and granular cells derived from normal anterior pituitary. Posterior pituitary resembles normal glia in smear preparations.

Even if identification of adenoma and normal pituitary is not required during the operation, some difficulty may be encountered in distinguishing normal tissue from adenoma in paraffin sections, especially if the tissue is fragmented and distorted. The grouping of cells and their cytoplasmic granularity exhibited both in H & E and in PAS Orange G stains may be of considerable assistance in identifying normal pituitary even if it is compressed and fibrosed.

One feature that is not infrequently seen in tissue removed at trans-sphenoidal hypophysectomy is the extension of adenoma into or through bone. However, this does not appear to indicate malignant change.

Although electron microscopy of pituitary adenomas is not as specific as immunoperoxidase techniques for identifying hormones secreted by the tumour cells, ultrastructural examination can be useful particularly with small fragments of tumour which are otherwise difficult to identify. This is particularly the case when adenomas spread around the base of the brain and their origin from the pituitary fossa is uncertain. Electron microscopy will reveal densely staining granules within most pituitary adenomas (Fig. 8.5).

Craniopharyngiomas and suprasellar cysts

These tumours arise from squamous epithelial elements associated with the pituitary. They are the commonest pituitary tumours in children but are also found in later life. Most lie above the pituitary fossa and their mode of presentation depends upon the age of the patient. *Symptoms* of raised intracranial pressure with headache, vomiting and papilloedema may predominate but endocrine disturbances also occur with diabetes insipidus and stunting of growth in children. *Hypogonadism* is frequently seen in young adults whereas psychological disturbance, including aggression and dementia may be seen in older patients. As with

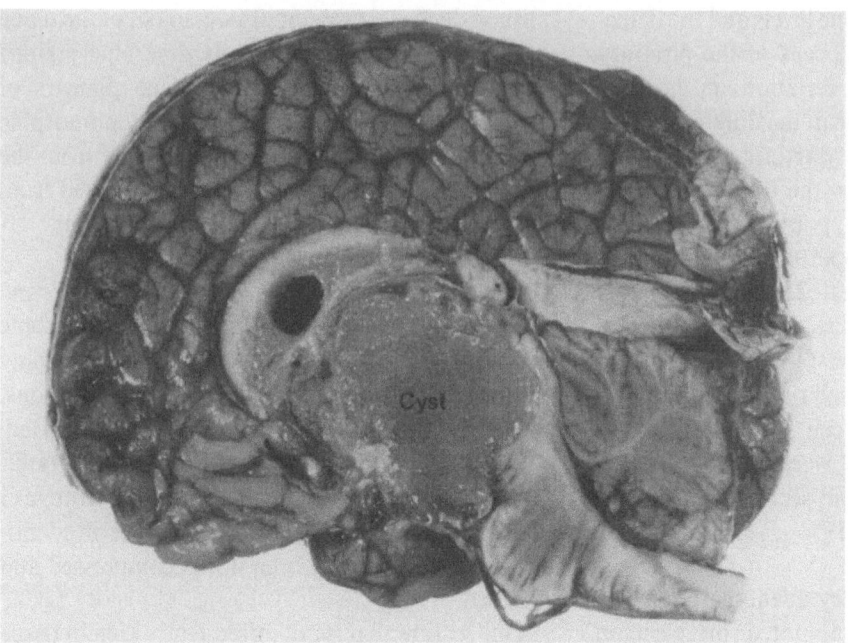

Fig. 8.6. Craniopharyngioma with an enormous cyst extending into the third ventricle.

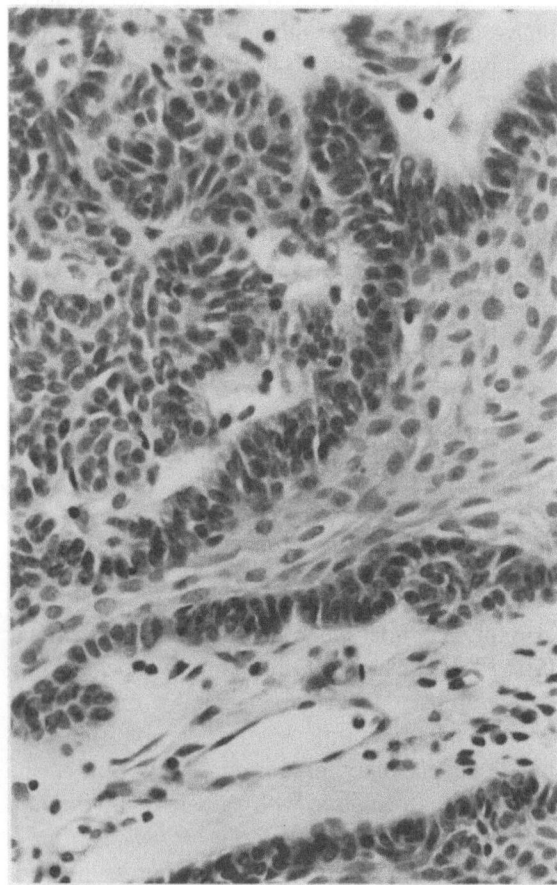

Fig. 8.7. Craniopharyngioma showing squamous, ameloblastoma pattern. (H & E × 330)

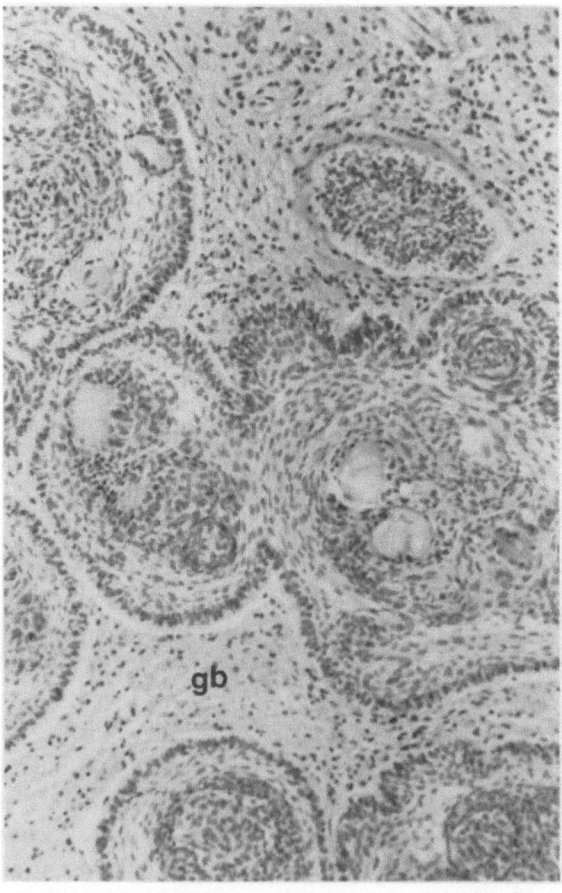

Fig. 8.8. Craniopharyngioma invading brain tissue. Gliotic brain (*gb*). (H & E × 125)

pituitary adenomas, the optic chiasm may be compressed and severe visual disturbance may ensue.

Radiological investigation may reveal enlargement of the pituitary fossa and calcification within the tumour. An enhancing tumour mass may be revealed on CT scan as may hydrocephalus resulting from the tumour's interference with CSF drainage.

Radical excision of craniopharyngiomas with postoperative radiotherapy seems to produce the best therapeutic results. Nevertheless, the tumour may recur and may enlarge rapidly due to the filling of cysts.

Pathology

The majority of craniopharyngiomas are cystic (Fig. 8.6) and may extend from the suprasellar region into the hypothalamus and the third ventricle. Frequently, the fluid within the cysts is brown and contains shimmering cholesterol crystals. Solid areas of the tumour are, in many cases, composed of sheets of squamous cells enclosing a fibrous stroma (Fig. 8.7.). The appearances resemble those seen in certain types of basi-squamous carcinoma of the skin and ameloblastoma of the jaw. Necrotic areas within the tumour may contain cholesterol crystals, the impressions of which remain as clefts in paraffin sections. In some cases the squamous elements in the tumour are confined to a stratified squamous epithelium lining a cyst.

Craniopharyngioma tissue is often stuck firmly to the brain and clumps of squamous epithelium may be seen extending into gliotic hypothalamus (Fig. 8.8). A layer of dense fibrous tissue may form as a result of leakage of cyst contents and separate craniopharyngioma tissue from the adjacent brain.

Surgical pathology. There is usually little diagnostic difficulty when classic squamous epithelium is present in the specimen removed at surgery, but occasionally much of the material is necrotic and is only recognisable as probable craniopharyngioma by the presence of cholesterol crystals and clefts. Similarly, fluid drained from a suprasellar cyst may be identified by detecting cholesterol crystals within it by polarised light.

Further reading

Adams J H, Graham D I, Doyle D (1981) Brain biopsy: The smear technique for neurological biopsies. Chapman and Hall, London

Collins W F (1978) Adenohypophyseal tumours. In: Matthews W B, Glaser G H (eds) Recent advances in clinical neurology, No. 2. Churchill Livingstone, Edinburgh, p 91

Currie A R, Wyllie A H (1978) The pituitary gland. In: W St C Symmers (ed) System pathology, 2nd edn, vol. 1. Churchill Livingstone, Edinburgh, p 1863

Hartog M (1978) Pituitary tumours. In: O'Riordan J H L (ed) Recent advances in endocrinology and metabolism. Churchill Livingstone, Edinburgh, p 17

Lawton N F, Evans A J, Weller R O (1981) Dopaminergic inhibition of growth hormone and prolactin release during continuous in vitro perfusion of normal and adenomatous human pituitary. J Neurol Sci 46: 229

McGregor A M, Ginsberg J (1981) Dilemmas in the management of functioning pituitary tumours. Br J Hosp Med 25: 344

Martinez A J, Lee A, Moossy J, Maroon J C (1980) Pituitary adenomas: Clinicopathological and immunohistochemical study. Ann Neurol 7: 24

Chapter 9

Virus Infections
of the Nervous System

Clinical aspects and pathology

Viruses cause neurological disease either as the result of *cytopathic effects* from direct invasion of the nervous system, or as a consequence of an accompanying or delayed *immunological response* to virus invasion of the nervous system (post-viral encephalitis or polyneuropathy). Viruses may enter the nervous system by one of a number of routes, but it is uncommon for there to be clinical evidence of the mode of entry. During viraemia, viruses may penetrate the CNS, usually causing viral meningitis or viral encephalitis. Invasion of the nervous system through the nasopharynx and the olfactory nerves, or by passage of viral particles along peripheral nerves, e.g. the trigeminal nerve, is also recognised. Furthermore, some viruses such as rabies virus may enter the nervous system after inoculation through a bite on an extremity and subsequent passage along periperhal nerves. Invasion during viraemia is probably the commonest of these routes of infection.

Viral meningitis

Usually acute in onset, viral meningitis presents with headache, fever, stiff neck, drowsiness, nausea and vomiting. The accompanying viraemia is usually manifest by a systemic illness, such as diarrhoea, pneumonia, fever, or diffuse myalgias. Apart from drowsiness and meningism there are no neurological signs; recovery occurs in a few days and is almost invariably uneventful. This clinical syndrome results from infection by one of a large number of different viruses. Clinically, it resembles a bacterial infection and the differential diagnosis is made on lumbar puncture. The *CSF* in viral meningitis may be under increased pressure with a raised cell count consisting entirely, or almost entirely, of lymphocytes. The protein is usually normal but it may be raised to about twice the normal level in some cases. CSF sugar levels are normal or may be slightly increased; this indicates a disturbance of the blood–brain barrier. Blood sugar levels should be estimated at the same time to exclude anomalous results due to hyperglycaemia. Microscopic examination and culture of the CSF reveal no evidence of bacterial infection. It is uncommon for virus particles to be detected in CSF by electron microscopy but they may be isolated by culture.

Sequential lumbar punctures may be used to demonstrate rising titres of antibodies in the 3 weeks after the initial infection; it is much more usual, however, to perform these tests on blood. Culture of throat washings or faeces may reveal a virus, often an enterovirus, in cases of viral meningitis.

Pathology. As viral meningitis is rarely fatal, there are few data regarding its pathological features. However, patients occasionally die in status epilepticus with viral meningitis and in these cases infiltration of the leptomeninges by mononuclear cells has been detected together with perivascular lymphocytic cuffing in the superficial layers of the underlying cerebral cortex.

Viral encephalitis

Direct invasion of the brain by virus is common in the exanthemas, particularly measles. Patients show symptoms and signs of viral meningitis together with signs of involvement of the CNS. These may include generalised or focal seizures, and focal signs of neurological disturbance such as hemiparesis, or signs of brain stem involvement, particularly ocular palsies and ataxia. Drowsiness or coma is usually a feature. Recovery is frequently complete but there may be residual brain damage

with impaired intellectual function, seizures or residual hemiparesis or other focal neurological signs.

The *CSF* in viral encephalitis shows changes reflecting the degree of damage to the CNS. Lymphocytes are usually the predominant cell type in the CSF but polymorphonuclear leukocytes are also seen and the CSF protein is higher than is found in uncomplicated viral meningitis. CSF sugar levels are normal or slightly increased and the CSF pressure is usually raised.

The clinical features and CSF findings in viral encephalitis may closely resemble those of pyogenic disease of the CNS, particularly cerebral abscess or parameningeal sepsis (Chap. 10). Viral encephalitis is thus difficult to define; it is an illness, usually of rapid onset and progression, with signs of diffuse or multifocal involvement of the CNS and of inflammation of the brain. Other causes of the illness must be excluded.

Pathology. Despite the very large number of different viruses that may cause encephalitis throughout the world, the general pathological features of viral infections of the CNS are very similar. However, the severity of the pathological changes and their distribution throughout the CNS depend to some extent upon the infecting virus. For example, in *herpes simplex encephalitis* the major damage is to the temporal lobes and adjacent areas of the cerebral hemispheres whereas in *poliomyelitis* severe damage may occur in the spinal cord or brain stem. In severe forms of encephalitis, as in herpes simplex infection, there may be extensive destruction of brain tissue with oedema and widespread invasion by macrophages. Pathological evidence of other viral infections, on the other hand, may be restricted to small foci of inflammation and cell destruction.

Lymphocyte and *plasma cell infiltration* of the brain is characteristic of viral infections of the nervous system (Fig. 9.1). Often the inflammatory cells are restricted to perivascular regions but they may spread into the adjacent brain (Fig. 9.2). Plasma cells can be identified by staining sections with methyl green pyronin or by staining for immunoglobulin by immunoperoxidase or immunofluorescence techniques. The presence of plasma cells suggests that there is local production of *viral antibodies*. In addition to the invasion by inflammatory cells, there is widespread proliferation of *microglial* cells recognisable by their rod-shaped nuclei (Fig. 9.1). Microglia are also seen in

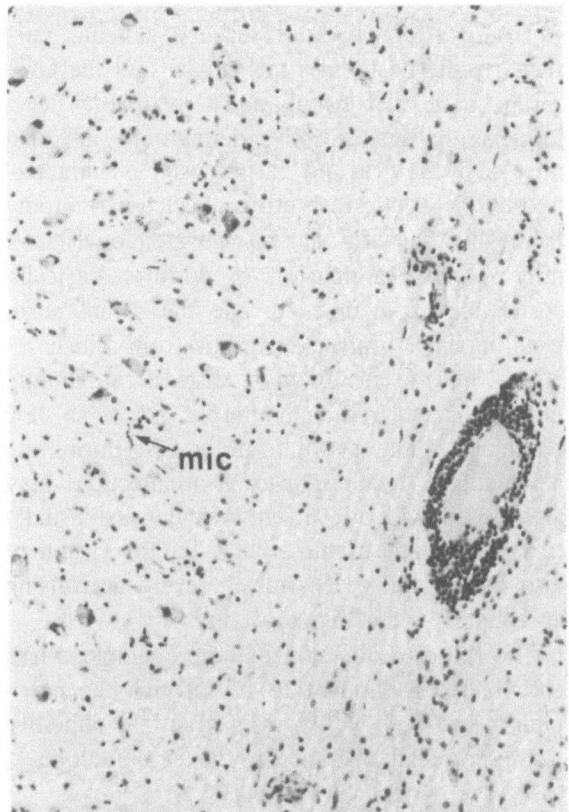

Fig. 9.1. Viral infection of brain stem. There is lymphocytic cuffing around a small blood vessel and microglial proliferation (*mic*) away from the vessel. (H & E × 135)

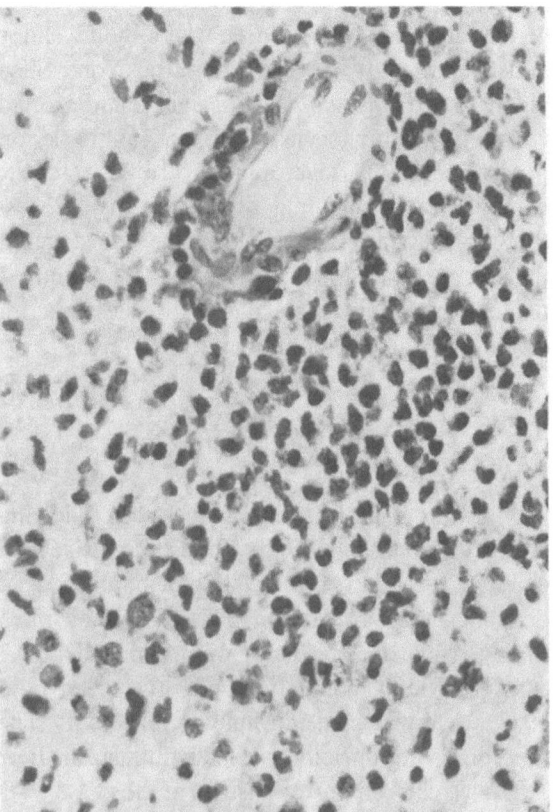

Fig. 9.2. Herpes simplex encephalitis. Lymphocytes, plasma cells and macrophages have spread into the tissue from the perivascular region. (H & E × 385)

groups forming 'microglial stars'. At a later stage in the encephalitis, foamy macrophages are much more prominent in the damaged tissue.

Neurons and other cells infected by virus may be killed by antibody-dependent or direct lymphocyte cytolysis and the remains of the cells ingested by microglia and macrophages. Phagocytosis of individual neurons, the process of *neuronophagia*, is typical of many viral encephalitides but also occurs following hypoxic damage to the brain.

Viral inclusions within glia and neurons are a prominent feature of some acute viral encephalitides. DNA viruses such as herpes simplex replicate in the nucleus and a large part of the nucleus may be replaced by an eosinophilic inclusion. Electron microscopically, partially formed virus particles may be identified within these inclusions. The presence of specific viruses may be detected within cells by immunofluorescence or by immunoperoxidase staining.

Patients dying some years after an acute viral encephalitis often show focal loss of tissue over a wide area. Following herpes encephalitis, the temporal lobes may be largely destroyed but in other viral encephalitides the scarred areas may be scattered in a distribution which often depends upon the type of virus involved in the primary infection.

Post-infectious encephalitis

Most cases of encephalitis occur during or shortly after a viral infection. In post-infectious (post-viral) encephalitis, sometimes referred to as allergic encephalomyelitis, the cerebral illness occurs in patients who have sustained a viral infection, usually sparing the nervous system, some days or up to 3 weeks before the development of the cerebral illness. The encephalitis may follow vaccination, measles, varicella or influenza virus infection; it is characterised by fever, seizures, and focal neurological disturbances. Despite the severity of the clinical disorder, the prognosis for recovery is usually excellent.

Pathology. Histologically, post-infectious encephalitis is characterised by widespread small foci of perivascular tissue destruction where the myelin is destroyed to a greater extent than the axons. Such plaques of *demyelination* are usually found around vessels with lymphocyte cuffing and as the lesion progresses foamy macrophages are seen in the damaged areas ingesting degenerate myelin. Astrocyte proliferation is also seen in the later stages of the disease and, following removal of damaged tissue, perivascular gliosis may be the only indication of damage that remains.

Reye's syndrome

This distinct acute encephalopathy is seen following viral infections and occurs almost exclusively in children. It is now considered to be a major cause of death in virus-associated CNS disease in the United States, where the incidence was estimated at 0.7 cases per 100 000 population under the age of 18 in 1977, a year with epidemic influenza B activity. The preceding viral infection is usually influenzal (B or A H_1N_1), chicken pox or gastro-enteritis.

Clinically, the viral infection is interrupted by the sudden onset of persistent vomiting followed by a rapidly evolving acute encephalopathy with initial lethargy and delirium followed by coma. The mortality rate is around 40% unless specific measures are employed to manage the rising intracranial pressure and metabolic changes associated with this acute, but reversible, toxic encephalopathy of unknown pathogenesis.

Pathology. Pathological changes seen in the mitochondria, and microvesicular fat droplets found in hepatocytes confirm the diagnosis on liver biopsy. There is evidence of cerebral oedema but without inflammatory changes. Severe fatty change is seen in the liver with elevated liver transaminase levels, hyperammonaemia and prolonged prothrombin times.

Viruses with specific neurotropic characteristics

A number of viruses, e.g. poliomyelitis, herpes simplex and varicella zoster have characteristic clinical effects on the nervous system. *Poliomyelitis* virus enters the CNS during viraemia and in particular it invades anterior horn cells in the spinal cord resulting in paralysis and neurogenic atrophy of muscles innvervated by the affected neurons. *Varicella zoster* invades sensory ganglia, particularly the posterior root ganglia and the Gasserian (trigeminal) ganglion. The peripheral nerve branches in the respective dermatomes are also infected by the virus and 'herpes zoster' is characterised by a vesicular rash in the affected dermatome from which the virus may be recovered for electron microscopic examination or culture. Varicella zoster may sometimes invade the spinal cord, resulting in a tranverse myelitis from which recovery may occur. In most cases of apparently uncomplicated radicular herpes zoster, a few lymphocytes may be found in the CSF during the acute stage. *Herpes simplex* virus infections may also present with a recurrent vesicular rash usually to be found in the mouth or vulva but this virus may also invade the CNS causing severe necrotising encephalitis with a high mortality.

The route of infection of herpes simplex virus encephalitis is thought to be through the nasopharynx possibly with passage along the olfactory nerves and olfactory tracts to the temporal lobe.

Viruses and polyneuropathy

There is some evidence that virus infection may precede polyneuropathies of the *Guillain–Barré* type; it has been particularly suggested that this disorder may be associated with infection by Epstein–Barr virus, and thus with infectious mononucleosis. However, epidemiological studies have failed to confirm a close relation between previous endemic viral infections and the development of this neuropathy. Guillain–Barré polyneuropathy seems to follow exposure to a number of different immunological stresses including viral infections, immunisations and vaccinations. The pathology of this condition is described in Chap. 16.

Slow virus encephalitis

Subacute sclerosing panencephalitis (SSPE) and progressive multifocal leukoencephalopathy (PML) are two examples of viral encephalitis which do not have an acute clinical course and differ in their pathological features from the acute encephalitides. Also included in the slow virus diseases are Creutzfeldt–Jakob disease and kuru. Although both these diseases are transmissible to experimental animals and to man, the nature of the transmissible agent is at the moment unknown. Scrapie, a disease of sheep, is similarly a transmissible encephalopathy in which the infective agent awaits identification.

Subacute sclerosing panencephalitis (SSPE)

This disease usually occurs in children and is characterised *clinically* by involuntary jerking movements of the limbs and deterioration of intellectual function. The disease may be present for several months before the patient dies and during this time there is a characteristic EEG picture with high voltage complexes which are usually synchronous with involuntary movements. High levels of oligoclonal immunoglobulin are found in the CSF.

Patients dying with subacute sclerosing panencephalitis show variable degrees of cerebral atrophy which is often severe. *Histologically*, there is perivascular accumulation of lymphocytes and plasma cells, proliferation of microglia and large viral inclusions in the nucleus and cytoplasm of neurons and glial cells (Fig. 9.3). *Electron microscopically*, the inclusions contain tubular structures resembling the nucleocapsid of paramyxovirus. Isolation of *measles virus* from SSPE brains usually requires co-cultivation techniques as the measles virus within the cells is incomplete. Widespread proliferation of astrocytes is also seen in SSPE and is responsible for the 'sclerosis' of the brain.

Progressive multifocal leukoencephalopathy (PML)

This is a rare disease which usually occurs in patients who are immunosuppressed, often in association with a lymphoma or chronic leukaemia. The disease is characterised *clinically* by progressive deterioration in intellectual function and by neurological signs and symptoms referable to various parts of the cerebral hemispheres, cerebellum and brain stem. Death usually occurs after 3–6 months, but survival of many years has been reported in patients with the disease who are not immunosuppressed.

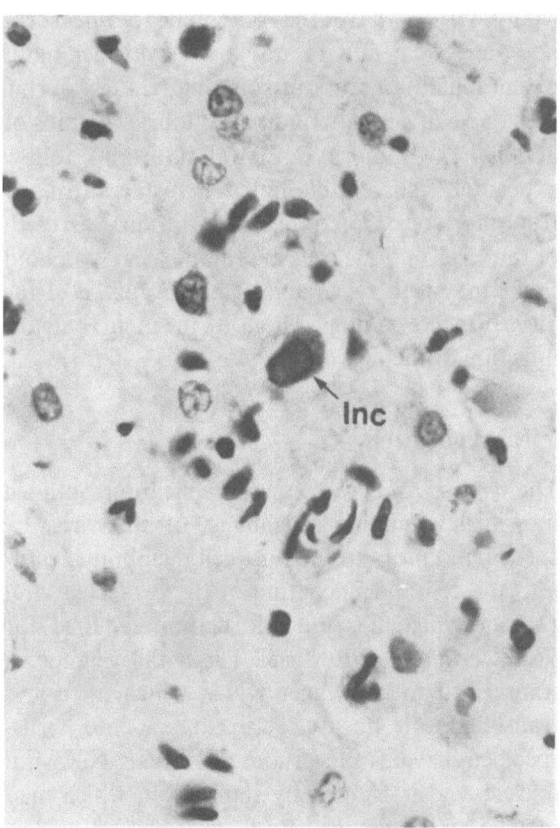

Fig. 9.3. Subacute sclerosing panencephalitis: nuclear inclusion (*Inc*) in a neuron. (H & E × 940)

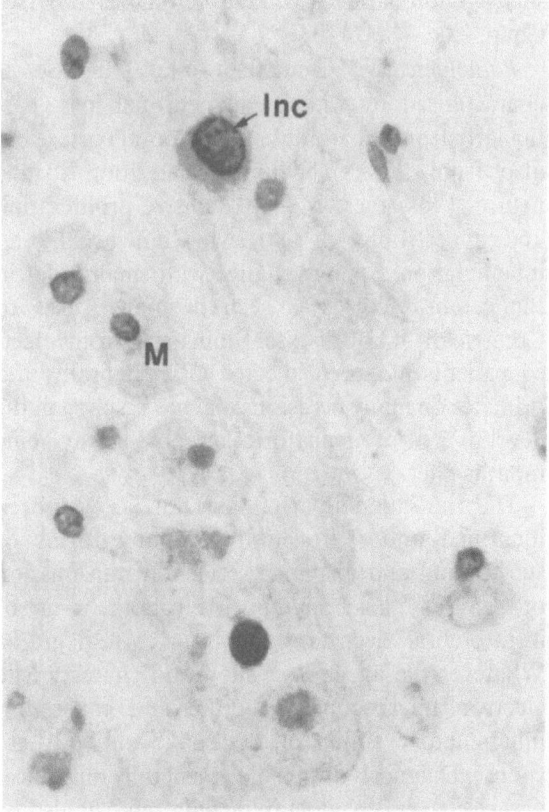

Fig. 9.4. Progressive multifocal leukoencephalopathy. Oligodendrocyte with an intranuclear inclusion and hyperchromasia (*Inc*). Macrophage (*M*). (H & E × 620)

The brain shows multiple areas of *demyelination* which are more irregular and 'fluffy' in their outline than those seen in multiple sclerosis. Prominent within the areas of demyelination are bizarre astrocytes which are large and often multinucleate. Many oligodendroglial cells show enlargement of their nuclei with hyperchromasia and the presence of intranuclear viral inclusions (Fig. 9.4). Electron microscopy, immunofluorescence and virological studies have shown that the inclusions contain *polyoma virus* usually of JC type, but occasionally SV40 virus is isolated from brains with progressive multifocal leukoencephalopathy.

Creutzfeldt–Jakob disease

In addition to the slow virus diseases where a definite causative agent, a virus, has been identified, there are transmissible diseases of the CNS in which the causative agent has not yet been fully character-ised. One such disease is a relatively rare progressive dementia, Creutzfeldt–Jakob disease, which has a course extending from several months to a few years before death. The *clinical* picture is variable; a progressive loss of memory and intellectual func-tion is usually accompanied by motor abnormalities such as choreoathetosis and myoclonic seizures (see Chap. 15).

Pathologically, Creutzfeldt–Jakob disease is characterised by widespread neuronal loss, par-ticularly from the frontal and temporal cortex, but also from the cerebellum. In addition to the neuronal loss there is very extensive proliferation and hypertrophy of astrocytes but usually no inflammation. Spongy change with small holes in the cerebral cortex is seen in many cases of Creutzfeldt–Jakob disease. Brain tissue from affect-ed patients has been injected intracerebrally into primates on many occasions and has resulted in the development of spongiform encephalopathy some months later.

The transmissible agent has not, as yet, been identified and is resistant to many forms of sterilisation and fixation. Accidental transmission of the disease has been reported from the re-use of intracerebral electrodes and from corneal grafts. Whatever the agent is, it shows no characteristic electron microscopic structure and causes no inflammatory action or detectable antibody re-sponse. Diagnosis during life is generally on clinical and electro-encephalographic data but can also be confirmed by cerebral biopsy. A code of practice for dealing with patients with Creutzfeldt–Jakob dis-ease has now been established owing to the danger of transmission of the agent which is resistant to destruction by conventional sterilisation techniques (see Appendix).

Kuru

Kuru is an encephalopathy which was discovered in a primitive tribe in New Guinea and appeared to be transmitted through the ingestion of infected brain tissue during funeral rites. *Intracerebral* injection of brain tissue from patients dying of kuru into primates causes an encephalopathy after a long incubation period of many months. Kuru in man has a long incubation period and the disease is protracted; it involves the cerebrum but mainly affects the cerebellum and histologically is characterised by loss of granule cells from the cerebellar cortex and by the formation of character-istic PAS-positive and congophilic plaques, some 30 μm in diameter.

Virology of nervous system infections

Many viruses have the potential to infect the nervous system, and it is not known why meningitis or encephalitis occurs in some individuals during the course of such common infections as mumps or herpes. The majority of viral infections follow exposure of susceptible mucosal surfaces (usually respiratory or oropharyngeal) to the virus. Growth of the virus in these cells and in the local lymphoid tissue may lead to viraemia and to uptake of the virus by nerve endings. These are the main routes of infection of the nervous system.

Viral replication

The *sequence* of events in viral replication, outlined in Fig. 9.5, entails attachment of the virus by specific receptors to the host cell membrane, entry into the cell and uncoating of the protected viral genome which has the information required for production of new virus. The viral genome is transcribed to messenger RNA, which in turn is translated, on host cell ribosomes, into virus-specified enzymes and structural proteins. New viral nucleic acid is formed by replication, which may involve viral enzymes. Viral proteins and nucleic acid are assembled into new virus particles and released from the cell; many viruses acquire an

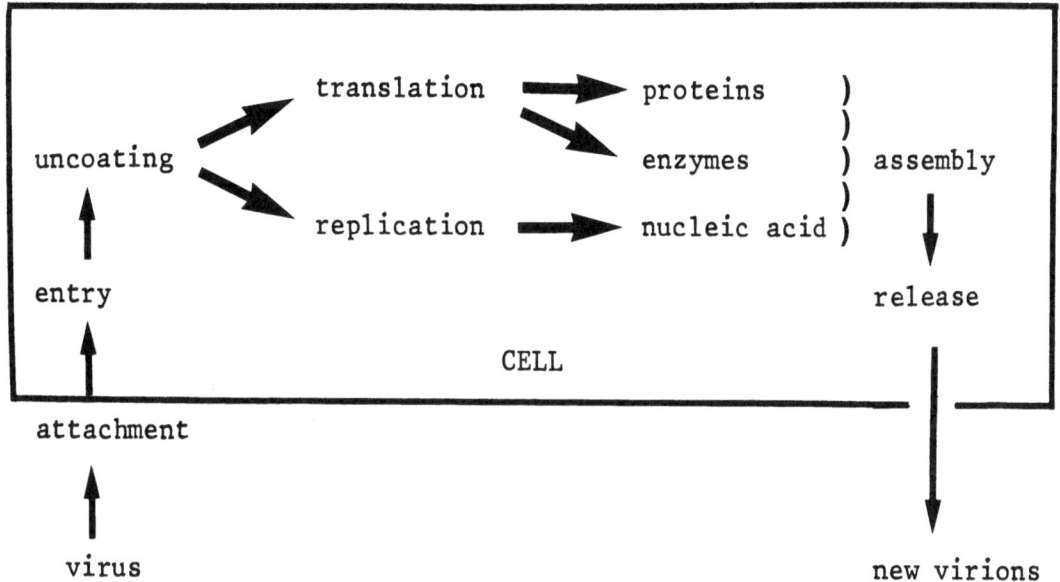

Fig. 9.5. The sequence of events in viral replication.

outer envelope by budding off from host cell membranes into which virus proteins have been inserted.

Defences against viral infection

The absence of specific receptors on nerve cells may determine whether a particular virus can infect the nervous system. If infection does occur, its progress may be halted by host defence mechanisms and the degree of damage to cells depends upon the rapidity with which virally induced cytopathic effects are prevented and upon the extent of the immunological destruction of infected cells. There is increasing scope for therapeutic interference with the natural sequence of events, although at present most of the agents used are experimental and of limited availability.

The routes of spread of virus infection within the cells of the nervous system are shown diagrammatically in Fig. 9.6 with indications of possible sites for natural and therapeutic intervention. The relative importance of these various natural defences in effecting recovery from infection varies with the nature of the infecting virus. Where viral antigens are not expressed on the infected cell surface and subsequent lysis releases many new free virions, as in enterovirus infection, *antibody* plays the major role in limiting the spread of infection to new cells. Thus individuals with hypogammaglobulinaemic disorders are particularly at risk from enterovirus infection. *Cell-mediated immune responses* are essential for recovery from infection with viruses that remain cell associated. Such viruses (e.g.

herpes) pass from cell to cell in the presence of circulating antibody. Infected cells exhibit new (viral) antigens on their surfaces and cell-mediated cytotoxic attack on these membrane antigens ends the infection. *Interferon* is the first available natural defence but it is not known whether any delay or deficiency of interferon production plays a part in determining infection of the nervous system in viral diseases.

Intervention in certain infections of the nervous system is possible when antiviral drugs, interferon, or specific antibody are available. Transfer factor (lymphocyte culture supernatant) has also been used in an attempt to stimulate cellular immune responses in viral infections. When planning *therapy*, it is necessary in each case first to establish the particular virus involved and to be aware of the natural history of that infection and the likely immunological competence of the individual patient.

Viruses associated with CNS infections

The viruses most frequently found in nervous system infections are listed in Table 9.1, as are the clinical conditions usually associated with them. A review of viral and mycoplasmal meningitis and encephalitis recorded in the United Kingdom in 1979 by Noah and Urquhart (1980) indicated that the enteroviruses and mumps virus were the commonest agents involved. *Echovirus* and *Coxsackie B* virus infections were the most common in infancy, *mumps* in the first decade, and *Echovirus* in the 15–44 age group. *Echoviruses* 7, 11, and 24 accoun-

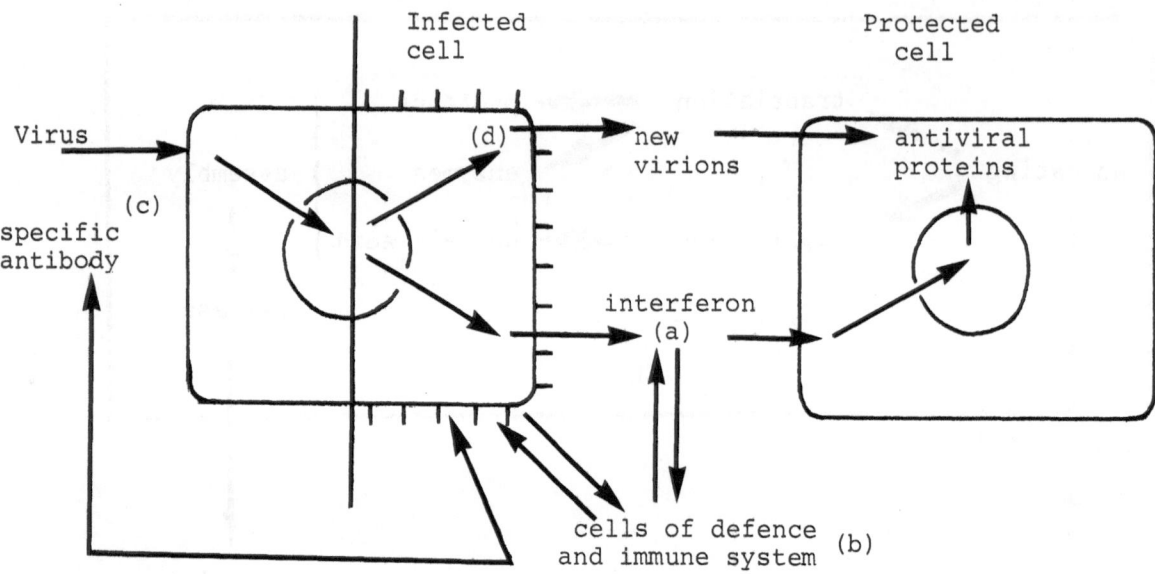

Fig. 9.6. Sites for interference in the spread of viral infection.

(*a*) Interferon. First defence: produced rapidly by any cell in response to virus infection and particularly by lymphocytes and macrophages; stimulates production of antiviral protein (interferes with subsequent viral replication).

(*b*) Cell-mediated immunity. Very important in recovery from infection especially with cell-associated viruses such as herpes, and measles. Responsible for recognising infected cells and destroying them.

(*c*) Specific antibody. Produced in late stage of infection, specific antibody neutralises free virions, prevents further infection and confers immunity. Important in antibody-dependent lymphocyte attack on infected cell membranes.

(*d*) Specific antiviral agents. Few are available. Ideally they act by inhibiting viral enzyme activity without host cell toxicity. Includes interferon.

Table 9.1. Viruses associated with acute infection of nervous system

Clinical presentation	Associated viruses	
	Common	*Rare*
Paralysis	Polio 1, 3	Other enteroviruses
Meningitis	Mumps Coxsackie B1-5, A9 Echovirus 4, 6, 9, 11, 30	Other enteroviruses Herpes simplex 2 Varicella zoster Lymphocytic choriomeningitis
Encephalitis	Arboviruses Enteroviruses Herpes simplex 1 Mumps Measles	Rabies Varicella zoster EB virus Adenovirus

ted for the majority of CNS cases recorded in England and Wales, but type 33 caused CNS infections in Scotland. Thirty-six cases of *herpes* encephalitis were reported; only three of these occurred in children under 15 years of age, and there was evidence of virus in the brain, or antibody in the CNS in only 23 cases. Fourteen of these 36 patients died.

Virological investigations in CNS infections

Meningitis and paralytic disease

Appropriate investigation of cases of meningitis ('aseptic' or non-bacterial), and of paralytic disease is likely to reveal the causative agent. Specimens for such virological study should include:

1) CSF
2) Acute and convalescent sera
3) Throat swab in viral transport medium
4) Faeces

In all *virological* studies, the *clinical* information supplied with the specimens is of great importance in guiding the laboratory towards the appropriate investigations. Rapid virus isolation can be expected with *enteroviruses* and *herpes simplex*; indeed, provisional results from the cytopathic effects in tissue culture may be obtained within 1–3 days. The most rapid results currently available, however, rely upon the identification of virus in the CSF by electron microscopy. *Mumps* infection can be recognised from a single serum sample examined during the initial stages of the disease and can be confirmed by a rising titre of antibodies in convalescence. Identification of an *enterovirus* in the CSF is strong evidence of its causative role in the nervous system infection, whereas isolation from throat or faeces may simply reflect a carrier state. Unfortunately, it is seldom possible to isolate *poliovirus* from the CSF in poliomyelitis.

Herpes simplex meningitis

While recognised as a consequence of neonatal infection, the occurrence of herpes simplex meningitis in other age groups is often overlooked. Herpes causes a lymphocytic meningitis, usually in young adults, and appears to accompany primary infection with herpes simplex type 2 (HSV 2), the strain responsible for the majority of herpes infections of the genital tract. As in the neonatal HSV 2 infection, the virus is readily isolated from the CSF. Recovery without specific treatment is usual in immunocompetent adults. Such infections may become more frequent as the incidence of genital herpes rises.

Investigation of encephalitis

Data from the United States for 1977 indicate that in 1553 cases of encephalitis, the aetiology was not determined in 70%. Encephalitis associated with viral infections may be classified either as encephalitis complicating a common system virus disease i.e. '*post-infectious*', or as acute encephalitis associated with a *direct virus infection* of the CNS.

Post-infectious encephalitis

Many cases of encephalitis fall into the 'post-infectious' category; they follow common infections such as the childhood exanthemas. A clinical history of the precipitating infection, and positive results of routine serology or virus isolation, should yield the diagnosis. The *incidence* of post-infectious encephalitis should fall as the associated virus infections become less frequent, and already the use of measles vaccine has resulted in a reduction in the incidence of measles encephalitis in young children in the United States. However, there may be a period when an increasing number of cases occurs in young adults who have escaped both natural measles and immunisation in childhood. Adults who contract measles infections have a higher incidence of encephalitis than children.

There is evidence that *demyelination* in post-infectious encephalitis is an auto-immune process involving antibodies to myelin basic protein, and the cell-mediated destruction of myelin sheaths. Experimental studies have shown that myelin antigens and antibodies are present in the serum and CSF from such cases. *Therapy* should thus be directed towards control of the immune reaction. Currently, *diagnosis* rests with identifying the precipitating infection since there are no practical clinical tests for recognition of the immune reaction.

Mycoplasma pneumoniae infections

Neurological complications may accompany *M. pneumoniae* infection. The organism is an antibiotic-sensitive microbe, but serological tests for *Mycoplasma* infection are usefully included in a virological service. Tests for cold agglutinins are positive in only half the cases. If there is evidence of an appropriate clinical illness such as an atypical pneumonia, treatment with erythromycin or tetracycline may be considered. The neurological syndromes associated with *Mycoplasma* infections are meningoencephalitis or transverse myelitis. *Mycoplasma* has been detected in the brains of fatal cases but as *Mycoplasma* antigens cross-react with human tissues, including brain and red blood cells, destruction of brain tissue may be due to immunologically mediated damage rather than to the direct action of the *Mycoplasma*.

Acute encephalitis

Acute viral encephalitis is characterised by widespread death of brain cells infected by virus. Severe encephalitis may occur during *arbovirus* or *enterovirus* epidemics but may also present sporadically due to infection of the brain by one of a number of viruses. The most commonly recognised severe sporadic encephalitis is due to *herpes simplex* virus infection.

Demonstration of a virus in brain tissue is the ultimate proof of its causative role in encephalitis but if biopsy or autopsy tissue, or ventricular CSF is not available, diagnosis must be based upon the detection of a specific antibody response within the CNS. In some cases, a serological response confirming a current viral infection is sufficient evidence, as with encephalitis due to an epidemic arbovirus. Particular diagnostic problems arise, however, with common virus infections, especially with herpes simplex, because this virus is frequently reactivated during intercurrent disease.

Specimens obtained for investigation of encephalitis should, if possible, include:

1) Brain tissue (biopsy or autopsy material)
2) CSF ⎫ in the acute and convalescent phases
3) Serum ⎭ of the illness

In addition, virus isolation may be attempted from throat swabs, faeces or from blood mononuclear cells.

Antibody may be present in the serum when encephalitic symptoms first appear and can give a presumptive diagnosis which may be confirmed later by a further rise in antibody titres in serum and in CSF. In this way prompt and early diagnosis of arbovirus encephalitis, for example, should lead to public health control measures to contain epidemics such as the one in the United States in 1975, when encephalitis occurred at three times the usual annual rate and nearly 2000 cases of St Louis encephalitis were documented.

The early recognition of severe sporadic herpes simplex encephalitis is also particularly important as effective antiviral agents for the treatment of herpes infection are being developed. It is for this reason that the following section deals in some detail with the current methods of diagnosis and therapy of herpes encephalitis.

Herpes simplex encephalitis

When strict diagnostic criteria are applied to reported cases, it appears that up to 50 cases of severe herpes encephalitis occur in the United Kingdom annually. In the period April 1979–April 1980, 45 cases of herpes encephalitis were recorded in reports to the Communicable Disease Surveillance Centre (Table 9.2).

Acceptable diagnostic criteria are: (1) isolation of the virus from brain or CSF, or identification of

herpesvirus in brain tissue by immunofluorescence or electron microscopy, or (2) the appearance of specific antibody in the CSF. By these criteria there were 28 confirmed cases of herpes simplex encephalitis out of the 45 reported by virologists in England, Ireland and Wales over the 12-month period surveyed in Table 9.2.

Diagnosis

Demonstration of virus or antigens. Brain tissue or ventricular CSF is required to demonstrate the presence of virus or antigens.

Brain tissue obtained through a burr-hole biopsy, during decompressive craniotomy, or at autopsy, is divided into the following portions for examination:

1) For histopathology—fixed in formalin
2) For electron microscopy—fixed in glutaraldehyde
3) For virology; the tissue should be fresh and unfixed and it should be transported immediately to the laboratory for:

   a) Inoculation of tissue cultures for virus isolation

   b) Preparation of cryostat sections (or impression smears) for immunofluorescence

   c) Direct electron microscopy of negatively stained material for demonstration of herpesvirus particles

A diagnosis can be obtained within a few hours from immunofluorescence and from electron microscopy of negatively stained material. Isolation of the virus can be attempted in any virus laboratory, and the herpes simplex cytopathic effect may be recognised as early as 24h. Slides for immunofluorescence can be stored or sent to other laboratories for examination, as may material for electron microscopy. Details of techniques and reagents involved are given in standard laboratory reference texts.

Additional useful techniques include a cell-spreading method for the preparation of grids for negative staining; this technique avoids centrifugation. The array of particles in Fig. 9.7 was prepared by this technique; the virus particles in this illustration are incomplete and probably derived from a disrupted nucleus. Complete herpesvirus with an outer envelope is seen in Fig. 9.8. Both complete and incomplete virus can be detected by

Table 9.2. Herpes simplex encephalitis. Cases reported in England, Wales and Ireland between 6th April 1979 and 4th April 1980.[a]

Total number reported	45	
Males	25	
Females	20	
Number known to be dead	15	(33%)
Diagnostic criteria reported:		
Herpes simplex virus (HSV) identified		
in CNS	20	
Herpes simplex antibody rise in CSF	8	
HSV in other sites, serum antibody	17	

[a]Data from Communicable Disease Surveillance Centre, PHLS, London (unpublished). Reproduced here by permission.

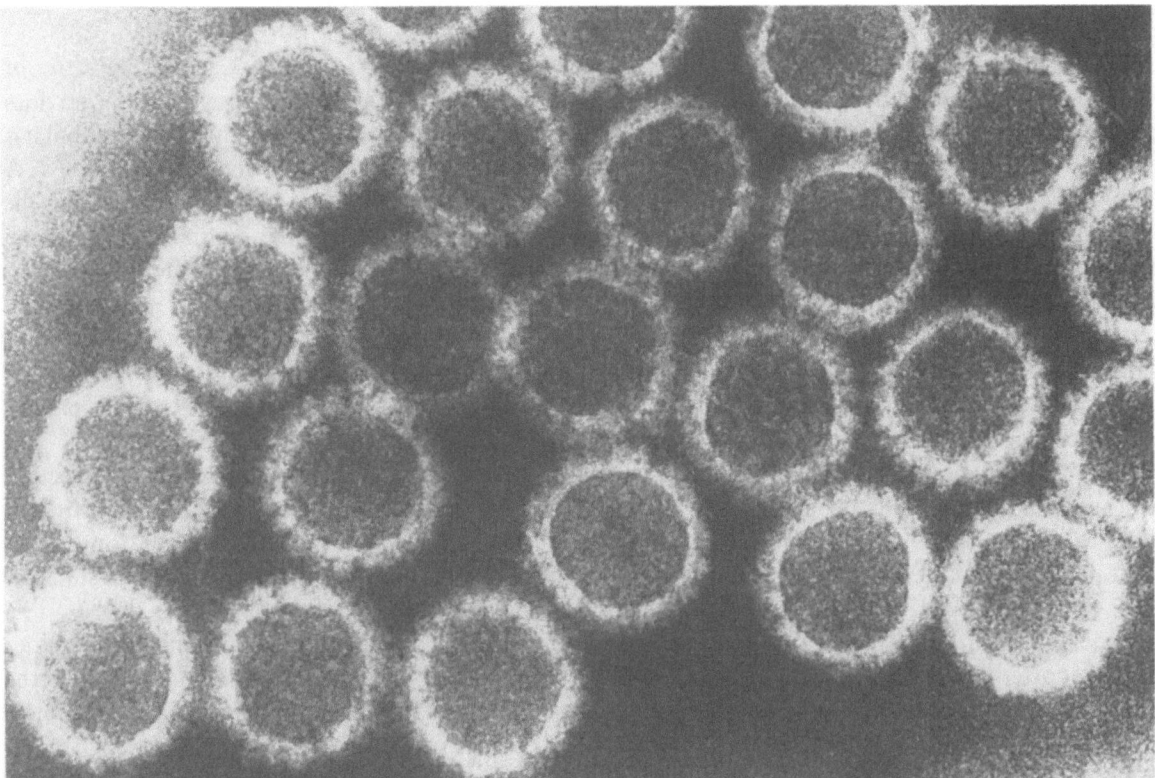

Fig. 9.7. Herpes simplex virus capsids released from brain biopsy tissue and negatively stained. (EM × 270 000)

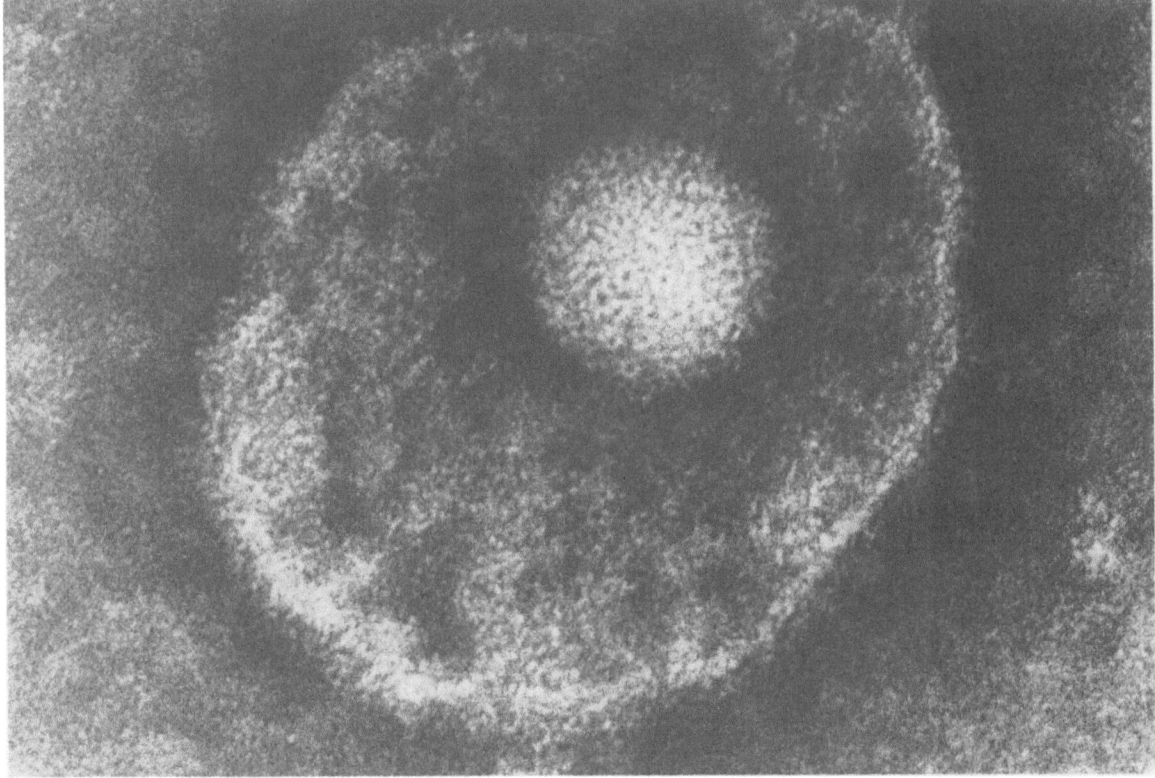

Fig. 9.8. Complete herpesvirus with outer envelope. Negatively stained. (EM × 378 000)

electron microscopy in sections of infected cells (Fig. 9.9).

When antibody is present, it may be difficult to isolate the virus, but prior trypsinisation of minced brain for some 30 min before inoculation into tissue culture improves the chance of successful virus culture.

Ventricular CSF may be used for culture and electron microscopy after ultra-centrifugation. Isolation of virus from lumbar CSF, however, has been reported only very rarely in cases of herpes simplex encephalitis. The failure to detect herpes antigens by immunofluorescence in cells from the CSF does not exclude the diagnosis. Electron microscopy of lumbar CSF should be undertaken but again, negative results do not exclude herpes encephalitis.

Tests for detecting specific viral antigens in the CSF of encephalitis patients are not yet available. The demonstration of soluble viral antigens has been reported, but this finding requires confirmation. Samples of CSF from cases of suspected,

or proven, encephalitis should be stored frozen for further study.

Demonstration of antibodies. A rising titre of antibody to herpes simplex virus in the serum does not constitute proof of herpetic encephalitis, but it is a useful adjunct to other diagnostic methods. A diagnosis based solely on antibody tests requires the demonstration of specific antibody production within the CNS, and this can be demonstrated in all cases during convalescence. Conventional complement-fixation methods will not detect antibody before the 10th day of the neurological illness, although more sensitive techniques such as passive haemagglutination and radioimmunoassay can reveal antibody by the 7th day. Antibody detection by immunofluorescence has advantages also; it is more often available in virology laboratories. IgM can be detected by this technique and the results can be made available within a few hours.

Antibody production within the CNS is demonstrated by the presence of IgM antibody in the CSF, or by a significant lowering of the serum to

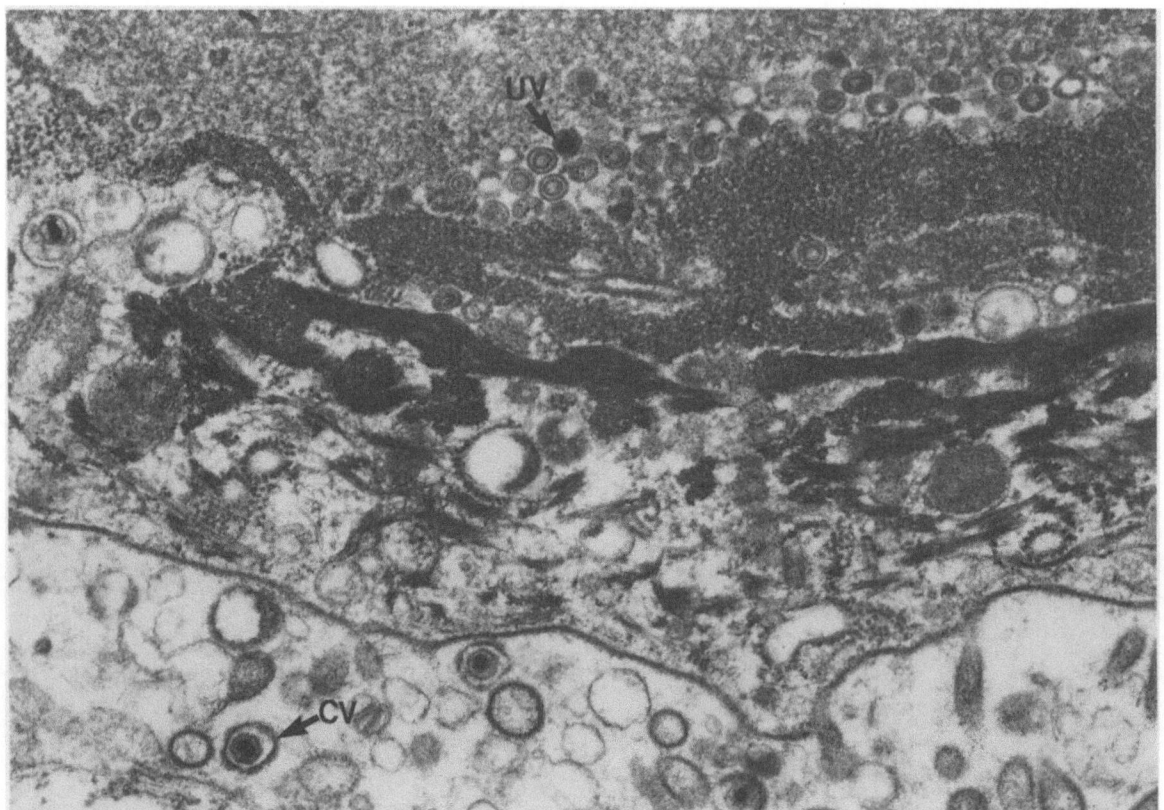

Fig. 9.9. Herpesvirus in an electron microscope section. The nucleus (*top of picture*) contains uncoated virus particules (*UV*). Coated virus particles (*CV*) have been released into the extracellular space at the *bottom of the picture*. (EM ×46000)

CSF antibody ratio. The normal ratio is $>200:1$; ratios $<40:1$ are considered to be diagnostic when the integrity of the blood–brain barrier is confirmed. IgM is a large molecule and does not easily pass across the blood–brain barrier, but IgG can be found in the CSF as a result of transudation across inflamed meninges. A simple control test consists of the parallel estimation of herpes antibody and an unrelated antibody, e.g. rubella in the serum and CSF. Another control is the IgG index in the CSF:

$$\text{IgG index} = \frac{\text{CSF IgG} \times \text{serum albumin}}{\text{serum IgG} \times \text{CSF albumin}}$$

(normal range 0.34–0.58).

An *increased* IgG index in the CSF indicates *local antibody production* in the CNS and if that antibody is shown to be herpes simplex antibody, the diagnosis of herpes encephalitis is confirmed.

Specimens of serum and CSF for antibody tests should be taken within 24 h of each other, and ideally, acute and convalescent samples should be tested. The optimum timing for the convalescent samples is 3–4 weeks after the onset of neurological signs. Blood-stained CSF cannot be used and further samples should be submitted to the laboratory as soon as practicable.

Typing of herpes simplex virus (HSV) in encephalitis

The majority of isolates from cases of acute herpetic encephalitis have been *HSV type 1* which is the type that usually infects the mouth, face and eyes. Encephalitis due to *HSV type 2*, the cause of most genital herpes, is usually confined to neonatal cases of disseminated infection acquired from the mother at birth. However, encephalitis due to HSV 2 has been described in immunosuppressed adults.

Genital herpes is a common sexually transmitted disease and in populations without prior experience of HSV 1, the primary disease is particularly severe. If HSV 2 meningitis develops in this group, encephalitis may also occur even in immunocompetent individuals. It is not current practice to use antiviral therapy to treat HSV meningitis, an uncommon disease with only four cases reported during 1979–1980 in the United Kingdom.

Specific antiviral therapy for herpes encephalitis

The original report of a collaborative trial in the United States of biopsy proven herpes encephalitis showed a mortality rate of 70 % (7/10) in a placebo group, and 28 % (5/18) in the group treated with adenine arabinoside (Vidarabine). Only patients treated early, before the stage of pre-coma, did well; this emphasises the importance of instituting early treatment. No antiviral drug can reverse extensive brain tissue damage, and although delayed treatment may allow the patient to survive, he may show severe residual neurological disability.

Acyclovir [9(2-hydroxyethoxymethyl)guanine] is an acyclic nucleoside (Fig. 9.10) which has little effect upon host cells but has a considerable inhibitory effect upon herpesvirus DNA replication. The compound enters virus-infected cells preferentially; as it enters the cells it is converted to a monophosphate by the viral thymidine kinase and subsequently to the triphosphate which is a potent

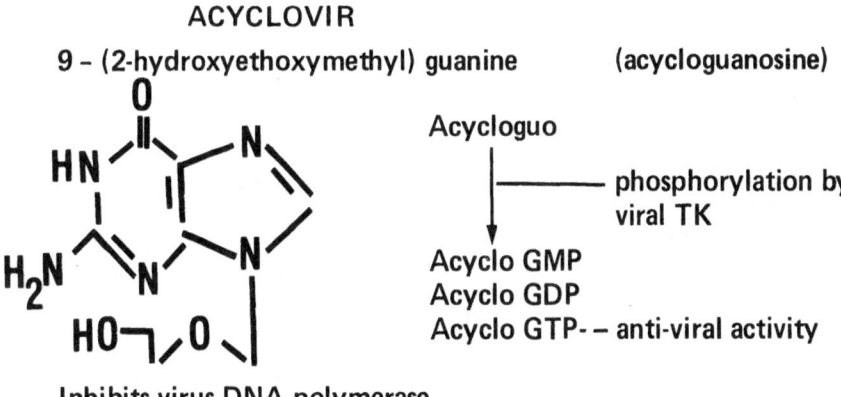

Fig. 9.10. The structure of Acyclovir [9(2-hydroxyethoxymethyl) guanine].

inhibitor of viral DNA polymerase. The sodium salt is used for IV infusion, 10 mg/kg given by slow infusion over 1 h, 8-hourly for 10 days. Providing renal function is monitored, the drug is remarkably non-toxic and has proved to be effective in muco-cutaneous herpes infections and in ocular infections. The results of treating individual cases of herpes encephalitis with Acyclovir have been sufficiently promising for a national trial to be organised.

Diagnosis of other viral encephalitides

There are no specific remedies, as yet, for any forms of viral encephalitis apart from herpes. When interferon becomes available, it may be useful in the treatment of encephalitis if it can be delivered to the brain tissue.

The approach to the diagnosis of other viral encephalitides, and the specimens required for identification of the causative virus, are similar to those set out in the section on herpes encephalitis. Brain tissue is seldom obtainable except at autopsy but as a wide range of antisera for immunofluorescent testing is held by many laboratories, examination of frozen sections by immunofluorescence is worthwhile in all cases. Unstained sections can be stored frozen or sent by post for examination at reference centres.

Where *rabies* infection is suspected, conjunctival cell smears can be examined by immunofluorescence for rapid diagnosis.

Slow virus encephalitis

Virological tests can confirm cases of suspected subacute encephalitis due to the measles virus (subacute sclerosing panencephalitis SSPE) or the human polyoma viruses (progressive multifocal leukoencephalopathy, PML). In SSPE, a high serum antibody titre to measles virus is found, with oligoclonal measles antibody in the CSF. If brain tissue is examined by special co-cultivation techniques, the virus can be isolated, and electron microscopy can reveal the typical paramyxovirus nucleocapsid tubules. Similarly, in PML, specific antibody may be found in the CSF and the polyoma virus may be cultivated by special techniques from brain tissue or identified by immunofluorescence. There is, as yet, no universally accepted therapy for these diseases.

Further reading

Clinical aspects of meningitis and encephalitis

Clyde W A (1980) Neurological syndromes and mycoplasmal infections. Arch Neurol 37: 65
Kennard C, Swash M (1981) Acute viral encephalitis. Brain 104: 129
Noah N D, Urquhart A M (1980) Virus meningitis and encephalitis in 1979. J Infect 2: 379

Reye's syndrome

Haller J (1980) Intracranial pressure monitoring in Reye's syndrome. Hosp Pract 15: 101
Trauner A (1980) Treatment of Reye's syndrome. Ann Neurol 7: 2

Pathology

Adams J H (1976) Virus diseases of the nervous system. In: Blackwood W, Corsellis J A N (eds) Greenfield's neuropathology, 3rd edn. Arnold, London, p 292

Herpes simplex

Longson M, Bailey A S (1977) Herpes encephalitis. In: Waterson A P (ed) Recent advances in clinical virology—1. Churchill Livingstone, Edinburgh
Longson M, Bailey A S, Klapper P (1980) Herpes encephalitis. In: Waterson A P (ed) Recent advances in clinical virology—2. Churchill Livingstone, Edinburgh

Antiviral chemotherapy

Bauer D J (1979) Antiviral chemotherapy. In: Heath R B (ed) Virus diseases. Pitman Medical, London
Whitley R J, Soong S-J, Dolin R et al. (1977) Adenine arabinoside therapy of biopsy-proved herpes simplex encephalitis. New Engl J Med 297: 289

'Slow virus' diseases

Masters C L, Richardson E P (1978) Subacute spongiform encephalopathy (Creutzfeldt–Jakob disease). Brain 101: 333
Walker D L (1978) Progressive multifocal leukoencephalopathy: an opportunistic viral infection of the central nervous system. In: Vinken P J, Bruyn G W (eds) Handbook of clinical neurology, vol 34, Infections of the nervous system, Part II. Elsevier/North-Holland Biomedical, Amsterdam, p 307

Standard laboratory virology texts

Grist N R, Bell E J, Follett E A C, Urquhart G E D (1979) Diagnostic methods in clinical virology, 3rd edn. Blackwell Scientific, Oxford
Lennette E H, Schmidt N J (eds) (1979) Diagnostic procedures for virus rickettsial and chlamydial infections, 5th edn. American Public Health Association, Washington

Chapter 10

Bacterial, Fungal and Parasitic Infections of the Central Nervous System

Bacterial infections

There are *acute* and *chronic* forms of bacterial infections of the CNS. The infection may be primarily localised in the subarachnoid space and ventricular system, i.e. bacterial *meningitis* and *ventriculitis*, or may involve the parenchyma of the brain itself leading to the formation of a cerebral *abscess*. On rare occasions, infections may cause subdural abscesses or involve the epidural spaces with secondary spread to the subarachnoid space or to the parenchyma of the brain. Bacterial infections may spread to the brain and spinal cord either by haematogenous routes or by direct spread from surrounding tissue. Thus bacterial meningitis or cerebral abscess may occur as complications of head injury when fractures at the base of the skull perforate the meninges or even perforate the brain itself. Furthermore, infection in the bones of the skull, as in chronic otitis media or chronic petrositis may lead to secondary invasion of the brain. Infection may also spread to the subarachnoid space from a primary site of infection in the paranasal air sinuses. In some cases, bacterial infections of the CNS are a complication of malignant disease in which erosion of the bones of the skull or spine has occurred; the infection thus enters the brain through a break in the meninges.

Bacterial meningitis

Bacterial meningitis is commonest at the extremes of life. Most cases thus occur in neonates and infants, and in the elderly. Epidemic meningitis, usually due to *Neisseria meningitidis*, however, may occur in young adults. The causes of bacterial meningitis differ according to the age of onset and susceptibility of the individual. Even with antibiotic treatment, bacterial meningitis is always a serious disorder but before the era of effective antimicrobial agents, there was a high mortality and a high incidence of disabling late complications in patients who survived the initial infection.

Clinical features

Although certain specific features may occur in association with different types of bacterial meningitis, the clinical picture is dominated by the signs of meningeal inflammation. The patients appear ill and may be comatose or stuporose with a high temperature accompanied by sweating and vasodilatation. Often the respiratory rate is increased, with deep sighing respirations, and the pulse is slower than expected in relation to the fever; this is an indication of raised intracranial pressure. The patient is irritable when disturbed and prefers to lie in a dark, quiet environment. In extreme cases, there may be a tendency to assume a hyperextended posture but most patients present before this late stage and may lie slightly flexed on their sides. There is marked neck rigidity. On ophthalmoscopy, the fundal veins appear engorged but it is unusual to find papilloedema in uncomplicated bacterial meningitis. Sometimes there is an accompanying pneumonia, and a skin rash is a prominent feature of meningococcal meningitis. There may be signs of recent cranial trauma. Examination of the external auditory meati may reveal pus, or septic perforation of the tympanic membrane with pus in the middle ear. There may be evidence of bacterial sinusitis, or of a recent upper respiratory tract infection. The history of the onset of the infection is often non-specific but may be quite brief with only a few hours of rigor followed by lethargy and stupor.

Even in the relatively *acute* stages, there is a risk that blood vessels in the subarachnoid space will become inflamed and thrombosed with consequent *infarction* of the brain. This usually presents with focal seizures and hemiplegia and is often followed by marked cerebral oedema, and by papilloedema. The prognosis in such cases is poor. Sometimes bacterial meningitis is itself a complication of cerebral abscess especially when the abscess is near the surface of the brain and the infection spreads to the subarachnoid space; similar spread of infection into the ventricles may occur from deep-seated abscesses. The prognosis in these cases is also poor and there is a risk that the abscess may actually rupture with the release of pus into the subarachnoid or ventricular fluid.

Chronic or subacute forms

Not all patients with bacterial meningitis exhibit a rapidly progressive course. This is particularly so in *tuberculous* meningitis where the onset of the disease is non-specific and subacute, sometimes extending over several weeks. Fever is not usually a major feature but the patient may complain of headache, stiffness of the neck, depressive symptoms, tiredness and malaise. The disease may not become apparent until signs of bacterial inflammation with neck stiffness, fever and changes in the CSF present. Sometimes, tuberculous meningitis occurs as a complication of tuberculous infection near the meninges. In Pott's disease for example, where there is tuberculous infection of the vertebrae and intervertebral discs, the infection may extend through the meninges to involve the spinal roots and lead intitially to localised spinal arachnoiditis. Later, the infection may become disseminated in the spinal and cranial meninges.

Fungal meningitis is a rare disorder in the United Kingdom but it is commoner in the United States and in warmer climates; it usually pursues a protracted course at onset, although some infections, for example mucormycosis, may present with an acute craniofacial cellulitis with involvement of the meninges.

Immunosuppressed patients, and patients in generally poor health are particularly prone to meningitis, both of acute bacterial and subacute tubercular types.

Late complications

In bacterial meningitis, there is an inflammatory response in the meninges, particularly involving the arachnoid. Organisation of the inflammatory exudate leads to fibrosis, thickening of the meninges, and a variable degree of obliteration of the subarachnoid space. This is often sufficient to interfere with the circulation of the CSF so that communicating or non-communicating hydrocephalus may develop. Cranial nerve palsies also occur, commonly involving those nerves, such as the sixth nerve, which have a long course through the subarachnoid space at the base of the brain; such palsies usually resolve. Facial weakness, deafness and blindness from the involvement of the seventh, eighth and optic nerves are rare complications now that treatment is more effective, but recovery from these disabilities is less likely to be complete. If the parenchyma of the brain is involved by infarction or by direct infection, then epilepsy, mental retardation or focal neurological disorders such as hemiplegia and spasticity may be evident.

CSF examination

As many as half of all patients admitted to hospital with meningitis have already been treated with antibiotics at home. This, however, has not altered the results of CSF examination as much as might have been expected. It has been shown that pre-admission antibiotic therapy does not significantly alter the results of total white cell counts, the percentage of polymorphonuclear leukocytes, or the protein and glucose levels in the CSF. However, antibiotic treatment does reduce the chance of finding organisms on Gram-stained films of CSF from about 98% in untreated patients, to 70%. In particular, the concentration of bacteria in the CSF, especially in the case of penicillin-resistant organisms such as *Neisseria meningitidis*, is reduced by previous antibiotic therapy, even when quite small doses are used.

Lumbar puncture is a pre-requisite for the diagnosis of meningitis, since only by examination of the CSF can the diagnosis be confirmed. The CSF pressure is increased and the CSF, in typical cases, appears cloudy and viscous. Slight cloudiness, or a slight increase in viscosity of the CSF may be significant abnormalities. The total *white cell* count in the CSF is increased and consists almost entirely of polymorphonuclear leukocytes (Fig. 10.1) in the case of bacterial meningitis, and of lymphocytes in the case of tuberculous or fungal meningitis. Even a few polymorphonuclear leukocytes in a lymphocytic exudate, however, should raise the suspicion of bacterial infection either within the meninges, or contiguous with them. A predominantly lympho-cystic CSF is a major feature of viral meningitic infections (see Chap. 9). The CSF *protein* in bacterial meningitis is greatly increased, often to levels of more than 5 g/litre. In tuberculous meningitis the increase in protein is much greater, and when the protein content of the CSF exceeds 20 g/litre a web-like clot may form within the fluid.

The diagnosis of bacterial meningitis rests not only upon determination of differential white cell

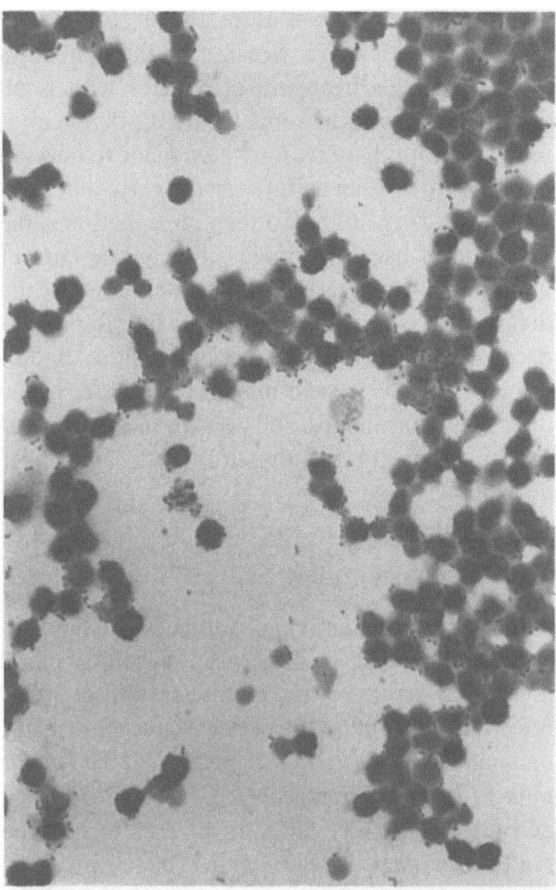

Fig. 10.1. Pneumococcal meningitis. CSF containing polymorphonuclear leukocytes and bacteria (*Strep. pneumoniae*) (Gram stain × 550)

counts in the fluid, but also upon the estimation of the *glucose* level in the CSF, and its comparison with the glucose level in the blood taken at the same time. In normal CSF, the glucose level is approximately two-thirds that in the blood; whereas in patients with bacterial, tuberculous or fungal meningitis the CSF glucose is reduced to less than half the level in the blood. Since there are fluctuations of blood glucose in normal subjects, and particularly in patients stressed by infection, or by diabetes, it is evidently essential to compare the levels in blood and CSF. Reduction in CSF glucose levels also occurs in patients with carcinomatous invasion of the meninges (carcinomatous meningitis) and to a very slight extent in patients with measles and mumps virus meningitis but not usually in the latter diseases to levels lower than 50% of that in the blood.

The CSF specimen should not only be examined for inflammatory cells and for biochemical abnormalities but should also be studied *bacteriologically* so that organisms present in the fluid can be identified by Gram stains of the deposit or by bacteriological culture. Because of the difficulties arising from the treatment of patients with small doses of antibiotics at home before the diagnosis is made, attempts have recently been made to develop methods other than culture for the early detection of causative organisms. Among these methods, the detection of bacterial antigens by counter-current immunoelectrophoresis is now widely used in the diagnosis of *Haemophilus influenzae* type B, pneumococcal and meningococcal meningitis. Estimation of CSF lactic acid may also be useful in the diagnosis of meningitis, and tests for the presence of endotoxin or for inflammatory cells are under development.

Bacteriology of meningitis

Although any organism may cause CNS infection in a susceptible host, few organisms regularly cause meningitis as a major manifestation of their infection. The important bacteria causing primary meningitis are *Neisseria meningitidis*, *Haemophilus influenzae* and *Streptococcus pneumoniae*. They account for 70% of all cases of meningitis. The relative frequencies with which these three organisms are found in cases of meningitis differ according to the age group. Between the ages of 2 months and 5 years, *H. influenzae* is the commonest infection followed by *N. meningitidis* and then by *S. pneumoniae*. From the age of 5 years to 30 years, *N. meningitidis* is the commonest cause of meningitis. After the age of 30–40 years, *S. pneumoniae* becomes the most common, and *H. influenzae* the least common infection.

Meningococcal meningitis

Neisseria meningitidis is a Gram-negative coccus occurring in pairs and is the commonest cause of bacterial meningitis in the United Kingdom. It can be divided into several serogroups. Group B predominates in children and is usually responsible for the sporadic cases, whereas groups A and C are commonly associated with epidemics. Meningococcal infection occurs sporadically throughout the year in the United Kingdom.

N. meningitidis is a parasite of the human nasopharynx in 2%–8% of healthy people. The incidence of carriage of an epidemic strain may be as high as 80%–90% in closed populations, e.g.

military camps. In each individual, natural immunity is reinforced and broadened by the intermittent carriage of different strains of meningococci throughout life. The unsuspected carrier of a virulent strain serves as a reservoir from which susceptible people may be infected. Secondary cases of meningitis may develop in as many as 5% of families in which an index case (the first diagnosed case) has occurred. The organism is transmitted mainly by droplet spread.

The meningococcus is sensitive to *penicillin*. Resistance to sulphonamide has been noted in nearly 50% of group A, 20% of Group C and 10% of group B strains in the United Kingdom.

Infection of the meninges forms part of a *septicaemic* process which may be overwhelming and associated with a petechial or purpuric rash in 50% of cases; disseminated intravascular coagulation may also occur. The Waterhouse–Friderichsen syndrome, with adrenal haemorrhage, circulatory collapse and cyanosis is a complication in some patients with *N. meningitidis* septicaemia.

Haemophilus meningitis

Haemophilus influenzae is a small pleomorphic Gram-negative rod, which is present in the nasopharynx as a commensal in some 50% of healthy adults, and in a large proportion of healthy children. It occurs mostly in the non-capsulated forms which cause acute and chronic secondary (endogenous) respiratory tract infections. Capsulated strains, which are more invasive and mostly of type B, are found only in 2%–4% of people at any one time.

Nearly all systemic infections of *H. influenzae*, half of which are accompanied by meningitis, are caused by type B strains. This organism is the commonest cause of meningitis in the United States and in Australia, and has its highest incidence in young children between the ages of 2 months and 5 years. There is a high frequency of nasopharyngeal carriage of type B organisms among the close contacts of children with illnesses caused by this serotype.

H. influenzae is generally sensitive to *ampicillin* and *choramphenicol*, but resistant strains, particularly to ampicillin, are becoming more frequent.

The mortality from *H. influenzae* meningitis approaches 10% and many of the survivors have residual brain damage.

Pneumococcal meningitis

Streptococcus pneumoniae is a Gram-positive coccus occurring in pairs. There are 84 different serotypes. The majority of cases of *S. pneumoniae* meningitis are caused by a limited number of serotypes; infection by type 3 is the commonest in the United Kingdom. Nasopharyngeal carriage of *S. pneumoniae* is common.

Not uncommonly, pneumococcal meningitis is associated with predisposing factors, which suggests that it occurs as an opportunistic infection. There may be a suppurative focus present in another part of the body, e.g. pneumonia, sinusitis or a structural cranial defect. Alternatively, there may be a systemic disorder which alters the patient's response to infection as occurs following splenectomy in childhood. *S. pneumoniae* is also an important agent in recurrent meningitis.

The organism is sensitive to *penicillin*, but a few penicillin-insensitive strains have been reported from Australia and South Africa, some of which may also show resistance to a number of other antibiotics.

Prevention of meningitis

Chemoprophylaxis is useful as a preventive measure in the families or close contacts of a case of primary meningitis. In meningococcal infections, sulphonamides can be given to individuals at risk if a sensitive strain is involved, or rifampicin can be administered. Similarly, prophylactic penicillin has been given to children after splenectomy. There is as yet no drug, or combination of drugs, that can be confidently recommended for this purpose for children who are the close contacts of a case of *Haemophilus* meningitis.

Vaccines prepared from purified capsular polysaccharides of *N. meningitidis* serogroups A and C are available and are effective in preventing meningococcal meningitis of similar serotypes. Polyvalent pneumococcal vaccines containing antigens of the major types associated with pneumonia and meningitis have been shown to give good protection in controlled trials. *H. influenzae* vaccine, prepared from the type B polyribose phosphate, is disappointingly ineffective in young children under 18 months of age, who constitute two-thirds of the cases of *H. influenzae* meningitis.

Gram-negative infections

Gram-negative bacillary meningitis, other than neonatal meningitis and meningitis caused by *H. influenzae*, is mostly acquired in hospital and has increased in incidence during the last 20 years. Nearly 80% of cases are associated with head injury and neurosurgery. *Klebsiella spp.* are the organisms most frequently involved followed by *E. coli* and *Pseudomonas spp*; these organisms are normally present in the bowel, on the skin, and in the environment. Indirect routes of infection from the hands of staff, or cooking utensils are important modes of transmission from patient to patient. These hospital organisms are often resistant to many antibiotics; they flourish in patients treated with broad-spectrum antibiotics.

Neonatal meningitis

A disease which occurs in babies under 2 months of age, neonatal meningitis has an incidence of 1 in 2500 live births. It is more common in babies of low birth weight and in those with congenital malformations or born with obstetric complications. The most important organism in this group is *E. coli*. Eighty percent of *E. coli* strains carry the capsular K1 antigen which appears to be associated with high morbidity and mortality.

Streptococcus agelactiae (group B streptococcus) is responsible for almost one-third of cases of neonatal meningitis. The major reservoir for this organism is the female genital tract from which it can be isolated in about 30% of normal women. Strains isolated from early onset infections are likely to be of maternal origin, whereas those causing late onset infections are probably acquired in hospital.

Other important organisms in neonatal meningitis include *Listeria monocytogenes* and *Salmonella spp*. The pathogens already described, *N. meningitidis*, *H. influenzae* and *S. pneumoniae* are less important in this period.

Pathology of bacterial meningitis

The macroscopic hallmark of pyogenic meningitis is pus in the subarachnoid space (Fig. 10.2). This is clearly visible at autopsy and is particularly prominent over the vertex and base of the brain. Microscopic examination shows that the pus extends into the superficial layers of the cortex along the perivascular Virchow–Robin spaces. In the early stages of bacterial meningitis, dilatation of meningeal vessels is a major feature. Later, the basal cisterns become filled with pus which extends over

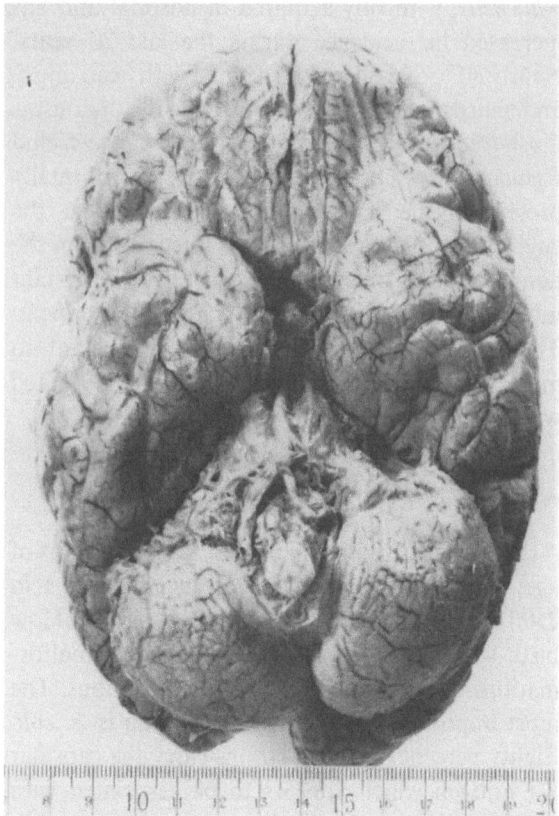

Fig. 10.2. Bacterial meningitis. Basal aspect of a brain from a patient with acute purulent leptomeningitis showing a thick layer of pus most prominent in the basal meninges. The meningeal vessels are prominent and dilated.

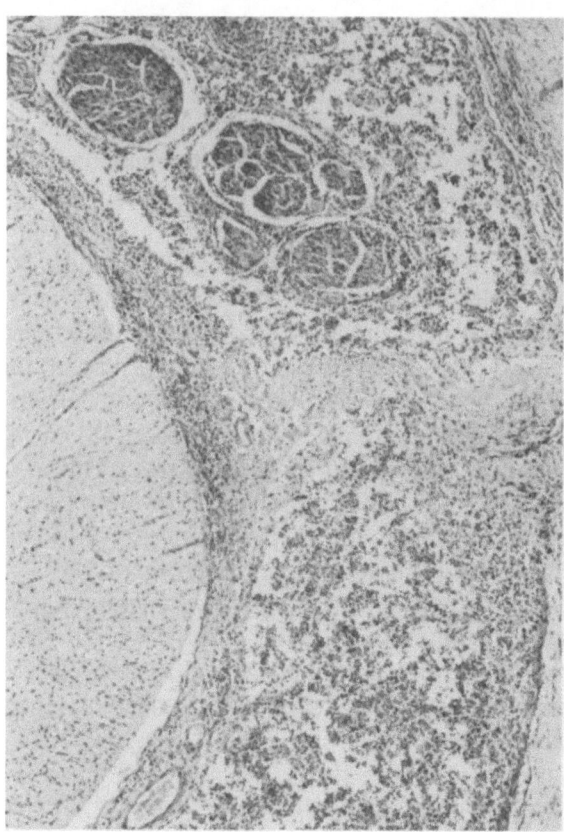

Fig. 10.3. A photomicrograph of the spinal cord and nerve roots in acute purulent meningitis. The subarachnoid space is filled with pus (H & E × 60)

the whole surface of the brain, filling the subarachnoid space and the ventricular system; at this stage, spasm and constriction of the major blood vessels in the subarachnoid space may occur. Pus may infiltrate the choroid plexus and also extend over the posterior aspect of the spinal cord, eventually involving the whole of its length.

Sections of the brain reveal pus in the depths of the sulci and, in many cases, extensive oedema of the hemispheres. Petechial haemorrhages in the grey and white matter are a feature of meningococcal meningitis and focal infarction may be seen in many cases of purulent meningitis. Meningeal vessels, bathed by pus in the subarachnoid space, are inflamed and may be occluded by thrombus. The infarction resulting from such vascular occlusion may be extensive if a large artery is involved or may be focal if it is the small surface-penetrating vessels which are blocked.

Microscopic examination of brain sections in the acute stages of meningitis show a subarachnoid space filled with polymorphonuclear leukocytes

(Fig. 10.3) with pus spreading into the cortex along the perivascular space. Small foci or microabscesses may also be seen within the white matter. At a later stage in the disease lymphocytes, plasma cells and macrophages appear in increasing numbers. The causative organism can sometimes be identified by Gram stains in autopsy sections.

Examination of the *skull* at autopsy is important as a septic focus may be found in the air sinuses or middle ear. Osteomyelitis of the *spine* may also be a focus from which infection has spread to the meninges.

In *partially treated* cases of meningitis and in some patients who have recovered, fibrosis of the meninges is common and is often associated with hydrocephalus, especially if the basal meninges are involved. Sometimes encysted collections of pus occur, particularly in the meninges around the spinal cord, resulting in damage to the cord from compression or infarction. Clinically, such patients may develop paraplegia.

Tuberculous meningitis and tuberculomas

Tuberculous meningitis (TBM) is always secondary to tuberculosis elsewhere in the body and is particularly common in the young and in the very old. It may be a complication of miliary tuberculosis, or the tuberculous infection may spread from active pulmonary tuberculosis, particularly in the adult. In addition to haematogenous spread, tuberculosis may invade the CNS from a tuberculous spine as in a patient with Pott's disease. *Clinically*, the onset of tuberculous meningitis is insidious but may be marked by cranial nerve palsies, and by rapid deterioration from cerebral infarction if the major cerebral arteries become thrombosed due to their involvement in the tuberculous process.

Although tuberculosis in the CNS is usually seen as meningitis in Britain, certain populations, particularly Asians, develop localised tuberculous lesions. These *tuberculomas* present as space-occupying lesions and show signs of a mass effect but rarely give rise to the clinical signs of meningeal inflammation. Tuberculomas may be single or multiple; they may be the sole sign of a tuberculous infection or may even develop during the treatment of tuberculous meningitis. Tuberculosis in the spine may be complicated by radiculopathies.

In the United Kingdom, TBM accounts for 7% of all non-pulmonary tuberculous infections.

Bovine types of tuberculosis are responsible for less than 5% of all cases of meningitis where *Mycobacterium tuberculosis* is isolated. The CSF in tuberculous meningitis has a high protein but the organisms are very scanty, and the chance of finding acid-fast bacilli by fluorescence microscopy in a centrifuged deposit of CSF from a patient with TBM is only about 10%–22%. Much better results are obtained by CSF cultures in which about 90% of cases are positive. Nearly 50% of all patients with TBM have positive tuberculous infections elsewhere in the body from which organisms can also be cultured.

At *autopsy* the brains of patients dying with tuberculous meningitis reveal thickening and fibrosis of the arachnoid (Fig. 10.4) particularly over the base of the brain (Fig. 10.5). In some cases small tubercles may be identified. Cerebral infarction may be seen as in pyogenic meningitis due to involvement of major cerebral vessels and intraluminal thrombosis (Figs. 10.5, 10.6).

Microscopic examination of the meninges shows caseating granulomas which may be in a miliary pattern. Cranial nerves and vessels may show partial destruction. Typical tubercles consisting of a central area of caseous necrosis surrounded by epithelioid macrophages and lymphocytes with prominent Langhans giant cells are seen in active tuberculous meningitis (Figs. 10.6, 10.7). Although the inflammation may spread into the superficial layers of the cortex and brain stem, most of the

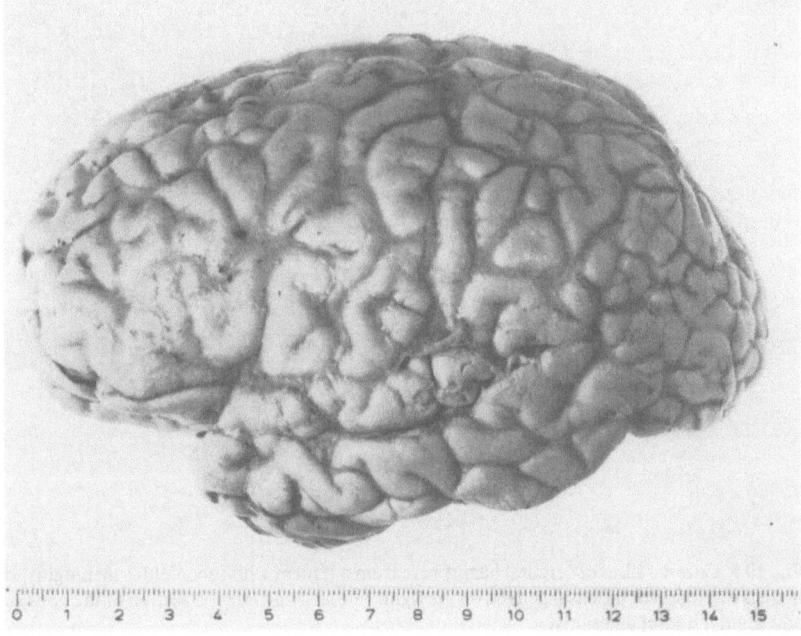

Fig. 10.4. Tuberculous meningitis. Brain showing granularity and thickening of the arachnoid over the frontal and parietal lobes.

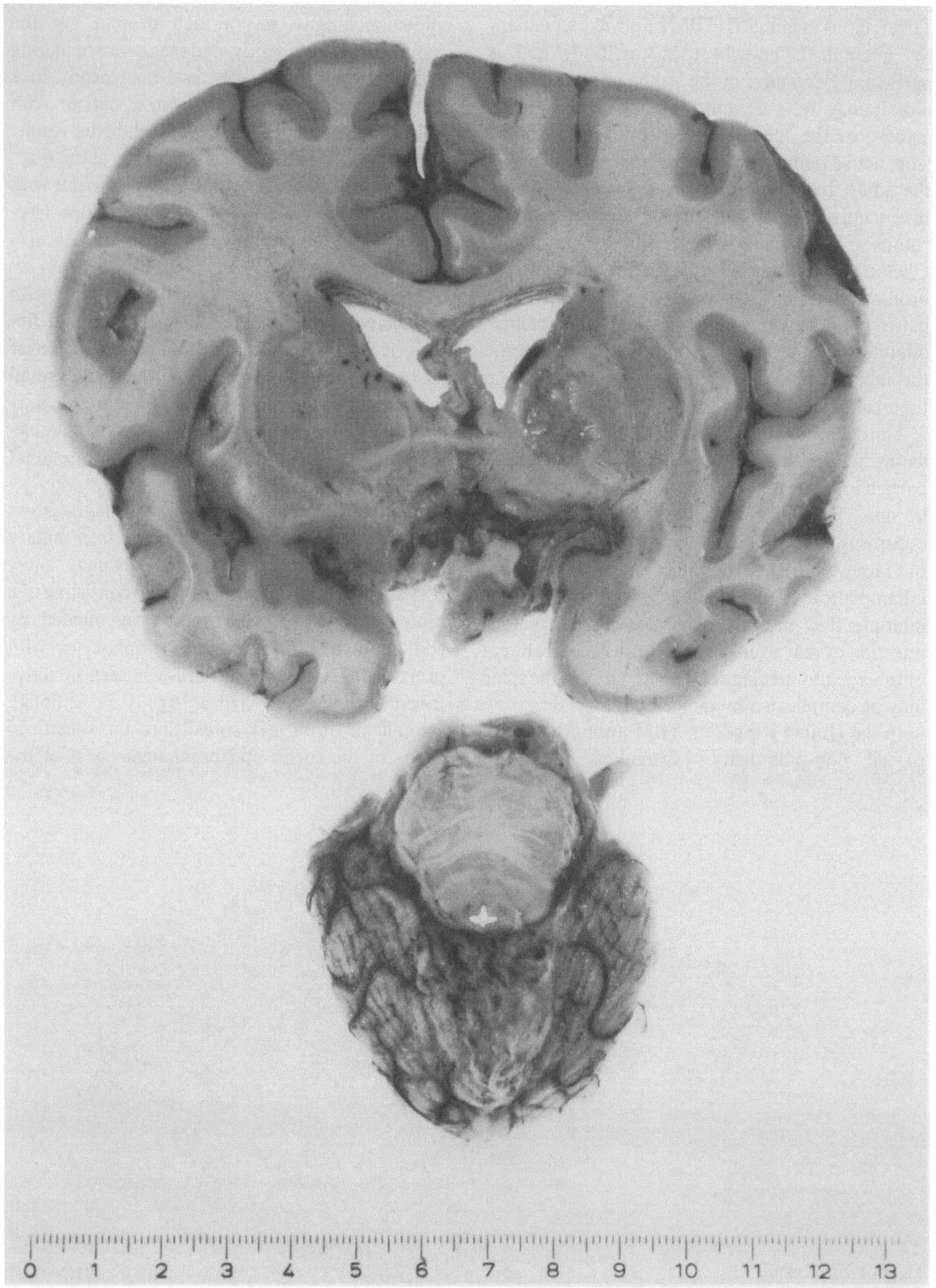

Fig. 10.5. Coronal slices of cerebral hemisphere from a patient with tuberculous meningitis, showing thickening of the basal meninges; there is infarction of the basal ganglia on the right. The *lower picture* is a section of the pons showing exudate in the subarachnoid space and a small infarct anteriorly.

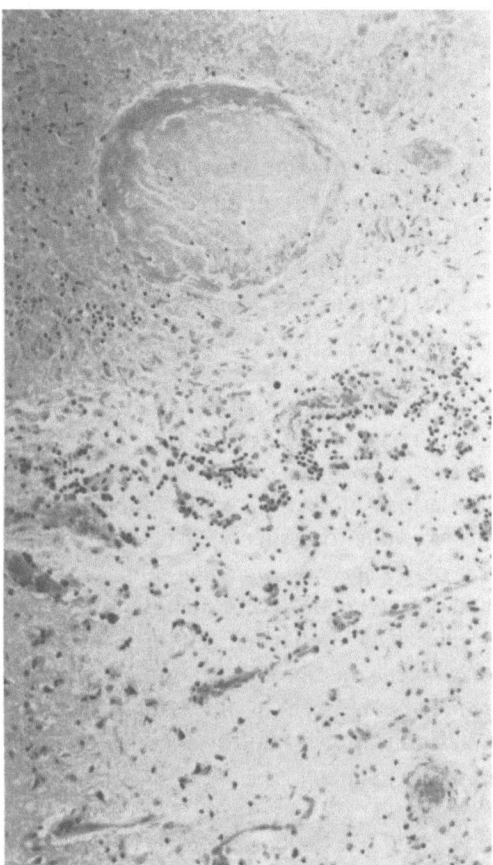

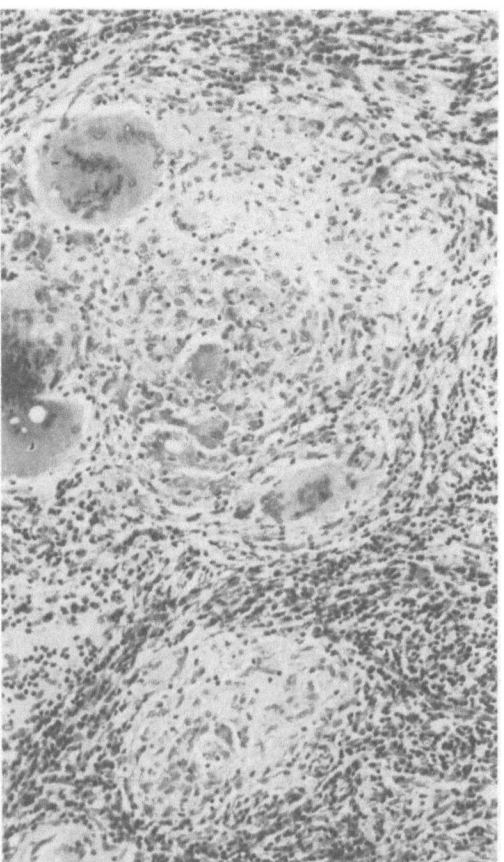

Fig. 10.6. Tuberculous meningitis. A thrombosed meningeal vessel is surrounded by caseous material (*top*). Inflamed and infarcted cortex is seen in the lower part of the picture. (H & E ×100)

Fig. 10.7. Tuberculous meningitis showing giant cell granulomas in the meninges. (H & E × 150)

damage to the brain is due to ischaemia from arterial thrombosis. Tuberculomas may be seen in the cerebral hemispheres or in the cerebellum; there is a mass of caseous necrosis surrounded by tuberculous granuloma. Frequently the tuberculoma has a fibrous capsule which may become calcified in older lesions. Acid-fast bacilli may be detectable in sectioned material from cases of tuberculous meningitis and in tuberculomas.

The intense fibrosis that occurs in tuberculous meningitis may lead, in treated cases, to obliteration of the subarachnoid space and to subsequent hydrocephalus.

Neurosyphilis

Treponema pallidum enters the site of primary infection and very quickly spreads via the lymphatics to the blood and is soon distributed throughout the body. In the *primary* and *secondary* forms of syphilis, invasion of the nervous system is not usually clinically apparent although there is sometimes a mild meningeal reaction with neck stiffness and fever persisting for a few days or weeks. At this stage the disease is curable. CNS complications are more a feature of the *tertiary* stage of syphilis when, as a rule, signs of meningovascular syphilis precede the development of parenchymatous neurosyphilis. However, parenchymatous disease, especially tabes dorsalis and dementia, may occur as the presenting feature of neurosyphilis. Meningovascular and parenchymatous forms of the disease almost never coexist.

Neurosyphilis may present *clinically* with a wide variety of neurological patterns and these are summarised in Table 10.1. The CSF in active neurosyphilis usually shows an increase in mononuclear cells and almost invariably gives a positive Venereal Disease Research Laboratories (VDRL)

Table 10.1. Classification of neurosyphilis

Primary infection: meningeal infection may occur
Secondary stage (latent neurosyphilis): inapparent
meningeal inflammation
Tertiary neurosyphilis;
A. Meningovascular syphilis (tertiary syphilitic meningitis)
    (i) Basal meningitis
    (ii) Syphilitic spinal arachnoiditis
    (iii) Pachymeningitis hypertrophica cervicalis (Charcot
       and Joffroy)
    (iv) Meningeal gumma
B Syphilitic arteritis
C Parenchymatous neurosyphilis
    (i) Tabes dorsalis
    (ii) General paralysis of the insane (paretic dementia)
    (iii) Syphilitic optic atrophy
    (iv) Syphilitic deafness
D Congenital syphilis

reaction. The Wasserman reaction, and the TPI and FTA reactions, confirm the diagnosis.

Meningovascular syphilis results in diffuse inflammation and thickening of the meninges around the base of the brain and around the spinal cord. Clinically the patient may present with confusion, headache, neck stiffness and gait disorder as hydrocephalus develops. The basal meningitis may also cause multiple cranial nerve palsies resulting in deafness, blindness with primary optic atrophy and oculomotor and abducens palsies. Spinal nerve roots may be affected when there is spinal arachnoiditis. Long tract signs may also develop due to intrinsic spinal cord damage.

Parenchymatous neurosyphilis occurs in two major forms. In one type, *tabes dorsalis*, the lesions are predominantly spinal. Clinical presentation is often with pain in the legs, frequently described as rheumatism or lightning pains. In the legs there is impairment of position sense and vibration sense, and of deep pain, and a sensory ataxia is common. A characteristic ptosis is seen with Argyll Robertson pupils; primary optic atrophy and deafness may occur as associated features. Tendon reflexes are usually absent in the legs. The syndrome is gradually progressive and dementia may occur in untreated cases in the late stages. *Pathologically*, the most striking feature of tabes dorsalis is degeneration of the dorsal columns of the spinal cord and in the dorsal roots. The exact cause of this distribution of damage is not fully understood.

General paralysis of the insane (GPI) is the other major type of parenchymatous neurosyphilis. Dementia presents at a late stage of tertiary parenchymatous neurosyphilis. The dementia begins insidiously and sometimes in conjunction with features of tabes dorsalis; it is accompanied by recurrent seizures, tremulousness and myoclonus, dysarthria, corticospinal signs and focal, stroke-like neurological symptoms. *Pathologically*, the frontal lobes are most severely affected by loss of neurons of all layers of the cerebral cortex and by proliferation of astroglia and microglia. Small blood vessels are thickened and frequently surrounded by cuffs of lymphocytes and plasma cells. The meninges also show prominent infiltration by lymphocytes and plasma cells. *Treponema pallidum* can be demonstrated in the cortex with appropriate silver stains. Patients with GPI thus show features of chronic meningoencephalitis with vascular involvement.

The *basic pathological mechanisms* involved in syphilitic lesions appear to be a combination of tissue necrosis due to tissue hypersensitivity to the presence of *Treponema pallidum* and of tissue ischaemia due to endarteritis obliterans in small vessels. Necrosis is particularly prominent in gummas whereas the signs of the immune response to *T. pallidum* are seen in the lymphocyte and plasma cell infiltration around arteries in most other types of tertiary syphilis.

Shunt-associated meningitis

Up to 20% of patients treated with ventriculo-atrial or ventriculo-peritoneal shunts develop meningitis. More than half these infections are caused by the coagulase-negative staphylococci which are part of our normal skin flora.

Fungal meningitis

In many cases fungal meningitis is associated with underlying conditions causing impaired cellular immune responses, e.g. Hodgkin's disease or non-Hodgkin's lymphoma. *Cryptococcus neoformans* is the most common cause of fungal meningitis in the United Kingdom. The organism can be seen as a spherical yeast in India ink preparations of CSF specimens in more than half the cases, but a much more reliable diagnosis can be made by the latex agglutination test which allows detection of the presence of cryptococcal antigen in CSF and serum in more than 90% of cases. Confirmation of diagnosis by culture of the organism is, nevertheless, mandatory and culture plates should be incubated for 5–7 days. *Pathologically* the meninges

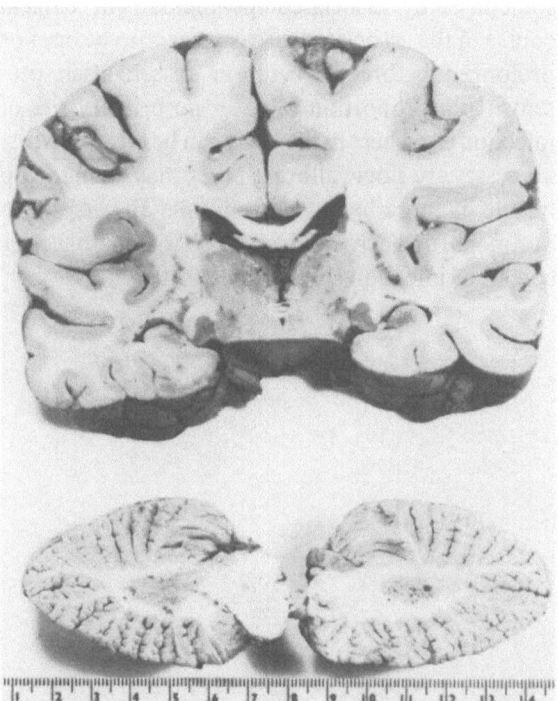

Fig. 10.8. Infection of the brain with *Cryptococcus neoformans*: slices of the brain show numerous cysts up to 3 mm in diameter both in the cortex of the cerebral hemisphere (*upper right*) and in the dentate nuclei of the cerebellum.

are thickened and opalescent. Brain slices show small cysts up to 3 mm in diameter both in the cortex and more deeply placed (Fig. 10.8).

Meningitis caused by *Candida albicans*, *Aspergillus* (Fig. 10.10) and *Actinomyces* is rare in Britain. Some other forms of fungal meningitis, e.g. histoplasmosis and mucormycosis, are well known in the tropics and in North America, but are not indigenous in the United Kingdom.

Other causes of meningitis

There are a number of other types of bacterial meningitis in which routine bacteriological examination of the CSF does not immediately reveal the aetiological agent. These include syphilis (see above), leptospirosis and mycoplasma (see Chap. 9) infections. In Mollaret's recurrent lymphocytic meningitis, repeated episodes of meningitis occur without evident cause. Meningeal inflammation is also a feature in some patients with sarcoidosis and Behçet's syndrome.

A chronic sterile meningitis may occur in patients when irritative material escapes from tumours into the subarachnoid space; this is particularly

characteristic of craniopharyngioma (see Chap. 8). Direct neoplastic invasion of the meninges occurs in metastatic carcinoma and lymphomas. In these cases there is rarely clinical evidence of meningitis but there may be cranial nerve palsies. The CSF contains lymphocytes, a few polymorphonuclear leukocytes, macrophages and often many neoplastic cells; thus the diagnosis is made by cytological examination of the CSF (see Chap. 7). In addition to the cytological abnormalities, the CSF glucose is low and the protein raised in carcinomatous meningitis.

Intracranial abscesses

Pus may accumulate in localised collections and form abscesses in extradural sites, in the subdural or subarachnoid spaces or within the cerebral or cerebellar hemispheres. Extradural abscesses are usually due to spread from surrounding bone and abscesses localised to the subarachnoid space are uncommon.

Subdural abscess

Thought to be due to spread of infection from the nasal sinuses, subdural abscess or empyema is usually caused by streptococcal or staphylococcal infection. *Clinically*, the patients usually present with high fever and seizures with hemiplegia developing in the later stages. Pus collects in the subdural space especially alongside the falx and over the convexities of the cerebral hemispheres. The underlying meningeal vessels become inflamed and there may be widespread cerebral infarction and oedema due to thrombosis of the cortical veins. Even early treatment by irrigation of the subdural space and antibiotic therapy may leave the patient with considerable neurological deficit.

Brain abscess

In some cases brain abscesses present as space-occupying lesions with progressive focal disorders of neurological function characterised by seizures and headache, suggesting raised intracranial pressure. Alternatively they may present clinically as expanding focal lesions complicated by inflammation of the brain and meninges. In the latter case, the clinical features of a focal mass lesion in the brain coexist with meningism and sometimes with fever. When signs of meningitis are part of the clinical presentation, the abscess has usually arisen by *direct spread* of infection from sepsis in structures adjacent to the brain such as petrous temporal bone, the middle ear cavity or paranasal air sinuses. Infection may also result from direct penetrating injuries of the brain in which meningitis coexists with a nidus of infection within the brain itself.

Abscesses arising from *haematogenous spread* of infection in patients with septicaemia, bacterial endocarditis or chromic pulmonary sepsis may also be accompanied by signs of systemic infection and sometimes by associated meningitis. The clinical course of the associated disease may thus be brief or prolonged before the cerebral abscess itself presents. In a proportion of cases no primary site of infection elsewhere in the body can be located. Most abscesses are single although they may be made up of one or more loculi, but multiple abscesses also occur, particularly as a result of haematogenous spread of infection (Figs. 10.9, 10.10).

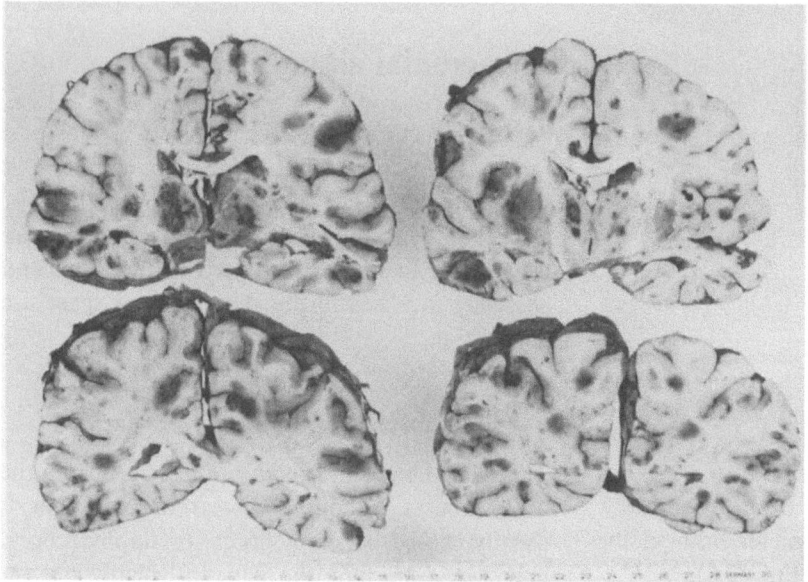

Fig. 10.9. Numerous haemorrhagic micro-abscesses in the brain due to *Aspergillus fumigatus*.

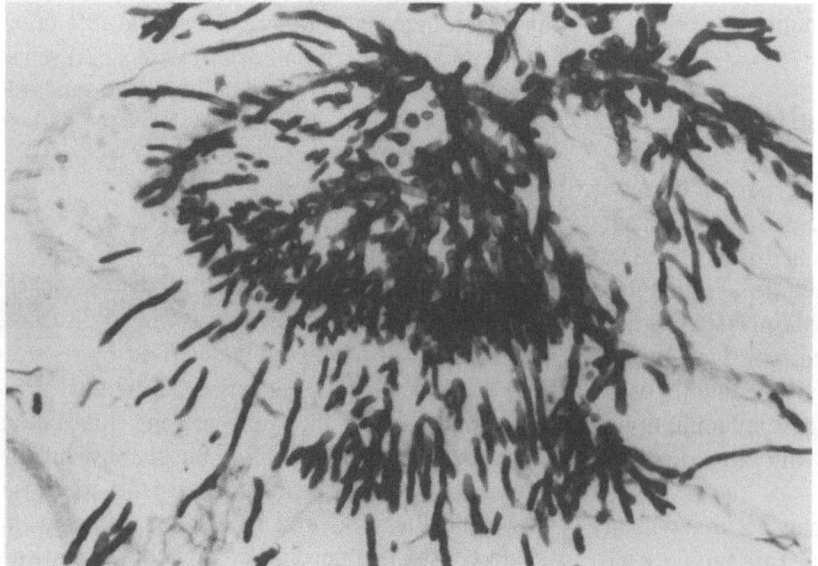

Fig. 10.10. Numerous branching septate hyphae of *Aspergillus fumigatus* from a micro-abscess in the brain. (Grocott stain × 350)

Bacteriology

Almost any organism may be found in a brain abscess cavity but certain organisms are particularly common. When the abscess arises through infection from a contiguous source in, for example, the middle ear, mastoid or paranasal air sinuses, the organisms in the abscess cavity reflect those found in the upper respiratory tract. Mixed infections are particularly common in this instance. Anaerobic organisms have recently been recognised as major agents in brain abscesses derived in this way from local infection within the cranial bones.

Bacteroides fragilis is the most common anaerobic organism isolated from those temporal lobe abscesses which are usually secondary to chronic middle ear infections. *Streptococci* (aerobic, microaerophilic and anaerobic) and aerobic Gram-negative rods of the Enterobacteriaceae are also found in these abscesses. In brain abscesses arising from the paranasal air sinuses, *S. pneumoniae*, *S. pyogenes* and *Haemophilus spp.* are particularly characteristic. Metastatic abscesses from the lung secondary to bronchiectasis, empyema or lung abscess are usually caused by organisms of oropharyngeal or tonsillar origin; *Fusobacterium spp.* are often found in these abscesses. *Streptococci*, *Staph. aureus* and *Bacteroides* are other organisms which are frequently isolated from metastastic brain abscesses. Fungi such as *Actinomyces spp.* and *Nocardia asteroides* may also be grown from pus aspirated from cerebral abscesses.

When abscesses develop in association with acute bacterial endocarditis or with congenital heart disease, they are usually due to the microaerophilic as well as viridans groups of streptococci, but *Haemophilus spp.*, *Staphylococcus aureus* and occasionally *Candida spp.* may also be important. *Staph. aureus* is commonly the organism in abscesses associated with trauma e.g. fracture or gunshot wounds, but aerobic Gram-negative rods and *Clostridia spp.* may also be involved.

The introduction of antibiotics seems to have made little difference to the incidence of cerebral abscess. Since many of the causative organisms discussed above can only be cultured with relatively sophisticated modern bacteriological methods, the possibility that antibiotic treatment of upper respiratory tract and ear infections might have led to a change in the bacteriology of cerebral abscess remains unresolved.

Pathology

The mortality in patients with cerebral abscesses remains high, approaching 50% if patients with acute cerebral abscess are included in the statistical analysis, but much smaller if patients presenting to neurosurgical units are studied. Abscesses occurring in the brain from haematogenous spread typically occur, like metastatic tumours, at the junction of the grey and white matter and are frequently multiple. Temporal lobe abscesses are usually the sequel of middle ear infection, following spread of infection through the petrous bone into the middle fossa. Cerebellar abscesses develop following mastoid infections but may also occur when the petrous bone is involved.

In its initial stage, an abscess consists of an area of vascular congestion associated with bacterial invasion in the white matter. Necrosis occurs in the infected part of the brain and there is invasion by polymorphonuclear leukocytes. A collagenous fibrous capsule, containing acute and chronic inflammatory cells, macrophages and fibroblasts, develops slowly around this nidus of infection and necrosis (Fig. 10.11). The abscess may then gradually increase in size if no treatment is given, finally rupturing into the lateral ventricle, or at the surface of the brain. Rupture of a cerebral abscess with discharge of pus into the subarachnoid space is often fatal within a few hours. Microscopically the central part of an abscess consists of necrotic brain, polymorphonuclear leukocytes and bacteria. At the periphery, granulation tissue forms and, particularly in the case of staphylococcal abscesses, a well-formed fibrous capsule develops with gliosis in the surrounding brain. The abscess cavity is itself often broken up into several different loculi, an important point to remember when a surgeon tries to drain an abscess cavity by needling the brain.

Since a cerebral abscess is a *mass lesion* acquired relatively quickly, and accompanied by marked white matter oedema, the brain becomes deformed and shifted within the cranial cavity. Transtentorial herniation of the parahippocampal gyrus on the side of the lesion is common and is often accompanied by herniation of the cingulate gyrus under the falx cerebri and sometimes by herniation of the cerebellar tonsils through the foramen magnum. Secondary vascular effects of the brain herniation may lead to further disability (see Chap. 4).

Epilepsy is a common feature in the clinical presentation of cerebral abscess and is a major complication of patients surviving the illness.

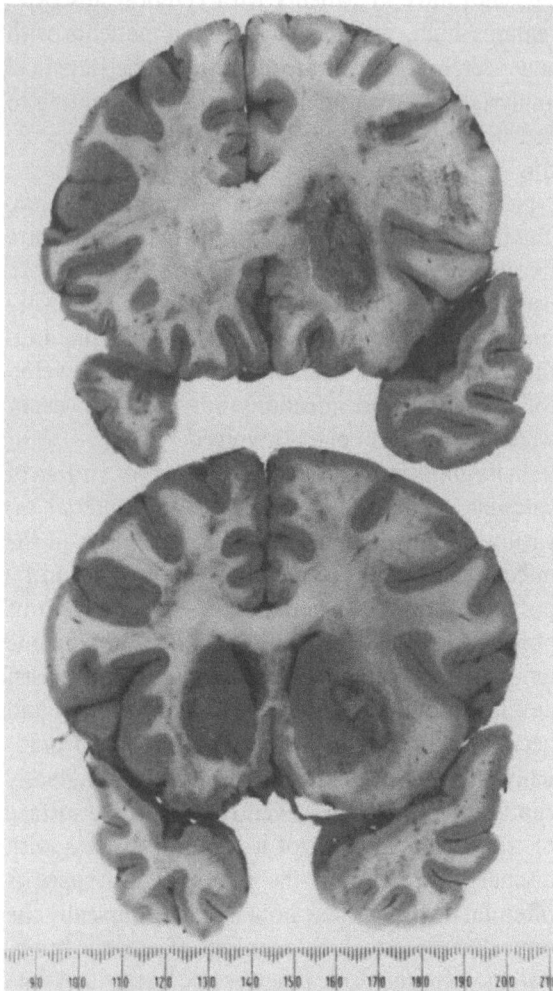

Fig. 10.11. Coronal slices of cerebral hemisphere showing metastatic cerebral abscesses due to *Staph. auereus*. In the *top picture*, there is diffuse oedema and necrosis in the right hemisphere; in the *lower picture* the abscess has become more circumscribed.

About 75% of those who survive a cerebral abscess develop epilepsy during the following 10 years. Focal neurological disabilities related to destruction of brain tissue by the abscess are also a major clinical feature in those patients who survive.

Mycotic aneurysms

Focal dilatations of intracranial or other vessels where an artery wall is weakened by necrosis and inflammation following bacterial invasion are known as mycotic aneurysms. They may be a result of infected emboli and if damage to the vessel wall is extensive, haemorrhage into the brain or subarachnoid space may ensue. Mycotic aneurysms are particularly common in patients with embolic septicaemia, as for example, in infective endocarditis.

Protozoal infections

Infestation of the CNS by amoebae and toxoplasma are recognised in the United Kingdom but are uncommon; cerebral malaria and trypanosomiasis on the other hand tend to be restricted to areas where these diseases are endemic.

Amoebic meningoencephalitis is a rare disease usually caused by the free-living amoebae of genus *Naegleria*. There is frequently a history of swimming or paddling in contaminated water followed by the development of a subacute meningoencephalopathy. The CSF shows an increase in lymphocytes and the protein is considerably raised. *Acanthamoeba spp.* have also been responsible for a few cases of meningitis in patients immunosuppressed by drugs or by lymphoma. Histological examination of the brains of patients dying with amoebic meningoencephalitis show amoebae not only in the subarachnoid space but also invading the brain. There is, however, little inflammatory reaction or tissue response to the presence of the amoebae. Such a picture may be confused, histologically, with carcinomatous meningitis. There is a high mortality rate in this disease but *Amphotericin B* appears to be an effective treatment.

Cerebral toxoplasmosis due to infestation by *Toxoplasma gondii* may be seen in neonates and immunosuppressed patients. The parasites appear as small haematoxyphilic dots in swollen cells which are probably macrophages (see Fig. 11.3). Granulomas are seen in the brain and may be associated with focal necrosis.

Cerebral malaria is associated with *Plasmodium falciparum* infection in areas of endemic malaria. In fatal cases, petechial haemorrhages are seen throughout the cerebrum and cerebellum and microscopically there are pericapillary haemorrhages and the accumulation of dark granules of malaria pigment within and around the vessels.

Trypanosomiasis with the clinical picture of sleeping sickness is seen with various species of trypanosome and a variety of intracerebral and meningeal lesions.

Metazoal parasites

Taenia solium (Cysticercosis) larvae may form cysts in the brain which may give rise, clinically, to epilepsy. Similarly, hydatid cysts from *Echinococcus granularis* may form in the brain. Schistosomiasis rarely gives rise to a cerebral infestation but when it does invade the brain is usually due to *S. japonicum*.

Further reading

Beller A J, Sahar A, Praiss J (1973) Brain abscess: a review of 89 cases over a period of 30 years. J Neurol Neurosurg Psychiatry 42:12

Beres D, Metzler T (1938) Tuberculous meningitis and its relation to tuberculous foci in the brain. Am J Pathol 14: 59

Dodge P R, Swartz M N (1965) Bacterial meningitis: a review of selected aspects. II. Special neurologic problems, post-meningetic complications and clinicopathologic correlations. N Engl J Med 272: 954–960, 1003

Freilich D, Swash M (1979) The diagnosis and management of tuberculous paraplegia with special reference to tuberculous radiculomyelitis. J Neurol Neurosurg Psychiatry 42:12

Ghaly A F, El-Banhawy A (1973) Schistosomiasis of the spinal cord. J Pathol 111: 57

Graber C D, Higgins L S, Davis J S (1965) Seldom-encountered agents of bacterial meningitis. JAMA 192: 956

Gray M L, Killinger A H (1966) Listeria monocytogenes and listeria infections. Bact Rev 30:309

Hardman J M, Earle K M (1967) Meningococcal infections: a review of 200 fatal cases. J Neuropathol Exper Neurol 26: 119

Kocen R S, Parsons M (1970) Neurological complications of tuberculosis: some unusual complications. Quart J Med 39: 19

Rich A R, McCordock H A (1933) Pathogenesis of tuberculous meningitis. Bull J Hopkins Hosp 52: 5

Chapter 11

Developmental and Neonatal Neuropathology

The morphological expression of abnormalities of development in the CNS is varied. The abnormality may be *anatomical*, i.e. structural, presenting as a developmental malformation or *biochemical*, presenting as a functional abnormality without structural change. Abnormal fetal development may thus result in a non-viable conceptus, leading to spontaneous abortion or stillbirth, to a dysraphic state, or to motor and behavioural retardation without specific clinical features. The viability of a conception depends on the nature and severity of the defect in the CNS and of any associated defects. Abnormalities of development of the CNS may be associated with defects in other organ systems. Gross defects result in spontaneous abortion, but some less severe anomalies may not become evident until late infancy or even adult life.

Some developmental abnormalities are due to a genetic defect, for example, the chromosomal disorders, which may themselves be inherited or acquired. However, most abnormalities arise as a result of exposure to extraneous factors, especially exposure to certain infections, toxins or physical injuries. In many instances the malformation produced by one of these factors is similar to that caused by another and it is only after cytological, bacteriological and biochemical study and a careful search for toxic agents that the cause may be identified.

The morphological expression of a developmental anomaly depends not only on the nature of the causative factor but also on the stage during development at which damage to the embryo occurs and at which abnormal development is initiated. This point is especially important in understanding the variety of abnormalities caused by exposure of the fetus to chemical toxins and in appreciating the specific susceptibility of the fetus to agents, such as rubella virus, at certain stages of development and the relative harmlessness of these agents at other times in development. The dysraphic states, for example, in which abnormalities of fusion of the neural tube result in characteristic and severe abnormalities, may result from a cytogenetic defect due to chromosomal or genetic abnormality or from exposure to one of a variety of extraneous toxic factors. This malformation only occurs however if the fetus is exposed to the teratogen at a specific stage during its development. The range of abnormalities which may occur is thus immense and only relatively few are compatible with life. The pathologist will therefore derive most of his experience of developmental malformations from spontaneous abortions or stillborn infants. The clinician will have a different experience, however, since those developmental abnormalities which are compatible with life are necessarily less severe.

Epidemiology

Antenatal factors

Spontaneous abortions occur in about 15% of recognised pregnancies and 90% of these occur in the first trimester. Many more spontaneous abortions are unrecognised or unreported. Genetic and chromosomal abnormalities are found in 85% of abortions. Of these 15% are due to *monosomies*, e.g. Turner's syndrome, and 50% are due to *trisomies*. A further 20% show *triploidy*, that is they have more chromosomal material in each nucleus (3n) than is present in a diploid cell (2n). In stillborn infants the incidence of genetic and chromosomal abnormalities varies from 30% to 60% in different series of cases.

Developmental abnormalities occur in 3% of all live-born infants and CNS malformations are common in these patients. Abnormalities attributed to genetic defects account for 40% of these malformations and a third of these are due to chromosomal abnormalities. In the remainder, extraneous environmental factors are important. With the decline in the incidence of death due to postnatally acquired infection since the early part of this century, malformations have become more important as a cause of death in the newborn and in infancy, accounting for about 20% of such deaths in the United Kingdom each year.

Perinatal factors

The prevalence of developmental disability due to brain lesions acquired in the perinatal period is difficult to assess. However, it is estimated that 3–4 per 1000 children in the age range 1–16 years have brain lesions acquired during the perinatal period; many affected infants die in the first few years of life. The brain lesions in this group are due to factors such as hypoxia, hypoglycaemia, seizures, infections, and physical injuries, especially intracerebral and periventricular haemorrhage, sustained at or shortly after birth.

Postnatal developmental disability

Developmental disability may be defined as a severe chronic disablement due to intellectual and physical impairment which affects the patient before the age of 18 years and is likely to continue indefinitely. Patients in this group are disabled in at least three areas of socio-economic activity which include self-control, reception and expression of language, learning, self-direction, mobility, economic self-sufficiency and the capacity to live independently. Such disability is seen in about 70% of all cases of cerebral damage acquired *before* birth; some 40% of these cases have a cytogenetic basis, the most important of which is Down's syndrome. Disorders of expression of single genes account for 7%. A further group results from prenatal infections, particularly rubella and cytomegalovirus infections. The role of teratogenic agents such as alcohol and other drugs and toxins is still poorly understood. Half of all patients with the motor defects of cerebral palsy (Little's syndrome) also show severe developmental disability.

In another large, but poorly documented, group of infants there is growth retardation. The infants are 'small for dates', thus showing impaired fetal growth. In many instances the functional anomaly may not manifest itself until postnatal life when physiological and psychological abnormalities become evident. This syndrome probably has many causes.

Pathogenetic considerations

Inherited or spontaneous genetic defects prevent normal genetic expression at a critical stage in development. Genetic defects may occur spontaneously in the parental germ cell, or they may be induced by chemical toxins or by ionising radiation. The genetic mutation results in alteration of the nucleotide sequence in such a way as to change the developmental potential of fetal cells. It must therefore occur at or before the zygote is formed. When such a mutation occurs in a germinal cell it is heritable, but this is not the case when it occurs in a somatic cell. An agent producing these changes in the genome is a *mutagen*.

Toxic effects which occur later than the zygote stage of development produce a phase-specific impairment of development. When a malformation is produced, the toxic agent is called a *teratogen*. The embryotoxic or fetotoxic effects leading to abnormal development depend on the nature of the agent, the stage during gestation at which it acts and the genetic background of the individual. The dose of teratogen is of less importance, although ex-

posure to large doses of a potent teratogen often leads to fetal death, rather than to a viable malformation. The agent thus acts at a critical period of development when biological development of the fetus is occurring rapidly. A quite minor change in the pace of development of a particular structure may thus produce a major structural abnormality.

At a subcellular level there are critical events in development which are particularly susceptible to derangement by teratogens. As a cell type proceeds in development, its potential is progressively restricted. It undergoes 'determination' as cells are selected and phenotypic characteristics are stabilised. Proliferating fetal cells are particularly vulnerable to injury at the G1 phase of the cell cycle, between mitosis and DNA synthesis. Following proliferation cells enter a migratory phase. If this is delayed or prevented the sequence of subsequent phases of development is disturbed and malformations may occur. The rate and direction of cell migration during the G1 'rest' phase is thought to be dependent upon binding between the cell surface and extracellular carbohydrate residues. Teratogenic agents may thus act at the cell surface or in the extracellular compartment.

When cell differentiation and migration is completed, some cells undergo programmed 'physiological' death, leaving the fetus with normal adult cell numbers in critical locations, as in the subependymal germinal plate. This stage of development is particularly vulnerable to cytotoxic teratogens, which may induce tumour formation and other abnormalities, such as hydrocephalus.

The teratogenic agent responsible for an anomaly may be absorbed by the mother and passed unchanged to the fetus or embryo. The toxicity of many such agents depends on the production of intermediary metabolites by the mother or fetus. Some teratogens produce highly specific and reproducible effects but many such agents cause widespread and non-specific abnormalities, some of which are relatively slight. Because of this, the damage induced by some teratogens may not be permanent, and the fetus is normal. Should it be irreversible a mild or severe anomaly results, or the fetus may even die.

Development of the human brain

Modern teratological studies and the examination of embryos have indicated the stages in development[1] when the nervous system is most susceptible to the action of teratogens. An appreciation of the embryology and postnatal growth of the brain is therefore essential for understanding the basis of developmental abnormalities of the CNS. The first major step is the establishment of the neural tube at *2 weeks* of gestation and its closure at *4 weeks*. At this stage the primitive circulation develops by the in-growth of blood vessels into the developing fetal nervous system. The cerebral ventricles appear at about *7 weeks'* gestation.

Brain growth is rapid between *10–18 weeks'* gestation. Neuroblasts migrate along ependymo-glial processes from the paraventricular region to form the cerebral cortex, where they undergo maturation. The second phase of brain growth consists of glial proliferation. This begins in fetal life but continues into the *2nd year* of postnatal life. It is accompanied by a phase of rapid myelination which continues into the *3rd and 4th years* of postnatal life. Myelination then continues more slowly, and is completed only in *late adolescence*.

The normal full-term infant brain weighs 350–430 g, about 25% of the adult weight. *At birth*, the primary cerebral gyri are well formed and all the important secondary gyri can be recognised. The brain is partially myelinated and all the major cell proliferation and migration processes are almost complete. A subependymal layer of germinal cells persists at the superolateral angle of each lateral ventricle well into the 1st year.

During the *1st year* of life, myelination of the white matter takes place, the brain reaches 75% of the adult weight and cell migration is completed. The external granular (germinal) layer of the cerebellum (Fig. 11.9) does, however, persist into the 2nd year. Groups of similar but heterotopic 'primitive matrix cells', may be found near the dentate nucleus of the cerebellum (Fig. 11.1).

Chromosomal abnormalities

Genetic abnormalities are present in 40% of patients with development malformations of the CNS, and *one-third* of these are chromosomal in type. The extent and severity of the malformation due to abnormalities of the chromosome groups

---

[1] The gestational age in weeks of a brain at birth can be estimated approximately by counting the number of convolutions crossed by a line extending from the frontal pole to the occipital pole along the insula, and adding 21.

13–15 (D), 17–18 (E) and 21, decrease with the size of the chromosome. This is probably an indication of the amount of genetic material involved in the abnormality. In addition to the malformation of the CNS found in these disorders, numerous other abnormalities occur. These include non-specific dysmorphic features, such as low-set or mis-shapen ears, hyper- or hypotelorism, anteverted nostrils, anomalies of digits and of skin creasing, and associated major developmental malformations of the heart and viscera. Some combinations are recognised as specific syndromes. However, many cannot yet be so characterised.

Microscopically the major abnormalities seen in the brain in the chromosomal disorders are mis-placed islands of neurons or primitive matrix cells which have not migrated to their normal positions. Such *heterotopias* probably represent neuroblasts which have failed to migrate normally into the cortex or deep nuclei, and have also failed to mature, although some mature neurons may be present. These features are commonly seen in patients with chromosomal abnormalities, and this probably indicates that in these disorders the defective genetic coding has been present from fertilisation. The morphological abnormality develops in the first trimester of fetal life when neuroblast division and migration normally take place. This causes secondary disturbances of brain development; malformations thus occur in the subsequent phases of rapid brain growth, and in the formation of primary and secondary cerebral gyral patterns.

Down's syndrome (mongolism)

Down's syndrome accounts for 30% of all cases of developmental abnormality due to chromosomal anomalies; its incidence is 1.4 per 1000 live births. There are three major types; *trisomy* 21 which accounts for 90%, *translocation* of chromosome 21 accounting for 4%, and *mosaicism* of chromosome 21, where the affected individual is a mosaic of normal and trisomic cells.

Down's syndrome occurs in a bimodal distribution in relation to maternal age. There is no relationship to paternal age. However one-third of cases occur between the two age peaks of maternal susceptibility. Down's syndrome in the children of mothers younger than 25 years is usually due to translocation of part of chromosome 21. This disorder is familial and all subsequent children of mothers with this translocation will also show the features of Down's syndrome. The second peak of incidence occurs in children born to mothers older than 40 years; in these cases the disorder is usually due to non-dysjunction of chromosome 21 leading to trisomy of this chromosome. The incidence of this form of disease increases with maternal age. It is 1 in 43 live births in mothers aged 40–44 years; and 1 in 21 live births in mothers aged 45–49 years. It has been suggested that metabolic or environmental factors in the mother's ovaries damage the oocyte during meiosis. Since the disorder can be recognised by chromosomal studies of fetal cells it is appropriate to consider diagnostic amniocentesis in all pregnant women aged 40 years or more.

Clinical features. Down's syndrome is usually recognisable, even at birth, by the characteristic facies. The face is flat and hypoplastic, with a short nose, a protruding tongue with a small mouth, and small rounded ears with a prominent antihelix. The eyes slant upwards and there are prominent epicanthic skin folds. A congenital malformation of the heart, usually consisting of atrial septal defect, occurs in half of all cases of Down's syndrome. The palmar creases are abnormal, with only one transverse crease which crosses the whole palm. There is mental retardation, but its severity varies from case to case. Life expectancy is reduced and death usually occurs before the 6th decade; many patients die from heart failure associated with the cardiac malformation but death may also occur in association with a progressive dementia which develops with increasing age. The clinical syndrome is identical in the three types of chromosomal abnormality, reflecting the specific abnormality of chromosomal material on chromosome 21.

Pathological features. Macroscopically, the brain weight is reduced, often to less than 1000 g, even in adults. The convolutional pattern of the brain is simplified, and there is a characteristic, unusually small and straight superior temporal gyrus. The occipital lobe is shortened. In the cerebral cortex there is a reduced neuronal density in all cortical layers but especially in layer 3, and there is an unusually prominent columnar arrangement of cortical neurons. The cerebellum is small and may show anomalies of development. These features all indicate impairment of brain growth and differentiation operating throughout gestation. Patients with Down's syndrome often have the histological features of Alzheimer's disease (see Chap. 15) by the time they die.

Pulmonary hypertension frequently develops leading to changes in the lung. Embolic infarction may occur in other organs, including the brain, from thrombosis or infection associated with the cardiac malformation.

Trisomy 17–18 (trisomy E; Edwards' syndrome)

This syndrome is due to an abnormality of group E chromosomes and is uncommon. It occurs in 1 in 6500 live births. As in Down's syndrome, cases of Edwards' syndrome born to young mothers may be familial. The disorder is also associated with increasing maternal age in mothers older than 40 years. In trisomy E, as in Down's syndrome, severe mental retardation is associated with facial dysmorphism, particularly malformed ears and micrognathia. Cardiac abnormalities also occur.

In the majority of cases the syndrome is due to trisomy of chromosomes in group E but mosaicism of these chromosomes has also been described.

Macroscopically, the brain shows gyral abnormalities, particularly affecting the superior tem-

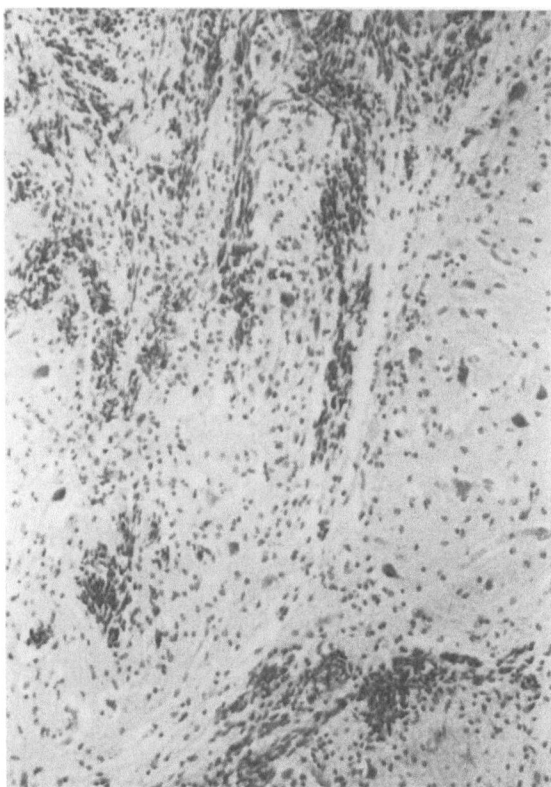

Fig. 11.1. Heterotopic primitive matrix cells of the external granular type in the dentate nucleus of the cerebellum in a neonate. (H & E × 200)

poral gyrus, the gyrus rectus and the pre- and post-central gyri. Hypoplasia or absence of the corpus callosum may be a feature, and heterotopias and nests of ectopic glial tissue commonly occur. 'Primitive matrix cells' are frequently found in the cerebellum (Fig. 11.1) and in the periventricular regions.

Trisomy 13–15 (trisomy D; Pateau's syndrome)

This trisomy has an incidence of about half that of trisomy E. The features of Pateau's syndrome have been reported not only with trisomy of chromosomes 13–15 but, as in Down's syndrome, also with translocation or mosaicism of these chromosomes.

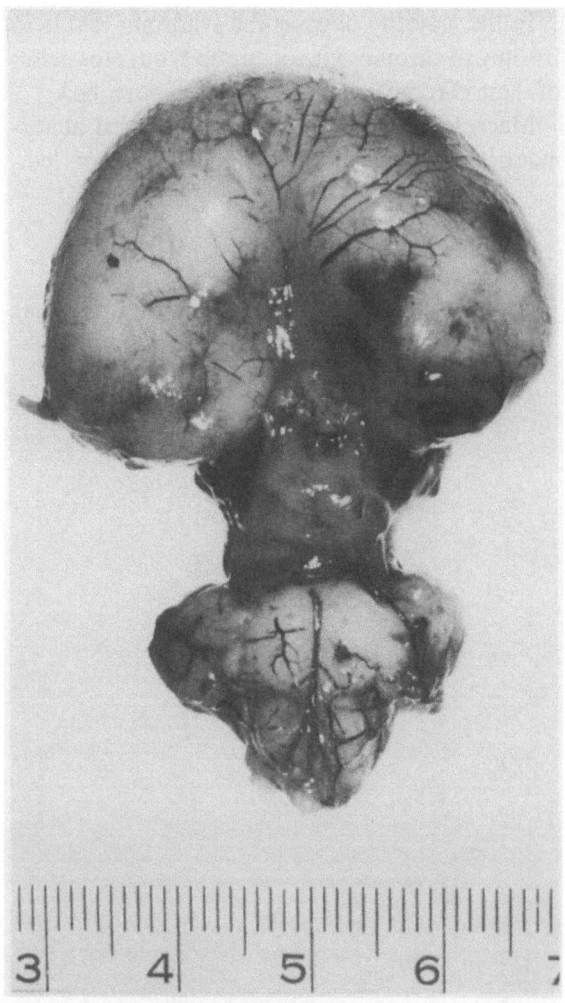

Fig. 11.2. Holoprosencephaly. There is no median division of the brain into two hemispheres; agyria and grossly abnormal cerebral vessels are also seen. The brain is from an infant with cyclopia, a median eye and a nasal proboscis. There was trisomy of chromosomes 13–15.

As would be expected in a disorder associated with abnormalities of large chromosomes, and hence of large amounts of genetic material, the abnormalities found in the syndrome are extensive.

The characteristic pattern of malformations includes microcephaly, micrognathia, webbed neck, low-set ears and congenital heart disease. Most of those affected die in early infancy, but a few survive till childhood with gross retardation.

The most severe intracranial manifestation is *holoprosencephaly* (Fig. 11.2) in association with cyclopia. In holoprosencephaly the brain is small, often weighing less than 100 g, the two hemispheres are fused and there is a single cerebral ventricle with a smooth non-gyral surface to the brain. This represents a very severe abnormality of neuroblast and glial migration. The third ventricle is present but the pituitary gland is absent and there is aplasia of the nasal bones and soft tissues with gross hypotelorism or even a single median eye (cyclopia). There are gross abnormalities of the cerebellum. The maturation defect is less severe in some cases, but abnormalities of gyral and basal ganglion development nearly always occur. In the least severe instances, the olfactory bulbs and tracts are absent, an abnormality termed *arhinencephaly*, but the remainder of the brain is normal.

Microscopical examination of the cerebral cortex shows gross hypoplasia with no discernible lamination. Massive neuronal and glial heterotopias occur in the cerebellum and in the brain stem.

Destructive lesions

Developmental malformations occur following injury sustained through the transplacental transfer of toxic chemical agents, or their metabolites, through infections and from ionizing radiation. Because of the extensive necrosis which characterises the reaction of the developing fetal brain to these noxious external agents, there may be a very severe malformation and it is often difficult to determine the nature of the agent responsible for the initial damage.

Infections

Toxoplasma gondii, cytomegalovirus and *herpesvirus hominis* infections may all affect the fetus, the infection being transmitted from the mother. Although the effect of these infections on the fetal brain is variable, in general the earlier in development the embryo or fetus is infected the more severe is the resultant damage.

Rubella infection has a teratogenic effect during a critical early period of development; infections after this period cause an inflammatory response without subsequent malformation. Cytomegalovirus infections may cause mental retardation without any grossly obvious malformations, but, when infection occurs at a critical period of cell migration and maturation it interferes with normal development, and a severe malformation, often including microcephaly, may result.

Toxoplasmosis

Toxoplasma gondii is a protozoan parasite. Fetal infection is likely to cause a malformation if it occurs at or after the 12th week of gestation. Maternal infection may already be present or may be contracted in the early stages of pregnancy. But, although maternal infection occurs in about 7% of pregnancies, fetal damage occurs in only about 40% of these cases. In most instances the maternal infection is not apparent; symptomatic toxoplasmosis occurs in only about 15% of infected mothers. The incidence of brain damage from fetal infection, often termed *congenital toxoplasmosis*, is 1 in 16000 in the United Kingdom as a whole, but in Scotland it is rather more common, occurring in 1 in 2000 births.

Abortion or stillbirth occur in about 20% of fetal infections with toxoplasmosis, but in many other instances no abnormality is apparent until early childhood, when hydrocephalus, epilepsy or mental retardation become apparent. The severity of the neuropathological damage can be related to the time of infection; generally, the earlier in fetal life the infection occurs, the more serious is the outcome.

Infection in mid-pregnancy is often associated with abortion or stillbirth, but later infections produce less severe abnormalities. Infected neonates show lymphadenopathy, hepatomegaly and chorioretinitis, and skull x-rays may reveal periventricular focal calcification. The Sabin–Feldman complement fixation dye test, or indirect haemagglutination tests, can be used to confirm the diagnosis of toxoplasmosis. The CSF is xanthochromic with a raised protein level and a lymphocytosis; CSF sugar levels may be low when the infection is active.

Pathology. At autopsy the brain is smaller than normal. Soft, yellowish, depressed areas several millimetres in diameter are seen in the cortex extending into the white matter; similar lesions are found in basal ganglia, cerebellum or brain stem. Polymicrogyria is often present. When the brain is hydrocephalic, the ventricular cavities are surrounded by friable necrotic tissue which frequently shows calcification (Fig. 11.3a).

Microscopic examination reveals areas of granulomatous inflammation or more diffuse inflammation with lymphocyte and plasma cell infiltration. The crescentic or oval parasite is an eosinophilic body, about $3 \mu m \times 2 \mu m$ in size, with a polar mass of chromatin. It may be found in an extracellular location or appear as an intracellular pseudocyst (Fig. 11.3b).

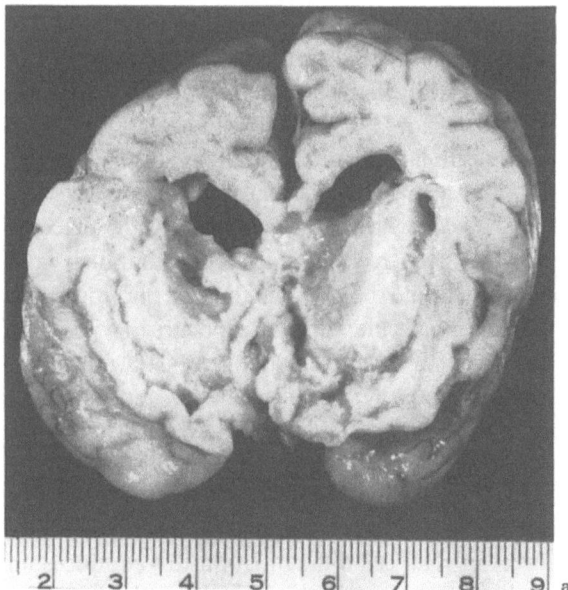

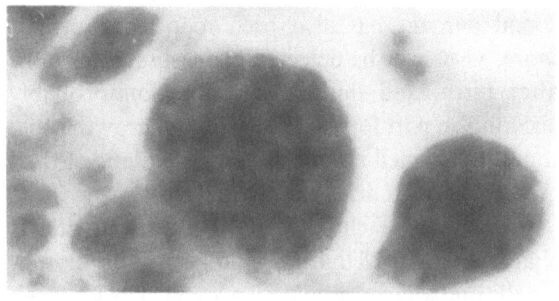

Fig. 11.3. a Coronal section of the brain from a still-born infant with generalised toxoplasmosis. The basal ganglia are soft and friable.
b Toxoplasma gondii in pseudocysts within the brain. (H & E ×2000)

Fetal rubella infections

The relationship between maternal rubella infection and the development of cataracts, patent ductus arteriosus and deafness in the child was first recognised in Australia in 1941. Additional abnormalities associated with maternal rubella have since been recognised. The syndrome is sometimes referred to as the 'congenital rubella' syndrome to indicate the fact that the infection occurs before birth. In the brain the major abnormalities consist of a *subacute* or *chronic encephalitis*, and *microcephaly*.

The risk of infection to the fetus when the mother has clinical rubella has been estimated at 50% in the *1st* month of gestation, 30% in the *2nd* and *3rd* months, and 10% in the *4th* month. The risk is thus greatest during the most vulnerable period of brain development. Rubella virus has been isolated from almost all fetal tissues in affected fetuses both at autopsy and at biopsy. While raised titres of rubella antibodies in the mother generally indicate maternal immunity and suggest that the fetus will be protected from infection, several recent cases of fetal infection in such circumstances have shown that this is not always the case.

The cellular immunity produced by the vaccine does not last as long as that produced by the wild virus. Vaccine virus is known to cross the placenta and has been recovered from the fetus, so conception should be avoided until 2 months after vaccination or, indeed, after exposure to wild virus. The vaccine is therefore best given during menstruation and the development of a satisfactory immune response should be checked since up to 5% of vaccinations fail to result in seroconversion.

In fetal infections the virus proliferates, producing cell necrosis. If the infection occurs in the early stages of fetal cell differentiation this produces an inhibition of cell replication which may have serious consequences for normal development. Chromosomal damage has also been reported. Furthermore, virus can be detected in the tissues months after birth, and this chronic infection probably accounts in part for the retardation of growth often found in affected infants. This delayed and slowed growth causes a delay in myelination.

Clinically the chronic meningo-encephalitis is characterised by lethargy, a bulging anterior fontanelle and an increased CSF protein. The CSF cell count may be raised and virus may be grown from the CSF. In some cases with active infection there may be an erythematous rash. Neurological abnormalities may be present at birth or become evident later. The main features are mental retardation and seizures. Cataract is also common. There is microcephaly, and the skull x-rays show intracranial calcification. Autistic behaviour patterns have been noted in children with the congenital rubella syndrome.

Pathology. At autopsy the brain may have a simplified gyral pattern. There is a chronic meningitis with an inflammatory reaction containing mononuclear cells, lymphocytes and plasma cells. Foci of necrosis are often found in the periventricular regions. The small blood vessels sometimes show intimal proliferation and this may be related to the presence of multiple small infarcts in the white matter. Many of these changes are non-specific effects which could be attributed to any inflammatory process, or even to neonatal asphyxia.

Cytomegalovirus infections

Many healthy persons excrete cytomegalovirus (CMV) and about 1% of all newborn infants excrete CMV in their urine. Most of these infants are otherwise normal and the infection is suppressed by the production of antibody as the immune system becomes competent. Infections of this type are usually acquired from the mother at birth. Active maternal CMV infection is usually suppressed in the early stages of pregnancy but may become reactivated later, despite the presence of circulating antibodies. Primary maternal infection during pregnancy is less common, probably occurring in only about 1 in 200 pregnancies. The fetus may, in rare instances, become infected by transplacental passage of virus and this may produce cerebral malformation, or a persistent infection with mental retardation and hydrocephalus, depending upon the stage of fetal development at which the infection occurs. It has been estimated that mental retardation due to CMV infection occurs at an incidence about half that of Down's syndrome.

The most severe abnormality, termed *cytomegalic inclusion disease*, consists of hydrocephalus and chronic meningoencephalitis with hepatomegaly, jaundice, anaemia, thrombocytopenia and diarrhoea. The CNS is involved in about 20% of such cases. The fully developed syndrome is rare, occurring in about 1 in 100000 live births. Death may occur a few days after birth. Survivors often remain retarded and spastic with deafness and choroidoretinitis.

Pathology. At autopsy, in severe cases, there is hydrocephalus and a widespread inflammatory response, especially marked in the periventricular white matter. This region contains focal zones of calcification. The teratogenic potential of the virus is low, but in a few cases polymicrogyria is found. The key to histological recognition of CMV infection is the presence of inclusions. These are round or oval, acidophilic intranuclear bodies, up to 15 μm in diameter, which are separated from the nuclear membrane by an unstained clear halo. They may occur in neurons or in glial cells.

In many instances macroscopic features consistent with CMV infection are seen but the characteristic inclusions cannot be found. In these cases the diagnosis can only be suspected.

Diagnosis can be made during the first weeks of life by isolation of virus from the urine. The demonstration of persistent circulating antibody during the first 6–9 months of life is also of diagnostic significance. Because hydrocephalus may develop insidiously, serial clinical assessments of children born with suspected CMV infection are important. The identification of infected women who risk producing damaged infants is particularly difficult as many infants of mothers with known, active CMV infection are normal.

Porencephaly and hydranencephaly

Porencephalic cysts are circumscribed, fluid-filled cavities (porus) with smooth walls in one or both hemispheres. The surrounding cerebral tissue is reduced to a thin layer of glia and the porus may or may not be in communication with the ventricles (Fig. 11.4). The frontal and occipital lobes are less commonly involved but usually show an anomalous arrangement of gyri around the porus itself with disruption of the normal laminar cortical architecture in this region. The term porencephaly should strictly be reserved to describe a congenital malformation in which parts of one or both cerebral hemispheres fail to grow and differentiate normally, resulting in a cyst-like enlargement of the lateral ventricle in the region of the malformation. The cyst in this form of porencephaly is thus lined by ependyma; in some instances it may communicate with the subarachnoid space. The term porencephaly is now generally extended to include cysts of similar appearance and location, not lined by ependyma. These probably form following infarction during fetal life and are seen mainly in a middle cerebral artery territory. It is thought that

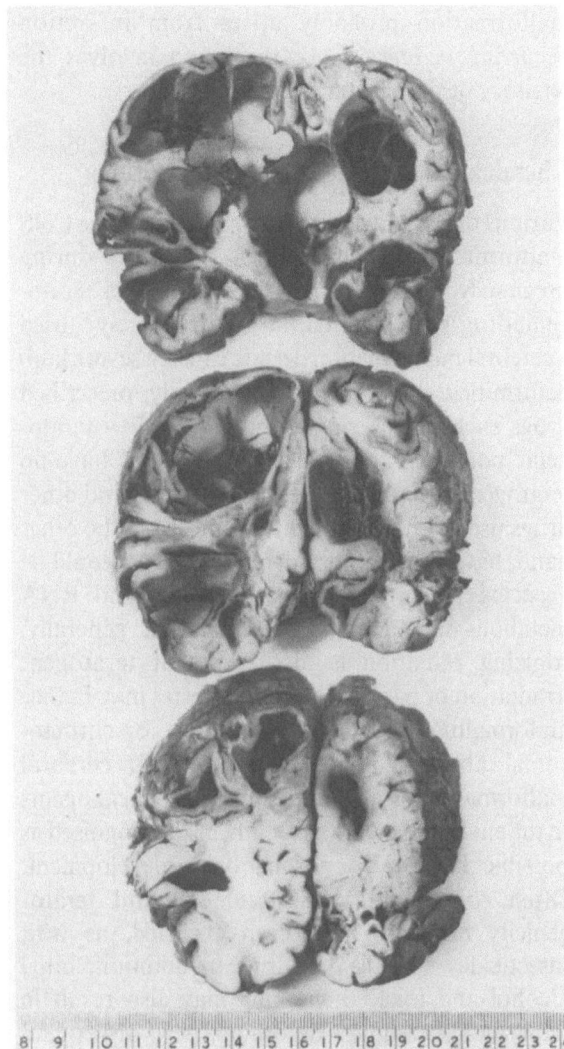

Fig. 11.4. Multiple porencephalic cysts in the brain of a severely retarded child. In the case illustrated here, the brain destruction is probably due to infarction in the perinatal period.

infection by toxoplasmosis or cytomegalovirus may cause this anomaly but it can probably also arise after birth, or from trauma sustained during birth. These forms of porencephaly, caused by damage later in development than the classic form, are not associated with microgyria or other cortical malformations. Clinically they are associated with spastic hemiparesis, epilepsy and mental retardation.

Hydranencephaly is a more severe malformation consisting of a large intracerebral cavity, which is commonly bilateral and often virtually replaces the hemispheres. The overlying skull and meninges are normal and there is a thin layer of superficial cortex in which an astroglial reaction is evident microscopically. This superficial layer is often adherent to the leptomeninges. The basal ganglia and hypothalamus are preserved and the cavity contains CSF, but is *not* lined by ependyma. This type of malformation probably arises from infarction occurring *in utero*, since the lesion involves the territory of the carotid circulation.

Chemical agents and CNS malformations

Various drugs and chemical agents may cause CNS malformations if injected or absorbed during pregnancy. The best known example of a teratogenic drug is thalidomide, but this drug rarely caused a cerebral malformation despite causing severe limb deformities. Most of the commonly prescribed drugs such as anticonvulsants have a low teratogenic potential, and many drugs seem to have no teratogenic effect at all. Alkylating agents and other drugs used in the treatment of cancer, on the other hand, have a potent teratogenic effect, as would be expected from their effects on DNA and RNA metabolism, and on protein synthesis generally. Ionizing radiation is also a potent teratogen; irradiation of parental ovaries or testes may induce abnormalities in DNA transcription, or chromosomal abnormalities leading to fetal cerebral malformation as a delayed effect. Chemical agents in the environment have recently been recognised as possible hazards to normal brain development. Often contamination is accidental and teratogenicity may not have been expected, as with insecticides such as Dieldrin. In addition, ethyl alcohol and tobacco smoking may also result in fetal malformations. Screening new drugs and chemicals for teratogenicity is a complex and time-consuming task, made more difficult by the fact that absence of teratogenicity in other species does not necessarily mean that the agent does not have teratogenic potential in man.

Ethyl alcohol

The specific syndrome of structural and functional abnormalities in the offspring of chronic alcoholic women is now well recognised. These abnormalities include prematurity, low birth weight and severe postnatal growth retardation usually accompanied by low intelligence. In addition, perinatal mortality is increased.

There is frequently a clinically apparent structural abnormality characterised by short palpebral fissures, prominent epicanthic folds, maxillary hypoplasia, cleft palate, micrognathia, and joint and cardiac anomalies. Striking abnormalities have been described in the brain in the most severely affected cases. These include microcephaly, ventricular enlargement and heterotopic islands of neurons forming subependymal nodules. Similar islands of displaced neurons are found on the cortical surface. Some degree of this *fetal alcohol syndrome* has been recognised in as many as 43 % of children of chronic alcoholic women, indicating that the teratogenic potential of ethyl alcohol may be quite high. The critical timing of exposure to ethyl alcohol during pregnancy is unknown.

Tobacco smoking

Several studies have demonstrated that infants of mothers who smoke tobacco during pregnancy have a reduced birth weight and that there is an increased incidence of abortion and perinatal death in such pregnancies. Several suggestions have been made to explain this finding. For example, impaired intrauterine growth could be secondary to reduced placental blood flow, possibly moderated by nicotine. Carboxyhaemoglobin formed from carbon monoxide absorbed from tobacco smoke might reduce the oxygen-carrying capacity of the blood of both the mother and fetus, and increased levels of thiocyanate in maternal blood might be toxic to the fetus. Despite these abnormalities in fetal growth a teratogenic effect of smoking has not, so far, been identified.

Radiation

Irradiation during pregnancy usually occurs during radiological investigation or treatment, but exposure of this type usually amounts to less than 1 rad. In recent years radiological investigations during pregnancy have been avoided and it is common practice to defer such investigations during the second half of each menstrual cycle in order to lessen the risk of accidental fetal exposure. Furthermore, exposure of gonads to irradiation in both men and women can be prevented by the use of suitable shields. Procedures involving the use of radionuclides are particularly dangerous in pregnancy since not only may the dose of ionizing radiation be rather larger but the radionuclide will cross the placenta and may then be selectively concentrated in certain tissues, e.g. iodine isotopes taken up by thyroid tissue.

The fetotoxic potential of x-rays has been known for several decades. It was first clearly recognised in the early years of this century when up to 350 rads of x-irradiation were given to produce abortion. When abortion was not produced by this procedure infants were born with microcephaly and mental retardation.

The major period of susceptibility of the developing fetal brain to radiation damage is in the *3rd* to *7th weeks* of gestation, during the period of organogenesis. Irradiation causes breaks in the DNA molecule, and impairs DNA repair processes so that defective genetic coding results, leading to developmental malformation. The malformation may be slight or severe, but only the latter can be recognised clinically and the possible hazards of exposure to small doses of irradiation are uncertain. Spina bifida and absence of the corpus callosum have been reported, but heterotopic islands of neurons may also occur. Down's syndrome has been reported following irradiation of the ovaries.

Dysraphic malformations

The dysraphic states consist of a group of disorders in which fusion of the neural tube has failed to occur. This may affect the whole neural tube so that the neural groove remains open throughout its length. There is thus a major abnormality of development of the brain, skull and spine; *craniorachischisis*. In *anencephaly* the neural groove of the brain (anterior neuropore) fails to close and in *spina bifida* the defect of neural tube closure is limited in extent, often affecting only the lumbosacral region. *Encephalocoeles* and *meningocoeles* represent limited forms of failure of closure of the rostral neural tube. Meninges and part of the brain project beneath the skin through a midline cranial bony defect in the frontal or occipital region. Dysraphic states thus result from failure of closure or from incomplete closure of the neural tube. The abnormality may also result from breakdown of the neural tube, but this mechanism is not easy to document.

Dysraphic malformations are induced by damage occurring during the 4th week of fetal development as a result of a combination of genetic and environmental factors. Numerous agents have been proposed as potential teratogens including tea, potatoes suffering from blight, nitrates and nitrites, but none of these suggestions have withstood investigation. However, these investigations do not preclude a commonly used agent, or a deficiency state which may act only in susceptible individuals. A genetic component is suggested by a higher risk in first-degree relatives, but the occurrence of areas of high incidence, such as Northern Ireland, suggests that environmental factors may be important.

Anencephaly

Anencephalic infants are usually born prematurely; 75% are female and up to 50% have polyhydramnios. Because of the gross nature of the defect, they rarely survive more than a few days.

The appearance of the anencephalic infant is typical. The head is retroflexed and appears to sit on the shoulders, the neck being shortened. All or most of the brain tissue is absent and the bones of the cranial vault are absent. The cranial cavity may thus be open without skin or meningeal covering. Clearly, therefore, anencephaly is always fatal. Because the orbits are shallow the eyes tend to protrude. The optic nerves end in the cranial cavity without entering the neural tissue. The base of the skull is flattened and the posterior fossa is small, but the lower cranial nerves are present. The cervical spine is abnormal, the neural arches having failed to fuse posteriorly, and the cord in this region may show failure of fusion of the lips of the neural tube. In severe cases this defect of the bony arches of the spine may also involve thoracic and lumbar segments, so that the defect is better classified as craniorachischisis. The spinal nerves, however, are always present. In many cases there are associated defects in other organs, especially the heart and adrenal glands. In most pregnancies in which the fetus is anencephalic there is pronounced hydramnios.

Microscopy of the small nodule of brain tissue in the malformed cranial cavity, the *area cerebrovascularis*, shows small vessels in a disorganised mass of glia and malformed brain. Choroid plexus may be present, and the characteristic hydramnios has been related to CSF secretion from this tissue. A portion of the anterior lobe of the pituitary is usually present, but the posterior pituitary is absent and the hypothalamus is abnormal. Most anencephalic infants are poikilothermic.

The *cause* of anencephaly is obscure. In rare instances the disorder has a familial basis but most cases are sporadic and it is assumed that an exogenous factor is responsible. It has been suggested that an abnormality of the developing craniobrachial vessels leads to infarction of the developing neural tube at a critical stage in development. Anencephaly has been produced experimentally in animals by irradiation of the fetus.

Ultrasonic screening of fetal development has been used to detect anencephaly early in pregnancy. The disorder may be suspected when hydramnios occurs, and the diagnosis is supported by the finding of a reduced 24-h excretion of oestrogens in the maternal urine. Recently the demonstration of *alphafetoprotein* by screening of the maternal blood and, where positive, examination of the amniotic fluid obtained by amniocentesis before the 16th–18th weeks of pregnancy has been found to be the most reliable method of diagnosis of anencephaly and of other neural tube defects, especially spina bifida, but this procedure carries a small risk of inducing abortion.

Encephalocoeles

Consisting of superficial, midline projections of displaced brain tissue and meninges, encephalocoeles are less common than anencephaly and spina bifida. Girls are more commonly affected than boys. The commonest type affects the occipital lobe (Fig. 11.5). There is a defect in the squamous occipital bone and in the basi-occiput in the midline through which a soft sac of brain tissue and meninges projects. The encephalocoele may be large or small. Small lesions are usually covered by skin but large encephalocoeles may have only an incomplete covering of skin, and these lesions are

usually fatal. Frontal encephalocoeles project through a cranial defect at the nasion or forehead, and the encephalocoele usually includes olfactory tissue and a portion of frontal lobe. There is usually an associated broadening of the face with hypertelorism. The brain tissue in the encephalocoele is usually abnormal, consisting of disorganised grey and white matter, without normal gyral development. Small vessels may be prominent.

There may be associated abnormalities in the cerebral hemispheres within the cranial cavity. These are partly mechanical, resulting from displacement as part of the involved hemisphere moves into the hernial sac. This stretches the cranial nerves, particularly the optic nerves. Other associated abnormalities include defective development of the corpus callosum, hydrocephalus, and distortion of the brain stem and cerebellum. The prognosis depends on the severity of these associated defects and on the extent of local tissue destruction at the site of the encephalocoele.

Spina bifida dorsalis

In spina bifida the defect is limited to the spine with failure of fusion of the neural arches; it most commonly affects the lumbosacral region, but extends rostrally to affect the thoracic, or even the cervical spine.

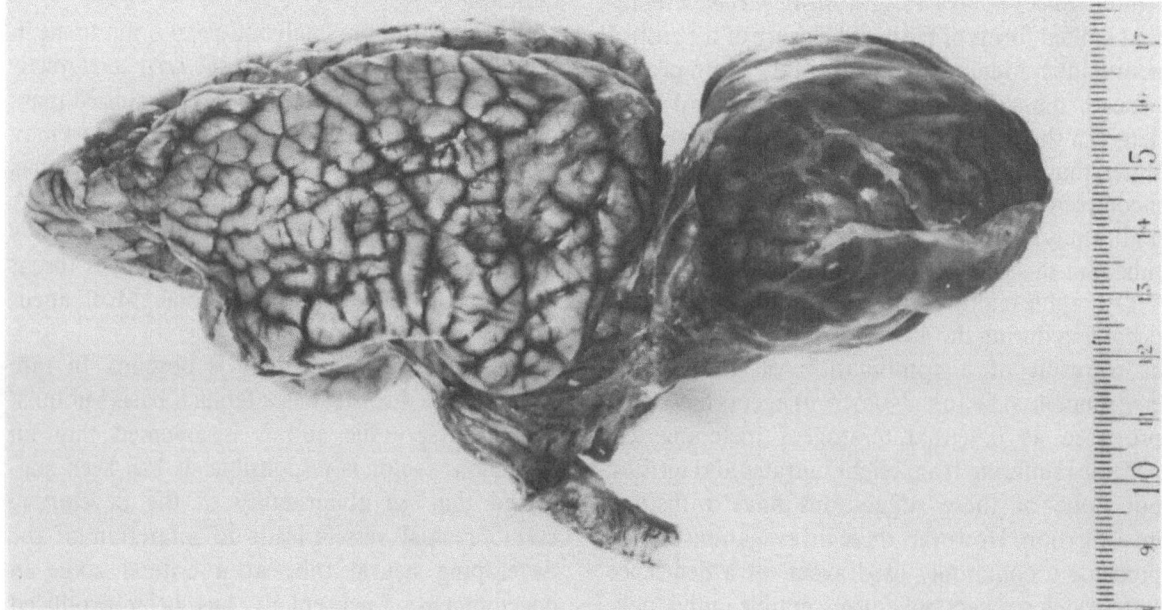

Fig. 11.5. Occipital encephalocoele. The cerebral hemispheres are on the left of the picture and a large encephalocoele containing brain tissue and coated by meninges has extended out of the cranial cavity posteriorly (to the *right* of the picture).

Spina bifida occulta

The commonest form of spina bifida is spina bifida occulta. The lesion consists of defective fusion of the posterior vertebral arches at one or more segmental levels, usually limited to the lumbosacral region. There is usually no abnormality of the overlying skin, or of the meninges and spinal roots, at the level of the developmental abnormality but in some patients the skin overlying the defective neural arches may be dimpled, abnormally hairy, or the site of a zone of *café au lait* pigmentation. Less frequently there may be a dermal sinus tracking inwards towards the malformation and, rarely, an intraspinal lipoma may be present in the defective spinal canal. All these cutaneous abnormalities are commonly associated with a localised spinal dysraphism, which is itself often asymptomatic. Indeed, spina bifida occulta is common, and is seen in up to 3 % of normal adults.

Neurological disturbances may present in adult life, but these are rare. Incontinence or retention of urine (neurogenic bladder) may occur as an isolated symptom. Occasionally the patient may present with slowly progressive numbness and weakness in the lumbosacral segments, with absent ankle jerks. In some patients these symptoms are found to be associated not only with spina bifida occulta but also with pes cavus. *Radiological investigation* shows that the spinal canal is larger than normal in the region of the spina bifida occulta, but the meninges are intact in this region. Frequently no other abnormality is discernible but sometimes an intraspinal mass, usually a lipoma, dermoid, granulomatous infection or rarely an ependymoma or glioma, can be identified. The filum terminale is sometimes tethered to the sacral theca in a more caudal position than normal and it has been suggested that this predisposes to the development of cauda equina or conus medullaris dysfunction.

Spina bifida occulta has also been associated with *diastematomyelia*, a disorder in which the cord is split into two slightly asymmetrical halves around a central, ventrally placed bony spur; the abnormality usually extends over several segments in the mid-thoracic region. The two hemicords are surrounded by their own dural and arachnoid tubes. Diastematomyelia may be asymptomatic or it may be associated with a spastic paraparesis, or with Arnold–Chiari malformation and hydrocephalus. There is usually a localised kyphoscoliosis at the site of the lesion, with fusion of adjacent vertebral bodies at this site. Spina bifida occulta itself is usually not associated with hydrocephalus.

Diplomyelia is a rare spinal dysraphism characterised by duplication of the spinal cord within a single meningeal tube.

Spina bifida cystica

There are two forms of spina bifida cystica. In one form a lumbosacral cyst is composed of meninges, contains CSF and is covered by skin. The spinal cord and roots within the cystic *meningocoele* are usually normal, but may be malformed, especially when associated with localised tumours such as lipomas and dermoids. *Myelomeningocoele* is the second, more severe form, where the cyst is covered at its edges by skin, but in the central part of the cyst the dermal covering is deficient, so that meninges are exposed. The meninges may also be deficient in some cases, so that the spinal canal is open, and may become infected shortly after birth. In this severe form of the disorder the spinal cord and roots lie open within the sac, and there is usually failure of closure of the neural tube in the region of the malformation. Many patients with myelomeningocoele are incontinent of urine and faeces and have flaccid, areflexic weakness of the legs, with sensory loss and lumbar kyphosis.

Myelomeningocoeles comprise about 80 % of cases of spina bifida cystica. The prognosis for function of the legs and sphincters is poor, even with attempted surgical closure of the defect, and most patients with the disorder die of infection in the first few weeks of life. There is a very high incidence of *Arnold–Chiari malformation* and of *hydrocephalus*; moderate or severe mental retardation is also common. Without treatment, survival at about 1 year is about 30 %, and at 2 years about 20 %. Only 3 % survive with minimal handicap and an IQ over 85. Early operation increases the number of survivors but most do not achieve a good quality of life. Delayed operation does not affect the number who survive but does improve their quality of survival. Most centres now adopt a selection policy in treatment and up to two-thirds of survivors have only mild to moderate neurological impairment.

The average *incidence* of spina bifida cystica in the United Kingdom is 2.5/1000 live births with the highest incidence of 4.5/1000 live births in Belfast. In addition to geographical differences in incidence of the disorder, racial differences have also been described. There is a higher incidence in Europeans than in Blacks, regardless of migration patterns or country of origin. Seasonal variations in incidence have also been described; the malformation is commoner in infants born in the winter months. A genetic factor is suggested by the high incidence, up to 10%, of the lesion in babies born to parents with a family history of the malformation. The risk increases with each additional child born with a neural tube defect. Prenatal counselling is now possible since in most pregnancies complicated by spina bifida cystica the alphafetoprotein level is raised in amniotic fluid.

Pathology. There is considerable anatomical variation in the arrangement of the cord, nerve roots, meninges and skin in spina bifida cystica. In *meningocoeles*, the cord is often intact and the cyst wall may be composed of skin and meninges; in some cases only the meninges are present. The central canal of the spinal cord is in communication with the sac of the meningocoele in one-third of cases.

Severe abnormality of the spinal cord may be seen in *myelomeningocoele*. Often the cord forms a flattened plaque at the base of the cyst and neural tissue may be incorporated into the skin and meningeal wall of the cyst. *Histological* examination of haematoxylin–van Giesen-stained sections of myelomeningocoele is particularly valuable for detecting the presence of neurological tissue in the wall of the cyst, as the cord tissue contains no collagen and can thus be easily distinguished from the overlying dermis. Granulation tissue may be present in the sac wall if it has been traumatised or infected. In some cases there is no sac and the plaque of neural tissue is exposed posteriorly.

The spinal cord is frequently abnormal above (rostral) or below (caudal) the level of spina bifida. Duplication of the cord (diastematomyelia or diplomyelia) commonly occurs rostrally, and may also be seen in the cervical region. Dilatation of the central canal (Fig. 11.6) (*hydromyelia*) may be seen in the cord, or duplication or extension of the canal into the surrounding white matter (*syringomyelia*) (Fig. 11.7) may be observed. Caudally, duplication of the cord with multiple canals is the commonest finding; the spinal cord is normal in only 15% of

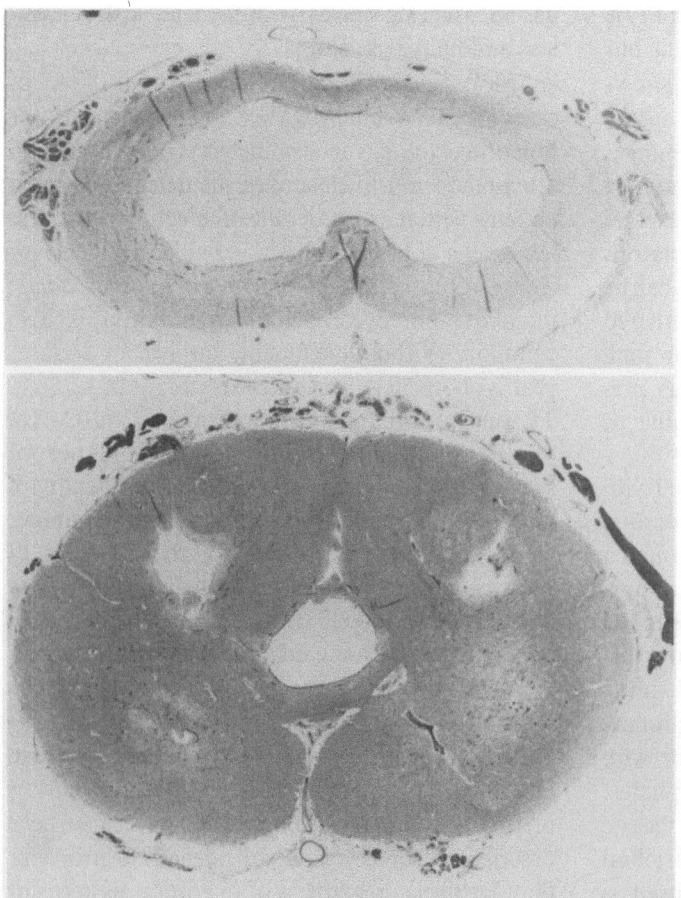

Fig. 11.6. Hydromyelia. A section of spinal cord rostral to a myelomeningocoele. There is gross dilatation of the central canal.

Fig. 11.7. Syringomyelia and hydromyelia. A section of the spinal cord caudal to a myelomeningocoele showing a dilated central canal and posterior laterally placed cavities (syringes).

cases. The Arnold–Chiari malformation, with hydrocephalus, is commonly found in patients with spina bifida.

Arnold–Chiari malformation

The association of the Arnold–Chiari malformation with spina bifida is particularly close in those patients in whom the myelomeningocoele is large and involves the upper regions of the spine. Arnold–Chiari malformations and spina bifida can occur independently, but both are associated with hydrocephalus. The hydrocephalus is frequently due to aqueduct stenosis and in these patients there may be other developmental abnormalities of the brain. Hydrocephalus may also occur as a complication of subacute or recurrent meningeal infections, especially in patients in whom a myelomeningocoele is open.

Chiari described three related combinations of malformation of the brain stem, cerebellum and base of the skull, which are often associated with severe, non-communicating hydrocephalus. In the mild, *type 1 form* there is herniation of the cerebellar tonsils through the foramen magnum. The cerebellar tonsils appear atrophic and sclerotic on microscopical examination. This mild form of the malformation is most commonly found in adults. In addition to tonsillar herniation there is elongation of the medulla, and the lower cranial nerves and upper cervical nerve roots project slightly upwards away from the caudally displaced medulla and cervical cord. These patients sometimes present with cerebellar ataxia or with signs of high cervical compression but the malformation is probably often clinically inapparent. Spina bifida is not usually present. Rarely, the type 1 Chiari malformation may present with hydrocephalus of communicating or non-communicating type. There is doubt as to whether this type 1 Chiari malformation is of developmental origin or whether it is due to a previous meningeal infection causing fibrous adhesions in the posterior fossa.

The *type 2* deformity, the *Arnold–Chiari malformation itself*, consists of herniation of the cerebellar vermis and tonsils through the foramen magnum

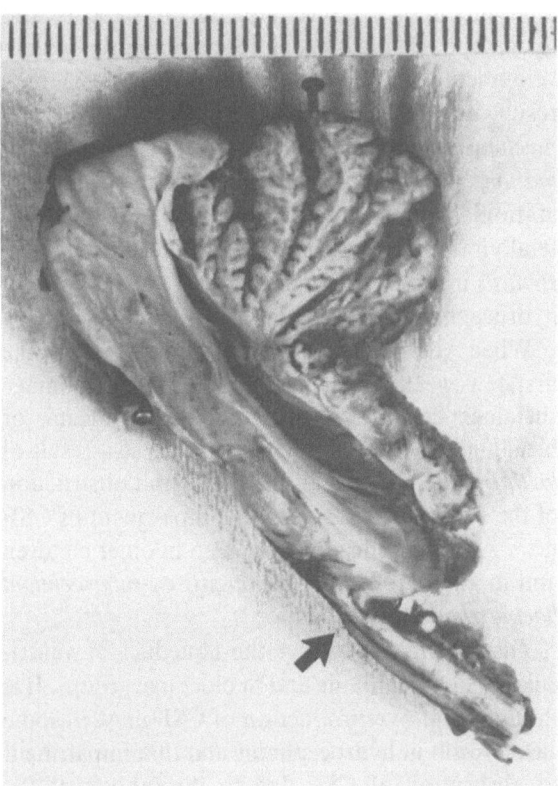

Fig. 11.8. Arnold–Chiari malformation. Sagittal section through the midbrain, pons and medulla showing elongation and herniation of the cerebellum through the foramen magnum. The medulla is elongated and *S*-shaped with a kink at the junction of the medulla and spinal cord (*arrow*).

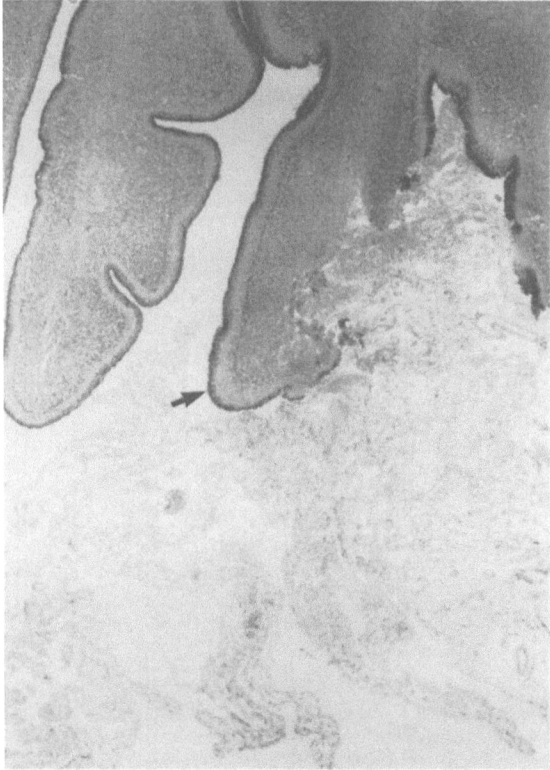

Fig. 11.9. Photomicrograph showing damage to the herniated tissue in an Arnold–Chiari malformation. The external granular layer of the normal neonate is well seen on the surface of the cerebellar folia (*arrow*).

into the upper cervical canal. In addition there is caudal displacement of the medulla, which appears narrow, *S*-shaped and elongated (Fig. 11.8). The cerebellar vermis and medulla show disorganisation of their nuclear structure and the herniated tonsils are often necrotic with meningeal adhesions (Fig. 11.9). As in the type 1 malformation, the cervical nerve roots run a cephalad course from their point of origin and craniolacunae may be found in the vault of the skull. In addition there is a shallow, malformed posterior fossa, with platybasia, basilar invagination and malformation of the craniovertebral joints. Obstructive hydrocephalus due to aqueductal stenosis is a major feature.

In the *third type* of Chiari's malformation the type 2 deformity, with hydrocephalus, is associated with spina bifida cystica. It has been suggested that the occipitocervical malformation in the various types of Chiari malformation might be due to tethering of the cord in the associated sacral malformation but this suggestion is not supported by the association with spina bifida, which would suggest that there is a developmental dysraphism at both sites.

Dandy–Walker malformation

In the Dandy–Walker malformation there is dilatation of the fourth ventricle and severe non-

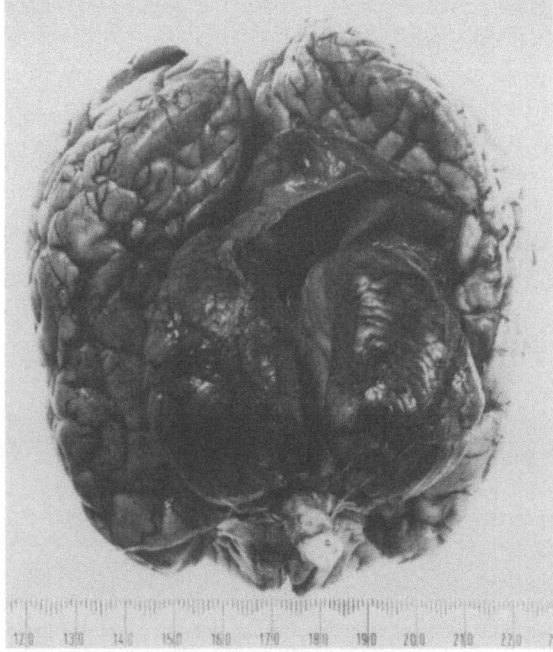

Fig. 11.10. Dandy–Walker malformation. There is deficiency of the cerebellar vermis; a cyst lined by meninges projects posteriorly and has been opened in this specimen.

communicating hydrocephalus. The foramina of Luschka and Magendie are closed so that the fourth ventricle does not communicate with the subarachnoid cisterns. The disorder is associated with agenesis of the cerebellar vermis (Fig. 11.10) and of the cerebellar hemispheres; and sometimes with agenesis of the splenium of the corpus callosum and with an occipital meningocoele. It thus appears to be a developmental malformation rather than an acquired disorder.

Hydrocephalus

Hydrocephalus occurs when there is an imbalance between secretion and absorption of CSF, usually due to blockage of the CSF pathways either within the ventricular system, the subarachnoid space or the arachnoid granulations. Dilatation of the lateral ventricles almost invariably occurs but an increase in the size of the third ventricle, aqueduct and fourth ventricle depends upon the site of the block.

In infants, hydrocephalus may be due to several causes. *Maldevelopment* of the aqueduct during fetal life may produce aqueductal stenosis and hydrocephalus in young children. Similarly, maldevelopments of the skull such as platybasia may result in hydrocephalus. As mentioned above, *myelomeningocoele* and the *Arnold–Chiari malformation* may be associated with ventricular dilatation. Damage to the aqueduct, possibly from fetal viral infections, may also result in *aqueductal stenosis* in the newborn and give rise to progressive hydrocephalus.

When ventricular dilatation occurs within the first few weeks of life, it may be due to damage sustained at birth. Tearing of the tentorium, or bleeding into the subarachnoid space as a result of *birth trauma* may result in fibrosis and obstruction of the subarachnoid space and impairment of CSF flow. A similar effect may be seen in older children and in adults following *meningitis* or *subarachnoid haemorrhage*.

Tumours may obstruct the aqueduct or ventricular system in infants and in older age groups. It is thought that overproduction of CSF may, in some cases, result in hydrocephalus and that impairment of absorption of CSF due to thrombosis of the superior sagittal sinus may also give rise to hydrocephalus.

As hydrocephalus develops in infants, the head circumference enlarges and the fontanelles become enlarged. The cranial sutures may also be separated. In very severe hydrocephalus the face appears small compared with the large head and the eyes are prominent. No enlargement of the head is seen in older patients when the cranial sutures are fused.

The *CSF pressure* is often increased in hydrocephalus but may be normal (see Chap. 4). During the acute stages of hydrocephalus, the patient may be drowsy, vomiting, and have a persistent downward gaze; weakness and spasticity of the legs may also be seen. Bilateral optic atrophy, deafness, facial weakness and sixth nerve palsies occur as complications of hydrocephalus.

Brain tissue damage has been difficult to detect in long-standing hydrocephalus but there is *clinical*

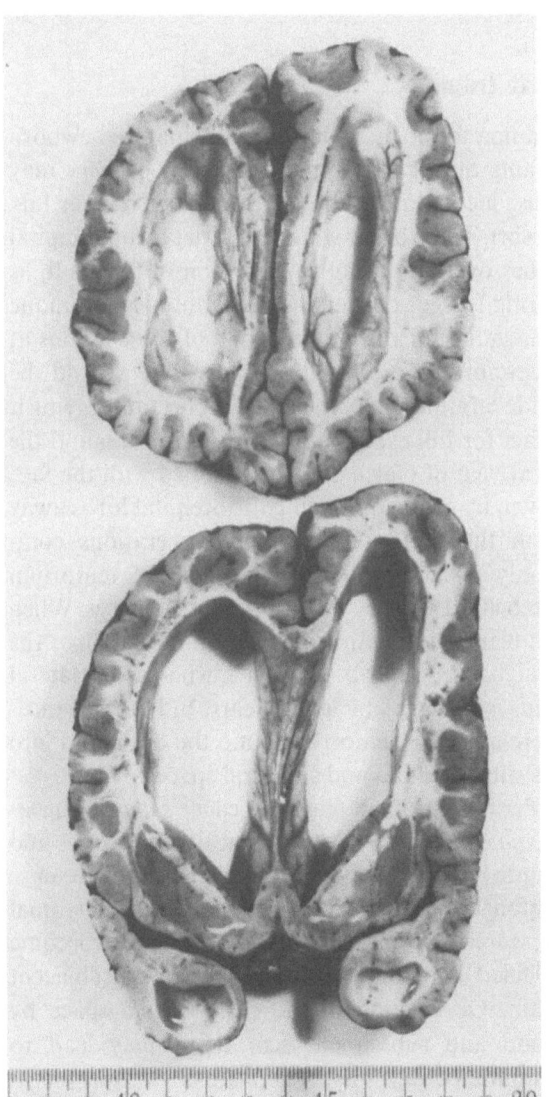

Fig. 11.11. Hydrocephalus: the lateral ventricles are grossly dilated and there is a marked reduction in the thickness of the cerebral mantle.

evidence in hydrocephalic children that delay in treatment by ventricular shunting results in brain damage which is reflected in low IQ scores and in poor school attainment. *Pathological* studies have shown that there is oedema of the periventricular white matter during the acute stages of hydrocephalus when CSF is forced into the periventricular tissue. Such oedema can be seen on CT scans. During this acute stage, there is destruction of axons in the periventricular white matter and progressive damage results eventually in gliosis. In untreated hydrocephalus, the cerebral mantle of the cortex and white matter may be very thin over the convexities of the hemispheres (Fig. 11.11). The ventricles may burst, particularly through the occipital lobe or through the lamina terminalis of the third ventricle and fluid may thus escape into the subarachnoid space.

Although *ventricular shunting* and the insertion of valves to drain CSF from hydrocephalic brains may be necessary to preserve brain tissue, the procedure is not without complications. Shunts may become infected and, if they are inserted into young children, they may need repeated revision due to the growth of the child. Nevertheless, clinical studies have shown that delay in the insertion of shunts results in a high incidence of mental retardation.

Syringomyelia

In this condition there is a cavity (*syrinx* = tube) in the substance of the cervical cord or lower brain stem (*syringobulbia*) which extends over a vertical distance of several centimetres, or at least several spinal segments. The cavity is situated more or less at the centre of the cord or brain stem, usually slightly posterior to the central canal, but it often extends eccentrically into one dorsal horn of grey matter. Syringomyelia only rarely involves the thoracic cord but lumbosacral syringomyelia has been reported. Sometimes the syrinx communicates with the central canal, or with the caudal part of the fourth ventricle, but more frequently no such communication can be demonstrated at autopsy. Despite this, it is apparent from neurosurgical and neuroradiological experience that the syrinx does communicate with the central canal at some point or with the fourth ventricle in as many as half the patients with syringomyelia studied in life. Furthermore, the cord may appear swollen in one position during myelography, and thin and collapsed in another.

Syringomyelia is an intermittent or progressive disorder starting in the *second* or *third decade*. It is characterised clinically by a combination of dissociated sensory loss, with selective loss of pain and temperature sensation, in a cape-like cervical segmental distribution, absent reflexes, and distal weakness and atrophy in the upper limbs. In the legs, there is usually a mild spastic paraparesis. Horner's syndrome and cranial nerve signs such as atrophy of half the tongue and facial hypoalgesia, with asymmetrical cerebellar ataxia and nystagmus, are features of brain stem involvement.

A proportion of patients with syringomyelia have been found to have mild non-communicating *hydrocephalus* but the relationship of this to the syringomyelia is controversial. Syringomyelia has been noted in the spinal segments adjacent to spina bifida cystica in the lumbosacral region, and adjacent to a localised diastematomyelia, and this relationship to spinal dysraphism has been mentioned above. A cystic cavity resembling syringomyelia may develop just rostral to a partial or complete *traumatic cord section* or in relation to a *glioma* of the spinal cord.

As the centrally located syringomyelic cavity with the spinal cord enlarges, the *spinothalamic fibres* crossing the cord at this level are damaged. This accounts for the selective loss of pain and temperature sensation in the affected segments of the upper cervical cord. Local damage to the descending tracts as they pass through the cervical region accounts for the corticospinal signs in the legs. The wasted hands result from local damage to anterior horns in the cervical cord.

Histologically, the syrinx is lined by glial tissue; a few macrophages are often present reflecting the damage to cord tissue. In some areas there are nests or rosettes of ependymal cells in the glial tissue which is further evidence of communication of the syrinx with the central canal of the cord.

Brain stem involvement is usually limited to the medulla and pons. The syrinx may be anterolateral to the fourth ventricle, in the midline, or anteriorly placed between the inferior olives and the pyramids. Syringomyelia is thus a disorder of the lower brain stem and of the cervical and upper thoracic cord. Lumbar syringomyelia is uncommon and cord enlargement in this region, with or without cyst formation, is more commonly associated with astrocytoma or ependymoma of the cord than with syringomyelia. Cervicomedullary syringomyelia is often associated with cerebellar ectopia, recognised at myelography by tonsillar herniation (the Chiari type 1 malformation) and with widening of the cervical spinal canal in the lateral plane. The CSF is normal in syringomyelia.

Perinatal brain injuries

The CNS is especially susceptible to damage during birth or in the neonatal period and it is often difficult to distinguish clinically between malformations arising in utero from those due to perinatal brain damage. Perinatal brain injuries may arise from trauma of hypoxia during birth, or from infection. In addition, seizures due to metabolic disorders, especially hypoglycaemia and hypocalcaemia, may also lead to brain damage. Bilirubin encephalopathy (kernicterus) is now less common than formerly.

Birth trauma

Trauma to the brain sustained by mature newborn infants during precipitate or breech delivery may cause lacerations of the tentorium cerebelli or falx cerebri. These occur when the parietal and occipital bones overlap during compression of the skull, as during forceps delivery. Careful autopsy technique is essential for the identification of these lesions at post-mortem examination. Incisions should be made on either side of the falx cerebri thus leaving it intact for full examination. The tentorium and the great vein of Galen can be examined with the face down, by gently displacing the occipital lobes away from the tentorium cerebelli. Lacerations commonly occur at the free edge of the tentorium cerebelli where they involve the dural sinuses. When the tear in the tentorium is near the midline, the straight sinus may be damaged, whereas the lateral sinus is damaged by lateral tears. In both instances there may be haemorrhage into the brain and into the subarachnoid and subdural spaces.

Perinatal trauma may also cause *subdural haematoma*, which may present clinically as seizures and failure to thrive. Later, suture diastasis and a tense fontanelle betray the presence of raised intracranial pressure. Chronic subdural haematomas become calcified, and interfere with growth of the subjacent brain. Obstruction of the *subarachnoid* space by blood and subsequent scar tissue may lead to communicating hydrocephalus. *Intracerebral* haemorrhages are less common than subdural haemorrhage, and are associated with very severe cranial trauma.

Haemorrhage into the subependymal plate (Fig. 11.12), a region in the lateral wall of each lateral ventricle which is still actively involved in the maturation of the developing brain even at birth, has recently been recognised as a feature of hypoxia or traumatic brain injury in neonates, especially in premature infants. Such lesions can be detected by CT and ultrasound scanning of the head and are obvious at autopsy. Haemorrhage in this site carries a poor prognosis and is particularly associated with failure to thrive, hydrocephalus and subsequently with mental retardation.

Cranial fractures are uncommon but may occur when delivery is forceps-assisted, and in breech deliveries. In the latter situation separation of the occipital squames (osteodiastasis), or fractures of the occipital bones occur.

Spinal cord trauma, like trauma to the head, occurs more frequently in full-term infants than in premature infants, particularly in the case of breech delivery. The cervical cord, and to a lesser extent the thoracic cord, are the usual sites of injury. Paraplegia is noted at birth, with flaccidity, and areflexia in the legs. This is associated either with fracture of a vertebra or with separation of the epiphysis during hyperextension of the spine. The cord is crushed and disrupted, and there is often an intraspinal haematoma at the site of injury. During healing of the injury a gliomesodermal scar is formed and a cyst develops in the damaged cord. In cervical injuries there may be associated damage to the vertebral arteries, leading to the occipital or brain stem infarction.

Cerebral trauma in neonates

Accidental or deliberate trauma in neonates, often called the *battered baby syndrome*, can produce bilateral subdural haematomas often associated with fracture of a parietal bone. The subdural haematomas are not necessarily related to the point

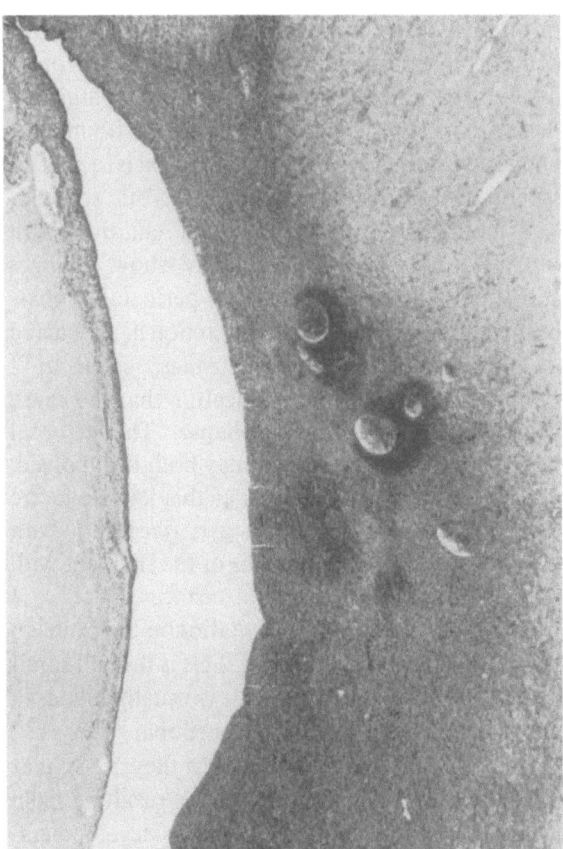

Fig. 11.12. Photomicrograph of the subependymal plate at the superior lateral aspect of the lateral ventricle in a premature infant. Two small haemorrhages are seen in the cellular subependymal plate to the right of the picture.

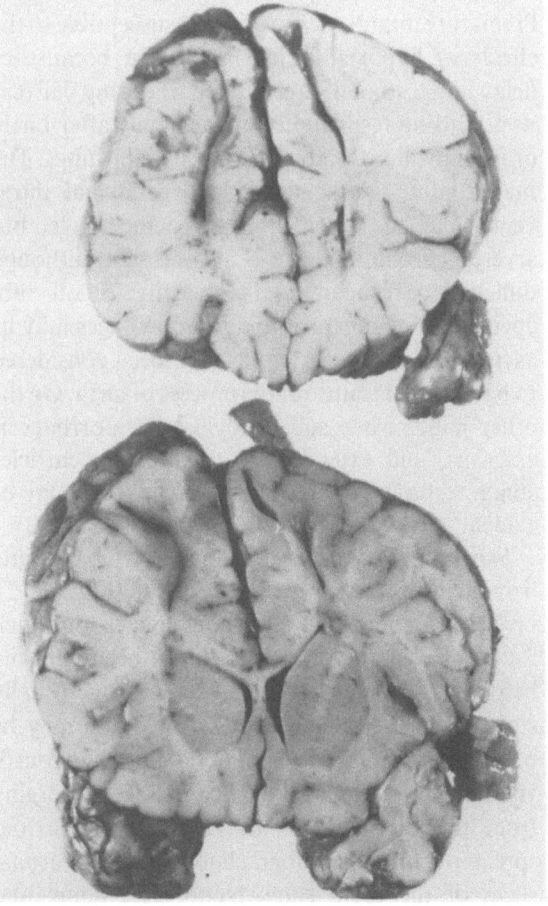

Fig. 11.13. Bilateral, symmetrical shearing clefts in the frontal lobe white matter of a 5-month-old infant. These occurred as a result of non-accidental injury (battered baby syndrome).

of impact; they can become chronic and act as a space-occupying lesion which gradually increases in size during a period of several weeks. In only half of the cases of infantile subdural haematoma is it possible to directly relate the haematoma to trauma. Retinal haemorrhages are seen in about two-thirds of all infantile subdural haematomas. In cases in which the trauma is deliberate, resulting from parent–infant stress, there are frequently multiple external bruises and multiple limb, rib or even pelvic fractures. The affected infant may appear poorly nourished and poorly cared for, and trauma is characteristically denied by the parents. Contusions are rarely seen in the brains of infants less than 9 months old because the floors of the anterior and middle fossae are smooth. In infants, shearing stresses act maximally in the white matter, producing clefts (contusional tears) extending from the frontal to the occipital lobes in the most severe cases (Fig. 11.13). These extensive tears may contain old or recent haemorrhage.

Hypoxia

Premature infants are particularly susceptible to the effects of hypoxia, which may occur because of delay in the second stage of labour, during delivery itself, during resuscitation immediately after birth, or from hyaline membrane disease of the lungs. The major pathological change is subependymal, intraventricular or leptomeningeal haemorrhage, but severe neuronal damage is also present, although difficult to recognise pathologically. Small subependymal or subarachnoid haemorrhages may be asymptomatic; the latter has even been considered to be a normal feature of the process of birth. On the other hand, when subependymal haemorrhage is extensive and extends into the lateral ventricles coma, respiratory arrest and quadriparesis may be evident.

Subependymal haemorrhage occurs from bleeding from veins in the subependymal plate (Fig. 11.12), probably secondary to the venous congestion which follows circulatory collapse. It can occur during, before or after delivery. The haemorrhage usually starts from the thalamostriate veins, and may be bilateral, spreading into the lateral, third and fourth ventricles. At autopsy, blood can be seen emerging from the foramina of the fourth ventricle and spreading into the subarachnoid space. Coronal slices of the brain show blood clot, filling and distending the lateral ventricles and occasionally rupturing into the brain through the ventricular

horns. In about one-quarter of cases there are secondary *periventricular infarcts*. Rarely, intracerebellar haemorrhage may also occur, and associated subpial haemorrhages sometimes disrupt the superficial cerebral cortex.

When infants survive the initial stage of the illness small brown streaks can be recognised in the subependymal zone and in the superficial layers of the cortex. In the case of larger haemorrhages small cysts are formed. Glial reaction is minimal, but there may be a local macrophage response. In the case of larger haemorrhages hydrocephalus may occur due to obliteration of the basal cisterns. Communicating hydrocephalus can also result as an acute complication arising from the large amount of blood obliterating the subarachnoid space and obstructing the arachnoid granulations.

Infarction of the *cortex* and *white matter* may occur in the neonatal period, particularly in the premature infant. It is found either in the distribuion of a major vessel, suggesting traumatic damage, or in the boundary zones between the territories of two vessels indicating circulatory failure. Infarction of the periventricular white matter may occur following severe hypoxia, for example in the respiratory distress syndrome of premature infants. Multiple sharply circumscribed pale areas are found in the subependymal white matter. Histologically these are zones of coagulative necrosis with macrophage invasion; astrocytic proliferation is seen after several days at the edges of these necrotic zones.

Examination of the brains of children with *cerebral palsy* and *epilepsy* may show changes consistent with the late effects of perinatal hypoxic brain damage. In most cases infarction has occurred in one or more boundary zones, often in a symmetrical distribution, indicating that the cause was hypoxic circulatory collapse. The cerebral hemispheres and cerebellum may both be involved. Characteristically the lesions at this late stage are seen as shrunken groups of gyri (*ulegyria*), with gliosis, especially in the depths of the sulci but with relatively well-preserved gyral surfaces.

Cystic degeneration or cavitation in the centrum semi-ovale may also be found. This is the end result of periventricular infarction. It is usually bilateral, and is sometimes called 'centrilobar sclerosis'. When cystic infarcts are very large they are similar in form to porencephalic cavitation resulting from infarction, or from failure of brain development, earlier in fetal life. *Status marmoratus (état marbré)* is a similar disorder, clinically manifest by double athetosis and mental retardation. Glial scars form in the corpus striatum following vascular or hypoxic damage and then the scars become *hypermyelinated*, producing a 'marbled' appearance in the affected areas.

Kernicterus: bilirubin encephalopathy

Infantile hyperbilirubinaemia results from poor conjugation of bilirubin. This may be due to inadequate uptake of bilirubin by the liver, poor conjugation of bilirubin due to reduced amounts of glucuronyl-transferase in the liver, or to reduced excretion.

Hyperbilirubinaemia is a normal phenomenon in neonates, partly because of physiological haemolysis occurring as red cells containing fetal haemoglobin are replaced by red cells containing adult haemoglobin, and partly because of immaturity of the neonatal liver.

The basal ganglia are especially vulnerable to damage from high levels of circulating bilirubin, presumably in part because bilirubin more easily enters these parts of the brain. This form of neonatal brain damage—kernicterus—is more likely to develop in premature infants than in fullterm infants. In the former it may occur with bilirubin levels somewhat lower than 20 mg/100 ml, but it is uncommon in full-term infants unless the bilirubin level is greater than 30 mg/100 ml. In premature infants, the blood–brain barrier is less mature, and the neurons themselves may be more vulnerable to the toxic effects of bilirubin. Since much circulating bilirubin is normally bound to albumin, drugs which themselves show affinity for albumin, such as anticonvulsants and sulphonamides, may displace albumin-bound bilirubin, thus increasing the amount of free, unbound circulating bilirubin and increasing the risk of kernicterus developing.

Since the brunt of the toxic effect of bilirubin falls on the basal ganglia, and to a lesser extent on cortical neurons, motor disorders are a prominent clinical feature. There is often bilateral athetosis and spasticity, with mental retardation and epilepsy. The condition can be prevented by avoiding high bilirubin levels, the commonest cause of which was formerly Rhesus iso-immunisation with profound haemolysis. This disorder can now itself be avoided by preventing the maternal sensitisation which occurs from transplacental bleeding of Rhesus-positive red blood cells during pregnancy and delivery. Due to this measure, kernicterus is now less common.

Pathology. The recently fixed brain of an infant dying of bilirubin encephalopathy shows a highly selective pattern of distribution of yellow bilirubin pigment. The commonest sites affected are the globus pallidus, subthalamic nucleus and hippocampus; the thalamic nuclei and corpus striatum are less prominently involved. Any focal areas of brain damage, especially coincidental infarcts in premature infants, take up the pigment preferentially. Histological examination shows neuronal loss, pyknosis and chromatolysis, with reactive astrocytosis in the affected areas. In cases surviving into adult life, brain shrinkage with neuronal loss and glial scars are the main features.

Neonatal infections

Neonatal meningitis usually occurs in the first few days of life. It is seen in about 40 per 100 000 live births, and in most cases involves premature infants. Because there is usually an accompanying septicaemia the mortality rate is high, and residual signs of brain damage are common in the survivors. Gramnegative organisms, especialy *E.coli*, are the commonest cause of meningitis in neonates in developed countries, but *streptococcal* infections are also common in the developing world. Tuberculosis of the CNS is uncommon in this age-group, but viral infections, particularly cytomegalovirus, herpes simplex and enterovirus infections may also lead to permanent brain damage.

The phakomatoses

A group of disorders with a familial basis, the phakomatoses are characterised by the presence of a malformation of the neuraxis, together with multiple small tumours which involve neuroectodermal structures. The nervous system, the skin, the eyes and some internal organs, for example the kidneys, are thus commonly involved. There are *five* relatively common phakomatoses (Table 11.1) of which von Recklinghausen's neurofibromatosis is the most important and the most frequent. The Sturge–Weber syndrome of encephalofacial angiomatosis is included in this group of diseases although true multi-ectodermal involvement is not a feature. Furthermore, multiple small tumours do not occur in this latter condition and it may therefore not be regarded as a phakomatous disorder.

Table 11.1. Major clinical and pathological features of the phakomatoses

	Neurofibromatosis	Tuberose sclerosis	Von Hippel–Lindau syndrome	Sturge–Weber syndrome	Ataxia–telangiectasia
Genetic pattern	Dominant with variable penetrance	? Autosomal recessive	Dominant with variable penetrance	?	Dominant
Mental retardation		+			
Epilepsy	+	+		+	
Skeletal malformation	+				
Areas of cutaneous pigmentation and depigmentation	+	+	+	+	+
Angiomas			+	+	+
Peripheral nerve tumours	+				
CNS tumours	+	+	+		
Tumours in other organs	+	+	+		
CNS malformations	+	+	+	+	

Neurofibromatosis

This disorder occurs in several forms of varying severity. In the mildest form there is a cutaneous abnormality without other stigmata of the disease. The cutaneous manifestations consist of areas of *café-au-lait* pigmentation (Fig. 11.14) which are often multiple and arranged in a slightly linear form within the boundaries of individual dermatomes. Smaller depigmented spots are also seen and pedunculated fibrous skin tumours occur which are usually small but are occasionally large. In addition, cutaneous neurofibromas may develop (Fig. 11.15); these can be very large, although soft, and are liable to undergo sarcomatous change. The cutaneous

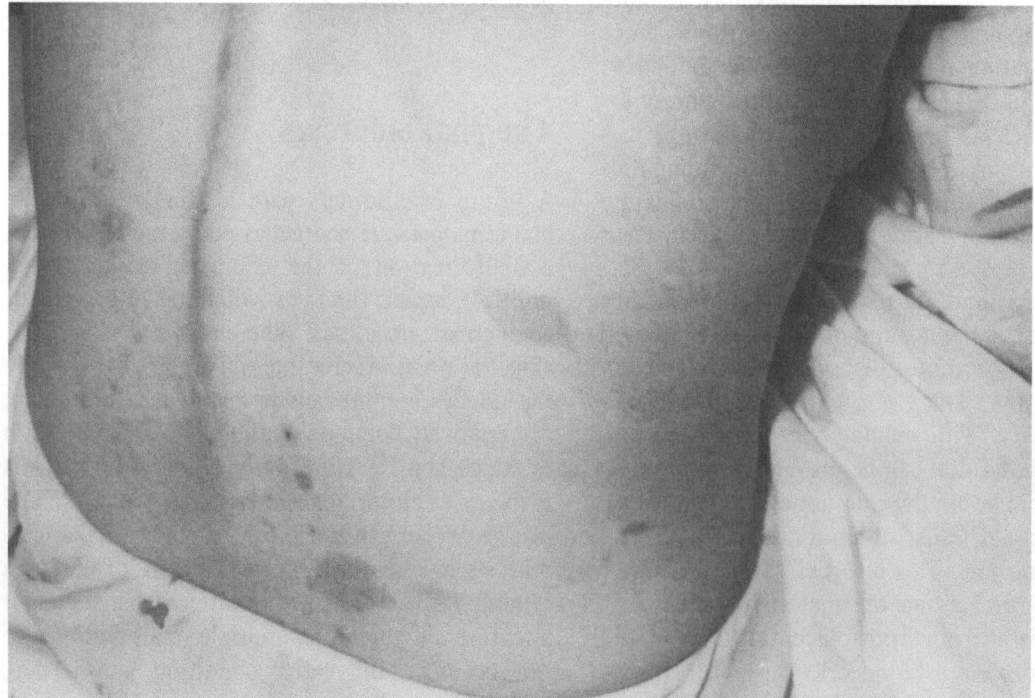

Fig. 11.14. von Recklinghausen's disease. Café-au-lait spots on the back with small, depigmented areas above.

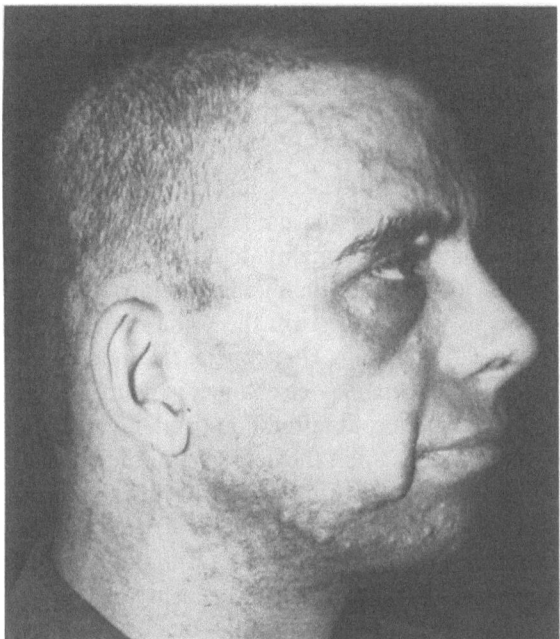

Fig. 11.15. von Recklinghausen's disease. Numerous facial neurofibromas.

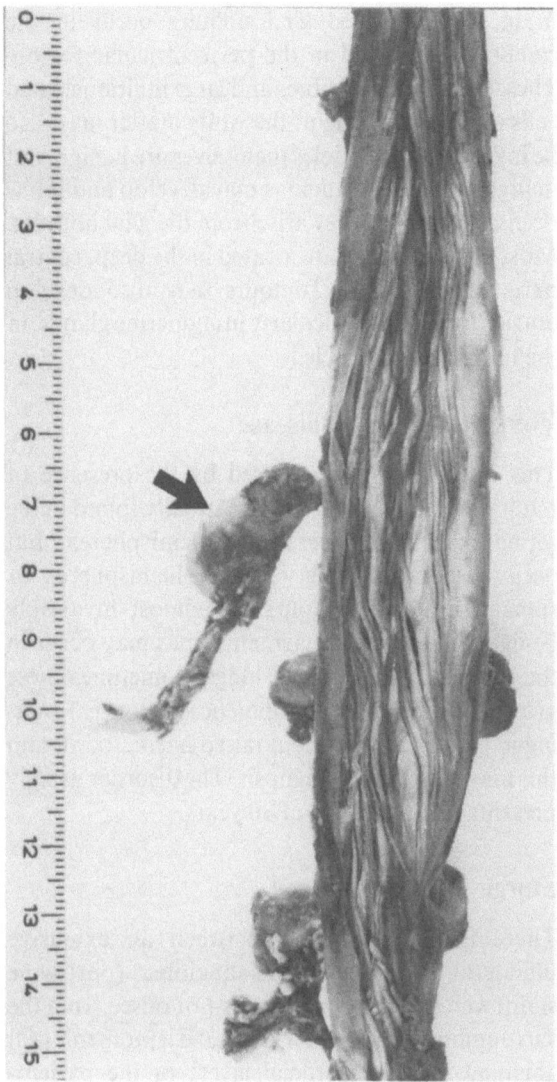

Fig. 11.16. von Recklinghausen's disease. Neurofibromas on lumbosacral nerve roots (*arrow*).

abnormality is often limited to a few moderate-sized (greater than about 5×2 cm) café-au-lait naevi, but in severe cases the cutaneous manifestations are both widespread and gross, resulting in the embarrassing deformity of *elephantiasis nervosa*.

In patients with CNS involvement, the cutaneous abnormality is often relatively slight, but this inverse relationship is not invariably true. Both malformations and tumours of the CNS may be associated with von Recklinghausen's disease. The malformations usually consist of heterotopias, zones of cortical dysplasia or polymicrogyria, syringomyelia, and hydrocephalus due to stenosis of the aqueduct of Sylvius. In patients with von Recklinghausen's disease these last two malformations are themselves commonly associated with malformations of the neural arches, vertebral bodies and the base of the skull. Other bony abnormalities occur, including dysplasia of the lateral walls of the orbits, and anomalies of the ribs and of the long bones.

The *most serious complication* of neurofibromatosis is the propensity to develop neural tumours. These most commonly involve nerve roots (Fig. 11.16) and peripheral nerves, but tumours of the CNS also occur and may be malignant. Schwannomas of the spinal sensory roots, of the vestibular part of the eighth cranial nerve, and of the sensory root of the trigeminal nerve are particularly common, but similar tumours may be found at multiple sites on the peripheral nerves themselves (see Chap. 7). Meningiomas are also a common feature of the disease, and these are often multiple. CNS tumours in this disorder include gliomas, both within the brain and in the optic nerves. Outside the CNS other neuroectodermal tumours may develop, including renal, pancreatic and suprarenal tumours. Phaeochromocytoma has been particularly associated with this disease.

Tuberose sclerosis

This is a relatively rare condition characterised by skin lesions, the classic *adenoma sebaceum*. These are small nodules in the nasolabial region. Cutaneous fibromas may be more widespread. In the brain, circumscribed glial nodules occur in the cerebral cortex and in the periventricular region. These consist of glial fibres and large multinucleated cells of uncertain origin; the white matter may also be involved. The nodules themselves are benign, but malignant cerebral gliomas may develop and it has been thought that they arise from the glial nodules. Most of the gliomas are located in the deep, central parts of the brain. Tumours may also develop outside the CNS, particularly in endocrine glands, in the lungs and in muscle.

Von Hippel–Lindau disease

This disorder is characterised by the presence of multiple haemangioblastomas, usually found in the retina and in the cerebellar hemispheres, but occasionally involving cerebral hemispheres or spinal cord. The tumours are almost invariably benign. Similar cystic haemangiomas may occur in the pancreas, kidneys and lungs. Sometimes these growths secrete an erythropoietic substance, resulting in erythrocytosis and a raised haematocrit, and this may be useful in diagnosis. The disorder usually presents before the age of 30 years.

Sturge–Weber syndrome

There is an association between an extensive unilateral facial cutaneous angioma (port-wine stain) which is characteristically not raised from the surrounding skin, and a widespread leptomeningeal angioma in the superficial layers of the parieto-occipital cortex on the same side of the body. The cerebral angiomatous malformation is often associated with loss and pyknosis of cortical neurons, and with glial proliferation; epilepsy is a common feature. Often the cerebral lesion is associated with calcification of the gyri, visible on x-rays and CT scans as linear bands of calcification.

Ataxia–telangiectasia

In this rare condition cutaneous vascular malformations resembling spider naevi are associated with retinal degeneration, ataxia and cerebellar malformation, epilepsy and visceral neoplasms. There is an associated deficiency of IgA.

Other phakomatoses

Other rare neuro-cutaneous syndromes, such as Marinesco–Sjögren syndrome, have been included in this group of disorders, but they are of uncertain origin.

Pathology of metabolic disorders of the brain

The severity of tissue damage and the degree of pathological abnormality in metabolic disorders varies according to the disease. In most cases, the main tissue damage is in the white matter, which often shows spongy change. Reactive astrocytosis occurs and there may be changes in neurons. There are few specific abnormalities and the diagnosis really depends upon the detection of the biochemical or endocrine disorder during life (Chap. 12). Nevertheless, a clear understanding of pathological changes that occur in the brain is important for planning the patient's management and, for the pathologist, for documenting the course of the disease at autopsy.

In neonatal *hypothyroidism* brain growth and development is retarded with hypomyelination of the cerebral white matter. This is reflected in the mental retardation and low IQ in affected children (see Chap. 12). Widespread calcification may also occur in the white matter.

The brain in children dying with *phenylketonuria* is generally small. In older, severely affected individuals, there is a generalised loss of white matter and gliosis. The spinal cord may also be involved with atrophy of the myelinated long tracts.

There is a characteristic appearance in the brains of untreated cases of *maple syrup urine disease*. The brain is heavy, enlarged and appears oedematous. Histologically, the cerebral white matter has a spongiform appearance and crystalline proteins may be detected in the cytoplasm of glial cells in alcohol-fixed material. Treated cases usually show no histological abnormality.

The brain damage resulting from the *urea cycle abnormalities* is variable and neurons are affected rather more than the white matter.

Two disorders of *glycogen metabolism* involve the brain. In von Gierke's disease repeated episodes of hypoglycaemia may lead to brain damage with loss of neurons. Glycogen may accumulate in the nervous system, producing little macroscopic change in the brain but, in tissue fixed in alcohol, glycogen can be demonstrated in almost all neuronal groups and in glial cells within the brain and spinal cord by the PAS technique. Glycogen is also present in cells in other tissues.

Ballooning of nerve cells is also seen in *mannosidosis* and *fructosidosis*, in which there is also neuronal loss and widespread damage to the white matter with reactive gliosis.

Pathology of inborn lysosomal storage disorders

Diagnosis of this group of disorders can usually be made in utero or in infancy by a combination of biochemical studies of plasma, leukocytes and cultured skin fibroblasts (see Chap. 13). Histological and histochemical examination of neural tissue from brain or rectal biopsy is now rarely necessary. The pathologists, however, may be confronted with the autopsy of a patient in whom the biochemical studies have not been completed. In such circumstances, a complete autopsy examination is valuable not only for clinico-pathological correlation but also for establishing a diagnosis for genetic counselling. The tissue examined should include the brain, peripheral nerves and reticuloendothelial system. Frozen sections of formalin- and dioxane-fixed material can be used for the histochemical demonstration of stored proteins and lipids. Electron microscopy of glutaraldehyde-fixed material from cortex, white matter and peripheral nerves may also be useful especially in diseases such as gangliosidoses, metachromatic leukodystrophy, and Krabbe disease where intracellular accumulation (storage) of material has a characteristic ultrastructure. Histopathological examination of autopsy material without the benefit of antemortem biochemical studies has limited usefulness and, in many instances, can only give a rough guide to the classification of the disorder.

Lysosomal storage disorders can be divided into two main histopathological groups: those that affect *neurons*, and those that affect the *white matter* (leukodystrophies). A third group of disorders, the *mucolipidoses*, show features of both neuronal storage disorders and leukodystrophy.

Neuronal storage disorders

Mucopolysaccharidoses (glycosaminoglycan storage diseases)

The major pathological changes in this group result from the storage of glycolipid, reflecting a disturbance of glycosaminoglycan metabolism. Connective tissue and bone are particularly affected but

myocardium and arterial intima are also involved. There is considerable overlap in the pattern of visceral involvement and in the pattern of brain involvement. In the *Hunter*, *Hurler* and *Sanfilippo* syndromes, meningeal thickening is often prominent and is sometimes so severe that the cerebral convolutions are obscured. Hydrocephalus due to meningeal and aqueduct obstruction may also occur. The blood vessels in the white matter are prominent with the accumulation of macrophages containing glycosaminoglycans and lipid expanding the perivascular spaces.

Microscopic examination of formalin-fixed brains shows widespread 'ballooning' of neurons with foamy or reticular cytoplasm displacing the nucleus. Although a small amount of PAS-positive material may be present in the neurons most is removed by processing for paraffin section. In frozen sections neurons and macrophages contain lipid and carbohydrate which is PAS positive and also stains with Sudan red and Sudan black. The intracellular lipid stored within the neurons and macrophages has been identified as *gangliosides*. Electron microscopy shows lamellated lipid bodies within the cytoplasm of affected cells; the lamellae are arranged in regular stacks with a periodicity of 5.5–6 nm and are referred to as 'zebra bodies'.

Gangliosidoses

The liver, spleen, reticulo-endothelial system and kidneys may be involved together with the brain in the gangliosidoses. In both the GM_1 and GM_2 gangliosidoses there is neuronal loss and the accumulation of stored material within the remaining neurons. Thus in the early stage of the disease the brain may be large, but it may be shrunken in the later stages. The gyral pattern is normal but, as in the glycosaminoglycan storage disorders, the meninges are thickened and the ventricles are often dilated.

Microscopically, neurons in the brain are distended and balloon-like with eccentric nuclei and fine granular cytoplasm. In paraffin sections of formalin-fixed material, the neurons stain only faintly with PAS but the glial cells and macrophages may contain more PAS material. In frozen sections, the stored gangliosides in the cytoplasm of neurons and glial cells stain intensely for PAS and with Sudan and other lipid stains. Electron microscopy of affected neurons shows the accumulation of spherical, lamellated structures (membranous cytoplasmic bodies) which are approximately 1 μm in diameter and have a periodicity of 5–6 nm; they differ in their appearance from the zebra bodies seen in the mucopolysaccharidoses.

Both central neurons and the peripheral autonomic neurons are affected in GM_2 gangliosidosis. Thus, the neurons in a rectal biopsy stain positively with PAS and lipid stains in frozen sections and show membranous cytoplasmic bodies in their cytoplasm.

Gaucher disease

The infantile and juvenile forms of Gaucher disease are characterised by hepatosplenomegaly as well as by bone involvement. Visceral pathology is characterised by the presence of Gaucher cells which are large, rounded cells 20–80 μm in diameter with a small eccentric nucleus; they show a strong PAS reaction in frozen sections, reflecting the accumulation of *glucocerebrosides*.

There is widespread neuronal loss in the brain in the rapidly progressive infantile form of Gaucher disease but with relatively little lipid storage within the neurons. The white matter shows no characteristic changes.

Niemann–Pick disease

There is widespread accumulation of large amounts of sphingomyelin within the viscera and brain in the classic infantile form of Niemann–Pick disease. Vacuolation of lymphocytes in the blood is also seen in this disease. Microscopy of the liver, spleen and lymphoid tissue shows massive accumulation of foam cells which, in frozen section, stain positively with Sudan black and with Baker's acid haematin method for phospholipids. PAS reaction is weak.

The brain is usually shrunken and on microscopy shows widespread storage of phospholipid in neurons. Cortex, basal ganglia and cerebellum may all be affected but the white matter usually only shows the secondary changes of neuronal destruction.

Ceroid lipofuscinoses

There are a number of disorders affecting infants, older children and occasionally adults, in which excessive amounts of ceroid material accumulate within the brain, usually within the cytoplasm of neurons. Although the high activity of lysosomal enzymes associated with the ceroid material sug-

gests that the ceroid lipofuscinoses are lysosomal storage disorders, evidence for specific enzyme deficiencies is scarce. No reliable biochemical diagnostic tests are yet available; the diagnosis is made on the clinical features of age of onset, pattern of mental deterioration and neurological defect. Pathologically, the various forms of the disease are recognised by the pattern of neuronal involvement in ceroid lipofuscin accumulation and to some extent by the electron microscopic appearance of the ceroid within the cells.

Leukodystrophies

The leukodystrophies are a heterogeneous group of diseases which are characterised pathologically by widespread demyelination involving the CNS white matter and in some cases the peripheral nervous system. The demyelination is often bilaterally symmetrical and may be due to degeneration or failure of maturation of the myelin. On examination of the brain, the white matter is often firm and gliotic but in advanced disease, the white matter may be spongy and soft.

There are several different types of leukodystrophy which vary in their pattern of onset and in details of their pathology. In many leukodystrophies the cause is unknown. Metachromatic leukodystrophy and Krabbe disease are both biochemical disorders of lipid metabolism and their biochemistry is discussed in Chap. 13.

Metachromatic leukodystrophy (sulphatide lipidosis)

As the name implies, there is an accumulation of metachromatic material within the central white matter and peripheral nerves. The term metachromasia refers to the brown staining of the abnormal lipid deposits when frozen sections are stained with acid cresyl violet. The *cerebroside sulphate* deposits can also be stained golden-yellow by Holländer's technique.

There may be little macroscopic abnormality in the brain of patients dying with metachromatic leukodystrophy but on microscopy, there is diffuse loss of myelin from the cerebral white matter. Astrocytes may be increased in number but oligodendrocytes are reduced. Granular masses of metachromatic lipid 15–20 μm in diameter are seen in the white matter. The cerebral cortex is usually well preserved and there is little accumulation of metachromatic lipid within neurons. The globus pallidus, thalamus and dentate nuclei tend to be involved in the disease.

Segmental demyelination occurs in peripheral nerves. The electron microscopic appearance of the metachromatic lipid in peripheral nerves in Fig. 16.19 is similar to the deposits in cerebral white matter.

Metachromatic lipid accumulates within cells of the gastro-intestinal tract, adrenals, ovaries and kidneys. Examination of early morning urine specimens may show metachromatic granules released from renal tubular cells shed into the urine.

Krabbe (globoid cell) leukodystrophy

The brain in globoid cell leukodystrophy is usually small and firm; in unfixed brain slices, the white matter is discoloured and usually grey. Microscopy shows an almost total loss of myelin from the white matter and a greatly diminished oligodendrocyte population; marked astrocytosis of the white matter is usually seen.

The diagnostic feature is the *globoid cell* which is large, 35–40 μm in diameter, and contains rounded cytoplasmic bodies. The cells are frequently multinucleate and the cytoplasm is clear or finely granular and stains diffusely with PAS. The abnormal cells are distributed throughout the dystrophic white matter and within the perivascular spaces. Electron microscopy shows characteristic angular crystalloid structures within the cytoplasm of the globoid cells.

Mucolipidoses

This group of disorders shows features intermediate between the mucopolysaccharidoses and the lipidoses. The brain is usually smaller than normal with marked loss of white matter. Various types of material may be stored for example, ganglioside, fructose and glycolipid (fructosidosis), and neuronal lipid.

Further reading

Emery J L, Lendon R G (1972) The local cord lesion in neurospinal dysraphism (myelomeningocoele). J Pathol 110:83

Friede R L (1975) Developmental neuropathology. Springer-Verlag, Wien New York

Hook E B, Fabia J J (1978) Frequency of Down syndrome in live births by single year maternal age interval with results of a Massachussetts study. Teratology 17:223

Karch S B, Urich H (1972) Occipital encephalocele: a morphological study. J Neuropathol Exptl Neurol 15:89

Krones S B (1976) Congenital rubella: an encapsulated review. Teratology 14:111

Loeser J D, Alvard L E (1968) Agenesis of the corpus callosum. Brain 91:553

Penfield W, Young A W (1930) The nature of von Recklinghausen's disease and the tumours associated with it. Arch Neurol Psychiatry (Chic) 28:320

Persand T V N (1977) Problems of birth defects. MTP, Lancaster

Reynolds D W, St Agno S, Alford C A (1978) Congenital cytomegalvirus infection. Teratology 17:178

Rokos J (1979) The pathogenesis of spina bifida and related disorders. In: Cavanagh J, Thames Smith W (eds) Recent advances in neuropathology. Churchill Livingstone, Edinburgh, p 224

Russell D S (1949) Observations on the pathology of hydrocephalus. Special report series. Medical Research Council, No. 265, HMSO, London

Schwetz B A, Smith F A, Staples R E (1978) Teratogenic potential of ethanol in mice, rats and rabbits. Teratology 18:385

Urich H (1976) Malformations of the nervous system, perinatal damage and related conditions in early life. In: Blackwood W, Corsellis J A N (eds) Greenfield's neuropathology. Arnold, London, p 361

Chapter 12

Metabolic Disorders Affecting the Nervous System

Inborn errors of metabolism make a considerable contribution to the morbidity and mortality of children in a Western population (Raine 1974), since there are so many different disorders, albeit each with a low incidence. Inherited biochemical defects have been reported for many groups of compounds including carbohydrates, amino acids, purines and pyrimidines, trace metals, lipids and mucopolysaccharides. The onset of clinical symptoms may not become apparent until adult life, but this is unusual, the majority appearing during childhood and frequently in the first few days of life.

This chapter refers to the biochemical aspects, diagnosis and treatment of some of the more important disorders which have consequences for the nervous system. Inborn lysosomal storage disorders affecting the nervous system are reviewed in Chap. 13, and the neuropathology of metabolic disorders is summarised in Chap. 11.

Neonatal hypothyroidism

The most important metabolic condition to affect the nervous system in childhood is hypothyroidism. Only a small proportion of cases will be due to inherited defects, but it seems appropriate to discuss neonatal hypothyroidism as screening programmes for the early detection of the condition are being introduced in conjunction with those for inherited disorders. Screening of neonates for congenital hypothyroidism was first introduced in Quebec in 1974 (Dussault et al. 1975) and since then programmes have been set up in many places. This has been done in the expectation that early diagnosis and treatment will improve the prognosis (Smith and Morris 1979).

In a retrospective survey of hypothyroidism amongst children in North London, only 40% of cases had been recognised before 3 months of age, about one-third of children with the condition required special schooling and one-quarter of them had an IQ of less than 70 (Hulse et al. 1980). In a pilot project in which 87 444 infants born in North London were screened, the incidence of the condition was 1 in 3363 births (Hulse et al. 1980). The *screening test* was a highly specific radioimmunoassay for thyroid-stimulating hormone (TSH) on single dried blood spots collected from heel-stabs during the 6th to 14th days of life. Of the first 26 infants detected, only 2 had been diagnosed before the screening test was available. An ectopic thyroid was the most common finding and 2 infants probably had inherited defects of thyroxine synthesis. Accumulating evidence from many centres is firmly supporting the belief that prognosis will be improved, but definitive evidence will not be available for some years.

The *TSH method* does not detect secondary hypothyroidism but this is uncommon (1 in 60 000 to 1 in 100 000 births) (Fisher et al. 1979) and there is no convincing evidence that these patients are at risk for mental subnormality.

Phenylketonuria

All infants are screened for phenylketonuria since this is one of the few causes of mental subnormality for which effective treatment is available. The children show adequate intellectual development, they attend normal schools and are strikingly different from untreated or late-treated phenylketonuric children, many of whom required permanent institutional care.

Screening

Early screening programmes depended on the detection of abnormal metabolites in urine (Fig. 12.1), but many cases were missed. In 1969 the Department of Health and Social Security issued a memorandum recommending the establishment of a screening programme relying on the detection of a raised concentration of phenylalanine in blood. The specimen is collected from a heel-stab between the 6th and 14th days of life. In many instances the Guthrie test (Guthrie 1961) is used, the blood being collected as spots on a special filter paper. Phenylalanine may also be determined by chromatography or fluorimetry using blood spots or liquid samples.

Experience has shown that phenylketonuria is not a single disease entity but encompasses a number of disorders of differing clinical and biochemical severity and the term 'hyperphenyl-

alaninaemia' is now more appropriate to embrace this heterogeneous collection of disorders. Indeed many other inherited disorders which used to appear to be single disease entities show genetic heterogeneity. Most patients with persistent hyperphenylalaninaemia have one of several defects of phenylalanine hydroxylase activity (Kaufman 1978; Güttler 1980).

In animals, excess phenylalanine interferes with the passage of other essential amino acids through the blood–brain barrier. Comar et al. (1981) have shown that this is true also for phenylketonuric children, especially in the first 2 years of life. They measured the brain uptake of ^{11}C-methionine in the presence of increasing concentrations of phenylalanine in the blood.

There is considerable geographical variation in the *incidence* of hyperphenylalaninaemia. For example, in a survey of three-quarters of a million infants born in North London from October 1969 to December 1978 the overall incidence of persistent phenylalaninaemia was of the order of 7 per 100 000 births (Walker et al. 1981). The comparable incidence for Northern Ireland was 28 per 100 000 births.

In the screening programme, false positives due to uncomplicated transient hyperphenylalaninaemia with or without tyrosinaemia were encountered and necessitated careful follow-up. During the study the incidence of such cases fell and the reduction coincided with a change in infant feeding practice in the United Kingdom which led to low intakes of protein and phenylalanine (Department of Health and Social Security, 1974).

Amongst the 51 infants with persistently elevated blood phenylalanine levels detected in North London, there were considerable variations in the amounts of natural protein which they could tolerate in their diets. Some were able to tolerate 10 g or more daily and others only between 3 and 6 g daily.

Treatment

The aim of treatment is to lower the circulating level of phenylalanine to a concentration just slightly higher than that found in normal subjects. The intake of phenylalanine is reduced by using a synthetic substitute for much of the protein in the diet (Francis 1975). This may be based on a hydrolysate (used in infancy) or on a mixture of synthetic amino acids excluding phenylalanine (used for all other ages). Since phenylalanine is an

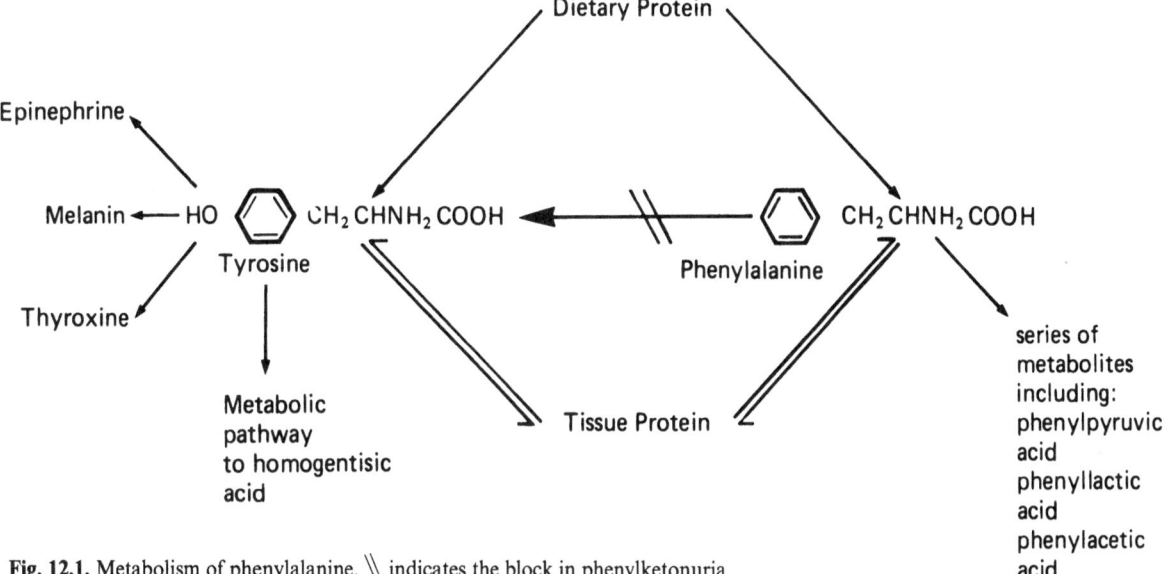

Fig. 12.1. Metabolism of phenylalanine. \\ indicates the block in phenylketonuria.

essential amino acid, regular monitoring of the level in the blood is essential so that the optimum amount of phenylalanine for an individual patient may be provided from natural foodstuffs. A number of manufactured foods are marketed, e.g. phenylalanine-free bread, and in the United Kingdom these are prescribable as drugs for patients with this disorder.

In the initial phases of phenylalanine deficiency there is failure to thrive and a characteristic skin rash which is likely to become infected; if untreated the deficiency is ultimately fatal. The diet must contain added minerals and also vitamins (including thiamine hydrochloride, riboflavine pyridoxine hydrochloride, nicotinamide, calcium, pantothenate, ascorbic acid, α-tocopheryl acetate, inositol, biotin, folic acid, acetomenaphthone, vitamins A and D, choline chloride and cyanocobalamin). Failure to provide the complete source of vitamins is potentially lethal.

Experience and knowledge of the diet has accumulated over some years. Poor nutrition due to inadequate dietary treatment has caused stunting of growth and impaired intellectual function (Smith et al. 1973). The principles of treatment by dietary restriction so well illustrated by phenylketonuria (Clayton 1975) are applicable to many other disorders, e.g. some other amino acid disorders, galactosaemia and Refsum's disease.

Disorders of biopterin metabolism

About 1%–3% of infants with hyperphenylalaninaemia have disorders of biopterin metabolism

(Kaufman 1980; O'Brien et al. 1980), and therefore fail to respond to a low phenylalanine diet (Fig. 12.2). The main clinical features seen in a number of such children have been summarised by Danks et al. 1978 (Fig. 12.3). They were generally similar to infants with other neurodegenerative disorders, although disturbances of tone and posture, myoclonic epilepsy and difficulties in swallowing were perhaps more frequent.

The deficiency of tetrahydrobiopterin may be caused by defective recycling of this cofactor due to deficient activity of dihydropteridine reductase, or by defective de novo synthesis (Danks and Cotton 1980). Tetrahydrobiopterin is the cofactor for phenylalanine hydroxylase, tyrosine hydroxylase and tryptophan hydroxylase, and is therefore of major importance in the ultimate production of neurotransmitters. The therapeutic response to the neurotransmitter precursors L-dopa and 5-hydroxytryptophan and to tetrahydrobiopterin and related compounds is encouraging (e.g. Butler et al. 1978; Curtius et al. 1979). Detailed investigation of biopterin metabolism should be performed in any infant with phenylketonuria detected on routine screening and developing suspicious features such as abnormal movements and hypotonia whilst on dietary treatment.

Termination of diet

Whether or not the low phenylalanine diet may be terminated or even relaxed as the child becomes older remains a controversial matter. Any diet during childhood produces psychological stress for

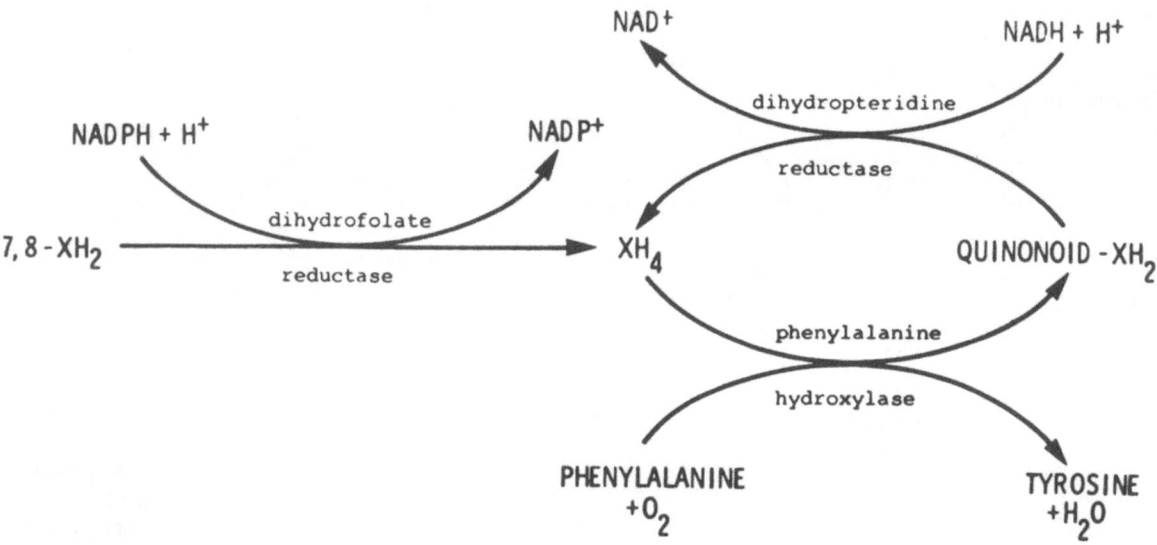

Fig. 12.2. Conversion of phenylalanine to tyrosine showing the biopterin pathway. XH_2 and XH_4, di- and tetra- hydrobiopterin.

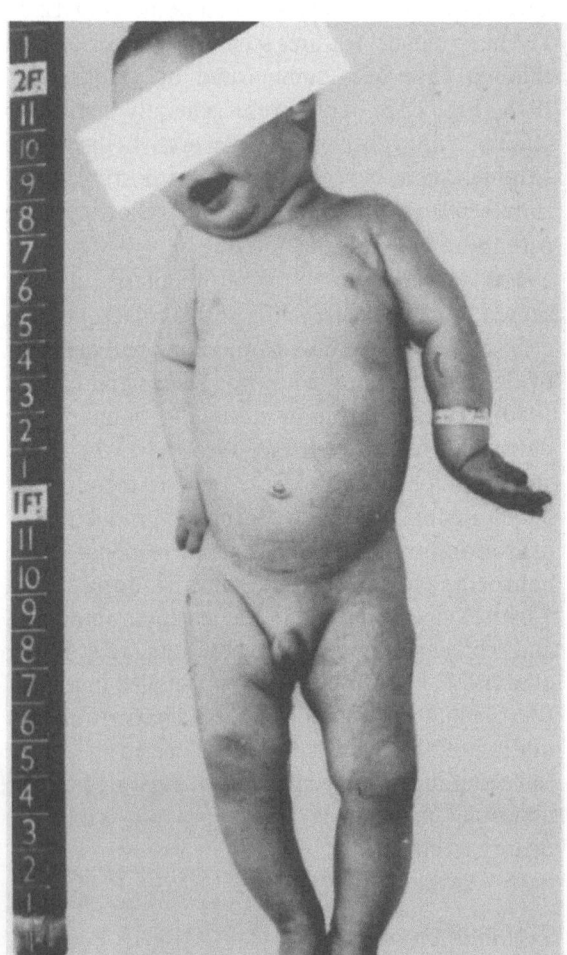

Fig. 12.3. Infant with hyperphenylalaninaemia due to a disorder of biopterin metabolism.
(Photograph kindly provided by The Department of Medical Illustration, Institute of Child Health, and the Hospitals for Sick Children, London.)

the child and his family, and Stevenson et al. (1979) found that treatment for phenylketonuria caused some of the highest levels of behaviour deviance in a group of children with various handicapping conditions. Against this must be set findings such as those of Sunderland et al. (1978), in which data from the National Phenylketonuria Register in the United Kingdom showed that there was an inverse relationship between IQ at 4 years of age and the mean phenylalanine concentration in the blood during the 4th year. A particularly good study concerned with terminating diet was that of Smith et al. (1978) in which early- and late-treated patients in London had the diet withdrawn at 8 years of age whereas those in Heidelberg continued the diet as long as possible and then had a relaxation of diet with the aim of keeping blood phenylalanine levels under 1200 μmol/litre. Cessation of diet resulted in some intellectual deterioration and there was probably some slowing of intellectual progress as the phenylalanine concentration rose in those on relaxed diet. As a result the patients in London now remain on a strict diet until 10 years old and then it is relaxed so that concentrations of phenylalanine are maintained between 900 and 1200 μmol/litre blood and a supplement of L-amino acids (1 g/kg body wt daily) is included.

Pregnancy and phenylketonuria

The successful *treatment* of children with certain inborn errors, in particular phenylketonuria, is now resulting in an increasing number of young women of reproductive age and of normal intelligence.

From reports in the literature on 50 mothers with phenylketonuria, Komrower et al. (1979) noted that these women had produced 163 children and had 27 known spontaneous abortions. Fourteen of their children died, 8 had phenylketonuria, 119 were of low intelligence and only 21 had a normal IQ. Many other congenital abnormalities were recorded including microcephaly, growth retardation, serious lesions of the cardiovascular system, skeletal system and gastro-intestinal tract, and also ocular defects. Komrower et al. suggested that phenylalanine to which the fetus was exposed was the most likely teratogenic agent.

Until recently there were no reports on the effect of diet reintroduced before conception, but results of dietary treatment instituted at varying times after conception have shown varied results and are confusing (Komrower et al. 1979; Scott et al. 1980). Successful outcome of pregnancy has now been reported in women who have conceived whilst on a low phenylalanine diet (Nielsen et al. 1979; Brenton et al. 1980). One of the mothers had already had a severely affected infant resulting from a pregnancy in which diet was not begun before conception (Smith et al. 1979). The use of synthetic diets in pregnancy poses fresh problems but so far the results are encouraging. Perhaps the administration of phenylalanine ammonia lyase may enable the pregnant woman to eat a more normal diet whilst maintaining satisfactory concentrations of blood

phenylalanine (Anonymous 1980). The Steering Committee of the MRC/DHSS Phenylketonuria Register has set up a national register of women of reproductive age with phenylketonuria. This will enable further study to be made of the problem, with the aim of improving the care which can be given. The problems have been discussed fully at a recent symposium (Bickel 1980).

The investigation of a child with microcephaly or of a mentally subnormal child who has a similarly affected sibling should include an investigation of the plasma amino acid pattern in the mother. Unrecognised phenylketonuria is occasionally found in adult women.

Disorders of the branched chain amino acids

The branched chain essential amino acids leucine, valine and isoleucine undergo a series of degradative steps involving transamination, oxidative decarboxylation of the resulting ketoacid to the homologous branched chain fatty acid and metabolism of the fatty acid (a simplified pathway is shown in Fig. 12.4). An inherited disorder involving each step in the degradation of leucine has been identified. Only maple syrup urine disease and β-methylcrotonyl CoA carboxylase deficiency will be discussed here.

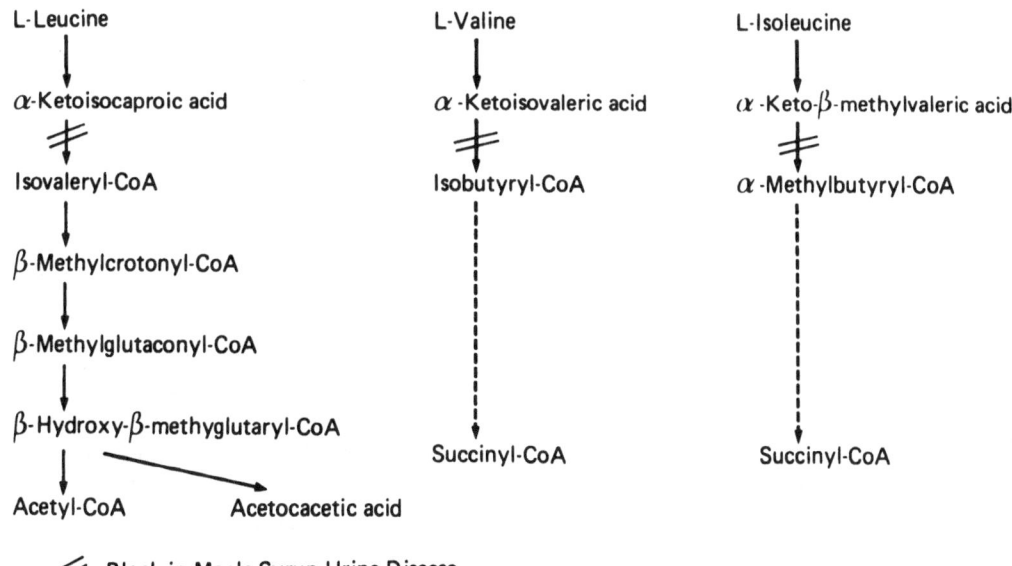

Fig. 12.4. Conversion of the branched chain amino acids.

Maple syrup urine disease

Maple syrup urine disease in its classic form (Menkes et al. 1954) presents within a few days of birth. There is usually failure to thrive, lethargy and vomiting. Convulsions and muscular hypertonicity may appear, there is profound acidosis and a characteristic smell is likely to be noted. The condition is usually lethal if untreated but if the patient does survive there is severe brain damage. Treatment which in the acute phase may include peritoneal dialysis, haemodialysis and exchange transfusion, is based on a diet low in branched chain amino acids. Control of the diet is very difficult and brain damage may occur consequent to the accumulation of metabolites. Acute episodes are especially likely with even minor infections.

There are also many reports of patients in whom the clinical manifestations have been variable and much less severe than in the classic form (Dancis et al. 1972). Very rarely, there may be a response to thiamine. Prenatal detection is possible for this disorder in families which have had an affected infant.

β-Methylcrotonyl CoA carboxylase deficiency

Patients with deficiency of β-methylcrotonyl CoA carboxylase present in the 1st year of life with varied clinical features (Leonard et al. 1981). Usually neurological signs predominate but occasionally acidosis is the striking feature. Neurological signs include floppiness and developmental regression, infantile spasms and convulsions. The condition does not have a single biochemical abnormality since biotin-dependent carboxylase arises by a series of complex steps.

These patients respond to large doses of oral biotin, as do patients with a combination of alopecia, skin rash and neurological features. Evidence so far suggests that the prognosis is generally good if treatment with biotin is begun at an early stage.

Disorders of sulphur metabolism

Methionine is converted by a series of steps to cysteine and two other metabolic sequences are intimately concerned: methionine is re-formed by the methylation of homocysteine, and the methyl group of methionine is ultimately transferred to many other methylated compounds by a number of transmethylation reactions. At least nine specific genetic disorders in these pathways have been described. Homocystinuria is of particular importance. There is considerable variation in the classic form of the condition which is due to deficient activity of cystathionine-β-synthase for which pyridoxal phosphate is a cofactor (Mudd et al. 1964). During the first 2 years of life the child frequently appears normal and gradually develops the characteristic features, comprising ectopia lentis; malar flush; skeletal abnormalities, which may include severe osteoporosis of the spine; abnormal gait and muscle weakness. Thromboembolic attacks are common, especially in the coronary, renal and cerebral arteries. Over two-thirds of them are mentally subnormal and even those of normal intelligence have swings of mood and behaviour abnormalities.

In some patients the biochemical findings revert to normal with pyridoxine alone, and in some with pyridoxine and a low protein diet. Others require a low methionine diet based on a mixture of L-amino acids with additional cysteine and enough natural protein to provide the requirement for methionine. Although the varied clinical course makes assessment of the efficacy of treatment difficult, it does appear to be worthwhile provided it is begun in early life. It is probably only worth screening infants for this condition in areas with a higher incidence such as Northern Ireland.

Excessive excretion of homocystine in urine may also arise from other rare enzymic defects associated with the metabolism of vitamin B_{12} and folic acid.

Urea cycle disorders

Five enzymatic steps are involved in the actual urea cycle which is the major pathway for ammonia detoxication. These include carbamyl phosphate synthetase 1, ornithine transcarbamylase, argininosuccinate synthetase, argininosuccinase and arginase (Snodgrass 1981). Although there are differences in the clinical features of inherited disorders of the urea cycle, patients characteristically have an intolerance of protein and hyperammonaemia. Irritability, lethargy and coma are common. If they survive, mental subnormality, cerebral atrophy and intermittent ataxia are usual, but the prognosis without treatment is generally poor.

In these disorders there is deficient regeneration

of the cycle intermediates and the uptake of ammonia is blocked. The synthesis of ornithine from glutamate is rate-limiting and thus arginine becomes an essential amino acid (Brusilow and Batshaw 1979). Treatment includes the use of low protein diets, additional arginine and ornithine, administration of sodium benzoate, and in some cases the nitrogen free ketoanalogues of essential amino acids. Treatment of acute hyper-ammonaemia and these urea cycle conditions generally is difficult; even minor infections may cause an acute crisis (Batshaw et al. 1981).

Carbohydrate disorders

Disorders involving carbohydrate metabolism include galactosaemia, hereditary fructose intolerance and glycogen storage disorders (some of which cause hypoglycaemia and severe acidosis leading to brain damage).

Galactosaemia

Infants with galactosaemia have deficient activity of galactose-1-phosphate uridyl transferase, which occurs in red cells (used for diagnosis) as well as in liver, kidney and small intestine (Fig. 12.5). As a consequence galactose-1-phosphate accumulates in the tissues provided galactose, i.e. lactose, is present in the diet. After appearing to be normal at birth these infants fail to thrive, develop vomiting and perhaps diarrhoea, and become jaundiced. They will be lethargic and floppy and hepatomegaly and cataracts develop. Such infants, if untreated, are susceptible to infection and it is likely that the diagnosis is sometimes missed since the course may be fulminant with early death (Lévy et al. 1977). If they survive without treatment they are likely to be mentally subnormal and show chronic liver damage (Fig. 12.6).

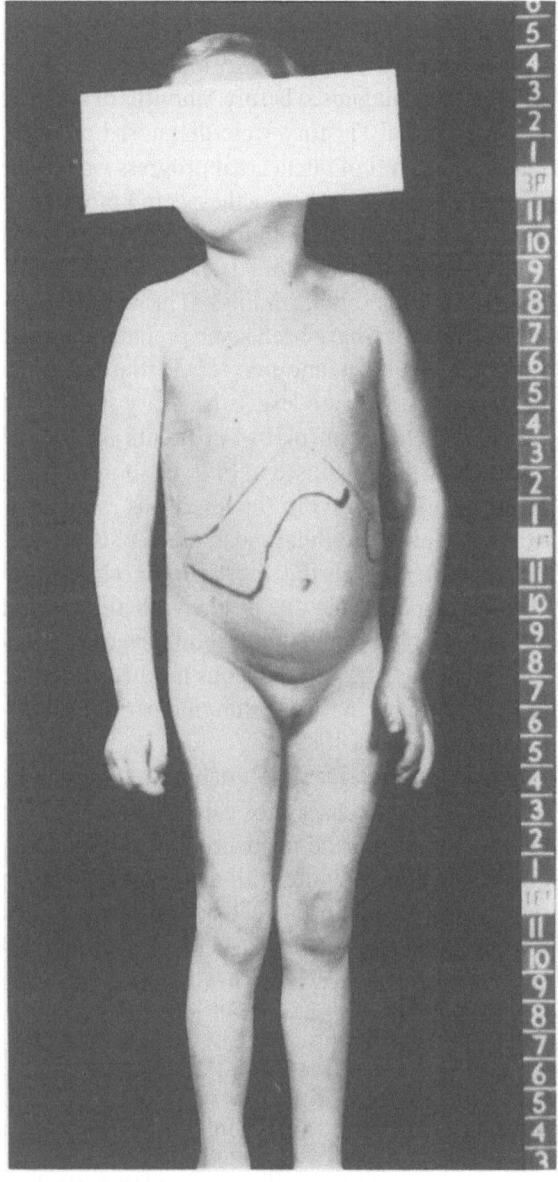

Fig. 12.6. Child with untreated galactosaemia. (Photograph kindly provided by The Department of Medical Illustration, Institute of Child Health, and the Hospitals for Sick Children, London.)

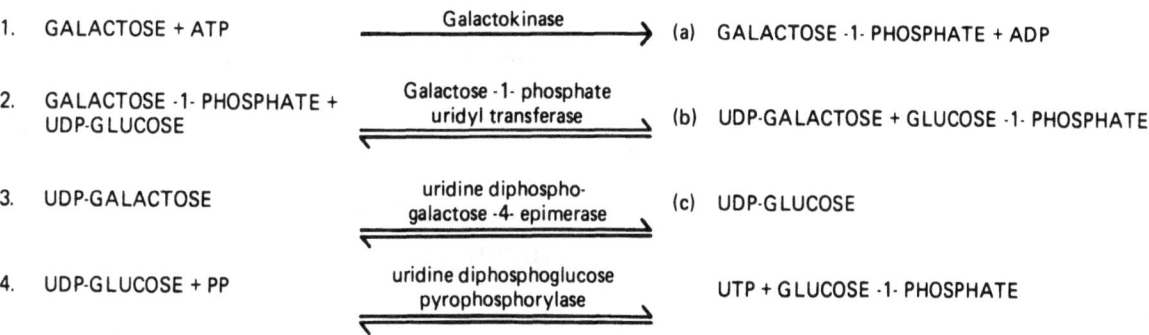

Fig. 12.5. Metabolism of galactose.

The only effective *treatment* is exclusion of galactose (and therefore lactose and milk) from the diet. Early treatment may affect the outcome as Fishler et al. (1980) have shown. Their longitudinal studies spanned 27 years and all except 4 of the patients were diagnosed before 4 months of age, and 11 with a family history were diagnosed at birth. The highest level of intellectual progress was in the 35 patients diagnosed before they were 1 month old. Their mean IQ was 95, but half of them showed abnormal visual–perceptual defects and about one-quarter had abnormal findings. The authors suggested there may have been some prenatal damage, albeit minimal. In another series (Sardharwalla 1980) the results were less satisfactory in spite of adequate dietary control. In 14 patients aged 15–27 years who were diagnosed at birth or soon after, all except two had an IQ in the lower 60s range. It is believed that intracellular galactose-1-phosphate is the toxic agent causing most of the changes in classic galactosaemia. It is likely therefore that galactose-1-phosphate in the homozygous galactosaemic fetus of a heterozygous mother is a cause of brain damage in the intrauterine period (Gitzelmann and Hansen 1980).

There is considerable debate about how worthwhile it is to screen for galactosaemia, taking into account both the incidence and the fact that affected infants may die with acute overwhelming infections with coliform bacilli before the result of a screening test is available (Lévy et al. 1977). Local circumstances concerning health care and the incidence of the condition will affect the decision about screening.

Disorders of fructose metabolism

Hereditary fructose intolerance arises from a deficiency of fructose-1-phosphate aldolase activity. Deficient activity of the enzyme can be demonstrated in a liver biopsy from an affected patient. The accumulation of fructose-1-phosphate and the depletion of inorganic phosphorus contribute to the complete failure of glycogen mobilisation during fructose-induced hypoglycaemia. If the diet does not contain fructose, as in a completely breast-fed infant, the disease does not manifest itself. With the introduction of sucrose in fruits, vegetables and table sugar, this condition, which may be life-threatening, produces symptoms and signs. These include failure to thrive, vomiting, jaundice and hepatomegaly, oedema, ascites and haemorrhages. Affected older children and adults

develop an aversion to sweet foodstuffs but infants are highly vulnerable. The diet is comparatively easy and the prognosis is good provided the condition is diagnosed early. Severe liver damage developing during infancy before the diagnosis is made, will not necessarily respond to treatment. An excellent account of this condition has been given by Baerlocher et al. (1980).

Fructose intolerance may very rarely be due to a deficiency of fructose-1,6-diphosphate aldolase (Baker and Winegrad 1970). Hypoglycaemia is associated with severe lactic acidosis. Acute attacks of acidosis and hypoglycaemia, shock, apnoea, lethargy, loss of consciousness and convulsions tend to occur with even mild infections.

It should be noted that there is a benign form of fructosuria in which there is a deficiency of fructokinase in the liver, kidneys and intestinal mucosa. Fructosuria is often discovered by chance.

Glycogen storage disorders

In glycogen disorders brain damage is most likely to occur in the type due to deficient activity of glucose-6-phosphatase, since severe recurrent hypoglycaemia and lactic acidosis are prominent features. The use of nocturnal gastric drips has been an advance in the management of this condition (Greene et al. 1980). Improvement has been reported in most of the metabolic and clinical abnormalities with catch-up growth occurring, liver size being reduced and hypoglycaemia and acidosis being controlled. Prior to such feeding regimes the patients are often relatively resistant to the effects of low blood sugar. A dangerous side effect of the treatment is the return of sensitivity to low blood sugars; precautions to avoid hypoglycaemia going unnoticed in a patient receiving drip feeds or frequent carbohydrate feeds from a cup are essential (Leonard and Dunger 1978). Retarded motor development in the first years of life, in addition to occurring in children with glucose-6-phosphatase deficiency, is also a feature of children with a deficiency of the debranching enzyme system (amylo-1,6-glucosidase) or of phosphorylase (Fernandes 1980).

Inherited disorders of trace metal metabolism

Inherited disorders affecting the nervous system and involving trace metals include Wilson's disease and Menkes' disease, the latter being very rare indeed.

Wilson's disease

In Wilson's disease the tissues, especially liver, kidneys, brain and cornea, show excess deposition of copper. There is considerable variation in the degree of liver damage and in the neurological symptoms and signs (Roche-Sicot and Benhamon 1977). Rarely, the condition may follow a rapidly fatal fulminant course.

Liver damage is a presenting feature in about half the patients, and they may die before any neurological changes are seen (Walshe 1962). Even presymptomatic patients may show abnormal tests of liver function (Wewalka and Wilson 1967). Perhaps the change from predominantly hepatic to predominantly neurological disease may be due to puberty.

The condition should be diagnosed as early as possible and all close relatives of an affected patient should be screened for the condition. The diagnosis can be a difficult one to make; although a whole-body distribution technique has been found valuable the equipment is not readily available (Walshe and Potter 1977). Gibbs et al. (1978) have provided most useful laboratory data to assist in making the diagnosis. They administered radioactive copper intravenously to patients with presymptomatic, symptomatic and treated Wilson's disease, to known heterozygotes, and to patients with neurological disorders mimicking Wilson's disease. Urine was collected for 24 h after the injection, a test dose of penicillamine was then given, and further urine was collected. Heterozygotes excreted less injected copper than controls both before and with penicillamine. Presymptomatic patients excreted less of the dose than heterozygotes after penicillamine, although their excretion during the basal 24-h period was very much larger. Patients with symptomatic Wilson's disease had the highest excretion of the dose both before and after penicillamine. A computer-based analysis of the data classified all but one of the subjects correctly. This would enable treatment to be given whilst the condition was presymptomatic and would avoid the risk of giving penicillamine treatment to a healthy heterozygote. Nevertheless the differentiation of chronic active hepatitis from Wilson's disease is not easy.

In children the level of caeruloplasmin and the 24-h urinary excretion of copper fails to provide ac-

curate discrimination. The most reliable index is the copper concentration in liver, provided it is related to dry weight (Perman et al. 1979). Those with Wilson's disease had concentrations greater than 400 μg/g liver, whilst children and adolescents with chronic active hepatitis had levels less than 300 μg/g dry weight. Serum caeruloplasmin concentration is very helpful in adults, but normal values are obtained in those patients presenting acutely with hepatic Wilson's disease (Perman et al. 1979).

The basic defect is unknown but chelation of copper with British anti-Lewisite (BAL), penicillamine or triethylene tetramine produces marked clinical improvement (Walshe 1973).

Menkes' disease

A very rare disorder, Menkes' disease is characterised by retardation of growth, kinky hair and focal cerebral and cerebellar degeneration (Menkes et al. 1962; Danks et al. 1972). Some of the findings are similar to those seen in copper-deficient animals (Hall and Howell 1973). The condition, which is fatal by about 3 years of age, usually presents with seizures at about 3 months of age, although developmental delay may have been suspected already. Serum concentrations of copper and caeruloplasmin are abnormally low. The defective intestinal absorption of copper observed by Danks et al. (1972) is only part of a more widespread disorder. It is not yet clear whether the basic defect is in membrane transport of copper or is related to an intracellular storage protein which has an increased affinity for the metal (Lott et al. 1979).

Diagnosis of inherited disorders of sick infants

Many inborn errors of metabolism lead to clinical manifestations within a few days of birth. Their symptomatology is not specific and the diagnosis is easily missed. Moreover, the laboratory facilities necessary to enable a definitive diagnosis to be made, require a high degree of sophistication. Particularly important features are jaundice, diarrhoea, vomiting, hypoglycaemia, disturbances of electrolyte and acid–base balance, convulsions and coma.

Infection is often the precipitating factor for seizures. Most useful summaries have been given by Aleck and Shapiro (1978), Chalmers et al. (1980) and

Chalmers and Lawson (1982). Many of these disorders result in mental subnormality, especially if they are untreated.

Prenatal diagnosis for an increasing number of metabolic disorders is now possible. Diagnosis may depend on the prenatal detection of abnormal metabolites in amniotic fluid, but more usually relies on demonstrating that a specific enzyme present in normal amniotic fluid shows deficient activity in cultured amniotic cells from an affected fetus. Miles and Kaback (1978) list many examples and describe some of the problems. An accurate diagnosis is essential in the first affected sibling in a family. If it is likely that a neonate is going to die and if an inherited metabolic disorder seems to be a likely diagnosis, samples of plasma and urine should be stored in a deep freeze. A skin biopsy should be placed in a culture medium and the nearest laboratory with tissue culture facilities should be contacted. If an accurate diagnosis is not made, prenatal detection during a subsequent pregnancy will be impossible.

For all the inherited disorders genetic counselling is essential. It may be necessary to offer this to members of the extended family.

References

Aleck K A, Shapiro L J (1978) Genetic–metabolic considerations in the sick neonate. Pediatr Clin North Am 25: 431–451

Anonymous (1980) Dietary promise for PKU patients. Medical Research Council News, No. 8, p 3

Baerlocher K, Gitzelmann R, Steinmann B (1980) Clinical and genetic studies of disorders in fructose metabolism. In: Burman D, Holton J B, Pennock C A (eds). Inherited disorders of carbohydrate metabolism. MTP, Lancaster, pp 163–190

Baker L, Winegrad A I (1970) Fasting hypoglycaemia and metabolic acidosis associated with deficiency of hepatic fructose-1,6-diphosphatase activity. Lancet ii: 13–16

Batshaw M L, Thomas G H, Brusilow S W (1981) New approaches to the diagnosis and treatment of inborn errors of urea synthesis. Pediatrics 68: 290–297

Bickel H (ed) (1981) Maternal phenylketonuria—an International workshop held in Frankfurt/Main April 22, 1980. Pentadruck, Eppingen

Brenton D P, Cusworth D C, Garrod P et al. (1980) Maternal phenylketonuria treated by diet before conception. Paper presented to the British Paediatric Association, York, April 15–19, 1980. (Abstract published in *Archives of Disease in Childhood*.)

Brusilow S W T, Batshaw M L (1979) Arginine therapy of argininosuccinase deficiency. Lancet i: 124–127

Butler I J, Koslow S H, Krumholz A, Holtzman N A, Kaurman S (1978) A disorder of biogenic amines in dihydropteridine reductase deficiency. Ann Neurol 3: 224–230

Chalmers R A, Lawson A M (1982) Organic acids in man. Chapman and Hall, London

Chalmers R A, Purkiss P, Watts R W E, Lawson A M (1980) Screening for organic acidurias and aminoacidopathies in newborns and children. J Inher Metabol Dis 3: 27–43

Clayton B E (1975) The principles of treatment by dietary restriction as illustrated by phenylketonuria. In: Raine D N (ed) The treatment of inherited metabolic disease. Medical and Technical Publishing, Lancaster, pp 1–32

Comar D, Saudubray J M, Duthilleul A et al. (1981) Brain uptake of ^{11}C-methionine in phenylketonuria. Europ J Pediatr 136: 13–19

Curtius H C, Niederwieser A, Viscontini M et al. (1979) Atypical phenylketonuria due to tetrahydrobiopterin deficiency. Diagnosis and treatment with tetrahydrobiopterin, dihydrobiopterin and sepiapterin. Clin Chim Acta 93: 251–262

Dancis J, Hutzler B S, Snyderman S E, Cox R P (1972) Enzyme activity in classical and variant forms of maple syrup urine disease. J Pediatr 81: 312–320

Danks D M, Cotton R G H (1980) Early diagnosis of hyperphenylalaninaemia due to tetrahydrobiopterin deficiency (malignant hyperphenylalaninaemia). Pediatr 96: 854–856

Danks D M, Campbell P E, Stevens B J, Mayne V, Cartwright E (1972) Menkes's kinky hair syndrome. An inherited defect in copper absorption with widespread effects. Pediatrics 50: 188–201

Danks D M, Bartholomie K, Clayton B E et al. (1978) Malignant hyperphenylalaninaemia—current status (June 1977) J Inher Metabol Dis 1: 49–53

Department of Health and Social Security, National Health Service (1969) Screening for early detection of phenylketonuria. HM(69)72, HMSO, London

Department of Health and Social Security (1974) Present day practice in infant feeding. Reports on Health and Social Subjects, No. 9. HMSO, London

Dussault J H, Coulombe P, Laberge C et al. (1975) Preliminary report on a mass screening program for neonatal hypothyroidism. J Pediatr 86: 670–674

Fernandes J (1980) Hepatic glycogenosis: diagnosis and management. In: Burman D, Holton J B, Pennock C A (eds) Inherited disorders of carbohydrate metabolism. MTP, Lancaster, pp 297–312

Fisher D A, Dussault J H, Foley T R P Jr et al. (1979) Screening for congenital hypothyroidism: results of screening one million North American infants. J Pediatr 94: 700–705

Fishler K, Koch R, Donnell G N, Wenz E (1980) Developmental aspects of galactosaemia from infancy to childhood. Clin Pediatr 19: 38–44

Francis D E M (1975) Diets for sick children, 3rd edn. Blackwell Scientific, Oxford

Gibbs K, Hanka R, Walshe J M (1978) The urinary excretion of radiocopper in presymptomatic and symptomatic Wilson's disease, heterozygotes and controls: Its significance in diagnosis and management. Q J Med 47: 349–364

Gitzelmann R, Hansen R G (1980) Galactose metabolism, hereditary defects and their clinical significance. In: Burman D, Holton J B, Pennock C A (eds) Inherited disorders of carbohydrate metabolism. MTP, Lancaster, pp 61–101

Greene H L, Slonim A E, Burr I M, Moran J R (1980). Type 1 glycogen storage disease: five years of management with nocturnal intragastric feeding. J Pediatr 96: 590–595

Guthrie R (1961) Blood screening for phenylketonuria (Letter). JAMA 178: 863

Güttler F (1980) Hyperphenylalaninaemia. Acta Pediatr Scand [Suppl 280]

Hall G A, Howell J M C (1973) Lesions produced by copper deficiency in neonate and older rats. Br J Nutr 29: 95–104

Hulse J A, Grant D B, Clayton B E et al. (1980) Population screening for congenital hypothyroidism. Br Med J 1: 675–678

Kaufman S (1978) The enzymes for the hepatic phenylalanine hydroxylating system. J Inher Metabol Dis 1: 63–65.

Kaufman S (1980) Differential diagnosis of variant forms of

hyperphenylalaninaemia. Pediatrics 65: 840–842

Komrower G M, Sardharwalla I B, Coutts J M J, Ingham D (1979) Management of maternal phenylketonuria: an emerging clinical problem. Br Med J i: 1383–1387

Leonard J V, Dunger D B (1978) Hypoglycaemia complicating feeding regimes for glycogen storage disorders. Lancet ii: 1203–1204

Leonard J V, Seakins, J W T, Bartlett K et al. (1981) The clinical spectrum of inherited disorders of 3-methyl crotonyl CoA carboxylation. Arch Dis Child 56:53–59

Lévy H L, Sépe S J, Shih V E, Gordon F V, Klein J O (1977) Sepsis due to Escherichia coli in neonates with galactosaemia. N Engl J Med 297: 823–827

Lott I T, Dipaola R, Raghavan S S et al. (1979) Abnormal copper metabolism in Menkes' steely-hair syndrome. Pediatr Res 13: 845–150

Menkes J H, Hurst P L, Craig J M (1954) New syndrome. Progressive familial infantile cerebral dysfunction associated with an unusual urinary substance. Pediatrics 14:462–466

Menkes J H, Alter M, Steigleder G K, Weakley D R, Sung J H (1962) A sex-linked recessive disorder with retardation of growth, peculiar hair and focal cerebral and cerebellar degeneration. Pediatrics 29: 764–779

Miles J H, Kaback M M (1978) Prenatal diagnosis of hereditary disorders. Pediatr Clin North Am 25: 593–618

Mudd S H, Finkelstein J D, Irreverre F, Laster L (1964) Homocystinuria: an enzymatic defect. Science 143: 1443–1445

Nielsen K B, Wamberg E, Weber J (1979) Successful outcome of pregnancy to phenylketonuric woman after low-phenylalanine diet introduced before conception. Lancet i: 1245

O'Brien D, Berlow S, Donnel G et al. (1980) New developments in hyperphenylalaninaemia. Pediatrics 65: 844–846

Perman J A, Westlin S L, Grand R J, Watling J R (1979) Laboratory measures of copper metabolism in the differentiation of chronic active hepatitis and Wilson's disease in children. J Pediatr 94: 564–568

Raine D N (1974) The need for a national policy for the management of inherited metabolic disease. J Clin Pathol 27: [Suppl 8] 156–163

Roche-Sicot J, Benhamon J P (1977) Acute. intravascular haemolysis and acute liver failure associated as a first manifestation of Wilson's disease. Ann Intern Med 86: 301–303

Sardharwalla I B (1980) In: Burman D, Holton J B, Pennock C A (eds) Inherited disorders of carbohydrate metabolism. MTP, Lancaster, pp 151, 152

Scott T M, Morton Fyfe W, McKay Hart D (1980) (With comment by Farquhar J W) Maternal phenylketonuria: abnormal baby despite low phenylalanine diet during pregnancy. Arch Dis Child 55:634–649

Smith I, Lobascher M, Wolff O H (1973) Factors influencing outcome in early treated phenylketonuria. In: Seakins J W T, Saunders R A, Toothill C (eds) Treatment of inborn errors of metabolism. Churchill Livingstone, London, pp 41, 49

Smith I, Lobascher M E, Stevenson J E et al. (1978) Effect of stopping low-phenylalanine diet on intellectual progress of children with phenylketonuria. Br Med J ii: 723–726

Smith I, Erdohazi M, Macartney F J et al. (1979) Fetal damage despite low-phenylalanine diet after conception in a phenylketonuric woman. Lancet i: 17–19

Smith P, Morris A (1979) Assessment of a programme to screen the newly born for congenital hypothyroidism. Community Medicine 1: 14–22

Snodgrass P J (1981) Biochemical aspects of urea cycle disorders. Pediatrics 68: 273–283

Stevenson J E, Hawcroft J, Lobascher M et al. (1979) Behavioural deviance in children with early treated phenylketonuria. Arch Dis Child 54: 14–18

Sunderland I, Hudson F P, Hawcroft J (1978) MRC/DHSS Phenylketonuria Register Newsletter No. 5. MRC/DHSS, London 1978.

Walker V, Clayton B E, Ersser R S et al. (1981) Hyperphenylalaninaemia of various types amongst three quarters of a million neonates tested in a screening programme. Arch Dis Child 56: 759–764

Walshe J M (1962) Wilson's disease: The presenting symptoms. Arch Dis Child 37: 253–256

Walshe J M (1973) Copper chelation in patients with Wilson's disease. A comparison of penicillamine and triethylene tetramine dihyrochloride. Am J Med 42: 441–452

Walshe J M, Potter G (1977) The pattern of the whole body distribution of radioactive copper (^{67}Cu, ^{64}Cu) in Wilson's disease in various control groups. Q J Med 46: 445–462

Wewalka, F Von (1967) Morbus Wilson. Einführung in die aktuellen Probleme (Frühdiagnose und Therapie). Wiener Zeitschrift fuer Innere Medizin und ihre Grenzgebiete 48: 461–467

Chapter 13

Inborn Lysosomal Storage Disorders Affecting the Nervous System

Lysosomes and lysosomal storage disorders

Lysosomes are membrane-bound cytoplasmic bodies involved in the degradation of material or debris resulting from autolysis, phagocytosis or other metabolic processes. They contain numerous degradative enzymes which are most active in an acid environment such as that found within the lysosome. Lysosomal enzymes are classified according to their functions; for instance, glycosidases remove specific sugar residues from complex carbohydrates or glycolipids, cathepsins (proteinases)

degrade protein and the sulphatases remove ester sulphate groups which are covalently linked to organic residues (e.g. sugars).

A large proportion of the known inherited lysosomal storage disorders are associated with deficiencies of specific glycosidases which normally remove specific sugar residues from one end (the non-reducing terminal) of a series of linked residues. Specific deficiencies of this type can lead to the storage of poorly degraded material within lysosomes (Fig. 13.1). Initially there was uncertainty about the nature of the engorged inclusion bodies in cells affected by these 'storage diseases' but the demonstration that the storage material was

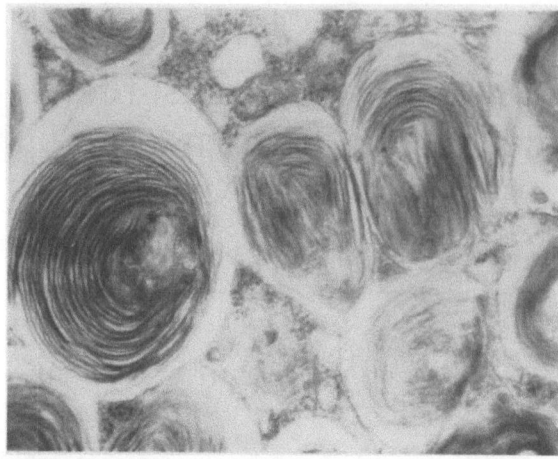

Fig. 13.1. Electron micrograph showing lipid storage in neurons in G_{M2}-gangliosidosis—the lipid is in the form of membranous cytoplasmic bodies. ($\times 30000$)
(Reproduced by kind permission of Dr. B. D. Lake, Hospital for Sick Children, London.)

contained in membrane-bound vesicles which also contained acid phosphatase activity (a lysosomal enzyme), and the demonstration of corresponding deficiencies of specific lysosomal enzymes helped to confirm that the cytoplasmic bodies were indeed lysosomes. In some inborn lysosomal disorders (e.g. the mucopolysaccharidoses) the stored material is water soluble so that large vacuoles may appear in the cells after preparation for microscopy. Storage material is not always confined within the cell but may also accumulate in the intercellular matrix, e.g. in Hurler disease. The finding of material in lysosomes does not automatically point to a specific enzyme deficiency. Material might also accumulate because of inability of the body to degrade or remove all remnants of foreign material or end products of metabolism that arise during the lifetime of an individual. Lipofuscin granules found in the cells of normal individuals, particularly the elderly, might arise in this way.

A few years ago the diagnosis of some specific lysosomal storage disorders could only be satisfactorily established by studying tissue obtained from open biopsy of major organs; sometimes this included brain biopsy. In many cases, diagnosis was only made after death by histological and histochemical study of the brain at autopsy (see Chap. 11). Today a specific diagnosis can be made in most instances by the assay of relevant lysosomal enzymes in blood leukocytes, plasma, cultured skin fibroblasts or urine. When measuring the activity of a leukocyte or fibroblast enzyme, it is necessary to relate the results to the protein content of the preparation or to a second enzyme. Sensitive techniques are required for the assay of some lysosomal enzymes and synthetic substrates with adequate sensitivity have been made in which the appropriate glycoside residues are linked to fluorogenic compounds such as 4-methyl-umbelliferone. Sometimes synthetic substrates are hydrolysed by irrelevant enzyme activity in which case suitable separation techniques are required as part of the diagnostic procedure.

Lysosomal disorders affecting the nervous system

A classification of lysosomal storage diseases affecting the nervous system is given in Table 13.1. For convenience, the diseases have been grouped into the mucopolysaccharidoses, the lipidoses, the mucolipidoses and a fourth group encompassing other disorders of glycoconjugate metabolism. The term glycoconjugate includes mucopolysaccharides, glycolipids, glycoproteins and other complex molecules containing carbohydrate residues. Although lysosomal storage disorders can now largely be classified according to the nature of the specific biochemical defect it is important to remember that a particular enzyme deficiency may manifest itself as more than one clinical phenotype.

The mucopolysaccharidoses

Mental retardation is encountered after infancy in Hurler and Sanfilippo diseases and sometimes occurs in Hunter disease. Other types of mucopolysaccharidosis are not usually associated with mental retardation although bone and connective tissue abnormalities can occasionally give rise to neural compression syndromes (e.g. carpal tunnel, compression of cervical cord). Although the pattern of distribution of different types of glycolipid (e.g. the gangliosides) in the brains of affected individuals is often abnormal, these diseases are now regarded primarily as disorders of *glycosaminoglycan* (GAG) metabolism (glycosaminoglycan is the more accurate modern term for mucopolysaccharide). Excessive somatic storage and urinary excretion of acid GAG is a characteristic feature of this group of disorders.

Table 13.1. Inborn lysosomal diseases affecting the nervous system

Classification	Alternative names and subtypes
Mucopolysaccharidoses	
MPS IH	Hurler disease
MPS II	Hunter disease: severe form, milder forms
MPS III	Sanfilippo disease: biochemical subtypes A, B, C and D
Lipidoses	
G_{M1}-gangliosidosis	Type I; Pseudo-Hurler; Norman–Landing disease
G_{M2}-gangliosidosis	Type II; juvenile form; Derry disease
	Type I; Tay–Sachs disease
	Type II; Sandhoff disease
	Type III; juvenile form
Gaucher disease	Type II; infantile acute neuronopathic form
	Type III; juvenile subacute neuronopathic form
Krabbe disease	Early onset. Late onset
Metachromatic leukodystrophy	Infantile form
	Juvenile form
	Adult form
Niemann–Pick disease	Type A; acute infantile form
Farber disease	
Fabry disease	
Mucolipidoses	
Multiple sulphatase deficiency	Austin-type metachromatic leukodystrophy
ML II	I-cell disease
ML III	Pseudo-Hurler polydystrophy
ML IV	
Other disorders of glycoconjugate metabolism	
Mannosidosis	
Fucosidosis	
Aspartyl-glycosaminuria	

Clinical features

Hurler disease (Fig. 13.2) is the severest form of mucopolysaccharidosis but characteristic features do not usually appear until after 6 months of age. Early features are large head, inguinal and umbilical hernias and recurrent chest infections. Manifestations of the full syndrome include coarse facies, multiple skeletal deformities, kyphosis, thickened spade-like hands, widely spaced peg-like teeth in thickened gums, large tongue, corneal opacities, hepatosplenomegaly, cardiovascular lesions (which include thickening of mitral and aortic valves and infiltration of the intima of the coronary, aortic and pulmonary arteries) and mental retardation. Most children with this disease die in their first decade from heart disease or respiratory tract infections. General anaesthesia can be hazardous because of deformities or obstruction in the respiratory tract.

Hunter disease resembles Hurler disease but is generally less severe. Unlike Hurler disease the cornea remains clear. Sometimes small hard nodular lesions are found in the skin over the scapulae. Mental retardation is variable and may be minimal in the milder forms. Hunter disease is the only known X-linked recessive mucopolysaccharidosis; the other types have an autosomal recessive inheritance.

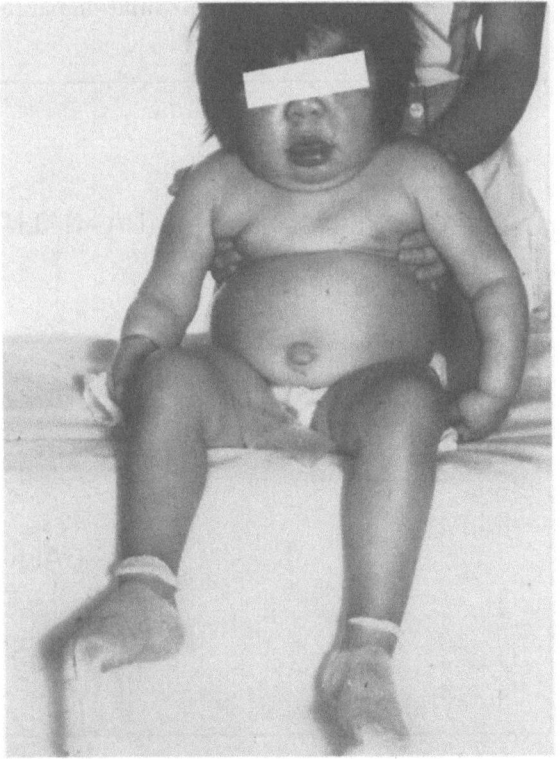

Fig. 13.2. A patient with Hurler disease. (Reproduced by permission of Department of Medical Illustration, Institute of Child Health, London.)

Sanfilippo disease presents mainly as progressive mental retardation, the onset of which may not become apparent until after the 1st or 2nd year. Somatic abnormalities may be present but they are less obvious. The cranial vault is thickened and the head may be enlarged. Whereas dwarfism is associated with many of the other types of mucopolysaccharidosis, some children with Sanfilippo disease are big and strong. Corneal opacities do not occur in Sanfilippo disease. These patients eventually develop severe neurological degeneration and most die in their second or third decade.

A classification of the mucopolysaccharidoses and detailed clinical descriptions have been given by McKusick (1972).

The biochemical abnormality in the mucopolysaccharidoses

The structural chemistry of GAGs is complicated but the enzyme abnormalities in the mucopolysaccharidoses can be easily understood by reference to Figs. 13.3 and 13.4, which indicate only the relevant parts of the molecules concerned. Dermatan sulphate and heparan sulphate are the two GAGs which are incompletely degraded in Hurler and Hunter diseases. Sanfilippo disease is associated only with defective heparan sulphate degradation. Dermatan sulphate and heparan

sulphate are both carbohydrate polymers consisting mainly of repeating disaccharide units, each unit containing a hexosamine and a uronic acid residue. The molecules are polyanions because of the carboxylate groups on the uronic acids and the presence of covalently linked sulphate groups.

Hunter disease is due to a deficiency of the enzyme idurono-2-sulphate sulphohydrolase (Bach et al. 1973) which is required for removing covalently linked ester sulphate groups from iduronic acid residues. *Hurler* disease is due to a deficiency of α-L-iduronidase (Bach et al. 1972) which is necessary to remove iduronic acid residues from the end of dermatan sulphate or heparan sulphate chains. Both dermatan and heparan sulphates contain iduronic acid and sulphated iduronic acid moieties but to a different extent. Both these GAGs are excreted in excess in the urine of patients with Hurler and Hunter diseases. *Sanfilippo disease* is associated with defective degradation of heparan sulphate and deficiencies of any one of at least four different enzymes can give rise to the condition (Fig. 13.4). Clinical characteristics seem to be similar in the different types of Sanfilippo disease and an excessive excretion of heparan sulphate in the urine is a characteristic feature, even at birth (Whiteman and Young 1977). Type A Sanfilippo disease appears to be the commonest form in the United Kingdom and is due to a deficiency of

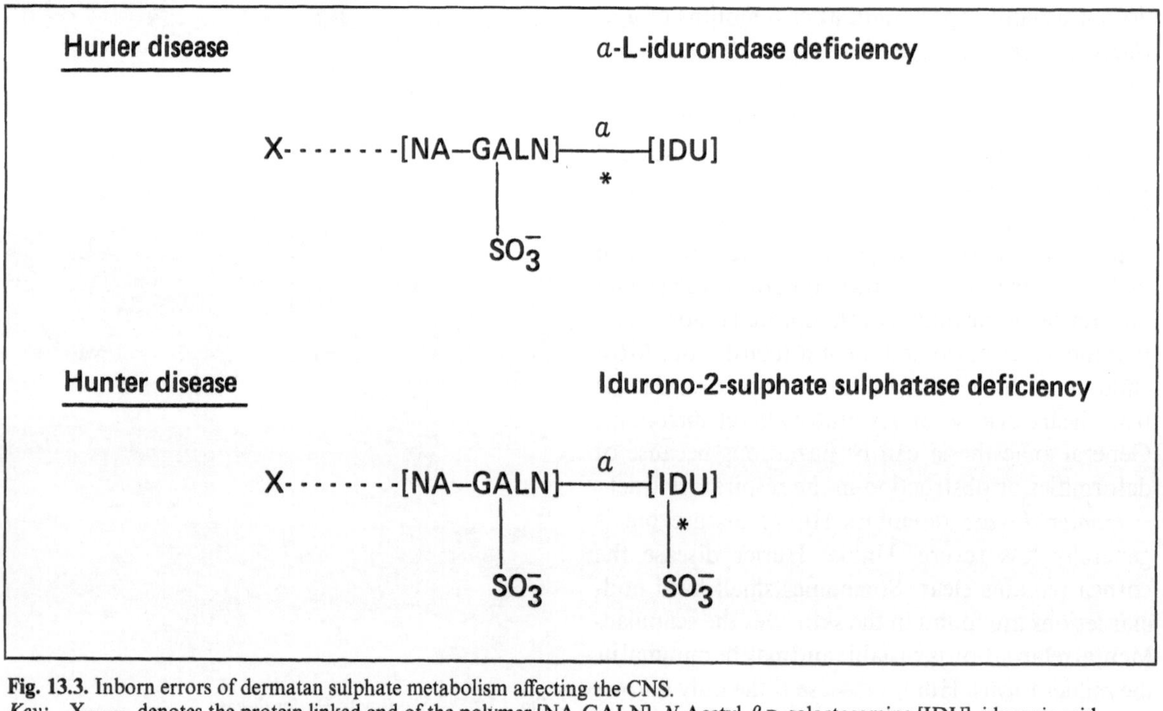

Fig. 13.3. Inborn errors of dermatan sulphate metabolism affecting the CNS.
Key: X------, denotes the protein linked end of the polymer [NA-GALN], *N*-Acetyl-β-D-galactosamine [IDU], iduronic acid
       *, indicates site affected by the enzyme deficiency.

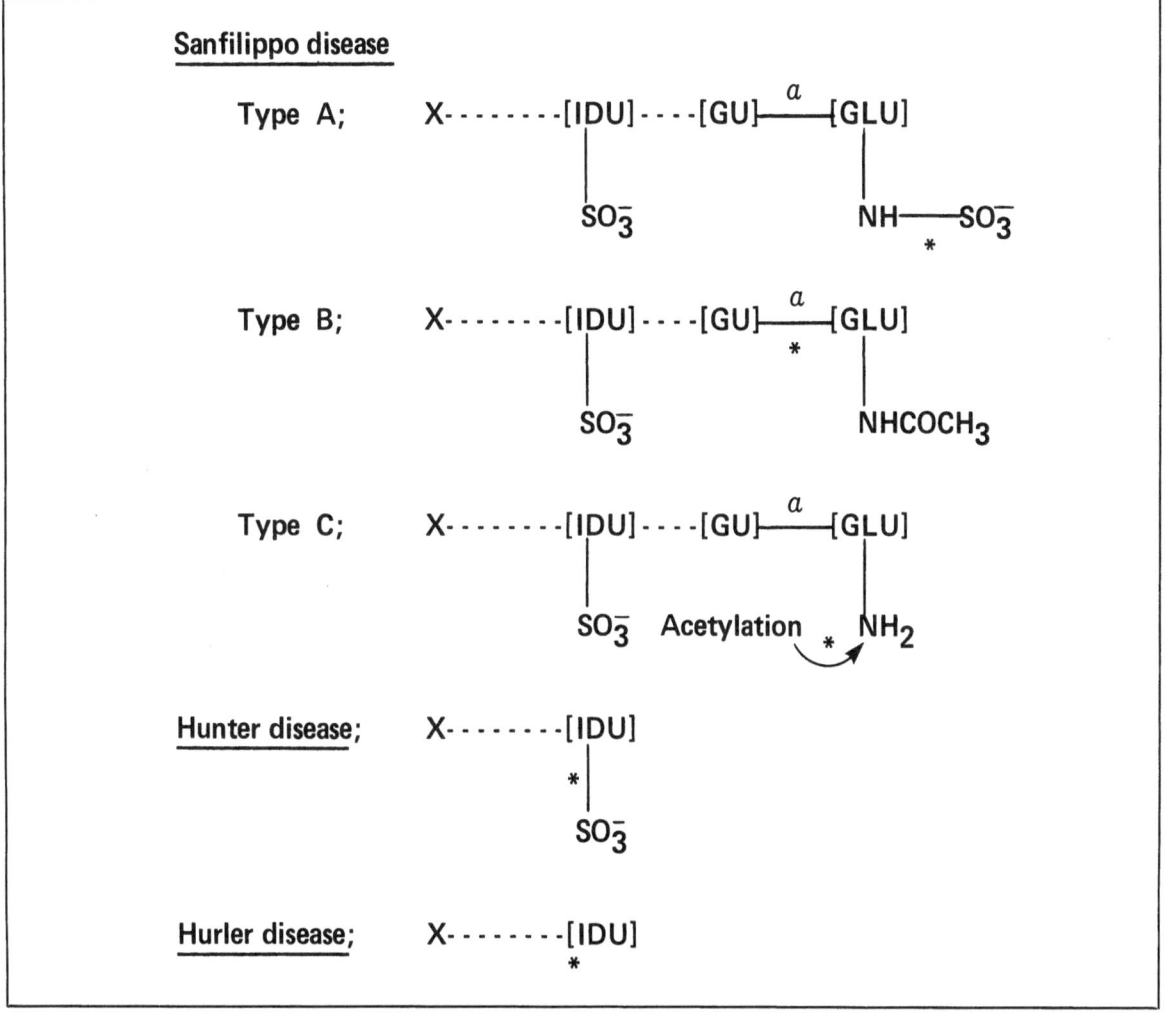

Fig. 13.4. Inborn errors of heparan sulphate metabolism affecting the CNS.
Sanfilippo disease; type A, heparan sulphate sulphamidase deficiency; type B, *N*-Acetyl-α-D-glucosaminidase deficiency; type C, ?Acetyl-CoA: α-glucosaminide *N*-acetyltransferase deficiency. Hurler and Hunter diseases; enzyme deficiencies as in Fig. 13.3.
Key: [IDU] iduronic acid; [GU], glucuronic acid; [GLU], glucose
          X------, denotes protein linked end of the polymer
          *, indicates site affected by enzyme deficiency
Note: Sanfilippo type D has recently been described in which there is a deficiency of a specific heparan sulphate, *N*-acetyl-glucosamine-6-sulphate sulphatase.

heparan sulphate sulphamidase (Fig. 13.4). Although α-L-iduronidase and idurono-2-sulphate sulphohydrolase are required for both dermatan sulphate and herparan sulphate degradation, the enzymes which are deficient in different types of Sanfilippo disease are not required for normal degradation of dermatan sulphate.

Laboratory diagnosis of mucopolysaccharidosis

Infants and children with mucopolysaccharidosis invariably have elevated urinary GAG excretion. The GAG/creatinine ratio is a useful index of GAG excretion but needs to be compared with an age-related control range (Fig. 13.5). Several methods are available for the analysis of urinary GAGs but since most of them have pitfalls they need to be carried out and interpreted in experienced laboratories. Now that *prenatal* diagnosis is often possible it is particularly important that these conditions are not missed due to inadequate screening methods. Most procedures for the quantitation and isolation of GAG from urine initially involve the formation of complexes between the polyanions (i.e. the GAGs) and organic cations which may be detergents such as cetylpyridinium chloride (CPC) and cetyltrimethylammonium bromide (CTAB) or cationic dyes such as Alcian blue 8G. Formation of the complexes is critically dependent on the electrolyte environment and the molecular weight and charge properties of the polyanion. For these reasons and

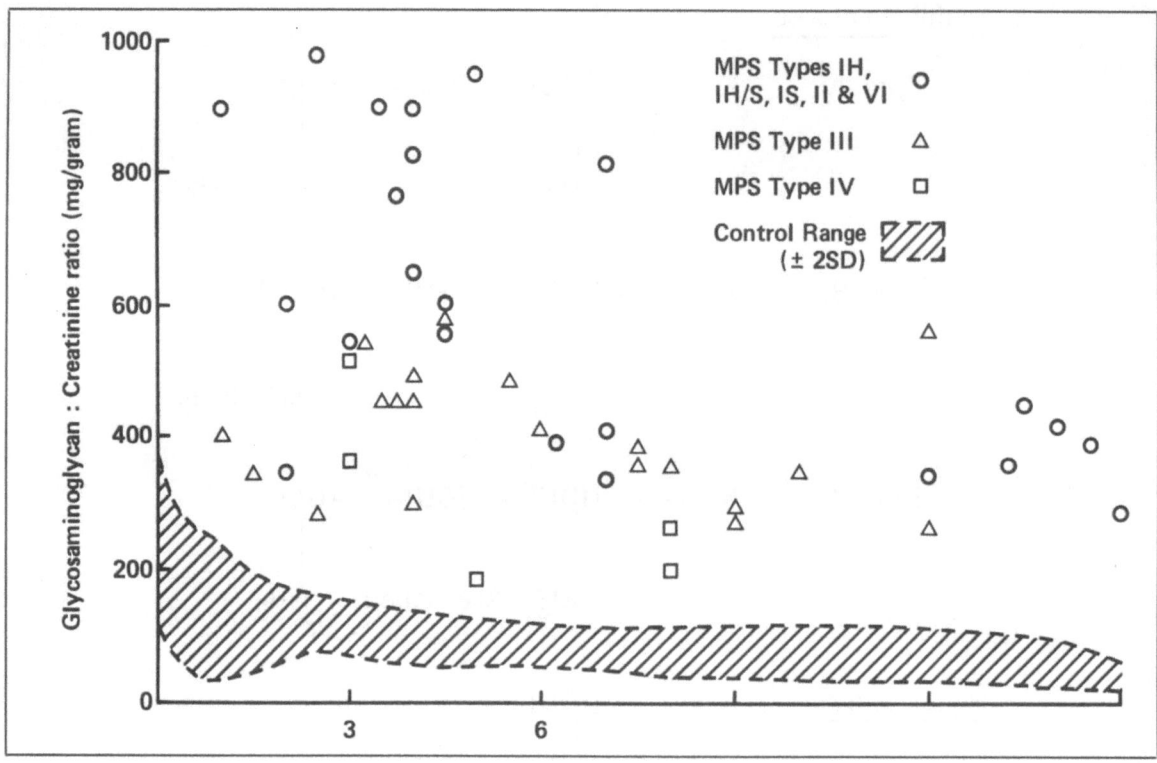

Fig. 13.5. Urinary glycosaminoglycan : creatinine ratio in children with mucopolysaccharidosis. MPS IH, Hurler; MPS II, Hunter; MPS III, Sanfilippo; MPS IV, Morquio; MPS VI, Maroteaux–Lamy.

because of the effects of renal concentration and dilution the use of simple spot tests and turbidity tests is not advised unless special precautions have been taken to allow for such factors. Urinary GAG can be determined quantitatively using Alcian blue 8G or by an estimation of the uronic acid content of precipitated GAG.

Qualitative analysis of urinary GAGs is a useful guide to the type of mucopolysaccharidosis (Fig. 13.6). Electrophoresis of isolated GAG in 0.1M barium acetate is probably the best simple method for distinguishing the types of mucopoly-saccharidosis associated with mental retardation. Once a probable diagnosis of mucopoly-saccharidosis has been established this should be finally confirmed when technically possible by relevant enzyme assays on leukocytes, cultured skin fibroblasts or plasma.

Abnormal inclusion bodies (e.g. vacuolated lymphocytes) can be demonstrated in the peripheral blood leukocytes in some types of mucopolysac-charidosis and cells in the bone marrow may also show abnormalities. Bone marrow biopsy is not necessary for the diagnosis of mucopoly-saccharidosis. Chemical and histochemical tech-niques relevant to the mucopolysaccharidoses and

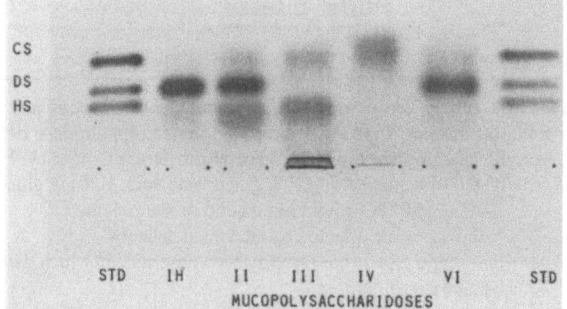

Fig. 13.6. Electrophoresis of urinary GAGs. Chondroitin sulphate is the main GAG component in normal urine.
Key: To MPS types—see Fig. 13.5
CS, chondroitin sulphate; DS, dermatan sulphate; HS, heparan sulphate.

other lysosomal storage disorders have recently been described by Lake (1981).

Prenatal diagnosis of mucopolysaccharidosis

In order to offer prenatal diagnosis during sub-sequent pregnancies, the biochemical diagnosis of mucopolysaccharidoses must be firmly established in the propositus. *Amniocentesis* is usually perform-ed as soon as possible after the 14th week of gestation. Laboratory methods involve either studies on cultured amniotic-fluid cells or an analysis of amniotic-fluid GAGs. When possible the activities of the relevant specific enzymes in cultured cells are determined (e.g. Harper et al. 1974). The first successful method used for prenatal diagnosis of Hurler and Hunter diseases involved measurement of the uptake and release of radiolabelled sulphate by cultured cells (Fratantoni et al. 1969); the method is still sometimes used when enzyme assays are not available. An inevitable delay occurs between receipt of amniotic fluid and the results from the laboratory studies on cultured cells; occasionally cell lines do not grow satisfactorily. Analysis of amniotic-fluid GAG offers a useful back-up for prenatal diagnosis but should not be used before the 14th week of pregnancy because the presence of an abnormal GAG pattern due to mucopolysaccharidosis probably depends on formation of fetal urine (Whiteman and Henderson, 1977). In the first half of pregnancy hyaluronic acid and chondroitin sulphate are the main GAGs in amniotic fluid. After the first trimester amniotic fluid contains, in addition, an abnormal amount of dermatan sulphate or heparan sulphate when the fetus is affected by Hurler disease or Sanfilippo disease, respectively. Earlier reports claimed that analysis of amniotic-fluid GAGs was unreliable for prenatal diagnosis but recent studies have suggested that some anomalous results may have been due to inadequate analytical methods.

The lipidoses

The gangliosidoses

Forms of lipidosis in which particular gangliosides accumulate in excess in the brain are designated as gangliosidoses. These diseases have an autosomal recessive inheritance. Gangliosides are glycosphingolipods containing sialic acid (N-acetyl neuraminic acid; NANA). G_{M1} and G_{M2} are two relevant gangliosides (using Svennerholm's nomenclature) which contain one sialic acid residue per molecule (M = mono); their structures are outlined in Fig. 13.7.

A detailed review of the gangliosidoses has been given by O'Brien (1978).

G_{M1}-gangliosidosis

Two types of G_{M1}-gangliosidosis are associated with psychomotor retardation. *Type 1* (infantile) displays mental and physical abnormalities at or soon after birth. Apart from the earlier onset, several features such as coarse facies, cranial

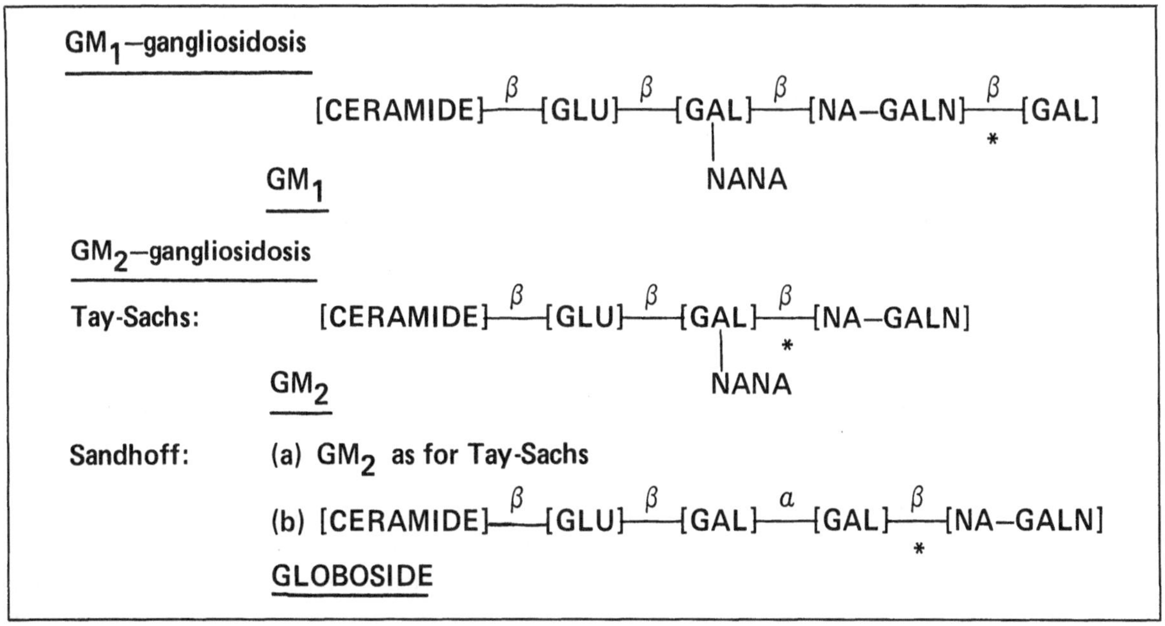

Fig. 13.7. Genetic gangliosidoses. β-Galactosidase is deficient in G_{M1}-gangliosidosis. Hexosaminidase A is deficient in Tay–Sachs disease and hexosaminidases A and B are deficient in Sandhoff disease.
Key: *, indicates site affected by enzyme deficiency
    [GLU], glucose, [GAL], galactose;
    [NANA], N-Acetyl-neuraminic acid;
    [NA-GALN], N-Acetyl-β-D-galactosamine—α and β indicate the type of glycosidic link.

bossing, thick gums, large tongue, hepatospleno-megaly and bone abnormalities, resemble those of Hurler disease. Psychomotor retardation is severe and progressive; the children have feeding problems and do not sit up or crawl. Half the children have a cherry-red spot in the region of the macula. Death occurs by about 2 years of age. *Type II* (juvenile) G_{M1}-gangliosidosis becomes apparent at about 1 year and progresses to spastic quadriplegia and death by about 10 years. Somatic changes are much less evident in this form and cherry-red spots are absent.

G_{M1} accumulates in the brain and viscera and foam cells can be found in bone marrow and urine. The disease is due to a deficiency of a specific β-D-galactosidase which is required for the conversion of G_{M1} to G_{M2} by the removal of a terminal galactose residue (Fig. 13.7). Mucopolysaccharide-like material has been found in the viscera of children with type I disease and there may be a slightly elevated urinary GAG excretion. However, the absence of excessive dermatan or heparan sulphate excretion excludes Hurler and Hurler diseases. Definitive diagnosis is made by demonstration of a marked deficiency of lysosomal β-D-galactosidase in leukocytes or cultured skin fibroblasts. Heterozygotes have partial deficiencies of the enzyme. Prenatal diagnosis is possible.

G_{M2}-gangliosidosis

There are two rapidly progressive forms of G_{M2}-gangliosidosis which are clinically similar but differ biochemically (type I and type II) and there is a juvenile form with a more protracted course. *Type I* (Tay–Sachs disease) and *type II* (Sandhoff disease) do not become apparent until about 6 months. Early features are hypotonia, feeding difficulties, failure to sit up, an exaggerated extension response to sound, visual disturbances and a cherry-red spot at the macula. Progressive psychomotor disturbance occurs and death ensues by about 3 years of age. The course of the juvenile form varies considerably; onset may be as early as 1 year and death as late as 15 years. Progressive psychomotor deterioration occurs and there may be optic atrophy or retinitis pigmentosa; cherry-red spots are occasionally found in this form.

G_{M2} storage occurs throughout the nervous system; this can be demonstrated with PAS and Sudan black staining techniques. Rectal biopsy may show the presence of typical membranous cytoplasmic bodies (Fig. 13.1) indicating neuronal storage

but this technique is unnecessary now that suitable enzyme studies can be carried out on blood. The disease arises from failure to remove the terminal N-acetyl-β-D-galactosamine residue from G_{M2} (Fig. 13.7). The lysosomal enzyme required for removal of this residue is commonly known as hexosaminidase A and is composed of α- and β-subunits (polypeptides) which can combine to form isoenzymes. Hexosaminidase A contains both α- and β-subunits whereas hexosaminidase B contains only β subunits. Hexosaminidase in the tissue and body fluids consists of a mixture of both the A and B isoenzymes. In *type I* (Tay–Sachs) there is an abnormality of the α-subunits so that a deficiency of hexosaminidase A results (but the total hexosaminidase activity may not be substantially diminished because of the presence of active isoenzyme B). In *type II* (Sandhoff disease) there is an abnormality of the β-subunits which leads to a deficiency of both isoenzymes and therefore a marked total hexosaminidase deficiency. Type II also differs from type I in that a glycolipid called globoside accumulates in the kidneys, liver and spleen (Fig. 13.7). Hexosaminidase A is inactivated by heat more readily than isoenzyme B. This provides one relatively simple method for determining the proportion of total activity due to hexosaminidase A. Biochemical diagnosis can be established using leukocytes prepared from a few millilitres of blood. Prenatal diagnosis (O'Brien et al. 1971) and carrier detection are possible for Tay–Sachs disease. Because of the high incidence of this disease among Jews of North-Eastern European origin (carrier frequency 1 in 30 compared to 1 in 300 for non-Jews) large scale population screening programmes have been undertaken in some countries. Such programmes have been very successful in parts of the United States but have not been generally enthusiastically received in the United Kingdom.

Metachromatic leukodystrophy (MLD)

The late infantile form of MLD becomes clinically apparent at about 3 years and is characterised by gait and speech disturbance with progression to dementia and quadriplegia. Eventually spontaneous movement ceases and death occurs in childhood. This form has a frequency of about 1 in 40000 and is commoner than many other types of lipidosis. A juvenile form of MLD is recognised with a later onset but the clinical course is otherwise similar. An adult form has also been defined with onset after 21 years. Such patients suffer from

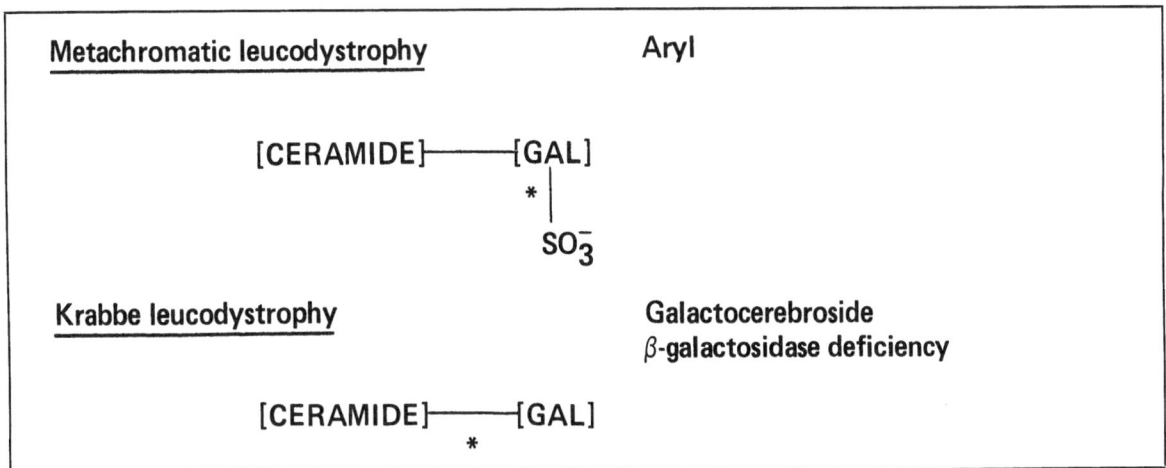

Fig. 13.8. Heritable lysosomal leukodystrophies. *, indicates site affected by enzyme deficiency.

dementia and psychosis. Mental, and eventually motor, functions gradually deteriorate but survival varies considerably—some live to middle age.

A specific sulphatase is deficient in MLD (Fig. 13.8) and excessive amounts of sulphatide can be found in the tissues and urine. The deposit from a fresh urine specimen contains metachromatic material. Metachromatic lipid accumulates in the white matter of the CNS and within Schwann cells and macrophages in peripheral nerves. Disintegration of the white matter occurs in the brain and there is segmental demyelination in peripheral nerves and slowing of conduction (see Chap. 16). The disease is confirmed by demonstration of the enzyme deficiency in leukocytes, urine or cultured fibroblasts. For convenience, a synthetic substrate, nitrocatechol sulphate, is used for the enzyme assay but this is hydrolysed by several sulphatases. Sulphatases acting on nitrocatechol sulphate are called arylsulphatases and in MLD one particular form is deficient, namely arylsulphatase A (see also Austin-type sulphatidosis). Prenatal diagnosis and carrier detection is possible.

The sulphatide lipidoses have been thoroughly reviewed by Dulaney and Moser (1978).

Krabbe leukodystrophy

This is a rapidly progressive disease with onset by 6 months and death by about 2 years of age. Infants present with irritability and sometimes with seizures. Mental and motor deterioration, deafness and blindness follow. Long tract signs are prominent and optic atrophy occurs. As in MLD, peripheral nerves are affected (see Chap. 16), but not usually as severely as the CNS.

Numerous globoid cells rich in galactocerebroside are found in the white matter of the brain but brain biopsy is no longer necessary to establish the diagnosis. There is a deficiency of the enzyme galactocerebroside β-galactosidase (Fig. 13.8). This enzyme is quite distinct from the β-galactosidase required for the conversion of G_{M1} to G_{M2} (see p. 222) and a radiolabelled natural substrate has so far been required for its accurate determination. Biochemical diagnosis can be made using leukocytes, serum or cultured fibroblasts. Prenatal diagnosis is possible.

Fabry disease (angiokeratoma corporis diffusum)

Fabry disease becomes apparent in infancy or childhood but is not associated with mental retardation (Desnick et al. 1978). However, the nervous system is affected and deposition of storage material in cerebral blood vessels can give rise to cerebrovascular complications in adult life. Lipid deposits also occur in the perineurial cells surrounding peripheral nerves and there may be an associated degeneration of axons within the nerve (see Chap. 16). The disease affects several systems but the most striking symptoms are crises consisting of excruciating pains in the hands and feet and sometimes abdominal pains which may mimic surgical conditions. These crises may be accompanied by fever and an elevated erythrocyte sedimentation rate. There are characteristic skin lesions, angiokeratomas, which are dark red networks of blood vessels found in clusters, particularly in the region of the buttocks. Eye lesions occur in the form of corneal opacities and abnormal

[CERAMIDE]—β—[GLU]—β—[GAL]—a—[GAL]
                                    *

Deficiency of a-galactosidase

Fig. 13.9. Fabry disease. The substrate shown is ceramide trihexoside
Key: [GLU], glucose; [GAL], galactose
        *, indicates site affected by enzyme deficiency.

[CERAMIDE]—β—[GLU]
                    *

Deficiency of glucocerebroside β-glucosidase

Fig. 13.10. Gaucher disease.
*, indicates site affected by enzyme deficiency.

networks of blood vessels in the conjunctiva and retina. Patients die in adult life from renal failure (extensive deposition of storage material in the kidneys), pulmonary disease (e.g. alveolar-capillary block) or from cardiac or cerebral vascular disease. Fabry disease is an X-linked recessive condition (unlike most other types of lipidosis which have autosomal recessive inheritance). Female carriers may also show some manifestations of the disease.

Trihexosyl ceramide (Fig. 13.9) accumulates in the tissues and in the plasma due to a deficiency of α-galactosidase (specifically isoenzyme A using synthetic substrate). Plasma ceramide trihexoside falls during crises. Lipid bodies can be demonstrated in urinary sediment (also in female carriers). Diagnosis is confirmed by the demonstration of α-galactosidase deficiency in leukocytes or cultured fibroblasts. In support of the Lyon hypothesis cultured fibroblasts from female carriers have been shown to contain two populations of cells, one with and one without the enzyme deficiency. Prenatal diagnosis is possible.

Gaucher disease

Type II (acute neuronopathic) Gaucher disease appears around 6 months and usually causes death before 2 years of age. Severe regression of motor function occurs and strabismus and spasticity are frequent features. Cranial nerves and extrapyramidal tracts are involved. There is hepatosplenomegaly and lymph nodes may be enlarged. In *type III* (subacute neuronopathic form) the onset is later and the course more protracted; seizures are common. Bone changes occur in this form as in the adult (non-neuronal) form with, typically, an expansion of the cortical bone at the lower end of the femur.

Glucosyl ceramide (glucocerebroside) accumulates in brain neurons. 'Gaucher cells' are found throughout the reticulo-endothelial system including the bone marrow. These cells are lipid-laden

histiocytes in which the cytoplasm has the appearance of crinkled tissue paper. There is an elevated serum tartrate-stable acid phosphatase in Gaucher disease. The basic defect is a deficiency of glucocerebroside β-glucosidase (Fig. 13.10). Diagnosis can be confirmed by determination of the enzyme activity in leukocytes using a synthetic substrate provided detergents are used in the assay mixture.

Niemann–Pick disease

Involvement of the CNS occurs in the acute infantile form of Niemann–Pick disease (*type A*). In the early stages, the disease is similar to the acute neuronopathic form of Gaucher disease. Hepatosplenomegaly, lymphadenopathy, pulmonary infiltration and progressive deterioration of motor and mental functions occur. A cherry-red spot may be found at the macula.

These patients store excessive amounts of *sphingomyelin*, which is a normal major component of the myelin sheath. Foamy histiocytes are present in bone marrow and vacuolated lymphocytes are seen in blood. The disease is due to a deficiency of sphingomyelinase, the enzyme necessary for the cleavage of sphingomyelin to form ceramide and phosphorylcholine (Fig. 13.11). Diagnosis can be confirmed by demonstration of the enzyme deficiency in leukocytes or cultured fibroblasts.

[CERAMIDE]————[PHOSPHORYLCHOLINE]
                *

Deficiency of sphingomyelinase

Fig. 13.11. Niemann–Pick disease.
*, indicates site affected by enzyme deficiency.

Ophthalmoplegic lipidoses

These conditions have been considered as variants of Niemann–Pick disease but the precise biochemical defect is not yet known. A characteristic feature is the development of vertical opthalmoplegia.

Farber's lipogranulomatosis

The striking clinical features of Farber disease are hoarseness, painful swollen peripheral joints and associated skin nodules. Onset is often in early infancy and death can occur in early childhood due to pulmonary involvement. Although storage material accumulates in nerve cells, as well as in other tissues, mental retardation has only been demonstrated in a few patients. Ceramide accumulates in the tissues and a deficiency of acid ceramidase has been demonstrated in cultured fibroblasts and white blood cells.

The mucolipidoses

A few conditions with features resembling both the mucopolysaccharidoses and the lipidoses have traditionally been classified under the heading mucolipidosis (ML). This classification is not entirely satisfactory but is convenient when considering differential diagnosis.

Austin sulphatidosis

This disease presents with features of metachromatic leukodystrophy, the physical features of mucopolysaccharidosis and an excessive excretion of sulphatide and GAG in the urine. There is a deficiency of arylsulphatases A, B and C. These isoenzymes act on specific natural substrates; the A form is deficient in MLD (see p. 222) and the B form is deficient in Maroteaux–Lamy disease (a mucopolysaccharidosis characterised by skeletal abnormalities, corneal clouding and an elevated excretion of dermatan sulphate).

I-cell disease

Also designated ML II, I-cell disease shows many of the features of Hurler disease but physical abnormalities appear earlier or may be present at birth. Psychomotor retardation develops and death occurs in early childhood. Urinary GAG excretion is not substantially elevated in this condition. The name 'I-cell' derives from the observation that cultured fibroblasts from these patients have striking inclusion bodies (seen with phase microscopy). Lymphocytes and bone marrow cells are vacu-

olated. The peculiar biochemical finding in this condition is a deficiency of several lysosomal enzymes in cultured fibroblasts (Leroy et al. 1972) together with an increased activity of these enzymes in the culture medium. Plasma acid hydrolase activities are also increased, particularly arylsulphatase A and α-mannosidase (the former is used as a screening test). However, the activities of these enzymes in leukocytes appear to be normal. I-cell disease appears to be due to defective phosphorylation of mannose residues present in the affected enzymes. Prenatal diagnosis is possible.

A milder variant of I-cell disease (also referred to as pseudo-Hurler polydystrophy or ML III) occurs, in which mental function may be normal. These patients can survive to adult life.

Mucolipidosis type IV
A disease characterised by psychomotor retardation and corneal opacities has recently been designated ML IV. A deficiency of a specific ganglioside sialidase has been proposed.

Other lysosomal disorders affecting the nervous system

Mannosidosis

Mannosidosis develops in infancy and can cause death in mid-childhood. Psychomotor retardation occurs and the physical manifestations resemble those of Hurler disease. One peculiar feature is the presence of cloudiness in the capsule of the lens (Milla et al. 1977). Biochemical features include a deficiency of α-mannosidase and excessive excretion of mannose-containing oligosaccharides of the type found in glycoproteins. Hypogammaglobulinaemia has been reported in these patients. Prenatal diagnosis is possible.

Fucosidosis

This disease is characterised by severe progressive cerebral degeneration culminating in decerebrate rigidity (intense spasticity is a prominent feature), cardiomegaly, thick skin and profuse sweating (the sweat has a high salt concentration like that in cystic fibrosis). Death occurs in early childhood. There is a deficiency of α-fucosidase and storage of fucose-containing glycolipid (Durand et al. 1969).

Aspartyl-glycosaminuria

This autosomal recessive condition is relatively frequent in Finland where its incidence is said to be 1 in 30 000 births. It has been diagnosed in children and adults. Psychomotor retardation occurs and physical features can resemble those of mucopolysaccharidosis (Isenberg and Sharp 1975). The patients excrete aspartyl-glucosamine fragments in the urine and have a deficiency of N-aspartyl-β-glucosaminidase.

Aids to diagnosis of lysosomal disorders

The following lists are presented as an aid to the diagnosis of lysosomal storage diseases affecting the nervous system.

Eye signs are numerous and can be of considerable value in diagnosis.

Cherry-red spots are found in G_{M1}- and G_{M2}-gangliosidosis and in Niemann–Pick disease; similar changes have been reported in metachromatic leukodystrophy but they are less distinct.

Corneal opacities occur in Hurler disease, ML IV and Fabry disease.

Optic atrophy occurs in Krabbe disease and lens opacities occur in mannosidosis.

Coarse facies and bone abnormalities are seen in:

Mucopolysaccharidosis
I-cell disease
Austin leukodystrophy
G_{M1}-gangliosidosis
Mannosidosis
Aspartyl-glycosaminuria

Hepatosplenomegaly occurs in:

The above six conditions
Gaucher disease
Niemann–Pick disease

Characteristic skin lesions are found in:

Hunter disease
Fabry disease
Farber disease

Leukocyte inclusions are found in:

Mucopolysaccharidosis
I-cell disease
Austin leukodystrophy
G_{M1}-gangliosidosis
Mannosidosis
Niemann–Pick disease

Analysis of urine reveals abnormalities in the following disorders although special techniques are required in some instances:

Mucopolysaccharidosis ⎫
Mannosidosis   ⎬ Abormality
Fucosidosis   ⎪ in supernatant
Aspartyl-glycosaminuria ⎭

G_{M1}-gangliosidosis ⎫
Austin leukodystrophy ⎪ Abnormality
Metachromatic leukodystrophy ⎬ in sediment
Fabry disease   ⎭

Neuronal storage may be demonstrated in rectal biopsy material in the following conditions (N.B. this procedure is not needed to establish diagnosis):

Mucopolysaccharidosis
G_{M1}-gangliosidosis
G_{M2}-gangliosidosis
Gaucher disease
Niemann–Pick disease

Management of lysosomal disorders

The first step in the management of inherited lysosomal storage disorders is to establish an accurate clinical and biochemical diagnosis. Advice on prognosis and good genetic counselling can then be given. Early diagnosis is particularly important now that prenatal diagnosis can be offered for many of these disorders. Although biochemical diagnosis ultimately rests on the determination of the specific enzyme deficiency it is important to remember that such tests are costly, time consuming and require skilled laboratory personnel, and that only limited facilities are available at present. Other simple investigations may help to narrow the differential diagnosis and therefore the choice of relevant enzyme studies. Improved methods for biochemical diagnosis should obviate the need for most of the biopsy procedures formerly used.

In general, only symptomatic treatment can at present be offered to patients with these storage diseases. Surgery has been undertaken for the treatment of corneal dysplasias and complications of skeletal and other connective tissue abnormalities but often this has been of very limited benefit. There is a risk from general anaesthesia in those conditions with respiratory tract abnormalities (e.g. Hurler disease). Appropriate drugs may be indicated for the treatment of disturbed behaviour, convulsions, heart failure and infections. Diphenylhydantoin has proved particularly effective in relieving the painful crises of Fabry disease (Lockman et al. 1973).

Recently, specific treatment of some lysosomal storage disorders has been attempted either by supplying exogenous enzyme or by transplantation of tissues or cells capable of supplying the missing enzyme. Several different approaches have been adopted and in some cases there has been biochemical evidence of increased degradation of stored substrate following treatment (e.g. in Gaucher and Fabry diseases and mucopolysaccharidosis). There have been few reports of significant clinical responses but these methods have so far been attempted mainly in patients with advanced disease. Some clinical improvement has recently been observed in patients with mucopolysaccharidosis following bone marrow transplantation. Possibly such an approach might eventually prove useful in preventing or ameliorating the onset of those diseases which manifest themselves after birth. The source of enzyme is important since particular chemical recognition groups need to be present on the enzyme molecules in order for them to be taken into cells by selective endocytosis. There are some formidable obstacles to successful enzyme replacement therapy. The plasma half-lives of exogenously administered enzymes tend to be short. The tissues or organs most affected by the disease may not be those which take up the enzyme most actively. Furthermore, the enzymes do not appear to cross the blood–brain barrier. Molecular engineering might eventually overcome some of these problems but it seems unlikely that the current experimental approaches to specific therapy will have any major impact on those disorders in which the CNS is severely affected.

References

Bach G, Friedman R, Weissmann B, Neufeld E F (1972) The defect in Hurler and Scheie syndromes: Deficiency of α-L-iduronidase. Proc Natl Acad Sci USA 69: 2048

Bach G, Eisenberg F Jr, Cantz M, Neufeld E F (1973) The defect in Hunter syndrome: Deficiency of sulfoiduronate sulfatase. Proc Natl Acad Sci USA 70: 2134–2138

Desnick R J, Klionsky B, Sweeley C C (1978) Fabry's disease. In: Stanbury J B, Wyngaarden J B, Fredrickson D S (eds) The metabolic basis of inherited disease. McGraw-Hill, New York, pp 810–840

Dulaney J T, Moser H W (1978) Sulphatide lipidosis: metachromatic leukodystrophy. In: Stanbury J B, Wyngaarden F B, Fredrickson D S (eds) The metabolic basis of inherited disease. McGraw-Hill, New York, pp 770–809

Durand P, Borrone C, Della Cella G (1969) Fucosidosis. J Pediatr 75: 665–674

Fratantoni J C, Neufeld E F, Uhlendorf B W, Jacobson C B (1969) Intrauterine diagnosis of the Hurler and Hunter syndromes. N Engl J Med 280: 686–688

Harper P S, Laurence K M, Parkes A et al. (1974) Sanfilippo A disease in the fetus. J Med Genetics 11: 123–132

Isenberg J N, Sharp H L (1975) Aspartylglucosaminuria: psychomotor retardation masquerading as a mucopolysaccharidosis. J Pediatr 86: 713–717

Lake B D (1981) Metabolic disorders; general considerations. In: Berry C L (ed) Paediatric pathology. Springer-Verlag, Berlin Heidelberg New York, Chap. 14

Leroy J G, Ho M W, MacBrinn M X, Zielke K, Jacob J, O'Brien J S (1972) I-cell disease: biochemical studies. Pediatr Res 6: 752–757

Lockman L A, Hunninghake D B, Krivit W, Desnick R J (1973) Relief of the pain of Fabry's disease by diphenylhydantoin. Neurology 23: 871

McKusick V A (1972) Heritable disorders of connective tissue, 4th edn. Mosby, St. Louis

Milla P J, Black I E, Patrick A D, Hugh-Jones K, Oberholzer V (1977) Mannosidosis: Clinical and biochemical study. Arch Dis Child 52: 937–942

O'Brien J S (1978) The gangliosidoses. In: Stanbury J B, Wyngaarden J B, Fredrickson D S (eds) The metabolic basis of inherited disease. McGraw Hill, New York, pp 841–865

O'Brien J A, Okada S, Fillerup D L et al. Tay–Sachs disease: Prenatal diagnosis. Science 172: 61

Whiteman P, Henderson H (1977) A method for the determination of amniotic-fluid glycosaminoglycans and its application to the prenatal diagnosis of Hurler and Sanfilippo diseases. Clin Chim Acta 79: 99–105

Whiteman P, Young E (1977) The laboratory diagnosis of Sanfilippo disease. Clin Chim Acta 76: 139–147

Chapter 14

Hereditary and System Disorders of the Nervous System

The hereditary system disorders of the nervous system form a large group of diseases in which the characteristic feature is degeneration of one or more systems of neurons, and of their interconnecting projections. In some the pathogenesis is relatively well understood, for example subacute combined degeneration of the spinal cord, but in others, for example motor neuron disease, the cause is obscure. The term 'system degeneration', which is often used to describe these degenerative disorders, indicates that certain functional groups of neurons and their axons are selectively affected, resulting in clearly recognisable patterns of abnormality.

Many of these disorders have a hereditary basis (Table 14.1). Although the pattern of inheritance is well documented in many, the underlying biochemical or metabolic cause has been determined in only a few. In many instances, particularly in the case of the spinocerebellar degenerations, classification therefore *depends on the clinical features*. However, the clinical features vary both within and between families, a phenomenon indicating variable penetrance and genetic heterogenicity. In an individual patient, it is often difficult to decide to which category a clinical disorder should be assigned. Pathological features, on the other hand, are more readily recognised and are characterised by selective neuronal loss, axonal degeneration and gliosis. In certain instances specific histopathological features are seen; inflammatory changes are not a feature. Greenfield devised a classification of the spinocerebellar degenerations, using *patho-anatomical criteria*, which forms the basis of most subsequent descriptions but, despite this, it has not proved easy to segregate the clinical features of these disorders, even knowing the pathological features found in other family members. In this chapter a clinically based classification of the degenerative disorders will be presented (Tables 14.1 and 14.2).

The *concept of system degenerations* arose from patho-anatomical studies in the 19th century in which the patterns of tract degeneration characteristic of certain clinical disorders, especially tabes dorsalis and subacute combined degeneration of the cord, were worked out. These studies, continued now in anatomical studies of cortical, brain stem and cerebellar connections (see Brodal 1981), were summarised by Greenfield (1954), who brought together the various familial and acquired cerebellar degenerative disorders described up to that time by employing the unifying concept of the spino-cerebellar degenerations. This term is still widely used in clinical practice but it is important to realise that it represents an attempt to simplify the clinicopathological basis of these disorders. When the biochemical lesion underlying a particular syndrome becomes elucidated the syndrome is better classified as a metabolic disorder, as in Chap. 12. It is thus apparent that the inherent difficulty in classification is due to imperfect understanding of the basic mechanism of so many of these disorders. Nonetheless it is implicit within the concept of hereditary and system disorders that the systems of neurons and pathways involved in each disorder are biochemically or otherwise related, and thus show differential susceptibility. Examples of this are common and include both acquired disorders, e.g. subacute combined degeneration of the cord and tabes dorsalis, and genetic disorders, e.g. Refsum's disease and Wilson's disease.

Clinical features

Since the concept of hereditary and system disorders excludes diseases with diffuse pathology, such as Alzheimer's dementia, the clinical features of these disorders show certain common features. These features have been used in Tables 14.1 and 14.2 as a basis for a simple clinical classification of the commoner acquired and hereditary system disorders. Some disorders in this group have been described in other chapters because their clinical and pathological features allow them to be related to other acquired disorders. Thus motor neuron disease, the spinal muscular atrophies and the

familial peripheral neuropathies are discussed in Chaps. 16 and 17 in relation to other neuromuscular diseases, and the dementias are considered as a group in Chap. 15.

The remaining disorders shown in Tables 14.1 and 14.2 present with signs of sensory or motor system disease, with cerebellar ataxia, with involuntary movement disorders, or with dementia, alone or in combination. In most there are features of involvement of more than one system, for example Friedreich's ataxia; but in some, for example familial spastic paraplegia, the clinical features are restricted to involvement only of a single system of neurons and their connections. *Familial* system disorders have an undefined onset and a slowly progressive course. Sporadic forms of the typical disorders often occur. *Acquired* system disorders usually present with a more rapid or even a subacute onset, as in subacute combined degeneration of the spinal cord, or alcoholic cerebellar degeneration. Other acquired disorders, such as tabes dorsalis, discussed in Chap. 10, present insidiously and pursue a relentlessly progressive course.

Familial spinocerebellar degenerations typically show features of multisystem involvement and this often extends beyond the features noted in Tables 14.1 and 14.2 to include retinitis pigmentosa, cardiomyopathy or deafness. Some of these associated features occur also in disorders in which the underlying biochemical defect is known, for example Refsum's disease and a-beta-lipoprotein-aemia, but this has not led to the establishment of any basic principles of pathogenesis for the whole group of disorders; thus classification rests, at present, on the clinical and pathological features of individual disorders. Indeed there may be minor differences between families affected by apparently similar disorders suggesting that in many instances, particularly in those disorders characterised by a dominant pattern of inheritance, polygenic inheritance with variable penetrance is a factor in the variable morphological expression of the disorder. Factors such as these have led to argument as to whether closely similar disorders should be regarded as the same, or different diseases: the 'lumping or splitting' argument. Such discussions do not add greatly to understanding these disorders. The prognosis of these diseases varies considerably; many progress slowly and are incapacitating but do not shorten life expectancy, while others are rapidly progressive. Death results from pneumonia or the secondary effects of inanition.

Table 14.1. Familial system degenerations of obscure cause

Spinal degenerations	
Sensory system disorders	Hereditary posterior column ataxia
	Hereditary sensory neuropathies (see Chap. 16)
Motor system disorders	Familial spastic paraplegia
	Motor neuron disease (see Chap. 17)
	Spinal muscular atrophies (see Chap. 17)
	Hereditary sensorimotor neuropathies, including Charcot–Marie–Tooth syndrome (see Chaps. 16 and 17)
Spinocerebellar degenerations	Friedreich's ataxia
	Mild, non-progressive, fragmentary, dominant Friedreich's-like ataxia
	Holmes cortical cerebellar atrophy
	Olivopontocerebellar atrophy (multi-system disease)
	Shy-Drager syndrome
	Other disorders with ataxia (Table 14.3)
Basal ganglia degenerations and dementias	Huntington's chorea
	Dystonia musculorum deformans
	Wilson's disease (see Chap. 12)
	Dementias (see Chap. 15)

Table 14.2. Acquired system degenerations

Spinal degenerations	
Sensory system disorders	Tabes dorsalis (see Chap. 10)
	Subacute combined degeneration of the spinal cord
	Carcinomatous sensory neuropathy (see Chap. 16)
Motor system disorders	Motor neuron disease (see Chap. 17)
	Motor neuropathies (see Chaps. 16 and 17)
Cerebellar degenerations	Alcoholic cerebellar degeneration
	Other drug-induced cerebellar degenerations, e.g. phenytoin, carcinomatous cerebellar degeneration, myxoedema
Basal ganglia degenerations	Parkinson's disease
	Post-encephalitic parkinsonism
	Other forms of parkinsonism
	Striato-nigral degeneration
	Progressive supranuclear palsy (Steele–Richardson–Olsjewski syndrome)
Cortical degenerations	Dementias (see Chap. 15)
Pathology obscure	Stiff man syndrome

Hereditary system degenerations

Hereditary spastic paraplegia (Strümpell)

A gradually progressive disorder beginning in adolescence or in adult life, hereditary spastic paraplegia is commoner in men than in women and usually shows a *dominant* pattern of inheritance. Cases beginning earlier in life develop more severe disability than cases beginning later. There is a spastic paraparesis with only slight involvement of the arms, or of speech. Sphincter involvement and sensory impairment are rarely found.

Pathology. At autopsy there is degeneration of the corticospinal tracts, most severe in the thoraco-lumbar cord. The posterior columns show degeneration in the gracile columns in the cervical region and the spinocerebellar tracts may also be affected. In some cases loss of motor neurons, with distal neurogenic muscular atrophy, has been recorded and optic atrophy may also occur. It has been suggested that the pathological features indicate a 'dying-back' or distal axonopathy (see Chap. 16) affecting central pathways.

Hereditary posterior column ataxia (Biemond)

A progressive ataxia with pronounced posterior column sensory abnormalities, sometimes associated with mild spasticity in the legs, are the features of hereditary posterior column ataxia. Examination of the spinal cord demonstrates axonal degeneration and loss of myelin staining in the posterior roots and posterior columns. This disorder is very rare.

Charcot–Marie–Tooth disease (peroneal muscular atrophy)

There are various forms of peroneal muscular atrophy. In the spinal form of the disorder, *degeneration of anterior horn cells* is the most prominent feature particularly in the lumbosacral region of the spinal cord. There may also be degeneration of the posterior root ganglia, which leads to severe axonal loss of the posterior nerve roots and posterior columns. Corticospinal tract degeneration is uncommon. Cranial nerve involvement, cerebellar atrophy with loss of Purkinje cells, and atrophy of the dentate nuclei have also been described, usually associated with axonal loss in the superior cerebellar peduncles. The disease runs a slow course, not usually shortening life but producing extensive deterioration and severe wasting of distal limb muscles. In another form of the disease there is a *distal axonopathy*, mainly affecting motor nerve fibres, and in a third form of the syndrome motor and sensory nerves are affected by a demyelinating neuropathy leading to *hypertrophic neuropathy* (see Chap. 16).

Friedreich's ataxia

An inherited progressive degenerative disease, Friedreich's ataxia shows an autosomal recessive mode of inheritance in most families, though a late-onset dominant form has been reported. Occasionally sporadic cases occur with a clinical and pathological pattern similar to that of the inherited form. Although Friedreich's ataxia is the commonest of the hereditary ataxias its incidence of 2/100 000 makes it an uncommon disease. It is commoner in families in which there have been consanguineous marriages and in genetically isolated populations.

Friedreich's ataxia usually presents before the age of 25 years with limb and trunk ataxia which

becomes progressively more severe. Dysarthria, signs of corticospinal tract dysfunction in the legs, and loss of joint position sense and vibration sense develop eventually in all cases and nystagmus is a frequent feature. Scoliosis and ECG evidence of cardiomyopathy occur in more than half the cases but primary optic atrophy, pes cavus and distal amyotrophy are less frequent. About 10% of patients develop diabetes mellitus, but this feature segregates within individual families.

Pathology. The major abnormalities are found in the spinal cord. There is marked loss of ganglion cells in the posterior root ganglia and this is accompanied by degeneration of the posterior spinal roots, and of the posterior columns of the spinal cord. The gracile columns are particularly affected, reflecting loss of afferent fibres, but the cuneate columns are less affected (Fig. 14.1). This may be due to a dying back axonopathy in the posterior columns, the largest and longest fibres being first and most severely affected. Similarly, the longest fibres in the corticospinal tracts are lost, so that corticospinal tract degeneration is most marked in the thoracolumbar segments of the cord (Fig.

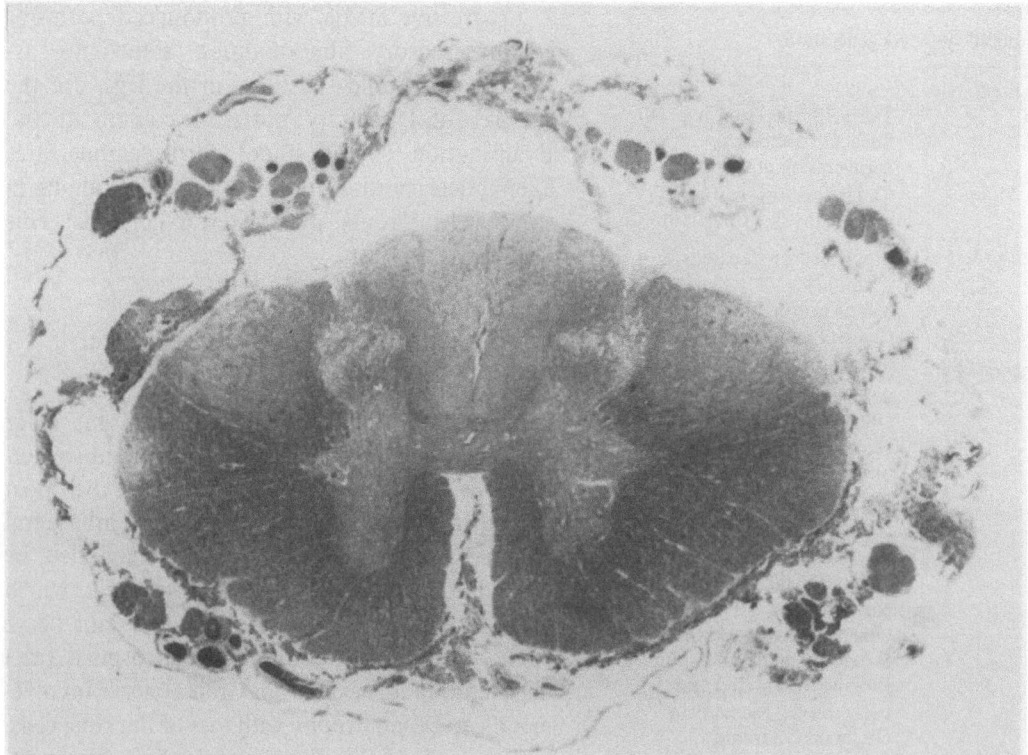

Fig. 14.1. Friedreich's ataxia. Transverse section of the spinal cord showing tract degeneration in the posterior columns, lateral corticospinal tracts, and the left dorsal spinocerebellar tract.

14.1). The peripheral nerves show very severe loss of the thicker myelinated fibres and teased fibre preparations show the features of an axonal neuropathy.

In the cord, the cells of Clarke's columns are lost and there is degeneration of the posterior spinocerebellar tracts and to a lesser extent, of the anterior spinocerebellar tracts. Gliosis is prominent in all degenerate tracts in the cord. The brain stem appears atrophic but the cerebral peduncles and cerebellar cortex are normal. However, there is atrophy of the superior cerebellar peduncles and of the dentate nuclei and cell loss and gliosis is also evident in the vestibular and cochlear nuclei. Loss of pyramidal cells in the cerebral cortex has also been reported, and there is loss of fibres in the optic tracts and of cells in the lateral geniculate bodies.

The heart shows muscle fibre degeneration in most cases, with focal or diffuse cellular infiltration, and fibrosis, consistent with a cardiomyopathy.

It has been concluded that the ataxia so characteristic of the disease is due to de-afferentation and the de-efferentation of the cerebellum, since the latter shows no signs of cortical atrophy.

Spinocerebellar atrophies

Classification within the group of spinocerebellar atrophies is controversial, mainly because there have been many reports of patients showing slight variations of a basically similar clinical picture without pathological study of the site and type of the degenerative process. Many of these disorders appear to be incomplete forms of Friedreich's ataxia, but the cortical cerebellar atrophies, and the syndromes of ponto-cerebellar atrophy are relatively well defined.

Cortical cerebellar atrophy

In this group of disorders the clinical presentation is variable. Marie described a group of patients with cerebellar and corticospinal signs, some of whom also had optic atrophy. In these patients there was cerebellar atrophy with degeneration of the spinocerebellar tracts, and to a lesser extent, of the corticospinal tracts (Marie's spastic ataxia), a disorder which clearly bears a fairly close relationship to Friedreich's ataxia. In the family reported by Sanger-Brown ataxia was associated with optic atrophy, ptosis, external ophthalmoplegia and mild

corticospinal signs. Pathologically there was atrophy of Clarke's dorsal nucleus, of the posterior columns, and of the posterior spinocerebellar tracts, but cerebellar atrophy was only slight. The Holmes type of cerebellar degeneration consists clinically of a severe, relatively pure cerebellar ataxia in which there is atrophy of all three layers of the cerebellar cortex, with atrophy and gliosis of the olives and of the inferior cerebellar peduncles. The spinal cord is normal. The cerebellar atrophy in the Holmes disorder is most marked in the superior vermis. Purkinje cells are almost completely lost and there is an increase in Bergmann glia, and gliosis of the molecular layer. The dentate nuclei are preserved.

Cerebellar degeneration with ataxia is a feature of a number of other rare disorders, in which the ataxia appears as one of several features suggesting multisystem involvement (Table 14.3).

Table 14.3. Familial multisystem disorders in which cerebellar degeneration is a feature

Refsum's disease
A-beta lipoproteinaemia
Dyssynergia cerebellaris myoclonica (Ramsay Hunt)
Cerebellar ataxia with slow eye movements
Marinesco–Sjögren syndrome
Sjögren–Larssen syndrome
Fahr's disease
Xeroderma pigmentosa
Kearns–Sayre–Shy syndrome [oculo-cranio-somatic syndrome ('ophthalmoplegia-plus')]

Olivopontocerebellar atrophy

Sometimes referred to as the Menzel, or Déjerine–Thomas type of cerebellar atrophy, olivopontocerebellar atrophy presents in several clinical forms. It occurs as a dominant or autosomal recessive condition, with or without dementia, or with prominent autonomic dysfunction, but these clinical distinctions do not correlate well with pathological differences.

The disease begins in late middle life with slowly progressive limb ataxia and dysarthria. Nystagmus is less frequent. The ankle jerks are lost and parkinsonian features develop, including bradykinesia, rigidity and slight tremor at rest. The plantar responses are often extensor, dementia may be evident and autonomic dysfunction, with incontinence or retention of urine, abnormal pupils, disordered sweating and postural hypotension may become disabling.

Pathology. The pons is atrophic and wedge-shaped with atrophy of the middle cerebellar peduncles, cerebellar cortex and olives (Fig. 14.2). The corticospinal tracts are normal but the tegmentum of the pons is markedly atrophic. The Purkinje cells are virtually all lost and there is marked cell loss in the inferior olives (Fig. 14.3) and pontine nuclei. In the dentate nuclei, neurons are relatively well preserved although this nucleus is gliotic. The spinal cord usually shows some degeneration of the posterior columns and corticospinal tracts; the cells of the dorsal nuclei and of the intermediolateral cell columns are usually virtually all lost, accounting for the autonomic disorder. In addition, there is gliosis and neuron loss in the putamen and in the substantia nigra, features which can be correlated with the extrapyramidal signs noted clinically.

Shy–Drager syndrome

In the Shy–Drager syndrome autonomic dysfunc-

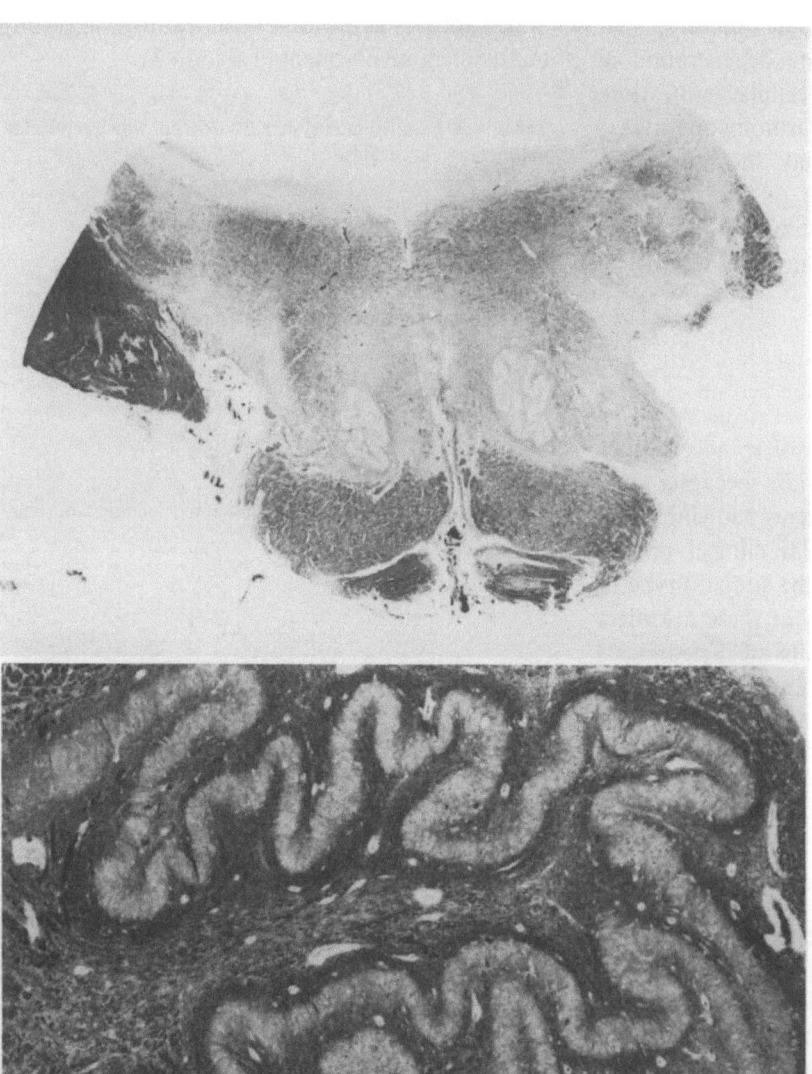

Fig. 14.2. Olivopontocerebellar atrophy. There is gross shrinkage of the olives with degeneration in the middle cerebellar peduncle. The inferior cerebellar peduncle to the left of the picture is normal.

Fig. 14.3. Photomicrograph showing one of the atrophic olives illustrated in Fig. 14.2; there is marked loss of olivary neurons.

tion is the major presenting feature, but extra-pyramidal signs may also be prominent and in some cases there may be additional cerebellar signs and evidence of a subclinical neuropathy.

Pathologically most of these cases fall into two groups; those in which the underlying disorder appears to be idiopathic Parkinson's disease associated with autonomic degeneration, and cases of olivopontocerebellar atrophy in which the autonomic features are unusually severe. Idiopathic postural hypotension is thus best regarded not as a distinct disease, but as a feature of some of the spinocerebellar degenerations, and of Parkinson's disease.

Basal ganglia disorders

Huntington's chorea (see also Chap. 15), *Wilson's disease* (see Chap. 12) and *dystonia musculorum deformans* are the best known examples of hereditary disorders involving the basal ganglia.

Dystonia musculorum deformans (torsion dystonia)

In this condition there is involuntary coactivation of antagonistic muscle groups in the limbs and trunk (dystonia). This presents in the patient as stiffness and the characteristic picture of distorted limb posture (dystonic posture). It is associated in many cases with chorea and athetosis (see Chap. 13). Some cases are hereditary and classically occur in families of Ashkenazi Jewish descent, while others are sporadic.

The disorder begins in the second or third decade, progresses for several years and may result in total disability; dementia, however, is not a feature. The cause is unknown and full pathological studies have failed to reveal a macroscopic or even a microscopic abnormality in the brain.

Increased plasma dopamine-beta-hydroxylase levels and noradrenaline levels have been recorded in patients with autosomal dominant torsion dystonia and in their unaffected relatives, but at present there is no proof of a causal relationship between these biochemical abnormalities and the disease itself.

The clinical disability of torsion dystonia overlaps with other diseases of proven basal ganglion origin, and it may be ameliorated by stereotactic thalamotomy. In recent years the group term *dystonias* has been widely adopted to include dystonia musculorum deformans or torsion dys-

tonia, together with more localised forms such as *spasmodic torticollis* and *dystonic writer's cramp*, both of which are now accepted as organic conditions despite the lack of histopathological defect.

Huntington's disease

An autosomally inherited disorder, Huntington's chorea has an almost 100% penetrance affecting half of any generation, with an incidence of 5/100000. It presents in the fourth decade, though commonly earlier when the father is the affected parent. The disease runs a course of 5–30 years, again more rapidly in male children.

Clinically there is a combination of initial spontaneous semi-purposeful movement with dementia. Either may dominate the clinical picture; indeed dementia sometimes occurs without movement disorder.

At *autopsy* the *brain* is generally small, less than 1000 g (Fig. 15.5, Chap. 15), but in many instances atrophy may not be marked. Cortical atrophy is variable but the most marked feature is atrophy of the caudate nucleus, particularly the head, and it appears as a brown concave ribbon on the lateral wall of the dilated lateral ventricle. The putamen and globus pallidus also shrink. While the corpus striatum and globus pallidus can shrink by up to 60% with loss of 40% of neurons, the cortex may only be reduced in volume by 20% with neuron loss in the 3rd, 4th and 5th layers. The subthalamic nuclei are also reduced in size and neuron number by one-quarter. Histological studies indicate that, in addition to the loss of small neurons, there is gliosis, but this is probably relative only and results from neuron loss and shrinkage in the size of the structure.

Neurochemical studies have shown a deficiency of gamma-aminobutyric acid in the substantia nigra, putamen and caudate nucleus in association with decrease in the synthetic enzyme glutamic acid decarbonylase. Choline acetyl transferase is considerably reduced while tyrosine hydrolase—the synthetic enzyme for dopamine—is not. These observations suggest that Huntington's chorea is associated with an imbalance between the gamma-aminobutyric acid, acetylcholine and dopamine-dependent neuron systems.

Acquired system degenerations

The acquired system degenerations are listed in Table 14.2. Several have been described elsewhere in this book, including tabes dorsalis (Chap. 10), motor neuron disease (Chaps. 16, 17), motor neuropathies (Chaps. 16, 17), sensory neuropathies (Chap. 16), and the dementias (Chap. 15).

Subacute combined degeneration of the cord

This acquired disorder is due to deficiency of vitamin B_{12}. The neurological disorder is usually, but not always, associated with megaloblastic anaemia. Vitamin B_{12} deficiency usually arises from impaired absorption due to absence of gastric intrinsic factor, itself secondary to an autoimmune chronic gastritis, but disease of the small bowel, or even dietary B_{12} deficiency in vegans, may also cause it.

The *neurological complications* of vitamin B_{12} deficiency occur mainly in the spinal cord, but the peripheral nerves, optic nerves and cerebral cortex may also be affected. Distal paraesthesiae are usually the earliest symptom, followed by tight feelings in the limbs, and by weakness and ataxia of the legs and, later, the arms. There is marked impairment of position and vibration sense, often extending into the trunk, with slight distal impairment of pinprick and touch. The plantar responses are extensor and the proximal reflexes brisk, but the ankle jerks are absent, reflecting involvement of peripheral nerves, and of the root entry zones in the cord. Sphincter disturbances and optic atrophy are relatively uncommon, and dementia may be a feature of some cases. The onset is usually insidious but it may be subacute. The prognosis with adequate treatment is excellent, but recovery may be delayed or incomplete in severe cases.

Pathology. Glossitis, megaloblastic anaemia, macrocytic hyperplastic marrow, slight enlargement of the spleen and a chronic gastritis with lymphocytic and plasma cell infiltration of the gastric wall and absence of gastric parietal cells, are the usual features in patients with idiopathic addisonian anaemia. Gastric parietal cell antibodies are usually detectable in the blood and antibodies to other tissues, especially to thyroid cells and to thyroglobulin and adrenal cortex, are also often present. The ESR is usually raised, and the CSF protein slightly increased.

In the *nervous system* the changes in the spinal cord are particularly characteristic. In the early stages there is ballooning of myelin sheaths and fusiform swelling of axons, in the mid-thoracic portions of the posterior columns and, to a lesser extent, in the corticospinal tracts. The axons then degenerate and it is the combination of degeneration in the posterior columns and lateral (corticospinal) columns that led to the term *combined degeneration*, a distinction which was important in neuropathology at a time when degeneration of the posterior columns was usually due to tabes dorsalis.

Later in the *untreated* disease, the cord lesion is most evident in the thoracic segments. In severe cases there may be degeneration of virtually all the white matter of the cord, sparing only the tracts close to the grey matter and those in the anterior part of the cord. In the cervical cord there is usually marked degeneration of the posterior columns, especially of the fasciculus gracilis, and of the spinocerebellar tracts. Degeneration of the corticospinal tracts is usually only slight at levels rostral to the cervical cord.

The axonal lesion leads to wallerian degeneration in distal parts of affected tracts, and gliosis of the damaged tracts. Scattered small zones of demyelination and axonal destruction may be found in the cerebral white matter, often in a perivascular location. In the peripheral nerves there is a mild loss of large myelinated axons, with some evidence both of axonal degeneration and of segmental demyelination. The changes in the optic nerves resemble those in the cerebral white matter.

The *pathogenesis* of the neuropathological change in vitamin B_{12} deficiency is not fully understood. It has been suggested that deficiency of this vitamin leads to the accumulation of neurotoxic radicles, for example cyanide, within the brain and spinal cord.

Acquired cerebellar degenerations (Table 14.2)

Cerebellar ataxia is a feature of acute intoxication with *alcohol*. A permanent cerebellar syndrome may also develop in alcoholics; the truncal musculature is predominantly affected, and thus the clinical disorder is most obvious when the patient is in the erect posture and walking. The cerebellar ataxia usually develops suddenly during a period of illness associated with a long-continued and severe alcoholic binge, and may therefore be seen during recovery from delirium tremens. It is thought to be a direct toxic effect of alcohol on the cerebellum.

Cerebellar ataxia is also a well-known sign of *phenytoin toxicity* and this may, in rare instances, be permanent, even when the drug is withdrawn. Although unsteadiness and nystagmus commonly occur with intoxication by other drugs, especially primidone, carbamazepine and diazepam derivatives, true cerebellar ataxia is not a feature of these drug-related syndromes.

Assessment of the role of phenytoin in epileptic patients with cerebellar ataxia is complicated by the occurrence of cerebellar atrophy, associated with loss of Purkinje cells, in patients with epilepsy not treated with phenytoin. This is probably due to recurrent episodes of hypoxia occurring during prolonged major convulsions. However, phenytoin has been shown to cause loss of Purkinje cells experimentally and after massive overdoses in man.

Myxoedema is a rare cause of cerebellar ataxia, and the pathological features of this syndrome are controversial. The ataxia resolves when the euthyroid state is achieved by treatment.

Cerebellar ataxia of subacute onset, with both limb and trunk ataxia, and sometimes with nystagmus, is a well-known but very uncommon *non-metastatic complication of certain neoplasms*, es-

pecially oat cell carcinoma of the bronchus. It is extremely rare with other tumours. The cerebellar syndrome is sometimes associated with other features of brain stem disturbance, such as signs of corticospinal tract dysfunction, and diplopia, and there may be a lymphocytic cellular response in the CSF. Investigation in these cases fails to disclose the presence of metastatic tumour in the posterior fossa.

Pathology. In *alcoholic cerebellar degeneration* the abnormality is largely restricted to the cerebellar vermis. Atrophy is most prominent in the superior vermis (Fig. 14.4) but the anterior lobe of the cerebellum is also affected. The folia are atrophic and the Purkinje cells in this region are almost totally absent. There is a slight increase in the Bergmann glia, with gliosis in the molecular layer and atrophy of the granule cell layer. The dentate nucleus, and the other deep cerebellar nuclei are preserved but there is secondary atrophy of the

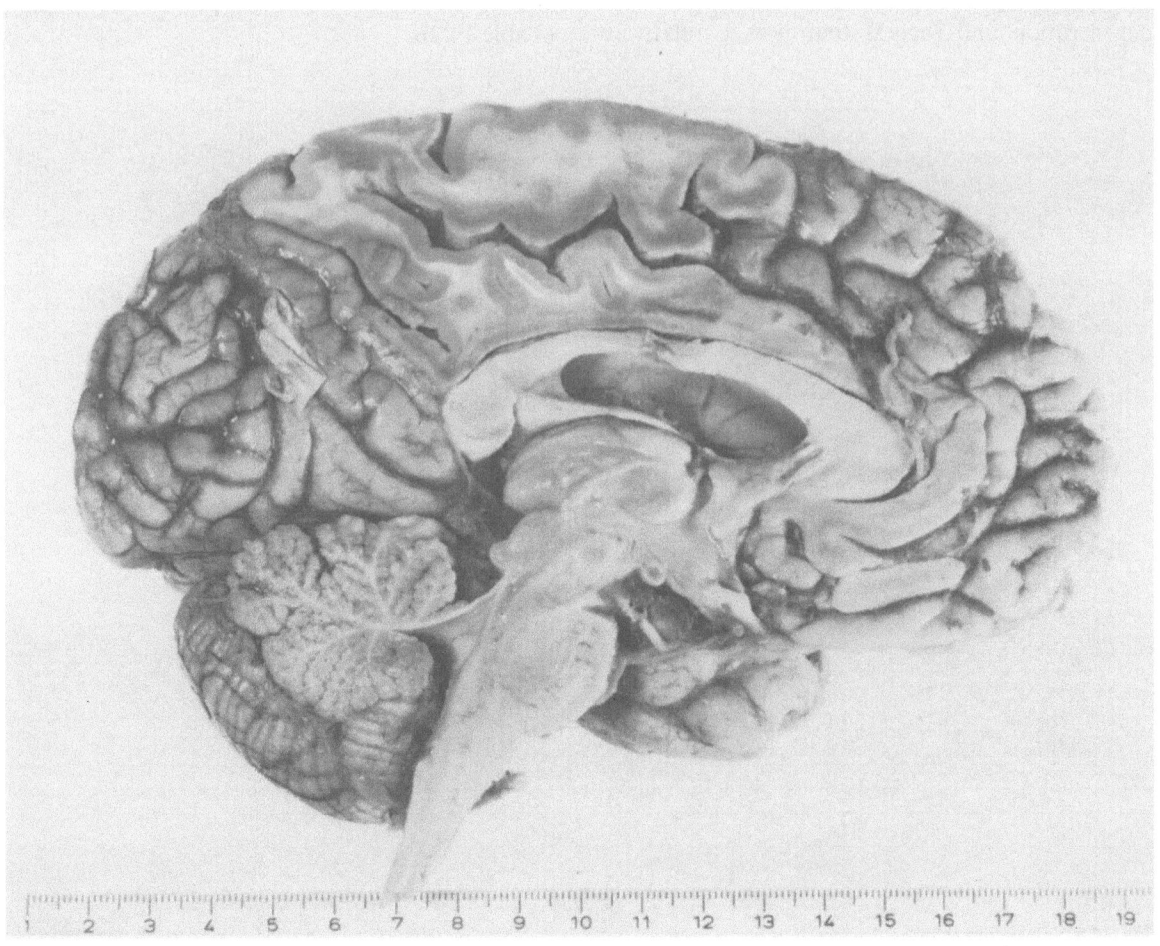

Fig. 14.4. Cerebellar atrophy due to alcoholism. There is marked atrophy of the vermis.

inferior olives, with loss of fibres in the inferior cerebellar peduncles. The middle and superior cerebellar peduncles are spared.

In *paraneoplastic cerebellar degeneration* the abnormality is widespread, involving all parts of the cerebellar cortex. The most striking feature is loss of Purkinje cells which is usually virtually complete. There is patchy loss of cells in the dentate nuclei and degeneration has also been reported in the olivary nuclei. The molecular and granular layers are both thinner than normal and gliosis occurs in the molecular layer. In the *spinal cord* there is usually degeneration in the spinocerebellar tracts, the posterior columns (Fig. 14.5), and in the lumbar part of the corticospinal tracts, suggesting that this is due to a distal axonopathy of 'dying back' type. Degeneration of cells in the posterior root ganglia is usually a feature of the syndrome. Meningeal and perivascular lymphocytic infiltration is almost invariably found and patchy demyelination and axonal loss in the white matter of the spinal cord and brain stem, with degeneration of motor neurons in the cranial nerve nuclei and in the spinal cord may also occur. These features indicate that this disorder is more than a restricted cerebellar degeneration and suggest that it is a relatively

diffuse encephalomyelitis. It has been presumed that this occurs as part of an immune response to the tumour, rather than an infective process.

The pathological features of cerebellar atrophy associated with *epilepsy* have been extensively discussed in the neurological literature but it is now generally accepted that the cerebellar damage is mainly due to episodic hypoxia. Purkinje cell loss in the depths of the cerebellar sulci is accompanied by gliosis in the molecular layer and by proliferation of the Bergmann glia. The abnormality is widely distributed. The cerebellum appears small, and may feel firmer than normal. There are associated changes in the cerebrum, especially in the hippocampus, amygdala and thalamus.

The morphological changes associated with the cerebellar ataxia found in *myxoedema* are poorly defined.

Acquired basal ganglia degenerations

The acquired degenerative disorders of the basal ganglia consist of the various forms of parkinsonism and rare syndromes such as striato-nigral degeneration and progressive pseudo-bulbar palsy (Table 14.2).

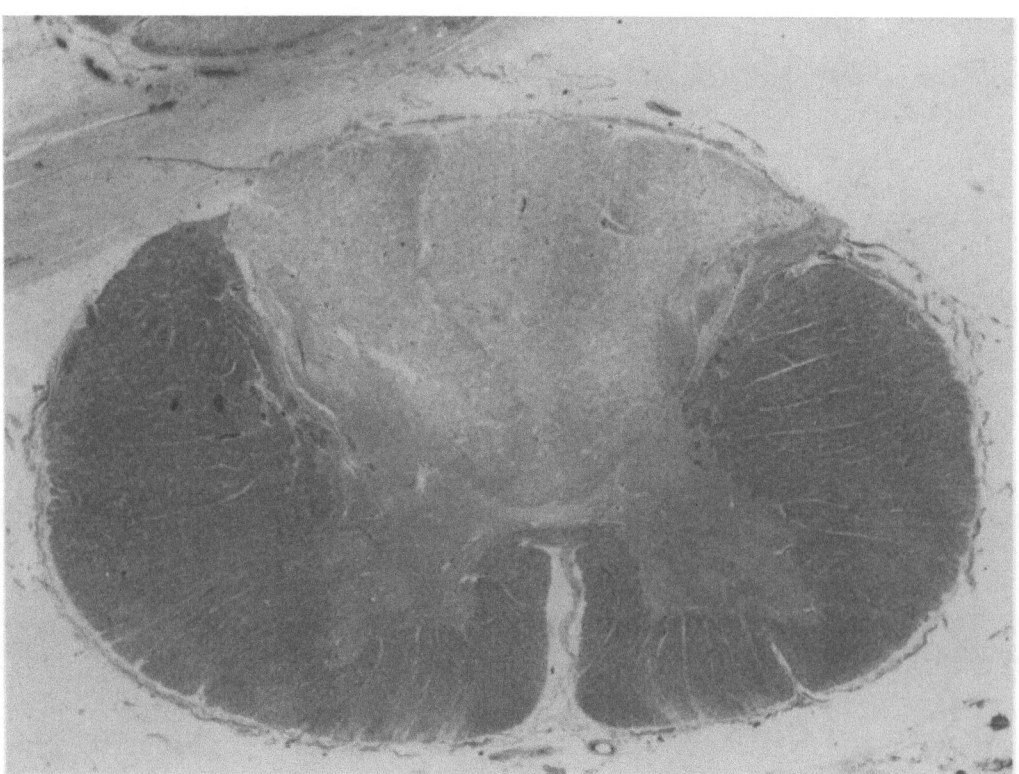

Fig. 14.5. Spinal cord showing degeneration of the posterior columns in a patient with an oat cell carcinoma of the lung.

Parkinson's disease

The term 'Parkinson's disease' (idiopathic parkinsonism or paralysis agitans) is used to describe the common idiopathic disorder, usually beginning in late middle life and showing a slowly progressive course. The disease is characterised by akinesia (the peculiar disinclination to move described by Parkinson himself in 1813), loss of normal balancing and righting reflexes, distal tremor at rest or during voluntary activation, a progressively flexed posture and a characteristic cogwheel increase in muscular tone during passive displacement of a limb. Various other features, such as salivation, greasy sweaty skin, postural hypotension and impotence, occur in some patients during the later stages of the disease. Dementia is a feature of about a third of patients surviving longer than 9 years after diagnosis. The rate of progression of the disorder is very variable; some patients show a relatively stable disability with little sign of progression over many years. The disorder is almost always asymmetrical.

About 10% of cases have a family history of parkinsonism and recent epidemiological surveys have suggested that these cases fall into two broad groups. In those presenting with rigidity and akinesia, the onset of the disease is later, but the course is more rapid and there is an increased incidence of hypotension and diabetes. In familial cases presenting with tremor, over 60% are males, the onset is earlier and the course more benign. In these patients there is an increased incidence of familiar idiopathic tremor and there may also be an increased incidence of thyrotoxicosis in the patients and their mothers. The juvenile form of familial parkinsonism is rare, being characterised by dystonic features and relatively mild tremor.

Pathology. In idiopathic Parkinson's disease (paralysis agitans) the characteristic lesion is loss of pigmented neurons in the substantia nigra (Fig. 14.6) and locus coeruleus. The pars compacta of the substantia nigra is most severely affected, and gliosis can be demonstrated in this region. Some remaining neurons contain hyaline cytoplasmic inclusions, *Lewy bodies* (Fig. 14.7). Similar Lewy bodies have also been found in the dorsal nucleus of the vagus, in the substantia innominata, in other brain stem nuclei and in the lateral cell columns of the thoracic spinal segments. They may also occur in the sympathetic ganglia.

The pathology of idiopathic Parkinson's disease is not restricted to the substantia nigra. De-generation and loss of neurons has often been observed in the striatum and globus pallidus, and to a lesser extent in the hypothalamus, but these changes are inconstant. In the cerebral cortex, features resembling Alzheimer's disease, including neurofibrillary tangles, granulovacuolar neuronal degeneration and senile plaques are frequently found, and these changes, when severe, can be correlated with the dementia (see Chap. 15). These Alzheimer-like abnormalities seem to occur more frequently in the brains of patients with Parkinson's disease than in an age-matched control population.

Dopamine and Parkinson's disease. Dopamine is synthesized in cells in the pars compacta (the middle zones) of the substantia nigra in neurons that project to the corpus striatum. Dopamine is an inhibitory neurotransmitter at the termination of this nigro-striatal pathway on cholinergic neurons. Striato-fugal pathways project to the ventrolateral nucleus of the thalamus and also descend into the substantia nigra, and to other sites in the brain stem; the striato-fugal neurons are probably GABAergic (gamma amino butyric acid). A large body of anatomical, physiological and biochemical evidence has led to the concept of an inhibitory nigro-striatal dopaminergic pathway that is functionally 'in balance' with the cholinergic neurons in the striatum upon which the output from the basal ganglia to the thalamus depends. The nigro-striatal pathway is modulated by the GABAergic feedback loop from the striatum.

The relative activity of these complex neuronal systems is important in determining mucle tone and motor activity. Relative deficiency in the dopaminergic system results in parkinsonism, and relative overactivity in this system may induce involuntary movement, e.g. iatrogenic L-dopa–induced dyskinesias. Chorea has thus been explained as an involuntary movement due to excessive dopaminergic neuronal activity, or to decreased cholinergic activity in the striatum. Recent clinical and experimental work, nevertheless, suggests that these concepts are too simple. Manipulation of the activity of dopaminergic and cholinergic neurons has a much more significant influence upon the clinical features of parkinsonism, chorea and athetosis than changes in GABAergic activity. However, this could be partly due to the lack of sufficient specificity in the drugs available to act on GABAergic neurons.

Treatment. Administration of L-dopa, a precursor

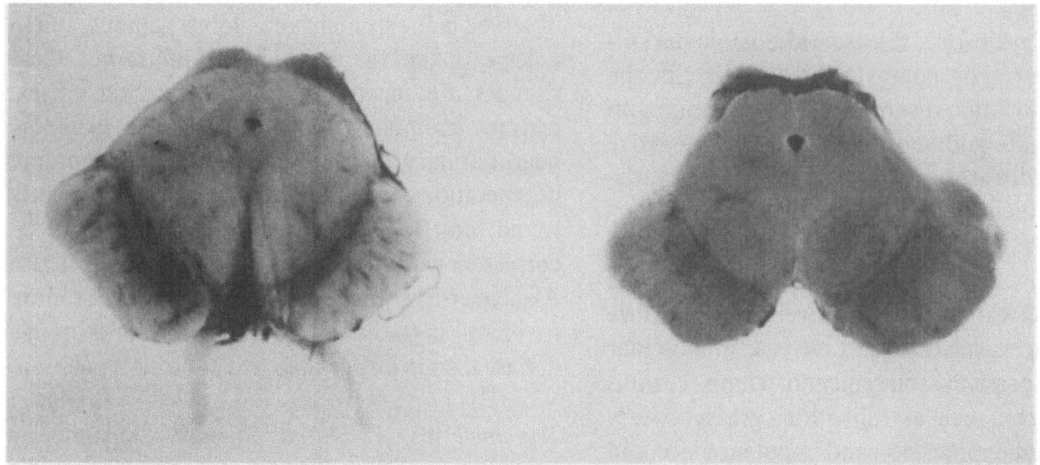

Fig. 14.6. Parkinson's disease. Section of midbrain showing depigmentation of the substantia nigra. (Normal control on the *left*).

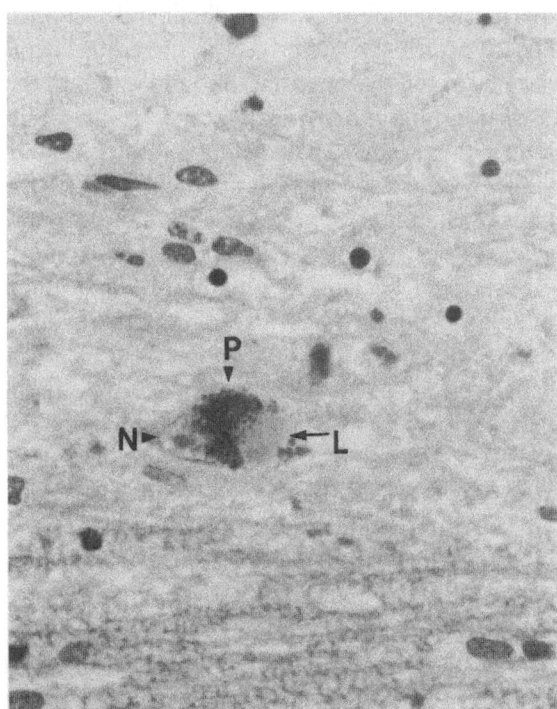

Fig. 14.7. Parkinson's disease. Lewy body (*L*) present in a neuron containing melanin pigment (*P*) in the substantia nigra. Neuronal nucleus (*N*). (H & E ×600)

of dopamine, produces the most striking results in the early stages of Parkinson's disease, especially in patients with bradykinesia and rigidity. Tremor responds less well to L-dopa therapy. The response to treatment is not directly related, however, to the extent of the changes in the substantia nigra, except in so far as patients in whom there has been very severe neuronal loss in this region usually fail to respond, as in the final stages of the disease. Drugs

that inhibit acetylcholinergic transmission in the striatum are also useful and indeed have been known for almost 100 years for their ability to suppress rigidity and tremor.

Post-encephalitic parkinsonism

Parkinsonism, in which features similar to those characteristic of idiopathic Parkinson's disease occur from other causes, must be distinguished from Parkinson's disease since the prognosis, and the underlying pathology may be different. The best known form is *postencephalitic parkinsonism*, a form of parkinsonism which followed the world-wide epidemics of encephalitis lethargica in 1918 and the early 1920s; only a few cases, almost invariably sporadic, have been reported in recent years. Cases with similar clinical features, although often with transient disability, have been described after illnesses that were probably viral encephalitides. In patients with encephalitis lethargica, characteristic upper brain stem features, notably athetosis and oculo-gyric crises, occur in the acute and convalescent phases of the illness.

Pathology. In the acute stages of encephalitis lethargica the brain showed the features of an acute encephalitis with perivascular infiltration by lymphocytes and plasma cells. Meningeal inflammation was not prominent. The substantia nigra was selectively affected, and there was marked destruction of neurons in this region (Fig. 14.8). In patients surviving the acute stage of the illness, but who developed parkinsonism in the convalescent phase or later, neurofibrillary changes were prominent in the remaining neurons in pigmented

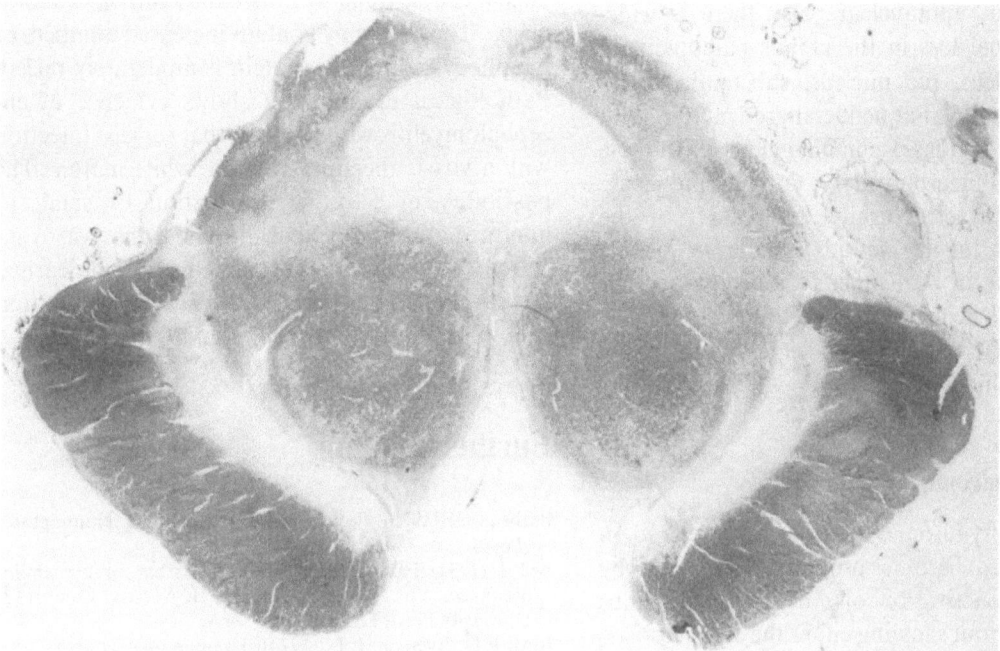

Fig. 14.8. Postencephalitic parkinsonism. Section of midbrain showing depigmentation of the substantia nigra due to almost total loss of melanin-containing neurons.

nuclei in the brain stem, especially in the substantia nigra. Glial scarring was found in this region and few neurons remained. Lewy bodies were not seen.

Other forms of parkinsonism

Drug-induced parkinsonism has increased in incidence because of the widespread use of phenothiazine derivatives in the treatment of the schizophrenias and of some affective disorders. *Calcification of the basal ganglia* most often occurs as a symptomless idiopathic phenomenon, but it is also associated with hypoparathyriodism when it may be accompanied by mild parkinsonism.

A combination of cogwheel rigidity and bradykinesia sometimes occurs in hypertensive patients when there have been multiple small *infarcts* in the basal ganglia and the adjacent white matter. The focal neurological signs resulting from these infarcts, especially pseudo-bulbar palsy, extensor plantar responses and dementia, usually suggest the diagnosis of 'arteriosclerotic parkinsonism'. *Carbon monoxide* poisoning may lead to necrosis of the globus pallidus in both hemispheres, cortical damage and widespread focal white matter necrosis, and so to a dystonic syndrome resembling parkinsonism. *Manganese* poisoning is also a rare cause of parkinsonism. On the island of Guam, a syndrome of parkinsonism and dementia, the *parkinsonism–dementia complex*, used to be endemic; this was probably due to a toxic substance occurring in flour prepared from cycad nuts.

Mild parkinsonism is a feature of *olivopontocerebellar atrophy*, and occurs in *striato-nigral degeneration* and in *progressive pseudo-bulbar palsy*. The latter consists of a progressive disorder characterised by inability to direct the gaze upwards, a hyperextended neck posture, impassive face and pseudo-bulbar palsy with parkinsonian features and dementia.

Striato-nigral degeneration

In this condition there is severe cell loss and gliosis in the corpus striatum, especially in the putamen, and in the substantia nigra, but Lewy bodies are not seen. Abnormal concentrations of neuromelanin and related pigments have been reported in the putamen. There are no diagnostic clinical features by which this disorder can be differentiated from idiopathic Parkinson's disease, but rigidity tends to be unusually prominent and tremor is mild or absent. There is little or no clinical response to dopaminergic drugs. Striato-nigral degeneration has been regarded by some authorities as a variant of multiple system atrophy, i.e. a form of olivopontocerebellar atrophy.

Progressive supranuclear palsy

In progressive supranuclear palsy there is widespread neuronal loss in the globus pallidus, subthalamic nucleus, red nucleus, substantia nigra, tectal nuclei and peri-aqueductal grey matter, with gliosis in these regions. Remaining neurons in these nuclei contain neurofibrillary tangles, but these tangles are ultrastructurally different from the neurofibrillary tangles found in neurons of the cerebral cortex in Alzheimer's disease. No other features of Alzheimer's disease are present. The disease is very rare, but presents as an easily recognisable clinical syndrome.

Stiff man syndrome

At least two syndromes have been described in which the patient becomes progressively disabled by involuntary coactivation of muscles in the limbs and trunk without showing either the characteristic changes in posture or the involuntary movements of torsion dystonia. The graphic term 'stiff man syndrome' is best reserved for a rare condition affecting adults of both sexes, in which there is gradually progressive and fluctuating rigidity of the trunk, limbs and face which may draw the head down between the shoulders and deform the spine. Painful and violent muscle spasms occur spontaneously and in response to fright or sudden movement. Sometimes there is a dramatic improvement in the stiffness with diazepam. A few of these patients also have nocturnal myoclonus and epilepsy. Several cases have come to autopsy but, as in torsion dystonia, no definite histological abnormality of the nervous system or muscles has been found. However, in many cases the pathological examination has been incomplete.

A second disorder, some cases of which have been described under the rubric of still man syndrome, is better termed 'progressive encephalomyelitis with rigidity'. This is an even rarer condition which progresses more rapidly, death usually occurring within 2 years. There is involuntary muscle contraction similar to that seen in the stiff man syndrome, together with other disorders that include sensory loss, incontinence, dysarthria, ataxia, coarse tremor of the hands and ophthalmoplegia. The CSF may contain increased numbers of lymphocytes and the protein is moderately raised. Pathological examination shows evidence of encephalomyelitis with features that suggest infection with a virus, affecting grey and white matter. The possibility of selective destruction of small to intermediate-sized spinal interneurons was suggested by one such case. Much remains to be learned about these disorders and very careful examination should be made of any case coming to autopsy.

Further reading

Barbeau A (1975) Progress in understanding Huntington's chorea. Can J Med 2: 81

Bell J (1934) Huntington's chorea. Treasury of human inheritance, Vol. IV part 1. Fisher R A (ed). Cambridge University Press, London

Bird E D, Iverson L L (1974) Huntington's chorea—post mortem measurement of glutamic acid decarboxylase, choline acetyl transferase and dopamine in basal ganglia. Brain 97: 457

Brain W R, Wilkinson M (1965) Subacute cerebellar degeneration associated with carcinoma. Brain 88: 465

Brodal A (1981) Neurological anatomy in relation to clinical medicine, 3rd edn. Oxford University Press, Oxford

Greenfield J G (1954) The spinocerebellar degenerations. Blackwell Scientific, Oxford

Hewer R L (1968) Study of fatal cases of Friedreich's ataxia. Br Med J iii: 649

Hughes J T, Brownell B, Hewer R L (1968) The peripheral sensory pathway in Friedreich's ataxia: an examination by light and electron microscopy of the posterior nerve roots, posterior root ganglia and peripheral sensory nerves in cases of Friedreich's ataxia. Brain 91: 803

Konigsmark G, Weiner L (1970) The olivopontocerebellar atrophies: a review. Medicine (Baltimore) 49: 227

Pallis C A, Lewis P D (1974) The neurology of gastro-intestinal disease. Thomas, London

Pearce G W (1979) The neuropathology of parkinsonism. In: Cavanagh J V, Thomas-Smith W (eds) Recent advances in neuropathology, Vol. 1. Churchill Livingstone, London, p 299

Rail D, Scholtz C, Swash M (1981) Post-encephalitic parkinsonism: current experience. J Neurol Neurosurg Psychiatry 44: 670

Walton J N (1977) The parkinsonism syndrome. In: Brain's diseases of the nervous system. Oxford University Press, Oxford, p 579

Whiteley A M, Swash M, Urich H (1976) Progressive encephalomyelitis with rigidity—its relation to 'subacute myoclonic spinal neuronitis' and to the 'stiff man syndrome'. Brain 99: 27

Chapter 15

Dementia

Dementia is a clinical concept which must be defined concisely in order to separate it from other disorders of cognition. Dementia is a global disturbance of higher mental functions occurring in an alert patient (Table 15.1). Other, less global

Table 15.1. Higher mental functions likely to be abnormal in a patient with dementia

Memory
    Personal events
    National events
    Formal tests of verbal and visual material
Orientation
Abstractional abilities
Calculation
Naming
Spatial percepts
Constructional tasks

disturbances of mental function must be categorised according to their underlying causation and localisation in the brain, as, for example, the characteristic syndromes attributed to frontal, temporal and parietal lobe lesions (Chap. 3). Dementia itself may be reversible or irreversible, static or progressive, depending on its causation.

The term *dementia* is usually reserved for *acquired* disorders of brain function. Impaired intellect arising from developmental malformation, or from brain lesions acquired in utero, in the perinatal period, or in early infancy, is usually termed mental retardation rather than dementia, although the latter term could equally well be used. Further, a distinction must be drawn between dementia and delirium. In the latter a similar global disturbance of higher mental functions is found, but it occurs in the context of a state of clouded consciousness, and visual hallucinations and restlessness are often features. *Delirium* is usually subacute or acute in onset and it may occur superimposed on an underlying dementia. A wide range of clinical data should therefore be available to substantiate a clinical diagnosis of dementia.

Epidemiology

Dementia has come to assume increasing importance not only in human terms as a serious disability leading to disruption of personal and family life, but also in economic terms. It has been estimated that as many as a quarter of beds in the National Health Service in the United Kingdom are occupied by demented patients. This figure includes beds set aside for long-term custodial care.

The frequency of dementia in the developed countries can be related to the longevity of the populations of these countries. About 5% to 8% of the population aged 60–70 years suffers from dementia, but in people aged 80 years and more the prevalence is much higher, approaching 25%. *Dementia is a syndrome*, not a disease and it must therefore be recognised that these figures include patients with a number of different disorders. Taken as a whole, dementia is slightly commoner among women than among men.

Causes

Dementia is a syndrome having many different causes (Table 15.2). However, many of these disorders, for example Wilson's disease, neurosyphilis, limbic encephalitis and porphyria, are rare and investigation of patients with dementia is often disappointing in that no potentially remediable cause is revealed. In any large group of patients with dementia, *Alzheimer's disease*, sometimes termed senile dementia of Alzheimer type, is the commonest cause, particularly in patients older than about 50 years. The distinction between senile and presenile dementia, on which great stress was laid in older text books, has little importance except that it serves to remind the clinician that younger patients with dementia, that is particularly people younger than 65 years, are likely to have a cause for their dementia other than Alzheimer's disease. The term Alzheimer's disease is now usually used to refer to any person with dementia with a particular clinical pattern and brain pathology regardless of age.

In *younger* people an identifiable cause for dementia other than Alzheimer's disease may be found, after investigation, in about 40% of patients. Huntington's chorea, post-traumatic dementia, dementia related to epilepsy, dementia following hypoxic encephalopathy and dementia following encephalitis, or occurring during the course of degenerative brain diseases such as the lipidoses,

Table 15.2. Causes of dementia

Primary cerebral degenerations
  Alzheimer's disease
  Multi-infarct dementia
  Pick's disease
  Huntington's chorea
  Creutzfeldt–Jakob disease
  Multiple sclerosis
  Spinocerebellar degenerations
  Wilson's disease
  Parkinsonism and its variants
  Post-traumatic encephalopathy
Cerebral infections and inflammations
  Neurosyphilis
  Cranial arteritis
  Disseminated lupus erythematosus
  Limbic encephalitis
  Progressive multi-focal leukoencephalopathy
  Post-encephalitic syndromes
Intracranial mass lesions
  Tumours
  Subdural haematomas
Hydrocephalus
Toxic and metabolic
  Hypothyroidism
  Hypocalcaemia
  Hypoglycaemia
  Porphyria
  Vitamin B_{12} deficiency
  Hepatic encephalopathy
  Renal dialysis
  Malabsorption syndrome
  Alcohol and other drugs

may be found in such patients. Multiple sclerosis is a relatively uncommon cause of dementia, although of course this disorder may cause severe physical disability. In younger people it is particularly important to search for metabolic and toxic causes, including chronic intoxications with drugs. Hydrocephalus is also an important cause of dementia in people in this age group; it is often related to previous subarachnoid haemorrhage, or to an unsuspected tumour.

The majority of *older* patients with dementia prove to have *Alzheimer's disease*, or a combination of Alzheimer's disease and *cerebral vascular disease*. As many as 80% of patients in older age groups fall into this category, and it is in these patients that investigation is so frequently unrewarding. Even if a metabolic cause for dementia is discovered in such patients, for example, myxoedema, or B_{12} deficiency, it is common to find that treatment of the metabolic abnormality does not result in improvement, an observation which suggests that the dementia and the metabolic disorder are unrelated. Dementia in *Parkinson's disease* has become a more important problem since the advent of L-dopa therapy for Parkinson's disease. Use of this drug has resulted in longer survival of patients with

Parkinson's disease and it has become apparent that dementia is seen in about 30% of patients who survive longer than about 7 years with the disease.

The *causes* of dementia shown in Table 15.2 can be reclassified according to the predominant site of the lesion in the brain responsible for the dementia, as in Table 15.3. In this classification the dementias

Table 15.3. Pathological classification of dementia (after Tomlinson 1980)

Diffuse cortical lesions
    Alzheimer's disease
    Pick's disease
    Creutzfeldt–Jakob disease
    Subacute sclerosing panencephalitis
    GPI (syphilis)
    Post-anoxic encephalopathy
    Hypertensive (small vessel) ischaemic disease
White matter lesions
    Multiple infarcts
    Multiple sclerosis
    Leukodystrophies
    Progressive multifocal leukoencephalopathy
    Post-traumatic dementia
Subcortical (nuclear) lesions
    Huntington's chorea (? cortical involvement also occurs)
    Wilson's disease (? white matter involved also)
    Wernicke–Korsakoff encephalopathy
    Progressive supranuclear palsy
    Parkinson's disease
    Striato-nigral degeneration
Widespread lesions
    Arteriosclerotic
    Post-traumatic
    Subarachnoid haemorrhage
    Meningitis
    Hydrocephalus
    Diffuse tumours
    Dementia pugilistica (boxer's encephalopathy)

associated with metabolic abnormalities are omitted because of the absence of morphological change in the brain (see Chaps. 11 and 12).

In *clinical* practice there is a particular difficulty in the recognition of the role of vascular factors in a patient with dementia. Since both Alzheimer's disease and cerebral infarction are common in patients in the senile and presenile periods of life it would not be surprising to find that these two disorders coexisted. However, dementia may occur in patients with vascular disease of the brain, without clinical or pathological evidence of Alzheimer's disease (Table 15.4).

One of the major components of dementia is *impairment of memory*, particularly memory for recent events. The amnesic syndrome (see later in this chapter) consists of loss of memory for recent events, and of impairment of short-term memory,

Table 15.4. Dementia associated with cerebral infarction (after Tomlinson 1980)

Arteriosclerotic or 'multi-infarct' dementia
Anoxic encephalopathy
Post-traumatic dementia
Subarachnoid haemorrhage
Meningitis and encephalitis
Congophilic angiopathy
? Myxoedema

so that the memory span may be of only a few seconds duration. It is seen particularly in patients with temporal lobe disease, such as herpes simplex encephalitis, and in other forms of encephalitis affecting the limbic system, bilateral hippocampal infarction, bilateral hippocampal trauma, or in bilateral temporal lobectomy. This amnesic syndrome also occurs as part of the Wernicke–Korsakoff syndrome seen in alcoholic patients, or in others subjected to profound thiamine deficiency. The pathological features of Alzheimer's disease may also be concentrated in the hippocampal region so that a disorder resembling the amnesic syndrome may occur as an early manifestation of Alzheimer's disease, and may lead to diagnostic difficulty.

Alzheimer's disease

The major clinical feature of Alzheimer's disease is dementia. It is a progressive disorder, and it occurs with increasing frequency with advancing age so that as many as 10% of people older than 65 years may have the disease. It was the first of the dementing illnesses to be recognised. Alzheimer's contribution was to associate two characteristic pathological changes, *senile plaques*, and intraneuronal *neurofibrillary tangles*, with a progressive dementia. Alzheimer's patient was a woman aged only 51 years, but the clinical and neuropathological similarities between this presenile disorder, and the more common senile psychosis, were evident to Alzheimer. He believed that presenile and senile cases, classified solely on the basis of an apparently arbitrary distinction based on age, were one and the same disorder. The dementia of Alzheimer's disease is not in itself specific in that there are no particular features in a patient with moderately advanced dementia which allow the disorder to be recognised on clinical criteria. However, the pattern of development of the disorder and the associated clinical features allow the diagnosis to be made, on clinical criteria, with a fair degree of confidence.

In *typical cases* of Alzheimer's disease there is a conspicuous early impairment of recent memory usually noted both by the patient and by the family. Loss of the ability to learn a new environment is also an early symptom and, in advanced cases, impairment of memory for previously familiar environments may be noted. Impaired judgement and reasoning, shown by failure to grasp the meaning of situations, results in abnormal behaviour. Disorders of speech and language, with gradual impairment of the ability to formulate new concepts and to understand or use abstractions are a characteristic feature which may occur as the first symptom in some patients, although loss of memory is a more usual early symptom. *Later* in the illness the patient's emotional life becomes disturbed, leading to changes in personality, delusions, carelessness in dress and carelessness in personal hygiene. In some cases these aspects are obvious early in the disorder so that the disease may present as a depressive illness, often with agitation. In this instance the diagnosis is particularly difficult and treatment of the depressive aspect of the illness may result in striking, if temporary, improvement.

Clinical features of involvement of *other systems* in the brain are also present. For example, signs of corticospinal tract disease may develop and there is usually impairment of the ability to follow a rapidly moving object with the eyes. The naturally smooth pursuit movement is interrupted by irregular saccadic jerks at velocities of pursuit (following) lateral gaze movements well within the range attained by normal subjects. Muscular tone may be increased in a plastic fashion, seizures occur in about a third of patients, and myoclonus may occur as a late manifestation. In the late stages of the disease these motor disabilities became prominent so that a form of flexion dystonia develops with profound dementia and double incontinence. Rapid weight loss is a common terminal event.

Most cases of Alzheimer's senile dementia are *sporadic* but the disease may occur in families, in a manner suggesting a dominant mode of inheritance. Such *familial* cases account for as many as 10 % of patients with senile dementia of Alzheimer type in some series of cases, but in most instances it is difficult to discover if there is a familial basis for the disorder.

Dementia due to Alzheimer's disease is a serious disorder with a high *mortality*. Fifty percent of patients die within 3 years and in the senile group 95 % die within 5 years of diagnosis. In younger patients the life expectancy is somewhat longer, a

phenomenon which probably reflects the lower incidence of other serious illnesses such as cancer and cerebral vascular disease in the younger group.

Pathology

The brain of a patient with Alzheimer's disease shows readily identifiable abnormalities on gross examination. The brain appears smaller than normal, with narrowing of the gyri and widening of the sulci (Fig. 15.1). These changes are often particularly evident in the frontal and temporal lobes, and least obvious in the posterior part of the brain, although the whole brain may be affected. There is often associated atrophy of the cerebellar hemispheres. The lateral ventricles are often symmetrically enlarged in Alzheimer's disease, an observation that can be made at autopsy (Fig. 15.1) and can be seen in CT scans of the brain during life. However, changes in ventricular size and configuration are quite variable in the disease and severe dementia may be present without ventricular enlargement. Similarly, the extent and distribution of cortical atrophy, especially when studied by CT scanning (Fig. 15.3a), is variable and not readily related to the severity, or type, of a patient's dementia.

The *weight* of the human brain is 1200–1300 g in the early 20s and decreases with increasing age so that the average brain weight of a group of subjects in their eighth decade is about 7%–10% less than that of a similar group of healthy subjects in their second decade. Such comparisons, however, are difficult to interpret because there is evidence that the human brain may have increased significantly in size, and in weight, during the last century. Comparisons in brain weight at autopsy thus tended to exaggerate any weight loss occurring in the process of normal aging. There is slight thinning of the cortex in advanced cases of Alzheimer's disease, but the difference between the thickness of the cortex in demented subjects, and in normal subjects of similar age, is slight. This radiological and morphological evidence of brain atrophy in Alzheimer's disease is accompanied by loss of weight of the brain, often to 1000 g or less, a degree of weight loss far in excess of that expected in normal age subjects.

It has often been stated that Alzheimer's dementia is associated with loss of neurons. However, recent quantitative studies have indicated that there is only a *small loss of neurons* in this disease. Increased numbers of hypertrophic fibrous as-

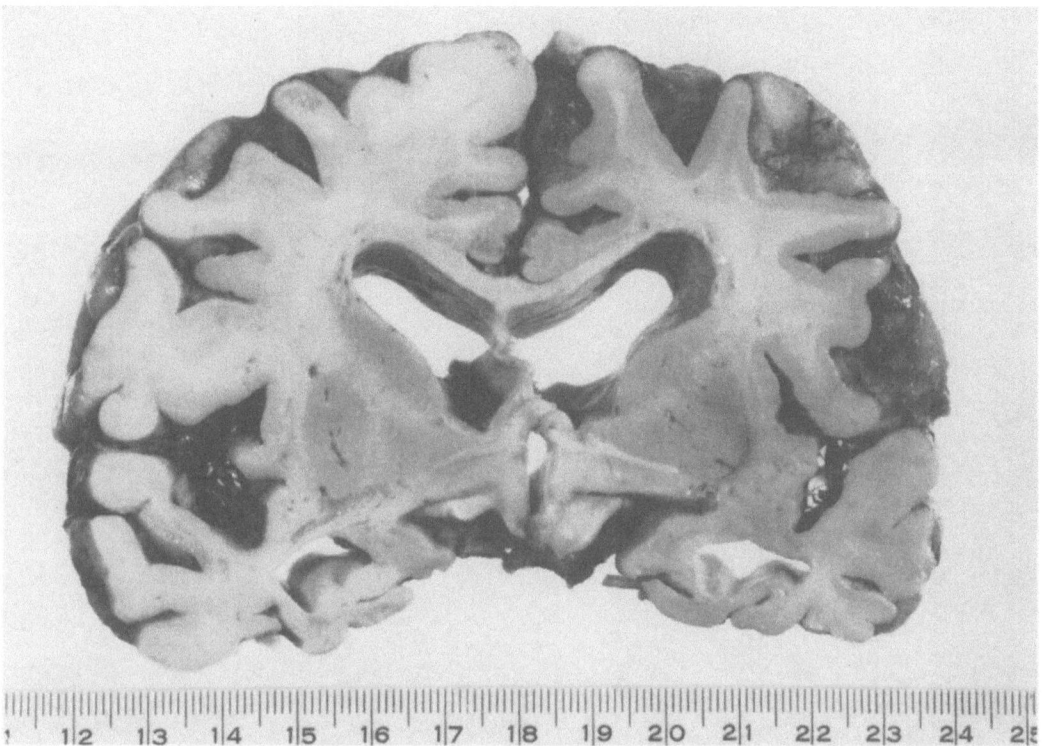

Fig. 15.1. Alzheimer's disease. Coronal slice of the cerebral hemispheres showing gross cortical atrophy with widening of the sulci. There is also ventricular dilatation.

trocytes with prominent processes are found and the number of neurons is slightly reduced, particularly in the temporal lobes. Dementia in Alzheimer's disease is thus not due to a severe diffuse loss of neurons, as was formerly thought. One difficulty in assessing quantitative studies of numbers of neurons in the brain in aged subjects is the lack of data about loss of neurons in normal aged subjects. There is evidence that there is considerable variability in neuronal stability with increasing age. For example, the facial nucleus, the sensory nucleus of the trigeminal nerve, the trochlear nucleus, the ventral cochlear nucleus, and the nuclei of the inferior olive show no loss of neurons with age. On the other hand, neurons in the locus coeruleus, the cerebral cortex, together with spinal anterior horn cells and Purkinje cells, are lost with increasing age, particularly after the age of 60 years. Loss of neurons from the temporal cortex is particularly prominent in normal aging.

Although neuronal loss may not be a major feature of Alzheimer's disease, at least in the tissues that have been studied by quantitative methods, reduction in the number and complexity of *dendritic arborisations* is seen in the normal elderly patient, but this reduction is more marked in Alzheimer's

disease. These studies have been carried out using modifications of the Golgi silver impregnation technique. The basilar and horizontal dendrites are particularly susceptible. These may be of great importance because they represent the receptors for intracortical neuronal circuits and their loss may thus greatly reduce the number of neuronal connexions available for normal brain function. Dendritic changes of this type are not limited to neurons in the neocortex as they are also seen in Purkinje cells. An increase in number and complexity of astrocytes and their processes in the cortex of patients with Alzheimer's disease seems to match the dendritic change.

Lipofuscin is a common feature of many tissues in aged people, but the amounts of lipofuscin found in the neurons in patients with Alzheimer's disease are not greater than those found in age-matched controls. Further, there is no evidence that accumulations of lipofuscin, when they occur, are neurotoxic. In advanced dementia the amount of lipofuscin found in neurons in the hippocampus may even be slightly reduced.

The main histological features of Alzheimer's disease are *senile (neuritic) plaques, neurofibrillary tangles*, and *granulovacuolar degeneration in*

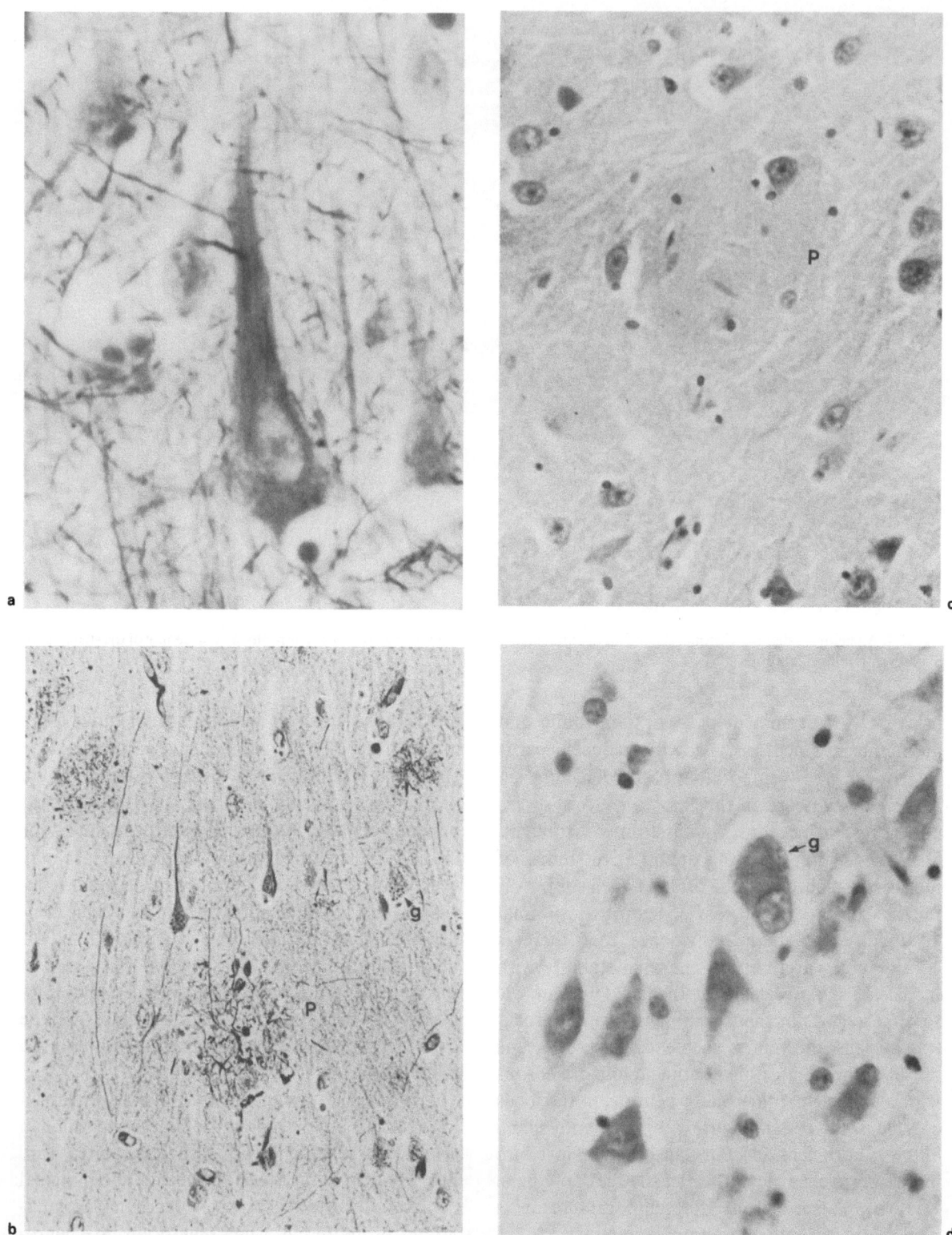

Fig. 15.2. Alzheimer's disease.

a A neuron containing neurofibrillary tangles (silver stain ×1200).

b Low power micrograph showing a senile (Alzheimer) plaque (*P*) and a neuron above it with neurofibrillary tangles. Granulovacuolar degeneration (*g*) is seen in other neurons. (Palmgren silver stain ×260).

c Senile plaque (*P*) in an H & E stained section appears as an amorphous eosinophilic area in the centre of the picture. (×500)

d Granulovacuolar degeneration in an H & E section. Small basophilic dots (*g*) surrounded by clear vacuoles are seen in the cytoplasm of the affected neuron. (×900)

neurons (Fig. 15.2). None of these three features are specific to Alzheimer's disease. Indeed, senile plaques and neurofibrillary tangles within the cytoplasm of neurons in the cerebral cortex are found in almost all elderly subjects over the age of 75 years, although usually in small numbers. Neurofibrillary tangles are found in a number of other disease processes (Table 15.5).

Table 15.5. Diseases associated with neurofibrillary tangles

Alzheimer's disease
Parkinsonism–dementia complex (Guam)
Progressive supranuclear palsy
Dementia pugilistica
Down's syndrome
? Dialysis encephalopathy
Subacute sclerosing panencephalitis

Neurofibrillary tangles. Found in the cytoplasm of medium and large pyramidal cells in the neocortex and palaeocortex (Fig. 15.2a), neurofibrillary tangles are less frequently present in the grey matter of the deep nuclei of the cerebral hemispheres and are almost never seen in cerebellar or spinal cord neurons. They are particularly prominent in neurons in the hippocampus (especially h1 and subiculum; see Fig. 4.1), and in the neocortex, particularly in the frontal regions. They consist of tortuous masses of thickened, coarse fibres running through the perikaryon of affected neurons and are best seen following silver impregnation, as in the Bielschowsky and Bodian techniques (Fig. 15.2a).

Electron microscopy shows that each neurofibrillary tangle is made up of clusters of paired helical filaments. Each member of the pair is a filament about 10 nm in diameter, resembling a normal neurofilament but without side arms. The pair of filaments measures about 22 nm at its maximum width and the helical twist has a period of about 80 nm. In affected neurons, clusters of these paired helical filaments fill the cytoplasm, displacing other cell organelles. They may be found in both myelinated and unmyelinated neuronal processes in the neuropil. The filaments are resistant to autolysis so that they are well preserved in autopsy material, even after formalin fixation. Normal microtubules quickly disappear after death and are not preserved by formalin fixation. The reason for the reactivity of neurofibrillary tangles to amyloid stains is uncertain but it is thought that this cross-reactivity indicates that some of the constituent proteins of the prepared helical filaments show beta-pleating of their helical strands similar to that found in amyloid

fibrils. There is immunocytochemical evidence that the neurofibrillary tangles in Alzheimer's disease originate from neurotubules.

Neurofibrillary tangles have not been found in other species, although prominent masses of normal neurofilaments can be induced in neurons by the administration of various mitotic inhibitors, including colchicine and vinblastine. Neurofibrillary tangles are also a feature of post-encephalitic parkinsonism and of Down's syndrome. In addition, similar, although unpaired, neurofibrillary tangles, with a different periodicity and of a slightly different thickness, are found in association with deposition of aluminium in the brains of patients with dialysis encephalopathy. These neurofibrillary tangles differ also in their distribution in that they are found in the spinal cord and in the cerebellum, sites at which it is rare to find neurofibrillary tangles in Alzheimer's disease.

Senile plaques (neuritic plaques). Senile plaques are found in the cortex in a similar distribution to that of neurofibrillary tangles. In silver-impregnated preparations senile plaques consist of irregular masses 15–200 μm in diameter (Fig. 15.2b) containing threads and granules and often with a more uniform and densely staining centre. The plaques are more difficult to identify in H & E-stained sections (Fig. 15.2c). Considerable variations occur in the numbers of plaques found in various parts of the brain, and even from gyrus to gyrus in the same area, but no part of the neocortex is free of plaques in patients with Alzheimer's disease, and usually all parts of the neocortex are heavily involved. The hippocampus, the amygdala and the neocortex are usually severely affected. Ultrastructural examination of the plaques reveals numerous greatly swollen nerve terminals, the majority of which are axonal in origin. These nerve terminals are filled with numerous laminated or dense, round or oval bodies and sometimes with abnormal fibrillary material. Normal cell processes, including microglia and astrocytes, may be found within the abnormal zone, but in large plaques the prominent feature is a central mass of *amyloid* fibrils situated among the neuritic processes and extending towards the periphery of the plaque. Amyloid is uncommon in very small plaques. Fibrous astrocytes are prominent in and around well-developed plaques and excess acid phosphatase, and oxidative enzymes, have been demonstrated histochemically in the plaques. The abnormal neuritic processes at the periphery of the plaque are themselves associated with intense *acetylcholinesterase* activity. These abnormal neurites contain lysosomes, degenerating mitochondria and numerous masses of neurofibrillary tangles.

Neuritic plaques have also been found in aged dogs and in primates. They are also a feature of the brains of animals dying of scrapie. The problem of the quantitative relation of senile plaques to normal aging, and to dementia, is discussed below.

Granulovacuolar degeneration of hippocampal pyramidal cells, like neuritic plaques and neurofibrillary tangles, is a feature both of normal aged subjects and of Alzheimer's disease beginning in the presenile period. Affected neurons contain vacuoles in their cytoplasm, approximately 5 μm in diameter, with a central haematoxyphilic and argyrophilic granule in the centre of each vacuole (Fig. 15.2b,d). Granulovacuolar degeneration is almost entirely limited to the pyramidal cells in the hippocampus and to the adjacent presubiculum and subiculum. In the hippocampus, it particularly affects the cells in the h1 and h2 segments although it may extend into the end-plate region (see Fig. 4.1). Involved cells may be swollen by the presence of several such vacuoles. Granulovacuolar degeneration is associated, in the same neurons, with numerous round, oval or rod-like eosinophilic bodies varying from 8 μm to 15μm across and up to about 30 μm long. In the larger, elongated forms faint longitudinal striations may be visible. These Hirano bodies usually occur in neurons but may also occur in other cells.

Nucleolar volume is reduced by about 40% in cells in the temporal cortex in Alzheimer's disease, particularly in those cells containing neurofibrillary tangles. This has been correlated with a reduction in RNA content in such cells and is thought to indicate a reduction in protein synthetic capability in these nerve cells. Recent studies of nuclei in biopsy samples of parietal cortex in patients with Alzheimer's disease have revealed linear nuclear inclusions of several types but the significance of these inclusions is uncertain.

Correlation of pathology with dementia in Alzheimer's disease

There is a highly significant relationship between clinical measures of intellectual decline in old people and in dementia, and quantified estimates of the severity of degenerative brain disease found at autopsy in the same subjects. In about 85% of patients with senile dementia 12 or more senile plaques per high-power field are found in the

hippocampus whereas in more than 90% of mentally normal subjects, or patients with functional psychoses, fewer than 12 such plaques are found per high-power field. Despite this statistical relationship in patients with Alzheimer's disease, considerable variations can be found in the number of senile plaques present in various lobes of the brain, and even in adjacent gyri, but no part of the neocortex is spared in such patients. Small numbers of plaques are found in the neocortex in about 15% of subjects in the fourth decade, in 50% by the seventh decade and in almost 80% by the tenth decade. Under the age of 60 years however, plaques are almost invariably few in number and widely scattered. In intellectually normal old subjects, plaques have been found in only about 65% of brains examined. However, in a few instances large numbers of plaques have been found in the brains of very old people known to have been intellectually normal. A major feature of Alzheimer's disease is the tendency for senile plaques to be concentrated more in the anterior temporal lobes than in any other part of the brain.

Neurons affected by Alzheimer's neurofibrillary degeneration can also be found in the majority of normal elderly subjects, particularly in the amygdaloid nucleus and the hippocampus, but such tangles are virtually absent in the neocortex in normal subjects younger than 65 years. Similarly, granulovacuolar degeneration occurs in only a very small number of subjects below the age of 60 years but with increasing frequency with increasing age. However, this abnormality is always much more frequent in patients with Alzheimer's disease than in subjects known to have been intellectually well preserved during their senility.

Other histological features. Amyloid is found in the centre of senile plaques, but it also occurs in the walls of blood vessels in some patients with Alzheimer's disease. This amyloid is probably formed inside the plaque itself. Sometimes it occurs in large amounts in blood vessels when it is termed *congophilic angiopathy*.

Biochemical features of Alzheimer's disease

Biochemical studies have shown a marked *deficiency* of *choline acetyltransferase* activity in whole temporal lobes, and in biopsies of temporal and parietal lobes, especially in the hippocampus in patients with Alzheimer's disease. This biochemical feature of the disorder suggests that Alzheimer's disease is a primary degenerative disease affecting cholinergic neurons more than other nerve cells. Indeed, a positive correlation has been shown between the degree of the reduction of choline acetyltransferase activity and the severity of the dementia in Alzheimer's disease. A particular feature of the *cholinergic* abnormality is that although the enzyme concerned with acetylcholine synthesis is reduced in amount, there is no abnormality of the binding of muscarinic receptor ligands. *Serotonin* receptor activity is also reduced and there is a reduction in *GABA* receptors. In some studies a reduction in *catecholamine* activity has been reported. These biochemical features have led to clinical trials of the effects of cholinergic therapy such as choline and physostigmine on memory in patients with Alzheimer's disease. The results of these experiments are encouraging but they have not yet led to practicable therapy.

Multi-infarct dementia

Patients with multiple strokes sometimes show dementia as a feature of their illness and, when the diagnosis of cerebral vascular disease is well established, this does not usually excite comment. However, sometimes dementia may be a presenting feature of patients with cerebral vascular disease, particularly those in whom multiple minor stroke episodes have occurred. Many of these small strokes may not be apparent without careful enquiry from the patient's family, or from the patient himself. Multi-infarct dementia thus typically presents with a relatively abrupt onset and with a fluctuating course. There is usually a history of stroke and of residual focal neurological symptoms. Examination reveals focal neurological signs with evidence of widespread atherosclerosis, often associated with *hypertension*. Deterioration in the illness is usually stepwise rather than steadily progressive. Nocturnal confusion with relative preservation of personality, together with fairly prominent depressive symptoms and somatic complaints are typical features. Emotional incontinence is also found more commonly in patients with multi-infarct dementia than in patients with progressive dementia due to degenerative disorders. Since aphasia and spatial disorientation are fairly common features of Alzheimer's senile dementia, symptoms and signs of cortical disease may be taken as clinical evidence of a neuronal degenerative disorder. Clinical features of white matter disease such as

spasticity and weakness, on the other hand, are features of multi-infarct dementia.

Dementia due to cerebral vascular disease is a feature of patients with both large and small infarcts (Fig. 15.3b). Large left frontal infarcts are associated with aphasia, and large parietal infarcts produce a complex disturbance of judgement and of orientation particularly involving multimodality sensory processing. These disabilities are often misinterpreted as dementia although a formal neuropsychiatric examination in such patients usually discloses that not all the mental processes listed in Table 15.1 are impaired. Although such patients are severely disabled, they are not demented in that they do not show global disturbance of function in the alert state. Delirium on the other hand is common in patients with large infarcts of this type.

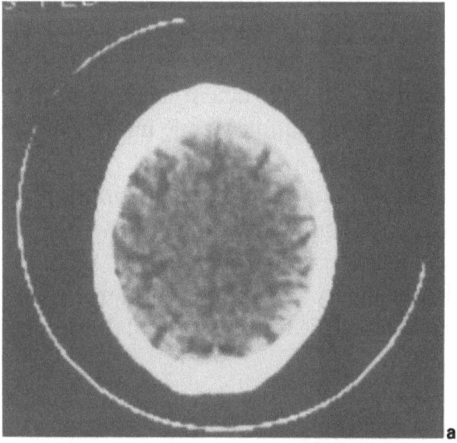

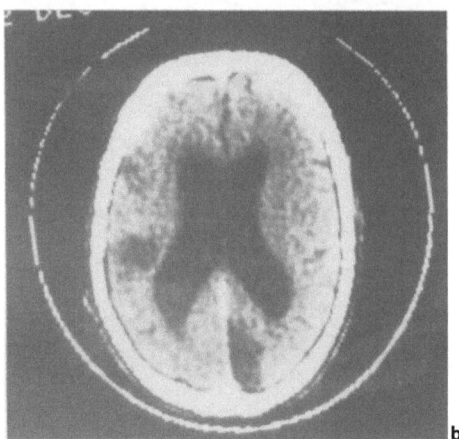

Fig. 15.3. CT scans in dementia.

a This cut shows cortical atrophy in a patient with Alzheimer's disease.

b Cerebral infarction and multi-infarct dementia. Two zones of cerebral infarction are seen, one in the left temporal lobe and the other in the right occipital lobe. The symmetrical ventricular dilatation suggests that infarction is more extensive than that detectable by CT scan.

Pathology

In patients with multi-infarct dementia there has usually been extensive infarction so that at least 100 ml brain tissue has been lost. If the corpus callosum and the temporal lobes are infarcted dementia may occur with slightly less marked loss of cerebral tissue. Since the small infarcts in patients with multi-infarct dementia are associated with hypertensive cerebral vascular disease many of the infarcts are found in the deep central white matter (Chap. 5), at sites which interrupt the ascending and descending pathways from the cortex to the deep grey matter and brain stem. The role of extracranial atherosclerosis and its relation to cerebral embolism has been discussed in Chap. 5. These factors are important in producing the multifocal distribution of cerebral infarction in patients with multi-infarct dementia (Fig. 15.4). As a rule the infarcts are bilaterally distributed; unilateral infarcts seldom if ever cause dementia. Boundary zone infarction due to hypotension may also cause dementia but parietal features are particularly common in such patients because of the particular susceptibility of the parietal lobes to boundary zone infarction (see Chap. 5).

Microscopical examination of the infarcts in patients with multi-infarct dementia shows that the infarcts are in varying stages of evolution. Some are fresh and others very old. There is often haemosiderin deposition in the walls of some of the infarcts

suggesting that haemorrhage may have been a feature, and strengthening the supposition that some of these infarcts are due to cerebral embolism, or even to primary small cerebral haemorrhages associated with hypertensive cerebral vascular disease.

The reduction of choline acetyltransferase activity in the temporal lobes in patients with Alzheimer's disease is not a feature of multi-infarct dementia. Multi-infarct dementia may be a feature of any form of vascular disease but it is only seen commonly in association with *hypertension* and *diabetic* vascular disease. Other forms of vascular disease are rare causes of dementia.

Coexistence of Alzheimer's dementia and multi-infarct dementia

Since both Alzheimer's disease and cerebral vascular disease are common in the later years of life, the brains of patients with dementia often show features of both disorders. This association depends simply upon the frequency of both conditions, and must be recognised in attempts to diagnose multi-infarct dementia and Alzheimer's disease during life (see Fig. 15.3). In surveys of patients with dementia it has been found that as many as 20 % or 30 % show features of cerebral vascular disease when the brains are examined at autopsy. In the converse situation, that is in the brains of patients dying with stroke,

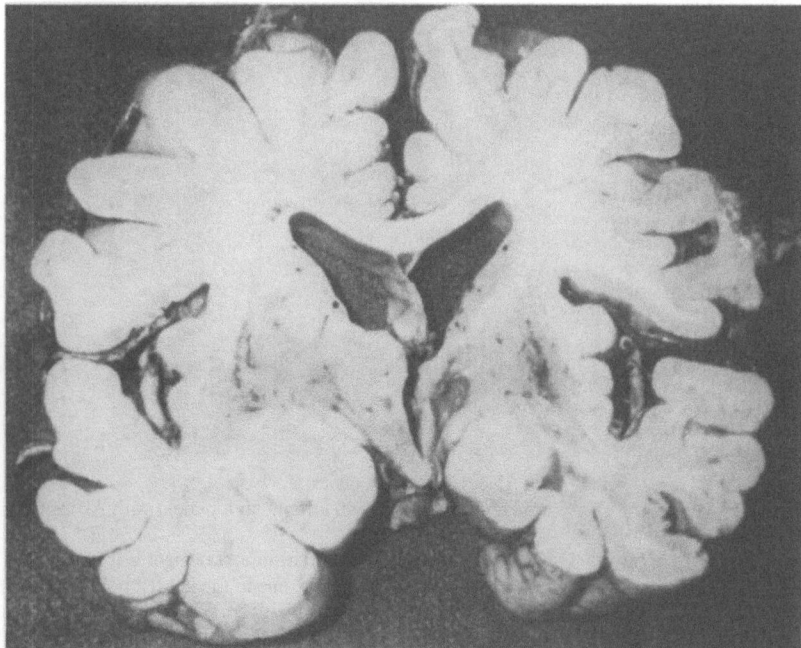

Fig. 15.4. Multi-infarct dementia. A coronal slice of the cerebral hemispheres showing multiple areas of softening; these are especially prominent in the basal ganglia on the right. Cerebral atrophy with widening of the sulci and lateral fissures is very noticeable.

senile plaques and neurofibrillary tangles are frequently found in the temporal lobes. However, in normal aged subjects the numbers of plaques and tangles are less than those ordinarily associated with Alzheimer's disease itself, although they are found in a similar location (see above).

Pick's disease

A rare disorder, Pick's disease has an incidence of no more than about 5% of that of Alzheimer's disease. Pick's original description of the condition was of macroscopic features only, and the disorder is now often known by the alternative designation 'progressive circumscribed cerebral atrophy'. The disorder begins most often during later middle life at about the age of 60 but cases beginning much earlier, or later, have also been described. The disorder probably has a genetic basis, being inherited as a *dominant* trait.

The illness begins with insidious intellectual deterioration, often presenting with difficulty in concentration and memory. The patient appears restless, apathetic and depressed, and behaves in a socially unacceptable manner without insight. Dysphasia, apraxia and alexia may occur and features of frontal lobe involvement, including repetitive utterances or actions, and perseverations, are a characteristic feature. Sometimes mutism develops. Disturbances of gait, with spasticity and rigidity, are prominent in the late stages of the illness but involuntary movements and seizures are uncommon. A number of cases have been described in which the clinical features were mistaken for those of a psychosis, the disorder being discovered at autopsy. Death usually occurs about 5 years after the onset.

Pathology

There is extreme atrophy of relatively circumscribed parts of both cerebral hemispheres (this is best seen after the leptomeninges have been stripped from the brain so that the underlying convolutions are exposed). The most affected gyri have a knife-like appearance, particularly in the fronto-temporal region so that widely gaping sulci can be seen. The atrophy is usually fronto-temporal in distribution and may selectively affect the frontal or temporal lobes. It is symmetrical in about a third of cases but in about a half the left hemisphere is more severely affected than the right. Parietal and occipital atrophy are very rare.

In the *frontal* lobe the atrophy is particularly marked in the medial orbital regions, including the gyrus rectus but extending along the inferior frontal gyrus towards the insula. The frontal convexity is less commonly involved but this may extend posteriorly to affect the precentral gyrus. In the *temporal* lobe atrophy is always most marked around the temporal pole; it extends back to involve the whole of the middle and inferior temporal gyri but the anterior third of the superior temporal gyrus is always more affected than the posterior part. This distribution of frontal and temporal atrophy has suggested to some pathologists that the disease tends to involve those parts of the hemispheres which have developed most recently in evolutionary terms. However, the hippocampus and the parahippocampal gyrus may also be considerably atrophied. The white matter is atrophic so that the junction between grey and white matter in affected areas becomes rather blurred and affected lobes feel rubbery. When the frontal lobes are severely atrophied the caudate nuclei and the thalamus are also usually atrophic but these regions are frequently spared.

The major *histological* features consist of loss of neurons, gliosis, and the occurrence of a characteristic cytoplasmic abnormality in neurons giving rise to the Pick cell. Neuronal loss is often greater in the outer cortical layers but the pattern is variable. In these regions there is marked cortical and subcortical gliosis which may be primary or secondary to the neuronal loss. Neurons near zones of cell loss may be smaller and stain less intensely than normal. The Nissl substance of these affected neurons is less prominent than normal.

The *Pick cell* is a swollen neuron which often takes a round or pear-shaped form. The Nissl substance disintegrates, the cytoplasm becoming homogeneous and acidophilic, while the nucleus is displaced towards the periphery of the cell. The abnormal zones of cytoplasm remain pale in PTAH stains and contain globular, homogeneous, well-defined masses of neurofibrils in silver impregnations and in electron microscope preparations. These features resemble to some extent chromatolysis which occurs following axonal degeneration and it has been suggested that the disease process may first affect the axon and other processes of the neuron rather than its cell body. There is astrocyte proliferation and gliosis but microglia and oligodendroglia play little part in the pathological reaction; in advanced cases, status spongiosis may be found in the cortex. The caudate nucleus and thalamus are often severely affected but the putamen, globus pallidus and pons are usually only slightly abnormal. Senile plaques, neurofibrillary changes, and granulovacuolar degeneration may be found in cases of Pick's disease, but it is probable that these represent chance associations rather than a related abnormality.

The aetiology of Pick's disease is not understood, and the difficulty in making a firm clinical diagnosis has not made it easy to study the condition.

Progressive subcortical gliosis

In this disorder there is an insidiously progressive dementia, resembling Alzheimer's and Pick's disease. There are usually prominent motor features including spasticity, tremulousness, and sometimes seizures. Perseverations and other features of frontal involvement are usually noted. *Histologically* there is pronounced subcortical gliosis and microglial proliferation with severe involvement of the cerebral cortex but with relatively little loss of myelin. The basal ganglia, brain stem and ventral

horns of the spinal cord may be involved. The condition resembles Pick's disease but differs in that the circumscribed atrophy of frontal and temporal lobes so characteristic of Pick's disease is not found at autopsy, and progressive subcortical gliosis is therefore classified separately.

Huntington's disease

This disorder is described in detail in Chap. 14; it usually presents with chorea. *Dementia* develops later in the course of the disease, but in some cases psychotic manifestions, or dementia, may be a presenting feature. The brunt of the pathological process falls on the nuclei of the basal ganglia (Fig. 15.5), particularly on the caudate nucleus and globus pallidus, but neuronal loss from the cerebral cortex is also a feature, first described by Alzheimer in 1911, and this probably accounts for the dementia. The frontal lobes are especially involved and this sometimes makes it difficult to delineate this condition from Pick's disease, particularly when the basal ganglia are involved in the latter condition.

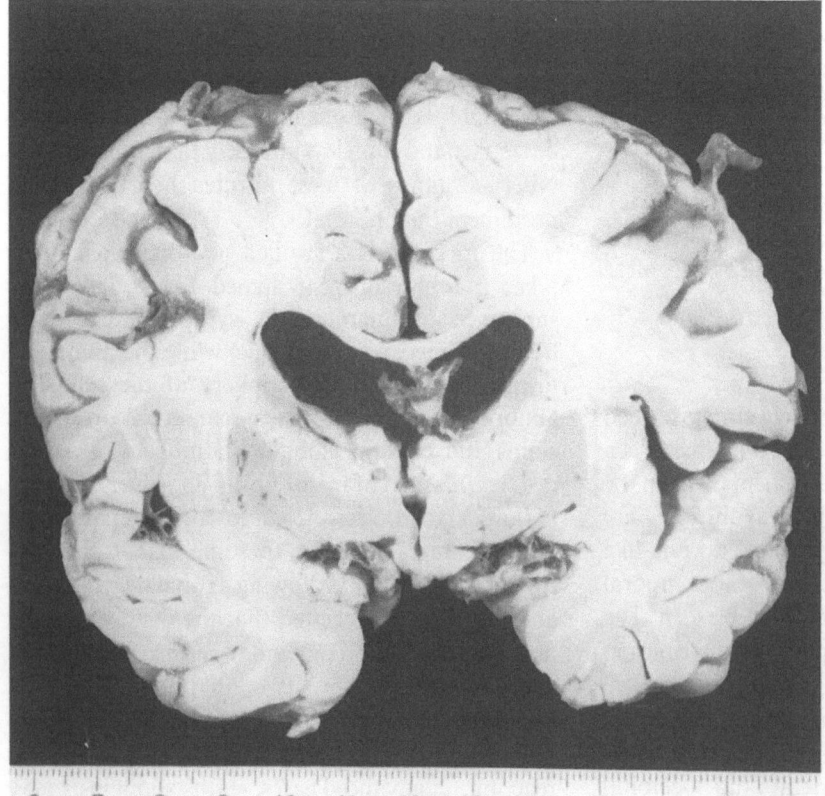

Fig. 15.5. Huntington's disease. A coronal section of the cerebral hemispheres through the frontal lobes. There is atrophy of the heads of the caudate nuclei on both sides (cf. Fig. 2.17). Due to the atrophy of the caudate nuclei, the anterior nuclei of the thalami are more prominent than usual as they project into the lateral ventricles.

Creutzfeldt–Jakob disease (subacute spongiform encephalopathy)

This condition is an acquired disorder with an incidence of about five cases per million per year. There are two main patterns of *clinical* presentation. In *one form* of the disease, usually beginning in middle age, dementia is the major feature. The illness runs a short course characterised by a rapidly progressive dementia, with myoclonus and spasticity. Extrapyramidal features may be observed during the early stages of the disease and seizures may also occur. Patients usually die within a few months of presentation. In the *second form* of the disease there is a more pronounced spastic quadriparesis and dementia is less evident until later in the course of the disease. The second form of the disorder runs a slightly longer course and usually affects somewhat older subjects. In the past, a clear distinction was drawn between these two forms of the disease, and other varieties were recognised with predominant frontal or occipitoparietal symptoms. Since the transmissible nature of the disease has been recognised by animal inoculation studies, however, these distinctions have become blurred and the subacute spongiform encephalopathies have been grouped together as a single disorder, usually called Creutzfeldt–Jakob disease.

The *diagnosis* of Creutzfeldt–Jakob disease can usually be readily suspected clinically. The EEG changes are particularly characteristic, consisting of a generalised, almost continuous, but irregular, spike-and-wave discharge, which is accompanied by irregular but virtually continuous myoclonus in all muscles of the body. A point of difficulty in the clinical diagnosis concerns the occurrence of myoclonus of similar type in some patients with a longer history in whom a diagnosis of Alzheimer's disease is suspected. It thus seems possible that there are cases of spongiform encephalopathy, presumably representing forms of Creutzfeldt–Jakob disease, in which the clinical features are not well formalised. This suggests that the disease may be more common than has been suspected.

Pathology

The brain may show atrophy, but this is a variable feature. The leptomeninges and blood vessels are normal. The ventricles may be slightly enlarged and there is usually some shrinkage of the deep nuclei. Cortical atrophy in some cases is very marked, and if there is extensive destruction of cortical neurons, laminar necrosis may be seen (Fig. 15.6). *Microscopically* there is loss of nerve cells, which is sometimes so marked that lamination of the cortex is lost. The grey matter of the basal ganglia is similarly affected. In the cerebellum the Purkinje cells may be lost. The neuronal loss is accompanied by striking astrocyte proliferation and hypertrophy, particularly in the cerebral cortex but also in the deep grey matter. There is accompanying microglial reaction with microglial clusters adjacent to small blood vessels, particularly in the deep layers of the cortex. Spongy change (Fig. 15.7) with large vacuoles in the grey matter is a feature of many but not all cases of Creutzfeld–Jakob disease. Sometimes perivascular lymphocytic cuffing is a feature.

Atypical cases

The various clinical forms of the disease described briefly above show a similar pathology to that of typical cases of *spongiform encephalopathy* but the distribution of the abnormality, and the degree of astrocyte proliferation and spongiform change, varies from case to case. These variants of the disease are therefore now usually regarded as part of the overall syndrome constituting Creutzfeldt–Jakob disease.

Pathogenesis

In 1968 Gajdusek et al. found that inocula of brain tissue from a cerebral biopsy, taken from a patient with Creutzfeldt–Jakob disease and injected into the brain of a chimpanzee, resulted in the development of a neurological illness resembling Creutzfeldt–Jakob disease in the chimpanzee about a year later. This observation has been confirmed in further inoculation experiments in other primates since that time. Indeed the disease has been transmitted accidentally from patient to patient via a corneal graft taken from a patient with the disease, and in a tragic series of cases the disease was transmitted by neurosurgical procedures in which the instruments had previously been inserted into the brain of a patient with Creutzfeldt–Jakob disease.

Despite this experience the *transmissible agent* has proved elusive. It has not been possible to visualise it by electron microscopy, or to develop any antiserum for its identification by immunofluorescence. Furthermore, the infective agent seems to be smaller than a virus and resistant to

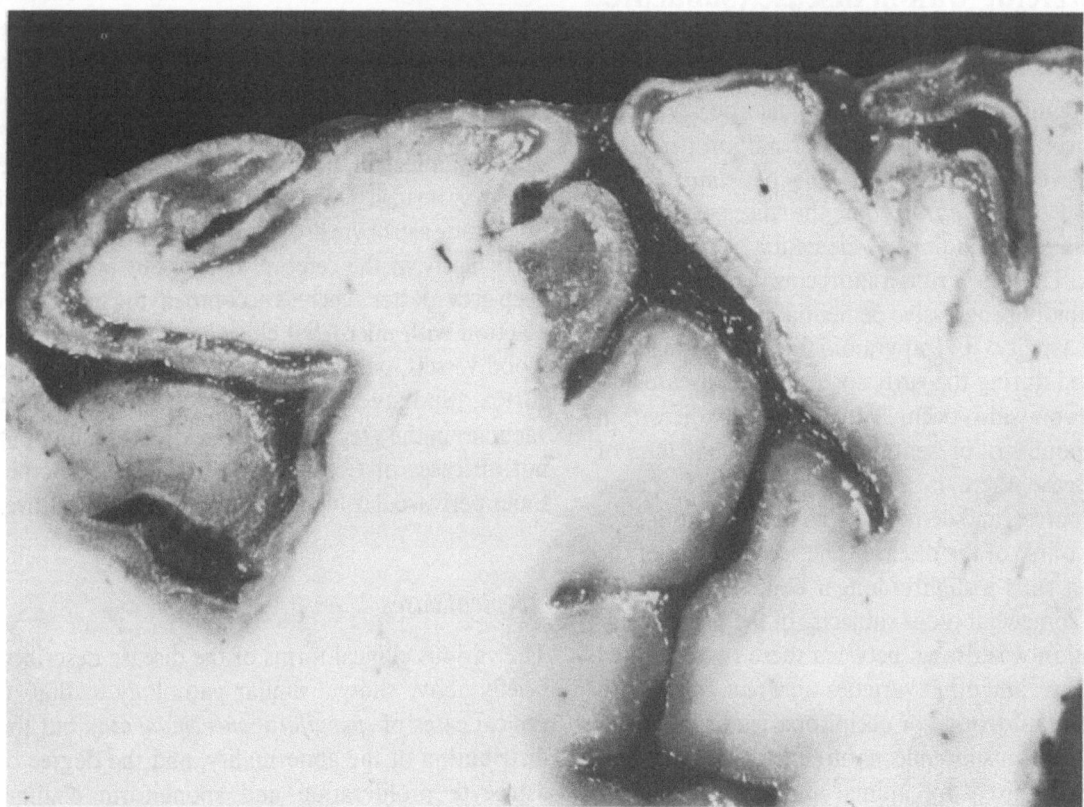

Fig. 15.6. Creutzfeldt–Jakob disease. An enlarged view of the cortex and white matter showing gross reduction in cortical thickness; at the *top* of the picture there is cavitation and laminar necrosis in the deep layers of the cortex.

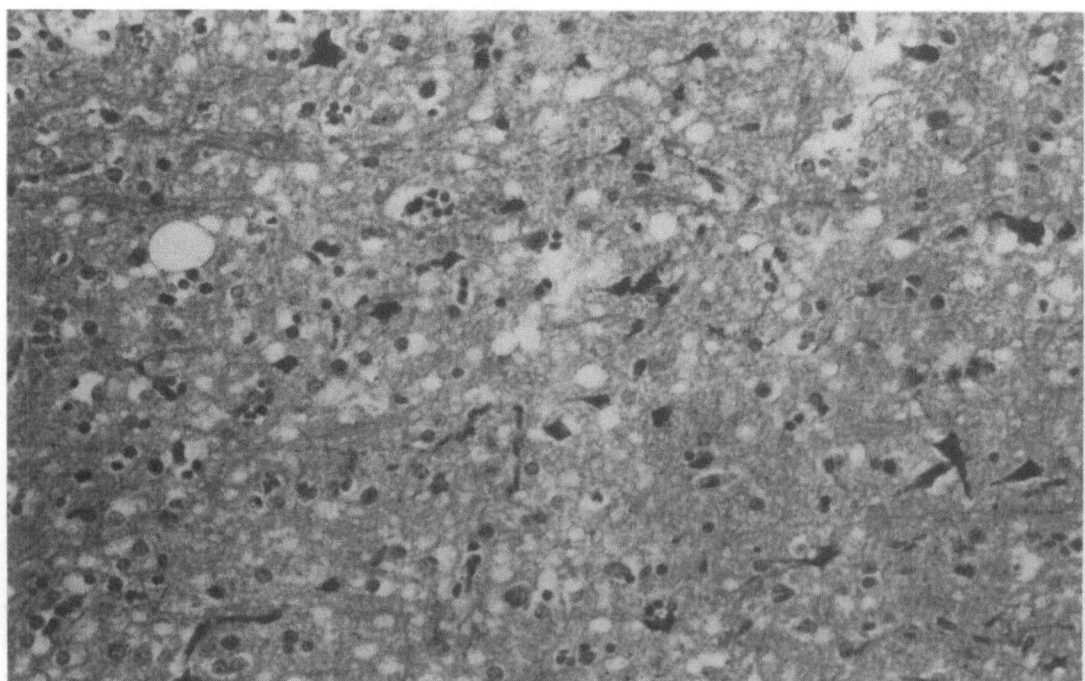

Fig. 15.7. Creutzfeldt–Jakob disease. A photomicrograph of cortex showing depletion of neurons and hypercellularity due to the increase in astrocytes. The microcystic appearance of spongiform change is seen throughout the picture. (H & E × 200)

inactivation by strong acids, alkalis or oxidizing agents, which normally inactivate virus particles. It is possible that the infective agent is membrane-associated (Spiroplasma). The infectious particle is not inactivated by formalin or by steam sterilisation unless high pressures or other special techniques are used (see Appendix p. 322).

The natural mode of spread and degree of infectivity of Creutzfeltd–Jakob disease are unknown but the disorder is rare and it must therefore be concluded that the natural infectivity of the condition is low.

Other spongiform encephalopathies

Spongiform encephalopathy is also a feature of kuru, a cerebellar degeneration found in the Highlands of New Guinea. This disorder is presumed to be acquired by contact with or even ingestion of infected brain. It consists of a progressive cerebellar ataxia with dementia, characterised pathologically by the development of mild spongiform change in the cerebral cortex, but the most characteristic and marked changes are in the cerebellar cortex with loss of granule cells and the appearance of PAS-positive 'kuru plaques' which are homogeneous and some 30 μm in diameter. Spongiform change is found in the cerebral cortex in some patients with Alzheimer's disease, particularly those observed to have prominent myoclonus during the later stages of their dementia but the relation between this disorder and Creutzfeldt–Jakob disease itself is controversial. There is no evidence, as yet, that Alzheimer's disease is transmissible by direct intracerebral inoculation. Spongiform change also occurs in two transmissible animal encephalopathies, scrapie and mink encephalopathy.

The amnesic syndrome

The amnesic syndrome consists of a profound impairment of recall for recent events, and of short-term memory, in an alert patient. The patient is aware of his personal identity and, usually, of details of his family, at least in relation to family events and family members of several months or years in the past. Memory for events during the immediately preceding weeks or months is usually absent or grossly impaired when formally tested. However, by recording a patient's conversation and his responses to questions it can be shown that

memories for these events are retained but are not accessible for recall. Items of information which are apparently not retrievable during testing are often produced later by the patient but in an irrelevant way. There is thus evidence that the disorder is due to impairment of recall rather than to ineffective establishment of memories, and that previously laid down memory traces are preserved but not retrievable from the memory store.

In the amnesic syndrome there is damage to the mesial parts of the hippocampal formations and usually also to the amygdala. There has been controversy as to the precise location of lesions necessary for production of the amnesic syndrome but it is clear that bilateral lesions are required and that the amnesic syndrome does not result after destruction of one hippocampus, even if it is extensive. A variety of disorders can thus cause the syndrome (Table 15.6).

Table 15.6. Causes of the amnesic syndrome

Wernicke–Korsakoff syndrome
Bilateral hippocampal infarction
Bilateral hippocampal surgery
Cerebral trauma
Encephalitis, especially herpes simplex encephalitis

Wernicke–Korsakoff syndrome

The onset of the Wernicke–Korsakoff syndrome is subacute. It usually occurs in heavy drinkers but also develops in people deprived of normal nutrition by starvation, or malabsorption syndromes. Vomiting and nystagmus are early symptoms. The patient may become confused, often in association with an acute febrile illness. Stupor and coma supervene and the mental changes of the Korsakoff syndrome, consisting of a defect in recent memory with confabulation, are noted as the patient begins to recover. Ophthalmoplegia, usually beginning with weakness of horizontal gaze movements, with nystagmus and with variable defects of conjugate gaze, is an early feature and this is usually accompanied by ataxia of the limbs and trunk. Korsakoff himself noted that peripheral neuropathy was a common associated feature but this is not always present. The disorder responds to treatment with intravenous or intramuscular thiamine; recovery occurs within a few hours, but is incomplete if the disorder is severe, and particularly if treatment is delayed.

Pathology

Symmetrical lesions are found in the paraventricular parts of the medial dorsal and anterior medial nuclei, and in the pulvinar of the thalamus. The mammillary bodies, periaqueductal region, floor of the fourth ventricle and anterior lobe of the cerebellum are also usually affected. The dorsal motor nuclei of the vagus, and the vestibular nuclei may show abnormalities. *Microscopically* the lesions are characterised by destruction of neuronal elements and by the proliferation of small blood vessels which may produce a haemorrhagic appearance in the affected areas. There is a marked infiltration by histiocytes and proliferation of astrocytes in the abnormal regions.

The location of these lesions is consistent with the clinical features of the disorder. The amnesic defect itself has been related to lesions in the diencephalon, particularly in the medial dorsal nuclei of the thalamus and perhaps in the medial parts of the pulvinar. In the past, it was thought that lesions in the mammillary bodies were critically placed and were responsible for interruption of the limbic system and so for the amnesia, but this appears not to be the case.

Intermittently raised pressure hydrocephalus (IRPH)

In a small number of demented patients, difficulty in walking, and incontinence are unusually prominent. These patients have large ventricles which can be demonstrated in life by CT scans, but cerebral atrophy is not a feature. It has been suggested that the dementia and ventricular dilatation results from communicating hydrocephalus.

This entity was formerly called *normal pressure hydrocephalus* because the CSF pressure measured by single lumbar puncture is usually normal. Ventricular pressure monitoring has established that patients with this syndrome develop periodic short-lived sharply peaked waves of pressure ('B waves'). Similar peaks occur in pressure recordings of patients with an enlarging intracranial mass especially when the mean pressure is also increased; the mechanism by which B waves are produced is unknown. In IRPH the ventricles of the brain, especially the lateral ventricles, progressively dilate and the subependymal tissue round the ventricles may become oedematous (see Chap. 4). This can happen as a delayed or late complication of subarachnoid haemorrhage, trauma or meningitis, but many cases give no such history and are termed idiopathic IRPH.

Pathologically the common findings are incomplete obliteration of the subarachnoid space by leptomeningeal fibrosis, sometimes accompanied by changes in the arachnoid granulations; there may be gliosis in the subependymal tissue with loss of axons and myelin. Some clinically similar cases have been described in which multiple small infarcts were found at autopsy in the deep cerebral and cerebellar grey and white matter without any obvious abnormality of the leptomeninges or arachnoid villi. Sometimes leptomeningeal fibrosis coexists with the pathological changes of Alzheimer's disease and these patients respond badly to shunting.

The *diagnosis* of IRPH is suggested by a combination of progressive gait disturbance, dementia and incontinence of urine. The gait disturbance may precede the dementia by 3 years or more and is often difficult to characterise: the steps are small and shuffling and balance is poor, but other pathognomonic features of parkinsonism, especially in the upper limbs, are lacking. The muscle tone in the legs is often increased in a manner that does not correspond precisely to spasticity or to the rigidity of parkinsonism. The patient is typically quiet and apathetic; the incontinence appears to reflect impaired voluntary control without any abnormality of reflex bladder responses.

These features are shared by many patients with other forms of dementia and investigation is required to identify the IRPH patients. The CT scan shows ventricular dilatation out of proportion to the degree of cortical atrophy; the diagnosis becomes very likely if the scan shows lucent areas round the ventricles with a radiological density similar to that of CSF oedema. IRPH is best confirmed by intracranial pressure monitoring which, it is claimed, predicts the results of ventricular shunting. The patients likely to respond are those in whom B waves of pressure occupy more than 5% of a 24-h period of monitoring.

The present evidence suggests that the *therapeutic* effects of shunting correlate with the results of pressure monitoring rather than with post-mortem histological appearances. In patients with IRPH where the aetiology is known—for example a previous subarachnoid haemorrhage—the insertion of a ventriculo-atrial shunt brings about improvement in up to 65% of cases and 30% can expect to recover completely. The results in the patients with idiopathic IRPH are probably worse, especially in those in whom the gait disorder is a late or minor symptom. The natural history of untreated IRPH has never been clearly delineated since positive identification by pressure monitoring inevitably leads to the insertion of a shunt. Most cases are characterised by progressive deterioration but some may stabilise; none has been reported to improve spontaneously. Although the ventricles often become smaller after shunting, some patients who respond very well to treatment show no alteration in the size of their ventricles after shunting and the clinical outcome does not correlate with the change in ventricular size that occurs after shunting.

Further reading

Blessed G, Tomlinson B E, Roth M (1968) The association between quantitative measures of dementia and of senile change in the cerebral grey matter of elderly subjects. Br J Psychiatry 114:797

Editorial (1977) Uncovering physical illness in elderly patients with dementia. Br Med J ii: 1499

Bowen D M, Smith C B, White P, Davison A N (1976) Neurotransmitting related enzymes and indices of hypoxia in senile dementia and other abiotrophies. Brain 99:459

Hachinski V C, Lassen N A, Marshall J (1974) Multi-infarct dementia. A cause of mental deterioration in the elderly. Lancet i:207

Mandybur T I (1975) The incidence of cerebral amyloid angiopathy in Alzheimer's disease. Neurology 25:120

Masters E L, Richardson E P (1978) Subacute spongiform encephalopathy (Creutzfeldt–Jakob disease). The nature and progression of spongiform change. Brain 101:333

Smith C M, Swash M (1980) Effects of cholinergic drugs on memory in Alzheimer's disease. In: Amaducci L, Davison A N, Antuono P (eds) Ageing of the brain and dementia. Raven, New York, p 295

Spillane J A, White P, Goodhart M J et al. (1977) Selective vulnerability of neurons in organic dementia. Nature 226:558

Tomlinson B E (1979) The ageing brain. In: Cavanagh J B, Thomas-Smith W (eds) Recent advances in neuropathology. 1. Churchill Livingstone, Edinburgh London New York.

Chapter 16

Diseases of Peripheral Nerve

Assessment of a peripheral neuropathy requires a firm understanding of the *clinical* and *electrophysiological* features of peripheral nerve diseases (see Chap. 3), in addition to an appreciation of the general and specific pathological reactions in peripheral nerves which are discussed in this chapter. Much of the present body of information regarding peripheral nerve pathology has been gathered from detailed examination of nerve biopsies, from autopsy material and from experimental studies.

Problems are often encountered in the pathological investigation of peripheral neuropathies due to artefact caused by incorrect handling of biopsy or autopsy material. In this chapter, therefore, the technique of nerve biopsy is briefly explained together with autopsy procedures for cases of peripheral neuropathy.

Since peripheral nerves exhibit only a limited range of pathological reactions interpretation of histological material often depends upon the balance of the different pathological features present in the nerve. For this reason, an account of the general pathology of nerves precedes a survey of specific peripheral nerve diseases.

Nerve biopsy

The main reasons for performing a nerve biopsy are (a) to obtain pathological information as an aid to diagnosis of a peripheral nerve disorder or (b) to assess the extent of nerve damage and to estimate potential for regeneration and recovery. It is usually possible in a nerve biopsy to distinguish between the primary pathological events of axonal degeneration and segmental demyelination. Furthermore, specific pathological patterns may be seen within the nerve which are characteristic of particular peripheral neuropathies. Structures closely associated with nerves such as epineurial blood vessels can also be examined in biopsy material. The investigation of peripheral nerve diseases by biopsy, however, is limited by the small amount of nerve that can reasonably be excised, by the restricted number of nerves which are suitable for biopsy, and by the exclusion of motor nerve biopsies on ethical grounds. Muscle biopsy may solve the problem of investigating motor nerves as examination of the small intramuscular nerve branches may reveal information of diagnostic value.

As nerve biopsy is an invasive procedure, it is usually not performed until a complete clinical history has been taken, the patient has been thoroughly examined, and nerve conduction studies performed. The choice of nerve for biopsy may be influenced by the clinical picture but for most purposes, the *sural nerve*, the *cutaneous branch of the radial nerve* on the dorsum of the hand, and the *lateral cutaneous nerve of the forearm* are most commonly used.

Technique. The general principles of nerve biopsy can be set out by considering the technique for obtaining tissue from the sural nerve. From sensory fibres supplying the lateral side of the foot and part of the lateral aspect of the leg, the sural nerve eventually joins the sciatic nerve and its fibres pass into the sacral plexus. The most convenient place to biopsy the sural nerve is just behind and just below the lateral malleolus at the ankle. At this site, the nerve may consist of several branches which are closely associated with the short saphenous vein in the subcutaneous tissue. Unfixed peripheral nerves are very fragile and *artefact* can very easily be induced in the nerve by stretching, by cleaning the fat away from the nerve or even by dabbing it with a swab. If possible, an experienced surgeon should take the biopsy and, following identification of the nerve, it should be removed with the *minimum of handling*. It should be gripped only lightly at one end of the specimen as it is cut from the subcutaneous tissue. A 2–3 cm length of nerve is usually enough for histological and histochemical purposes. The nerve should be laid gently upon a piece of dry card, to which it will stick and retain its orientation when placed in the fixative. Unless fresh, unfixed nerve is required, trimming and cutting the specimen should be avoided until the nerve is fixed.

Fascicular nerve biopsy, in which only part of the nerve is removed, is popular in some centres. Electrophysiological studies can be performed on the isolated biopsy before histological study.

Autopsy study of peripheral neuropathies

Autopsies on patients with peripheral neuropathies provide opportunities to examine the whole peripheral and central nervous system and avoids the sampling errors inherent in biopsy studies. One disadvantage, however, of an autopsy study is that the preservation of the nerve is less than ideal.

When a patient with a peripheral neuropathy dies the choice of nerves to be sampled should depend upon the clinical findings. For a complete picture, the brain together with the cranial nerves and the trigeminal ganglia should be removed; the spinal cord is best removed from the front so that the dorsal root ganglia may also be excised. If necessary, the brachial, lumbar and sacral plexuses can be removed in continuity with their roots. Similarly, the relevant nerve may be traced down to its muscle insertion or cutaneous branches. In a generalised symmetrical peripheral neuropathy, major nerve trunks can be sampled together with smaller nerves more distally placed in the limbs. The distribution of a motor neuropathy can often be determined by sampling muscles and examining them for changes of neurogenic atrophy.

Some neuropathies have a major autonomic component; the splanchnic nerves and sympathetic chains are easily identified at autopsy and can be sampled in these cases.

Techniques for peripheral nerve histology

Meaningful histological examination of orientated structures such as muscle, nerve, spinal cord and brain stem is only really possible if exact cross-sections or exact longitudinal sections are prepared. Many of the difficulties in interpretation of histological preparations arise because of the oblique plane of nerve sections. This general principle applies to both biopsy and autopsy material. Although only a small amount of nerve is usually available from a biopsy, it should be well preserved and well fixed so that it is ideal for examination by electron microscopy and by light microscopy as 1-μm resin sections. Portions of nerve can also be teased and, if required, other parts of the biopsy can be examined as paraffin sections. Due to its relatively poor preservation, autopsy material is usually best examined as paraffin sections or as teased preparations. A brief account of the histological techniques will be given in this chapter but more detailed accounts may be found in expanded texts on peripheral nerves (Weller and Cervós-Navarro 1977; Asbury and Johnson 1978).

One-micron resin sections and electron microscopy. As mentioned above, this technique is ideal for the examination of peripheral nerve biopsy histology. The nerves are fixed in glutaraldehyde for 4 h, then post-fixed in osmium tetroxide and embedded in araldite as for electron microscopy. Exact transverse sections of the nerve biopsy will reveal the detailed histology of the epineurium and its vessels, the perineurium and the contents of the nerve fascicles. Large and small myelinated fibres may be examined by the use of an oil immersion lens or enlarged photographs (Fig. 16.3). Abnormalities of endoneurial vessels can be detected together with abnormal deposits such as amyloid or lipids. Macrophages and other inflammatory cells can also be identified in these sections. A further advantage of the resin-embedded material is that electron microscopy may be performed upon selected areas of the nerve. Longitudinal sections are usually not as useful in evaluating the nerve as transverse sections but nodes of Ranvier are best studied in this orientation.

Teased preparations. Formalin- or glutaraldehyde-fixed nerve can be prepared for teasing in various ways. One of the standard methods is to fix the material in osmium tetroxide, having removed much of the surrounding fat from the nerve bundles. After soaking in 66% glycerine for 2 or 3 days, the nerve fibres may be separated sufficiently to follow individual axons through several internodes (Fig. 16.10). If the osmium tetroxide is omitted, myelin sheaths may be stained by Oil-Red-

O or Sudan black B before immersion in glycerine and subsequent teasing. Enzyme histochemical methods may also be applied to nerves before teasing and then the birefringent myelin can be identified by polarised light. Instead of teasing in glycerine, glutaraldehyde and osmium post-fixed nerves can be infiltrated with incomplete araldite and teased in the resin. Teased nerve fibres are particularly useful for detecting the nodal gap widening and internodal myelin breakdown in segmental demyelination (Fig. 16.10). Re-myelination may also be detected and, in chronic neuropathies, the differentiation between re-myelination and axonal regeneration may be evident in teased fibres. The disadvantage of teased preparations is that only a few fibres within the bundle may be examined at any one time and quantitative studies relating to the whole nerve may be difficult.

Paraffin sections. Nerves fixed in formalin or other fixatives can be embedded in paraffin and the sections stained with H&E, myelin stains (Luxol-fast blue or haematoxylin myelin stains), connective tissue stains (haematoxylin van Giesen) or with techniques to demonstrate axons (Glees or Palmgren). Although the degree of histological detail observed in resin-embedded sections cannot be resolved in paraffin sections, larger specimens of nerve can be examined in the paraffin-embedded material and is thus a more useful technique when studying autopsy cases. *Inflammatory* reactions within the nerves and thrombotic complications in the *vessels* are very well demonstrated in paraffin sections, as are *amyloid* deposits.

Sections of *spinal cord* obtained at autopsy are most satisfactorily examined in paraffin sections. Transverse sections of the spinal roots may either be viewed in sections of cord or the whole cauda equina may be embedded and cut as a cross-section.

The examination of *muscle* tissue at autopsy may be a valuable guide to the presence of peripheral nerve disease. Histochemical techniques similar to those applied to muscle biopsies (see Chap. 17) may be used for the examination of autopsy material as Myosin ATPase and mitochondrial oxidative enzymes are well preserved in muscle for 24–36 h after death. Group atrophy of muscle fibres indicating denervation may also be detected in paraffin transverse sections of muscle especially when the thin endomysial connective tissue is stained with the diastase-PAS technique.

Examination of *dorsal root ganglia* is also an

important part of the autopsy evaluation of a peripheral neuropathy. Selected ganglia can be removed from the spinal roots and processed whole until the paraffin-embedding stage; the ganglion and adjacent nerve can then be cut into several segments so that serial transverse sections through the ganglion and root may be obtained.

Anatomy of peripheral nerves

Motor nerves arise from anterior horn cells in the spinal cord. As the axons leave the cell body they are ensheathed in myelin formed by oligodendroglial cells. Upon passing into the anterior root, the axon becomes myelinated by Schwann cells. Anterior roots join the posterior roots and pass out of the intervertebral foramina to join plexuses and peripheral nerve trunks. At the end of their course the motor nerves form nerve terminals adjacent to motor end-plates.

Sensory nerves may supply various types of end organ, the most complicated of which are pacinian corpuscles composed of concentric cellular lamellae. Within a short distance of leaving the sensory end organ, the larger axons acquire a myelin sheath formed by Schwann cells; they then pass through the major nerve trunks and plexuses to a dorsal root. Cell bodies of sensory neurons are situated in the dorsal root ganglia of spinal nerves and their equivalents in the cranial nerves. Central processes from some sensory neurons pass into the spinal cord to continue their passage in the CNS in the dorsal columns (Fig. 16.13). Alternatively, dorsal root fibres may synapse with neurons in the cord, which may in turn contribute fibres to the spinocerebellar or spinothalamic tracts.

Autonomic nerves. Nerve fibres subserving the autonomic nervous system have a restricted exit from the CNS. Parasympathetic pre-ganglionic fibres pass out of the brain stem in the third, seventh, ninth and tenth cranial nerves and from the sacral cord in the second and third sacral nerves. Post-ganglionic neurons are situated near the final point of supply. Pre-ganglionic sympathetic fibres come from neurons in the lateral horns of grey matter in the thoracic spinal cord and pass out in the anterior roots of thoracic and first lumbar nerves. Many of the post-ganglionic fibres arise in neurons in the sympathetic chain which extends from the cervical to the coccygeal region stretched out along the side of the vertebral column. Other ganglia, such as the coeliac ganglia, are situated away from the vertebral column. Post-ganglionic sympathetic fibres usually travel with the blood vessels to their site of action.

Blood supply of peripheral nerves. Much of the blood supply of the spinal cord is through the radicular arteries which also supply the anterior and posterior roots. Small, muscular, longitudinal arteries accompany the nerve trunks within the epineurium and receive segmental branches from adjacent arteries. Similarly, branches from the epineurial arteries pierce the perineurium to supply the capillary plexus within the endoneurial compartment. Such an arrangement means that if the blood supply to one section of a nerve trunk is cut off the supply to adjacent regions of nerve is not necessarily jeopardised.

Histology of peripheral nerves

Gross and microscopic inspection of transverse sections of peripheral nerve trunks reveals multiple nerve fascicles bound together by the fibro-adipose tissue of the *epineurium*. Muscular arteries in the epineurium run parallel to the nerve fascicles and are accompanied by veins. Each nerve fascicle is surrounded by perineurium and the myelinated fibres can easily be identified within the fascicle in H & E-stained paraffin sections (Fig. 16.1). Axons can be specifically stained by silver techniques (Fig. 16.2). Longitudinal sections of paraffin-embedded nerve show the continuity of axons and myelin sheaths but may also show the considerable disruption of myelin which results from paraffin-embedding procedures.

A much clearer picture of peripheral nerve histology can be obtained from toluidine-blue-stained, 1-μm sections of resin-embedded nerve (Fig. 16.3). With high-power light microscopy, 1-μm sections can often give as much information as low-power electron micrographs.

The *perineurium* is seen to consist of eight or so thin cellular layers separated by collagen. It forms a barrier and prevents many substances, especially protein, from entering the nerve from the epineurium. Within the confines of the perineurium is the *endoneurial* compartment containing nerve fibres and capillaries. Large- and small-diameter *myelinated fibres* can be seen (Fig. 16.3); they range in size from 2 to 17 μm in total diameter (i.e. axon

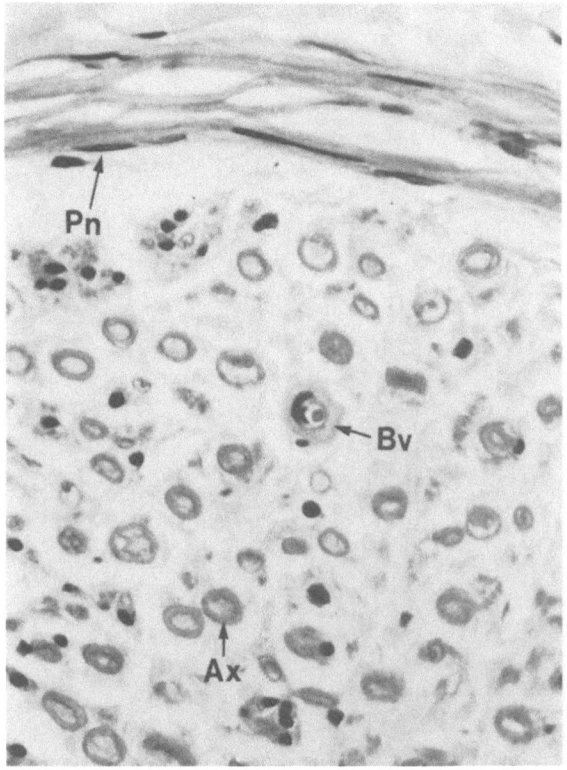

Fig. 16.1. TS normal nerve: perineurium (*Pn*), endoneurial vessel (*Bv*), myelinated axons (*Ax*). (H & E × 650)

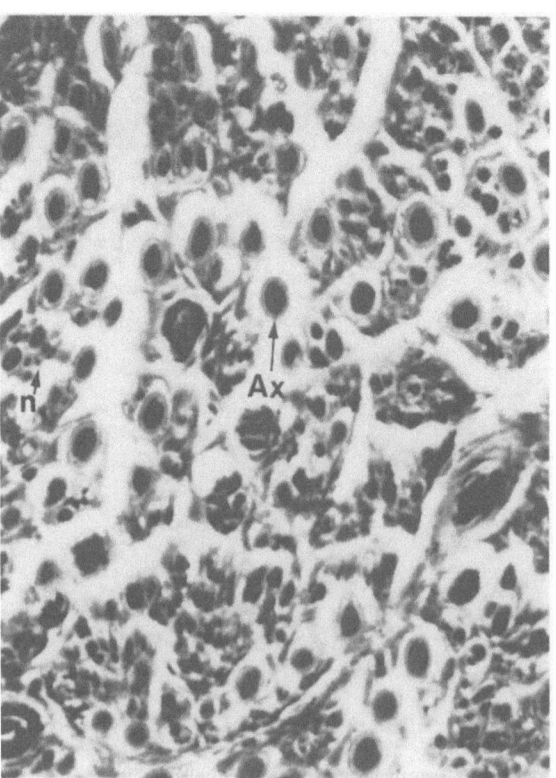

Fig. 16.2. TS normal nerve: myelinated axons (*Ax*), non-myelinated axons (*n*). Palmgren silver stain for axons and Luxol-fast blue for myelin. (× 650)

and myelin sheath) with peaks at 5 and 13 μm. The thickness of the myelin sheath is proportional to the diameter of the axon. The density of myelinated fibres in the sural nerve is approximately 8000 per square millimetre whereas the *non-myelinated* fibres, which are only 0.5–3 μm in diameter, are much more numerous at 30000 per square millimetre. Most of the nuclei, some 90%, are *Schwann cell* nuclei and only a few *fibroblasts* and *mast cells* are seen with a normal nerve

Electron microscopy (Fig. 16.4) reveals the microanatomy of the myelinated axons which contain numerous longitudinally orientated filaments and microtubules similar to those seen in CNS axons (see Figs. 2.8, 2.9). These structures together with the profiles of smooth endoplasmic reticulum are associated with axoplasmic transport (see Chap. 2). Mitochondria are also present within the axon. A 20-nm gap separates the axon from the surrounding Schwann cell, which forms myelin from compaction of its cell membrane. Continuity of the spiral membrane may be traced in some preparations from the internal mesaxon to the external mesaxon. Schwann cytoplasm is seen on the outer aspect of the myelin sheath, particularly in the perinuclear

region and at the node of Ranvier. A *basement membrane* coats the outer aspect of the Schwann cell membrane and separates it from the endoneurial collagen fibres. Fibroblasts within the endoneurium do not usually possess a basement membrane or surround axons. Mast cells can usually be identified by their complex intracytoplasmic granules.

Although each myelinated axon is surrounded by one Schwann cell forming its myelin sheath, multiple non-myelinated axons are associated with single Schwann cells (Fig. 16.4).

Endoneurial blood vessels are usually small and mainly the size of capillaries; they have tight intercellular junctions (zonulae occludentes) which are probably the basis of the *blood–nerve barrier*. They are surrounded by basement membrane which tends to increase in thickness with ageing.

Longitudinal sections of peripheral nerve cut both as 1-μm sections and as thin sections for electron microscopy are ideal for the study of the *nodes of Ranvier* where sequential Schwann cells meet. The myelin sheaths on each side of the node terminate as myelin end loops; Schwann cell cytoplasm fills the gap, often forming finger-like processes which are closely applied to the axon. The

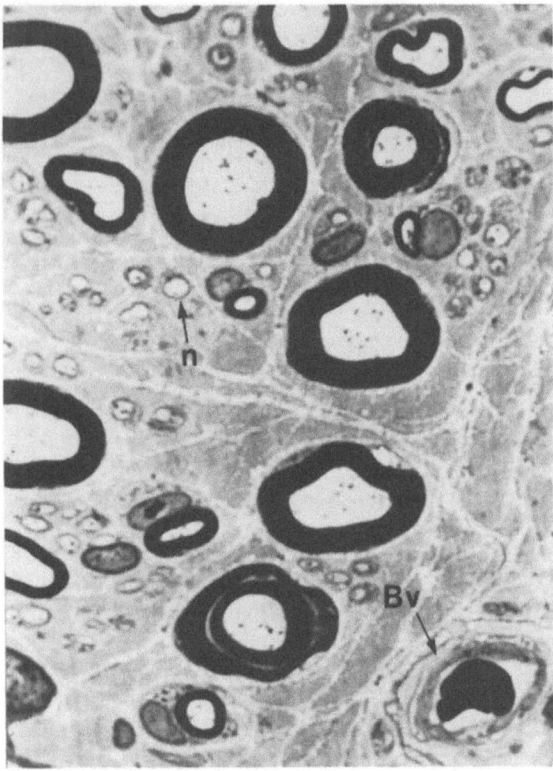

Fig. 16.3. TS normal nerve: large and small myelinated axons are seen together with non-myelinated axons (*n*). Endoneurial blood vessel (*Bv*). 1-μm resin section stained with toluidine blue. (× 1520)

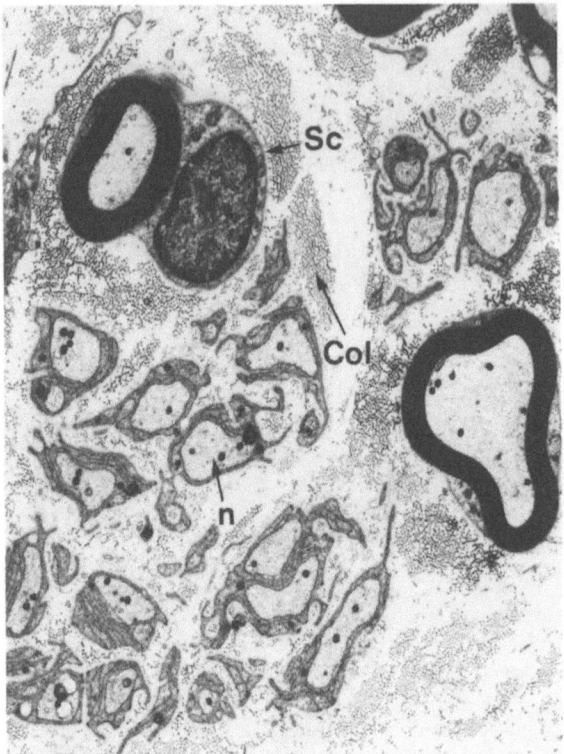

Fig. 16.4. Electron micrograph of TS normal nerve. Schwann cell (*Sc*) associated with a myelinated axon. Non-myelinated axons (*n*) surrounded by thin layer of Schwann cell. Collagen fibres (*Col*). (× 5000)

node of Ranvier has attracted a considerable amount of electrophysiological and anatomical interest as this is the zone of electrical activity during *saltatory conduction* of impulses along peripheral nerves. The myelin sheaths on either side of the nodes of Ranvier are often irregular in outline and there is an increased amount of Schwann cytoplasm, rich in mitochondria, associated with the sheath in this region.

Spiral cytoplasmic channels through the myelin sheaths away from the nodes of Ranvier may also be seen in longitudinal sections of nerve; these are the *Schmidt–Lantermann incisures*.

When myelinated nerve fibres are teased apart, the length of each individual Schwann cell and its myelin sheath can be estimated; this is the *internodal length*, i.e., the distance between each node of Ranvier. In an adult nerve, the internodal length is approximately proportional to the diameter of the myelinated fibre such that a 2-μm-diameter fibre may have an internodal length of 0.15 mm whereas a 12-μm fibre may have an internodal length of 1–1.2 mm (Fig. 16.10).

Development and ageing of peripheral nerves

As groups of axons grow from neurons into peripheral nerves during fetal life, Schwann cells insinuate their processes into the bundles of developing nerve fibres and those which are destined to be myelinated are singled out by single Schwann cells. Although each Schwann cell may have a standard internodal length as it starts to myelinate, this internodal length is considerably lengthened due to growth of the body. Thus the earliest fibres to be myelinated are the largest and they also attain the longest internodal length due to body growth. As the child grows, the thickness of each myelin sheath increases in proportion to the diameter of the axon it surrounds. Another feature of ageing nerves is an increase in the number of Schwann cell processes associated with the non-myelinated fibres.

Basement membrane thicknesses, particularly around the perineurial cells and blood vessels, also increase with age.

General pathology of peripheral nerves

Although there are many diseases of peripheral nerve, and a variety of histological appearances which may be of diagnostic value, there are only two basic ways in which peripheral nerve fibres themselves react:

1) Axonal (wallerian) degeneration and regeneration

2) Segmental demyelination and remyelination.

In most peripheral neuropathies, there is a combination of axonal degeneration and segmental demyelination. Except for a few uncommon diseases, e.g. amyloid neuropathy, the largest myelinated fibres are more sensitive to damage than the small myelinated fibres, and the non-myelinated fibres are the most resistant. Furthermore, severe damage to a nerve usually produces axonal degeneration whereas less severe damage from trauma or vascular disease may only result in segmental demyelination with little axonal damage. In some neuropathies, e.g. diphtheria, post-infectious polyneuropathy (Guillain–Barré syndrome), certain hereditary neuropathies, and lead neuropathy, segmental demyelination is the major pathological process.

Axon (wallerian) degeneration and regeneration

When a peripheral nerve is damaged by trauma or by ischaemia and axons are severed, the distal portions of the axons degenerate. This is most noticeable histologically when myelinated nerve fibres are involved because the myelin sheaths also degenerate (Fig. 16.5). *By 24 h* following nerve transection, the distal axon starts to disintegrate and the myelin sheath along its length forms round or oval globules. Both axon and myelin debris are largely broken down in cytoplasmic lysosomal vacuoles within the Schwann cells (Fig. 16.6B). Macrophages, however, do enter the nerve and assist in the process of myelin breakdown. *By 6 days* the lamellated myelin sheath debris is being transformed into amorphous globular lipid due to the esterification of cholesterol within the myelin. In addition to the infiltration of inflammatory cells, particularly macrophages, into the nerve, the

blood–nerve barrier is disrupted during the early stages of axonal degeneration so that fluid and protein enter the nerve, resulting in oedema of the most severely damaged fascicles.

Within the first *3 or 4 days* following transection of an axon, *regenerative* features are seen (Fig. 16.5C). The distal end of the proximal stump of the axon swells to form a regeneration bulb which is filled with neurofibrils and mitochondria. It is from this site that regenerating axon sprouts soon begin to grow distally at 2–3 mm per day. *Chromatolysis* of the neuronal cell body also occurs at this time reflecting the increased protein synthesis associated with axonal regeneration. Schwann cells in the distal stump of the nerve multiply (Fig. 16.5B) even while they are breaking down residual myelin debris. Bands of proliferating Schwann cells can be seen in the distal stump of the nerve and it is into these bands of Büngner that the multiple, thin, axonal sprouts (or neurites) grow from the expanded distal end of the proximal nerve stump (Fig. 16.5C). As the cluster of regenerating nerve fibres grows down the line of Schwann cells, *myelination* occurs and finally one or more of the regenerating axons may make contact with an end organ such as muscle (Fig. 16.5D).

Non-myelinated fibres regenerate in a very similar way but they do not become myelinated. As regeneration takes place and the blood–nerve barrier is re-established, fluid and protein no longer leak into the nerve. The damaged *perineurium* may partially or completely regenerate.

Factors influencing nerve regeneration

Although under ideal conditions axons may regenerate along the distal stump of the nerve and re-establish contact with an end organ, in many cases the conditions are not ideal. Severe damage to the nerve by trauma may break the continuity of the perineurium and the gap between the proximal and distal stump may be filled with haematoma and eventually by scar tissue. Under these circumstances regenerating axon sprouts may be unable to enter the distal stump and a disorganised tangle of nerve fibres forming an amputation neuroma may result (Fig. 16.5E). Infection of the wound in a nerve may similarly inhibit regeneration.

Axonal degeneration is a common feature of ischaemic neuropathy and the lack of a suitable blood supply to the nerve may also inhibit regeneration. Even if the continuity of the main nerve bundle is maintained, regeneration may bring poor functional results due to the distance and com-

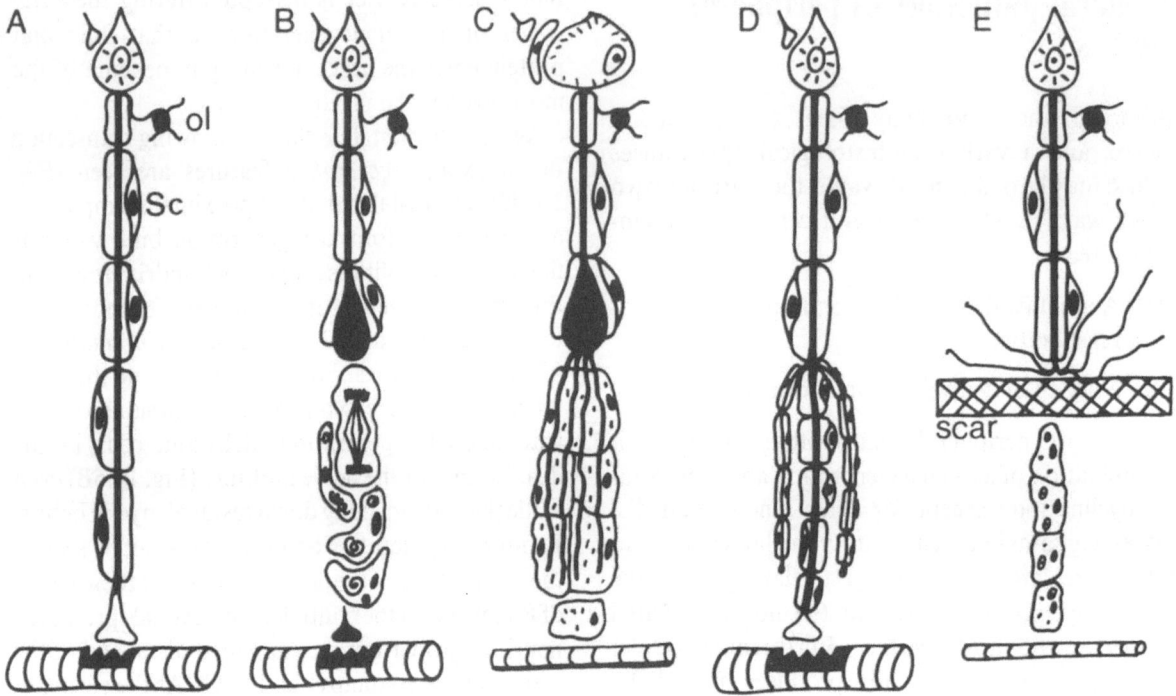

Fig. 16.5. Axon (wallerian) degeneration and regeneration. **A** Normal nerve and muscle. Schwann cell and myelin sheath (*Sc*), oligodendrocyte (*ol*). **B** 3-6 days following axonal section. **C** Regenerating nerve sprouts growing into the distal stump. Chromatolysis. Atrophy of denervated muscle. **D** Cluster of regenerating fibres: reinnervation of end organ. **E** Growth of regenerating axons into the distal part of the nerve is frustrated by the presence of scar tissue.

plexity of the anatomical pathway along which the nerve must regenerate; in these cases the nerves may be unable to reach their appropriate end organs.

Detection of axonal degeneration and regeneration

Electrophysiological studies in a patient with peripheral neuropathy may suggest that there is axonal degeneration. By histological means, it should be possible not only to confirm axonal degeneration but also to detect the presence of axonal regeneration.

In *1-μm transverse sections* of peripheral nerves embedded in epoxy resin, the early stages of axonal degeneration can be detected by the presence of myelin disruption or swollen axon profiles. At a later stage, myelin breakdown products may be seen in macrophages and in foamy Schwann cells; foamy macrophages may also be seen within the layers of the perineurium surrounding the damaged fascicle. If subsequent regeneration does not take place significant axonal loss may be detectable in the nerve distal to the site of injury. Many empty Schwann cell profiles may be seen electron microscopically, but no axons (Fig. 16.6). The presence of

clusters of 3 or 4 small myelinated fibres, however, is a good indication of *regeneration* within the nerve (Figs. 16.7, 16.5D).

Degeneration of nerve fibres can also be detected in *paraffin sections* by the fragmentation of myelin sheaths stained by Luxol-fast blue or by the fragmentation of axons stained by silver impregnation techniques. The changes that occur in the lipids during myelin breakdown also allow detection of nerve fibre degeneration by the use of lipid histochemical techniques. Oil-Red-O- or Sudan-positive globular lipid droplets may be seen in the distal stump of severed nerves especially during the 2nd week of axon and myelin degeneration. The Marchi technique (see Chap. 4) may also be used to detect myelin breakdown in peripheral nerves.

Although *teased preparations* of nerves are valuable in detecting the fragmented axonal and myelin debris following axonal degeneration, they are also particularly valuable in the detection of nerve fibres that have previously undergone regeneration following axonal degeneration. As mentioned previously, the internodal length along a nerve fibre is approximately proportional to the diameter of the myelinated nerve fibre. This is due to

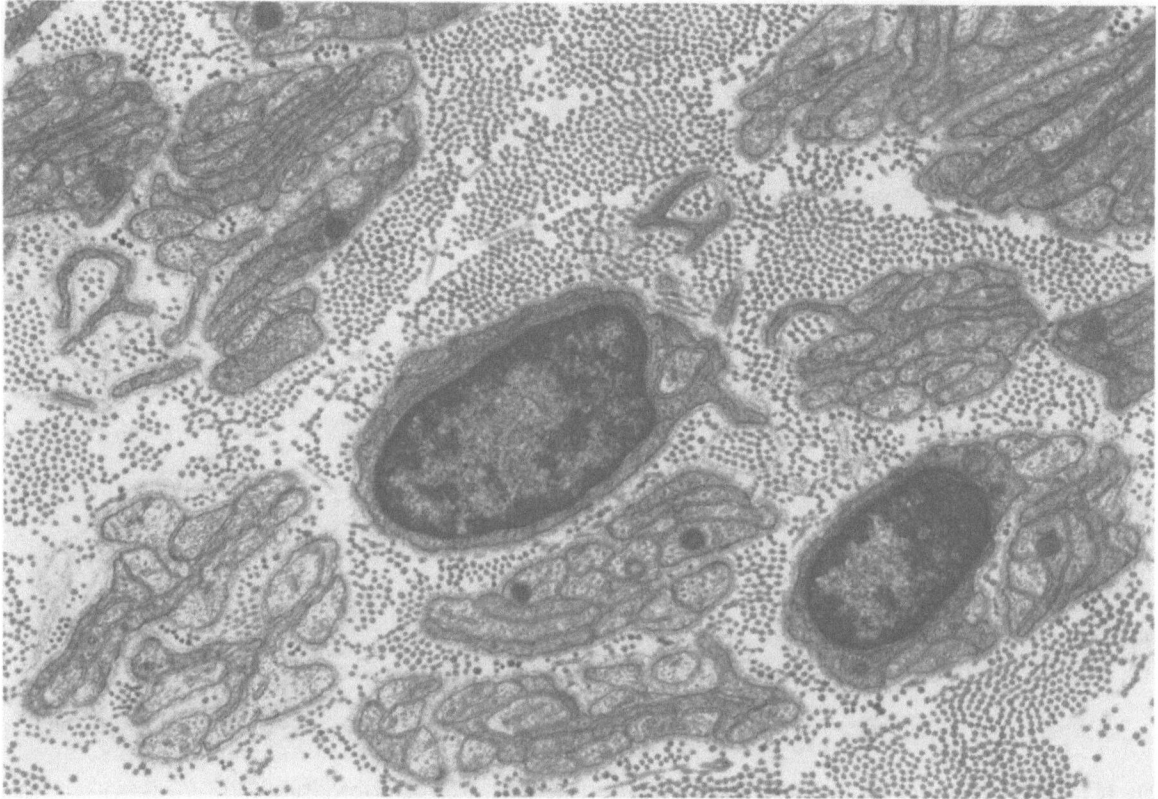

Fig. 16.6. TS. Distal end of transected nerve showing Schwann cells but no axons. (EM × 17 500)

the lengthening of the internode which occurs during growth of the individual. When a nerve degenerates and then regenerates, the internodal length returns to its embryonic proportion. Fibres which have undergone regeneration, therefore, have disproportionately short internodes throughout the length of the regenerated portion (Fig. 16.5D).

Segmental demyelination

When segmental demyelination occurs, the continuity of the axon is maintained but the myelin sheath is broken down over one or more internodes (segments) along the length of the fibre. Slowing of conduction of nerve impulses over the demyelinated segments can be detected electrophysiologically. Remyelination usually starts soon after the myelin sheath has been removed from around the axon, and often leads to good functional recovery especially in those cases of acute demyelinating neuropathy in which continuity of the majority of axons is maintained. Segmental demyelination is seen specifically in a small number of diseases including diphtheritic neuropathy, post-infectious

polyneuropathy, certain hereditary neuropathies and some cases of lead poisoning. Segmental demyelinating neuropathies may be divided into two main types: *primary* and *allergic* segmental demyelination.

Primary segmental demyelination

Primary demyelination occurs when Schwann cells are directly affected by toxic, ischaemic or metabolic insults and are thereby induced to destroy their own myelin sheaths without the intervention of inflammatory cells (Fig. 16.8). Such a process is seen in diphtheritic neuropathy, some hereditary neuropathies and lead poisoning, in addition to minor degrees in less severe trauma and ischaemia. Primary demyelination can also be induced experimentally by the injection of diphtheria toxin or lysolecithin into the nerve.

Allergic segmental demyelination

One example of allergic segmental demyelination is experimental allergic neuritis where an animal is sensitised to peripheral nerve myelin basic protein

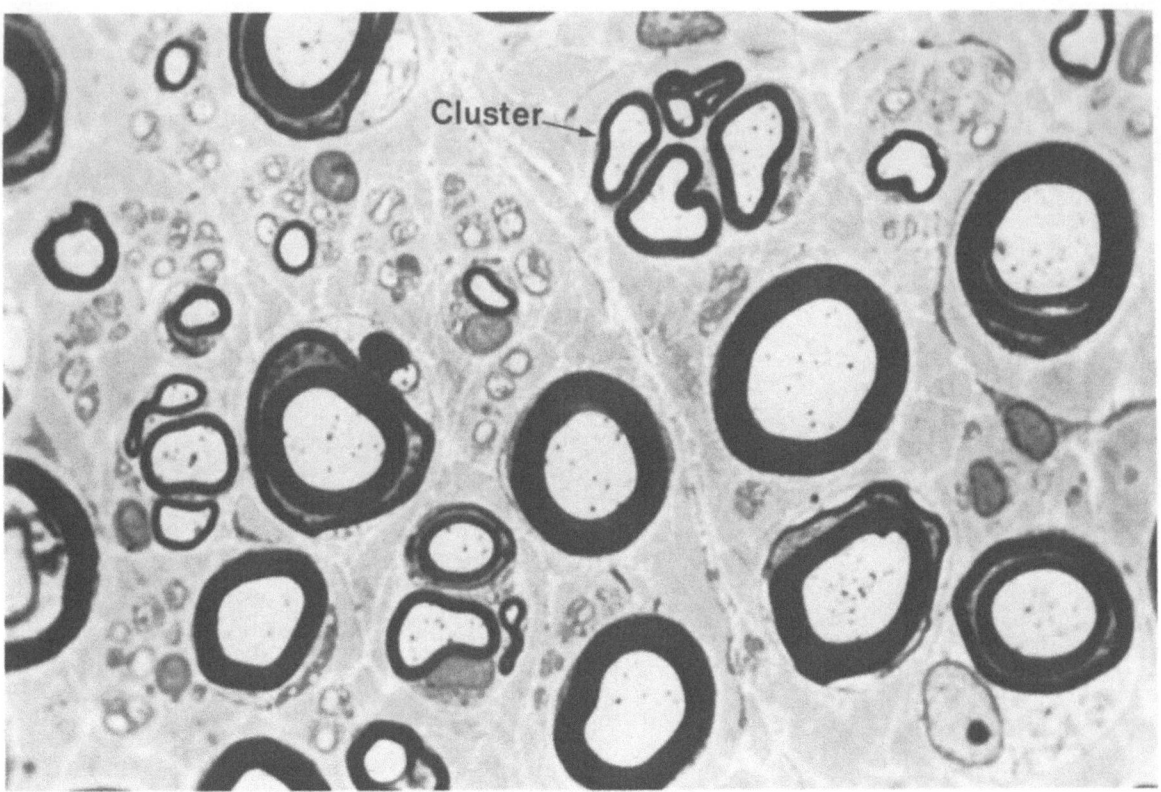

Fig. 16.7. TS of nerve showing clusters of regenerating myelinated fibres distal to the site of nerve damage. (1-μm resin section × 1860)

and the myelin sheaths are then attacked and broken down by activated macrophages in the presence of lymphocytes. The Schwann cells in this disease appear to play little part in the destruction of the myelin sheaths (Fig. 16.9) and the axons are for the most part preserved. *Acute post-infective polyneuritis* (Guillain–Barré syndrome) seems to be due to a similar mechanism of demyelination.

Detection of segmental demyelination and remyelination

Although the clinical onset and progression of the peripheral neuropathy with relatively early recovery of a severely affected patient may suggest that segmental demyelination is the major pathology, electrophysiological studies and nerve biopsy may be necessary to confirm the segmental demyelination.

Maximal nerve conduction velocities, when measured through the skin in a normal individual, are 58–72 m per second in the radial nerve and 47–51 m per second in the peroneal nerve. In demyelinating neuropathies, the conduction vel-

ocities may be severely reduced, often to below 20 m per second.

Histological verification of segmental demyelination may be obtained by nerve biopsy although this may not be possible if the affected regions of the nerve are inaccessible, for example when it is mainly the spinal roots that are involved, as in many cases of Guillain–Barré syndrome. Classically, segmental demyelination and remyelination are detected in teased nerve fibres. Widening of the node of Ranvier is usually the earliest sign of segmental demyelination; the myelin sheaths retract from the node and then demyelination may progress to involve the whole internode. In *primary* segmental demyelination, much of the myelin is broken down by the parent Schwann cells, which then undergo mitosis and begin the process of remyelination. When myelin breakdown is extensive, macrophages may also move into the nerve and become involved in myelin degradation. Myelin breakdown in *allergic* segmental demyelination is primarily by macrophages but prior to remyelination, Schwann cells in the affected internodes undergo mitosis.

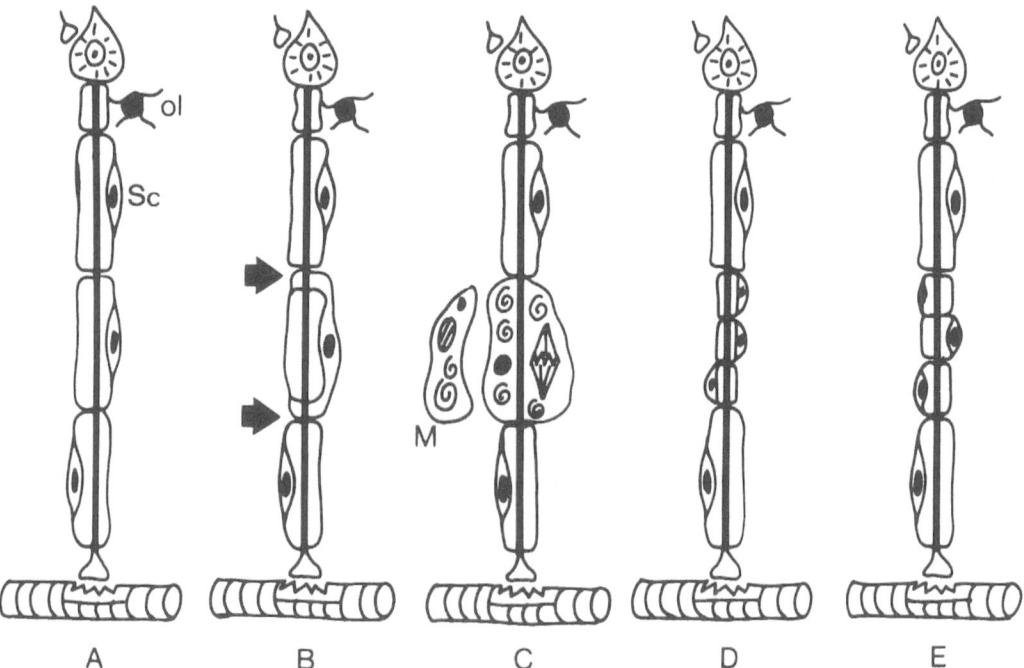

Fig. 16.8. Primary segmental demyelination.
A Normal nerve and muscle, Schwann cell and myelin sheath (*Sc*). Oligodendrocyte (*ol*).
B Early segmental demyelination with retraction of myelin sheaths from the nodes of Ranvier and widening of nodal gaps (*arrows*).
C Breakdown of a segment of myelin by the Schwann cell, shown here in mitosis. Axon preserved. Macrophage (*M*).
D Early remyelination.
E Reestablishment of normal myelin thickness but retention of short internodal lengths.

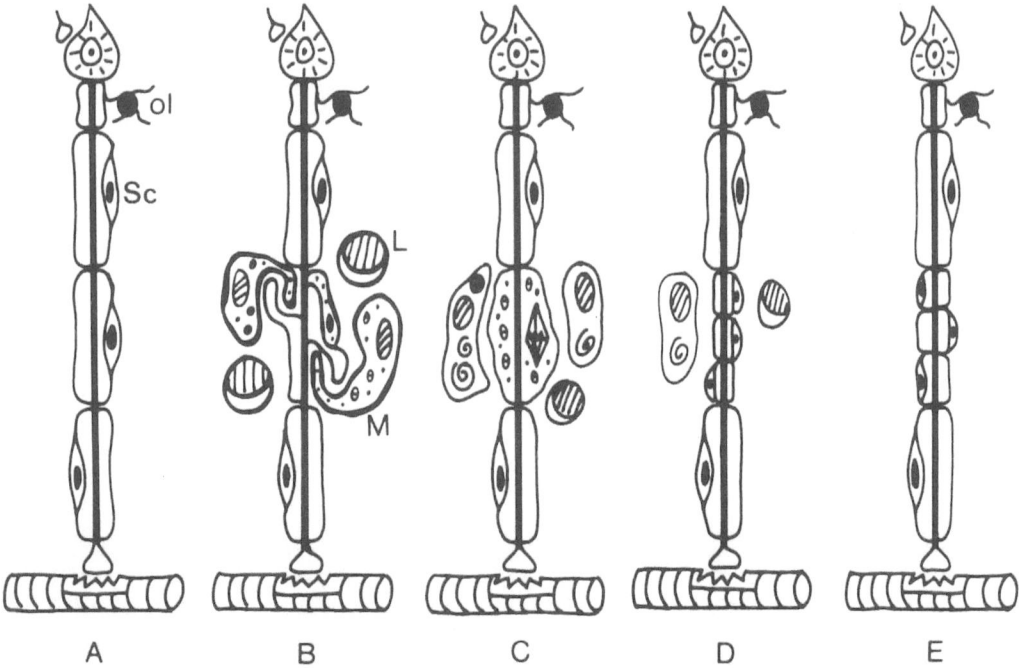

Fig. 16.9. Allergic segmental demyelination.
A Normal nerve and muscle. Schwann cells (*Sc*) and myelin sheath. Oligodendrocyte (*ol*).
B Destruction of the myelin sheath by macrophages (*M*) in the presence of lymphocytes (*L*). Axon preserved.
C Demyelinated segment of nerve. Schwann cell mitosis.
D Remyelination.
E Reconstitution of myelin sheath thickness but internodes remain short.

Remyelination begins within a few days of segmental demyelination. In some fibres, segmental demyelination may be limited to widening of the nodal gap, in which case remyelination may occur by extension of the myelin sheath back across the demyelinated zone. This only seems to occur, however, if the nodal gap widening is less than 15 μm. When the nodal gap is wider, up to 40 μm, a single Schwann cell migrates into the gap to myelinate the axon and form a short, intercalated segment (Fig. 16.10). In the more severely affected nerve fibres, myelin breakdown occurs throughout the length of the internode and remyelination of the whole segment is effected by two or three Schwann cells each reverting to the original embryonic length of 300–400 μm (Fig. 16.10a). In the early stages of remyelination, the myelin sheaths are very thin and they gradually increase in thickness as the recovery period progresses. Teased fibres, therefore, are ideal for detecting the various stages of demyelination ranging from nodal gap widening to longer lengths of demyelination. Remyelination can also be detected in teased fibres (Fig. 16.10). Conduction velocities across the remyelinating segments return towards normal as the myelin sheath thickens. Past episodes of segmental demyelination and remyelination can be detected in teased fibre preparations as the much shorter remyelinated internodes are intercalated between internodes of normal length. However, in nerves where regeneration following axonal degeneration has occurred, all the distal internodes are short and of the same length.

Although segmental demyelination may be difficult to detect in paraffin sections, examination of *1 μm resin sections* may be more rewarding. Widening of the gaps at the node of Ranvier, together with demyelinated and remylinating segments may be detected in longitudinal sections. Demyelination and the early stages of remyelination may also be observed in transverse sections of resin-embedded nerve. The presence of normal axons more than 4–5 μm in diameter with no myelin sheaths is an indication of demyelination, whereas a normal large-diameter axon surrounded by an in-

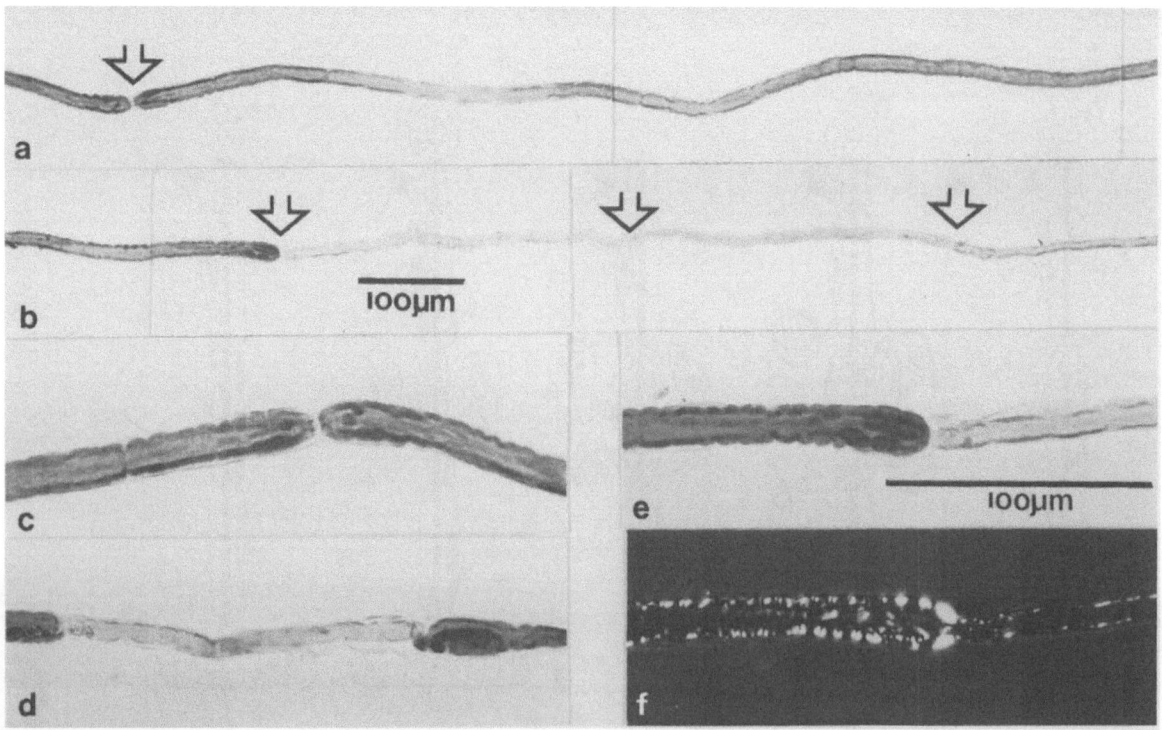

Fig. 16.10. Normal nodes of Ranvier and remyelination in teased nerve fibres stained with osmium tetroxide.
a and b A single fibre with arrows marking the nodes of Ranvier. The internodal length in the norml, thickly myelinated part of the fibre is 1150 μm whereas the thinly remyelinated segments are only 300μm in length. ($\times$47)
c Normal node of Ranvier. ($\times$352)
d Intercalated remyelinating segment 130 μm in length. (352)
e Node of Ranvier with a normal myelin sheath (*left*) and a remyelinating segment (*right*). ($\times$352)
f Same node as **e** viewed in polarised light showing birefringent myelin in normal and remyelinating segments. ($\times$352)

appropriately thin myelin sheath suggests re-myelination. Care must be taken to differentiate the normal axons in segmental demyelination from the swollen, densely staining axons just proximal to a site of axonal injury or at the site of axonal swelling in some toxic neuropathies; in these cases, focal swelling of the axon may cause thinning of the surrounding myelin sheath. Once remyelination is complete and the normal axon: myelin sheath ratio has been re-established, it may be difficult to detect evidence of past demyelination and remyelination in sectioned nerve.

In *allergic* segmental demyelination, associated with acute idiopathic (post-infective) polyneuritis (Guillain–Barré syndrome), there may be extensive lymphocytic and macrophage infiltration in the nerves. Electron microscopy has shown that the myelin sheaths are stripped from the axon and removed from the Schwann cell by invading macrophages in the presence of lymphocytes (Fig. 16.9). In this way allergic segmental de-myelination differs from primary segmental de-myelination in which disruption of the myelin sheath is effected by the Schwann cell alone. Remyelination following allergic segmental de-myelination follows the same pattern as described above.

Hypertrophic neuropathy

Hypertrophic neuropathies present with a distinctive picture of a chronic, disabling neuropathy, thickened nerves, gross slowing of conduction, often to 2–10 m per second, and a distinctive histological appearance of *'onion-bulb' whorls* in the affected nerves (Fig. 16.11). In teased preparations, evidence of extensive segmental demyelination and remyelination is seen, but the onion-bulb whorls are only truly appreciated in transverse sections of paraffin- or resin-embedded nerve. The whorls may be 30 μm or more in diameter and are formed from imbricated or interleaving lamellar Schwann cell processes encircling a central large-diameter axon. Frequently, the central axon is demyelinated and thus has no myelin sheath, or it is in the process of remyelination and is surrounded by only a very thin myelin sheath.

Experimental evidence suggests that hyper-trophic neuropathies are due to repeated de-myelination and remyelination either in response to an external insult or as a result of an inherent defect in Schwann cells. Nerves from patients with long-standing hypertrophic neuropathies may show very

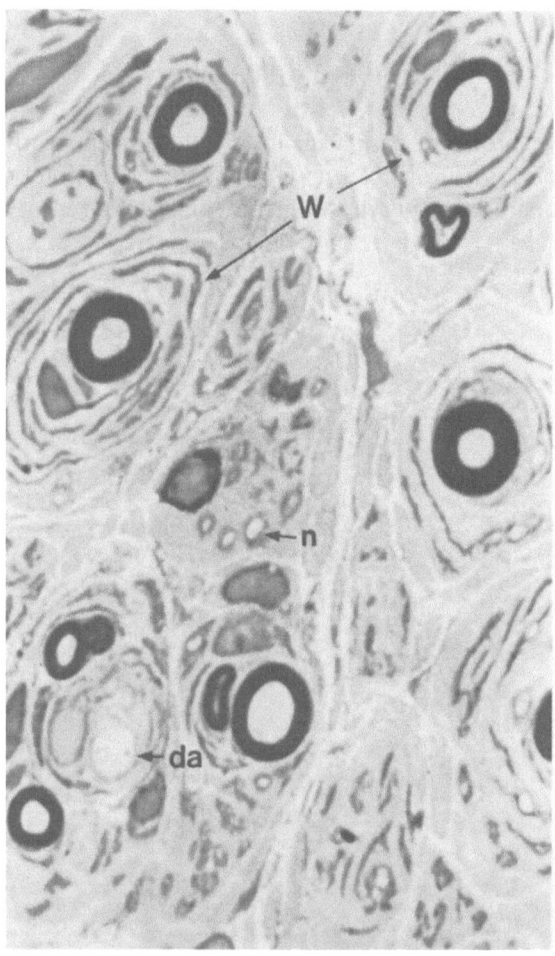

Fig. 16.11. Hypertrophic neuropathy. 'Onion-bulb' whorls (*W*) are composed of multiple Schwann cell lamellae surrounding a central myelinated axon. Demyelinated axon (*da*). Non-myelinated axons (*n*). Resin section stained with toluidine blue and basic fuchsin. (× 1370)

extensive axonal loss in addition to segmental demyelination.

The histological picture of hypertrophic neuro-pathy is found in a number of diseases; some are hereditary whereas others are due to relapsing segmental demyelinating neuropathies. For the most part, nerves throughout the body are involved in a symmetrical manner in hypertrophic neurop-athy. Localised swellings of peripheral nerve also form at sites of chronic peripheral nerve compres-sion and these lesions may superficially resemble the histological appearances of hypertrophic neuropathy. However, the cellular whorls in com-pressive lesions are due to perineurial cell migration into the nerve and compartmentation around the compressed axons. Unfortunately, this lesion has been referred to as 'localised hypertrophic neuropathy' when it bears no relationship to generalised hypertrophic polyneuropathy.

Peripheral nerve diseases

Disorders of peripheral nerve function and peripheral neuropathies may be due to destruction or malfunction of cells within the spinal cord, sensory neurons in the dorsal root ganglia, or lesions which affect the nerve roots, nerve trunks, or the terminal ramifications of motor and sensory nerves (Fig. 16.12). When either a motor neuron in the spinal cord or a sensory neuron in a dorsal root ganglion is destroyed, the axon degenerates and no regeneration of the cell occurs. If the disease process affects the neuron more peripherally, either by damage to the axon or by inducing segmental

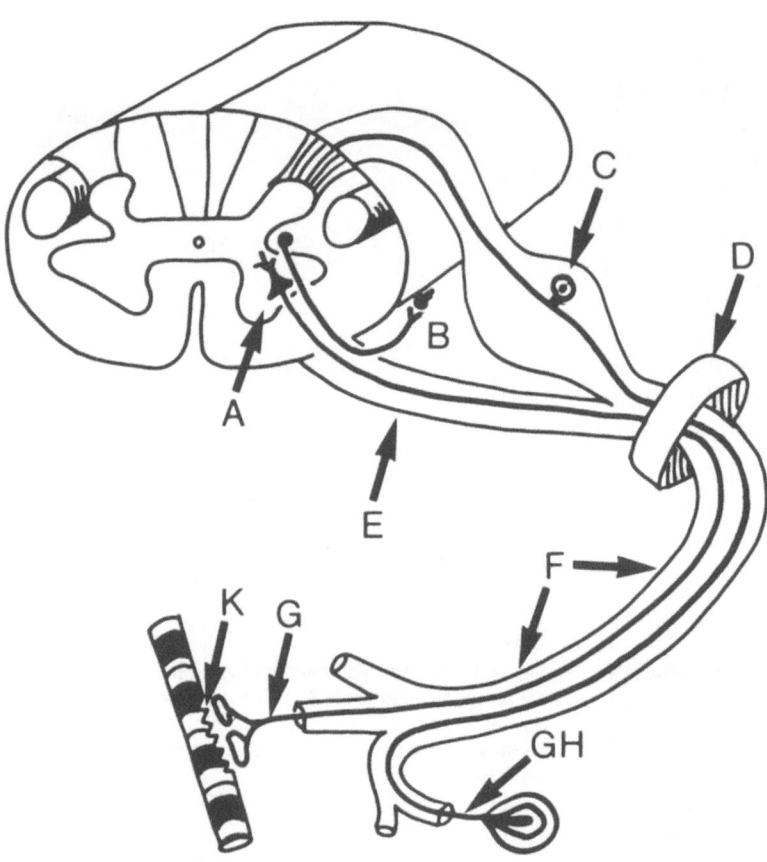

Fig. 16.12. Anatomical sites of damage in major disorders of peripheral nerves.

A *Anterior horn cells*
  Destructive lesions of the cord
  Motor neuron disease
  Spinal muscular atrophy
  Poliomyelitis
B *Autonomic neuropathies*
  Diabetes
  Amyloidosis
  Familial dysautonomia
  Fabry's disease
C *Sensory ganglia*
  Hereditary sensory neuropathies
  Herpes zoster
D *Spinal canal and intervertebral foramina*
  Trauma
  Nerve or root compression
E *Nerve roots*
  Post-infectious polyradiculopathy
  (Guillain–Barré syndrome)

F *Nerve trunks (with or without root involvement)*
  Trauma
  Compression
  Vascular disease
  Demyelination in toxic neuropathies
  Metabolic neuropathies
  Diabetes
  Amyloid
  Guillain–Barré syndrome
  Peroneal muscular atrophy
  Hypertrophic neuropathies
  Disorders of lipid metabolism
  Neuropathies in malignant disease
G *Distal axonopathies (dying-back neuropathies)*
  Toxic neuropathies
  Porphyria
  Vitamin deficiences
H *Leprosy*
K *Motor end-plate disorders*
  Myasthenia gravis

demyelination, then varying degrees of re-generation and re-establishment of function may occur. Good recovery from a peripheral neuropathy is more likely if the axon remains intact, as in segmental demyelination.

In some peripheral neuropathies, particularly those that affect the whole length of the nerve, information regarding the disease process may be acquired by peripheral nerve biopsy. However, in other cases in which the pathological lesion is restricted to an inaccessible part of the peripheral nervous system, such as a nerve root or dorsal root ganglion, nerve biopsy may be very unrewarding. In disorders which are predominantly motor neuro-pathies, nerve biopsy is usually not justified but information regarding the severity and chronicity of the disease process may be obtained from muscle biopsies.

Figure 16.12 summaries the anatomical distribution of lesions found in the major peripheral nerve diseases; it is upon this basis that this account of peripheral nerve disorders will proceed. A more detailed and comprehensive classification of neuromuscular disorders has been published by the World Federation of Neurology (1968) (see Further Reading) and a clinically orientated classification is given in Chap. 17 (Table 17.4).

Destructive lesions of the spinal cord

Localised damage to the spinal cord may occur during *trauma*, or may be due to compression by intrinsic and extrinsic cord *tumours*. *Multiple sclerosis* plaques or *infarction* of the cord following vascular occlusion may cause localised damage. In most cases, the more significant neurological signs arise from interruption of the long ascending sensory tracts and the descending motor tracts in the spinal cord. However, when the lower cervical or lumbosacral regions of the cord are damaged, destruction of anterior horn cells may lead to significant denervation, weakness and wasting of limb muscles. *Syringomyelia*, in particular, frequently affects the lower cervical cord and in addition to loss of pain and temperature sensation, there may be significant denervation and muscle wasting in either one or both arms as the syrinx expands in the centre of the cord and leads to anterior horn cell destruction.

Diseases affecting motor neurons

Motor neuron disease is a term usually reserved for a group of diseases with a wide spectrum of progressive upper and lower motor neuron para-lysis involving the limbs and, in some cases, the cranial nerves. Three clinical forms are described, namely, progressive muscular astrophy, amyo-trophic lateral sclerosis and progressive bulbar palsy. A familial form of the disease also occurs. Patients present, usually in adult life, with pro-gressive weakness and wasting of the small muscles of the hands, followed by atrophy of the proximal limb girdle muscles involving both shoulders and the pelvic girdle. Fasciculation is often seen in the affected muscles of the limbs and the tongue. Together with the obvious lower motor neuron lesion, there is evidence of upper motor neuron involvement with extensor plantar responses, re-tained or even brisk tendon reflexes and increased muscle tone.

Post-mortem studies show some reduction in the size of the spinal cord and more noticeably, atrophy of the anterior spinal roots. Motor neurons are lost from the motor cortex and axonal loss is seen in the corticospinal tracts, and to some extent in the spinocerebellar tracts in the spinal cord (Fig. 4.5). Examination of the anterior horns, particularly in the cervical region, shows a reduction in the number of anterior horn cells. The diagnosis of motor neuron disease may be confirmed clinically by electromyography and by muscle biopsy where there is evidence of denervation and reinnervation with widespread muscle fibre type grouping (see Chap. 17). As motor neurons disappear and their axons degenerate, collateral sprouting occurs from the surviving axons within the muscle. It is these collateral sprouts which reinnervate denervated muscle fibres. When the surviving neurons them-selves degenerate, in the later stages of the disease, the amount of denervation may be relatively greater, leading to rapid clinical deterioration.

In *spinal muscular atrophy*, the neuronal de-generation is usually confined to the anterior horn cells in the spinal cord. There is a wide spectrum of clinical presentation in this disease (see Chap. 17). The most severe form is Werdnig–Hoffmann disease in which affected infants are floppy at birth and usually die with extensive muscle denervation in the first year or so of life. Milder forms occur where the patient is not only less severely affected but the disease may only become obvious at a later stage. There are rarely any sensory signs in this disease and because spinal muscular atrophy affects proximal limb muscles among others, the differential diag-nosis is often between this condition and a muscular dystrophy. In both Werdnig–Hoffmann disease and the milder, later onset, Kugelberg–Welander form of spinal muscular atrophy there is an autosomal recessive pattern of inheritance. Electromyography may reveal the neurogenic nature of the muscle disease and denervation and reinnervation can be recognised on muscle biopsy (see Chap. 17).

Apart from the anterior horn cell degeneration that occurs in motor neuron disease and spinal muscular atrophy, widespread destruction of motor neurons may occur in *poliomyelitis*. In severe, rapidly fatal cases of poliomyelitis, phagocytosis of involved motor neurons may be seen and there may even be patchy necrosis within the cord. Those patients who survive show varying degrees of neurogenic atrophy in their muscles.

Diseases of sensory ganglia

Hereditary sensory neuropathies

This group of diseases is classified according to the pattern of inheritance, the clinical presentation and, to some extent, the pathology.

Many cases of chronic progressive sensory neuropathy with an autosomal dominant pattern of inheritance have been reported. There is dissociated sensory loss with impairment of pain and temperature sensation out of all proportion to the impairment of touch. Relapsing, painless ulcers appear on the toes and heels during the first two decades and may eventually lead to the loss of digits; the hands may be involved later. Motor function is not altered until later in the disease and death may result from uncontrolled infection or secondary amyloidosis. *Pathological* studies show degeneration and loss of sensory neurons in the posterior root ganglia and degeneration of axons in the sensory nerves. Sural nerve biopsies have shown that non-myelinated fibres are most affected in the dominant hereditary sensory neuropathies with some sparing of large myelinated fibres, but in recessive forms of the disease, myelinated fibres degenerate and large numbers of non-myelinated fibres are preserved. Vacuolated fibroblasts are seen in the endoneurium in many cases of hereditary sensory neuropathy.

Familial dysautonomia (Riley–Day syndrome) with widespread autonomic dysfunction and a deficiency of plasma dopamine beta-hydroxylase is an autosomal recessive condition occurring especially in Ashkenazi Jews. The cause of death is usually pulmonary infection, associated with scoliosis and acute disturbances of autonomic function

that are predominantly of central origin. An unusual type of sensory neuropathy is characteristically present. Sural nerve biopsies in this condition reveal a gross reduction of non-myelinated axons and no myelinated fibres above 12 μm in diameter.

Herpes zoster

One important viral disease which affects posterior root ganglia is herpes zoster due to infection by varicella zoster. A vesicular rash develops in the area of skin supplied by the affected neurons. Varicella zoster has been identified in the sensory neurons by immunofluorescence and virus particles can be isolated from the vesicular rash and from epidermal cells. The infection may be a recrudescence of the varicella zoster or due to reinfection. Autopsy studies show that the affected spinal or cranial nerve sensory ganglia are swollen, congested and haemorrhagic in the acute stages of herpes zoster. Individual sensory neurons may be shrunken, vacuolated or be in the process of destruction by phagoctyic cells. Perivascular cuffing by lymphocytes and plasma cells is also seen in the affected posterior root ganglia.

Traumatic and compressive nerve lesions

Peripheral nerves may be damaged by mechanical trauma or by compression in the spinal root zone and in the intravertebral foramina by prolapsed intervertebral discs, or by bony irregularities in spondylitic spines. Normal movements of the limb may traumatize peripheral nerves if they are dragged across an obstruction or their normal longitudinal mobility is restricted. Furthermore, nerve compression or entrapment occurs in relation to disordered joints, particularly at the elbow and knee; the median nerve may also be compressed in the carpal tunnel. Severe trauma to nerve trunks, often with complete transection, may complicate bony fractures, particularly in the limbs.

The effects of nerve trauma will vary according to the site and severity of the damage. When injury to the nerve is slight and short in duration, there may be only a temporary impairment of nerve conduction, and function may return to the nerve with no noticeable structural damage. *Mild trauma* may result in segmental demyelination; this occurs particularly in acute compressive lesions where the myelin sheaths are distorted and subsequent segmental demyelination ensues. Electrophysiologically, there is slowing of conduction in the affected region of the nerve but following alleviation of the compression, normal function may be restored. In the more *severe traumatic* lesions, axons are transected, the distal portions of the nerve degenerate and, clinically, the patients may have sensory loss and muscle denervation with weakness, wasting and fibrillation in the affected muscle groups.

Recovery of function depends on the ability of the nerves to regenerate and upon the proximity of the site of injury to the site of innervation. If, for example, there is complete transection of the sciatic nerve in the thigh with haemorrhage and scar tissue formation between the severed ends of the nerve, growth and regeneration of axons from the proximal to the distal stump of the nerve may be severely hampered. Functional recovery may then be poor or non-existent. However, when a relatively minor crush injury to a nerve occurs near its site of termination, regeneration of axons is often facilitated by the preservation of anatomical structures such as the perineurium. With axon growth rates of 1–2 mm per day, effective reinnervation may be rapid, especially when distances involved are short. Deep sensation and pain are usually the first modalities to return and the induction of vasodilatation and sweating in the skin may give some indication of recovery of autonomic function.

Histological examination of nerve biopsies distal to the site of injury may be useful in assessing the severity of a traumatic lesion, and the speed and degree of axonal regeneration. Following complete transection, there may be no myelinated or non-myelinated axons in nerves distal to the site of injury (Fig. 16.6). Regenerating myelinated axons may be detected, however, as they form small clusters of regenerating sprouts (Fig. 16.7).

Neuropathies due to vascular disease

Damage to peripheral nerves is usually due to disease of the small vessels. The blood supply of peripheral nerves is from the longitudinally orientated epineurial arteries which extend anastomosing branches through the perineurium into the endoneurial compartment of the nerve. Due to this anastomotic network and the frequent arterial contributions from larger vessels along the length of the nerve, occlusion of even the major epineurial arteries rarely causes complete infarction of the nerve. However, vasculitic lesions in polyarteritis nodosa, rheumatoid arthritis, and other collagen vascular diseases, cause extensive axonal degeneration in peripheral nerves.

Patients may present with a distal sensory neuropathy affecting the hands and feet or, if the vasculitis is severe, there may be a sensorimotor neuropathy. In *mild* cases, the major peripheral nerve lesion is segmental demyelination with slowing of conduction in the affected nerves. In more *severe* cases, however, there is axonal degeneration, and biopsy of a distal nerve may reveal varying degrees of nerve fibre loss. Large myelinated fibres are, in general, the first to be damaged, then small myelinated fibres and, lastly, the non-myelinated fibres. Clusters of small regenerating axons may be seen in less severe neuropathies but when involvement of the vasa nervorum is extensive, few, if any, myelinated axons may be preserved within the nerve. The distal distribution of the neuropathy may be due to the greater probability of a long nerve being damaged by ischaemia.

Toxic neuropathies

Many of the major cells in the central and peripheral nervous system have extended cytoplasm, often in the form of long processes. Such cells include neurons, oligodendroglial cells, astrocytes and Schwann cells. Protein synthesis and transport mechanisms are very important in these cells for the maintenance of cytoplasmic and membrane structure in the extended cell processes. A number of the toxic substances which cause peripheral neuropathies or long tract damage in the CNS may well interfere with either protein synthesis or transport systems within the cells.

To some extent the brain and peripheral nerves are protected from the actions of toxins by the presence of the blood–brain and the blood–nerve barrier, although such a barrier does not exist in the posterior root sensory ganglia. Nevertheless toxic agents do enter the central and peripheral nervous system; among these agents are drugs and many of the organic compounds used in industry and agriculture.

The main sites of toxic damage to nerve cells and axons in the spinal cord and peripheral nerves are illustrated in Fig. 16.13. Neuron cell bodies may be destroyed as in the neuronopathies affecting the posterior root ganglia due to Doxorubicin and mercury toxicity (Fig. 16.14a). The majority of toxins affect either the distal ends of central or peripheral axons, i.e. axonopathies, or they damage the Schwann cells and cause segmental demyelination.

Toxic Neuropathies – Central & Peripheral

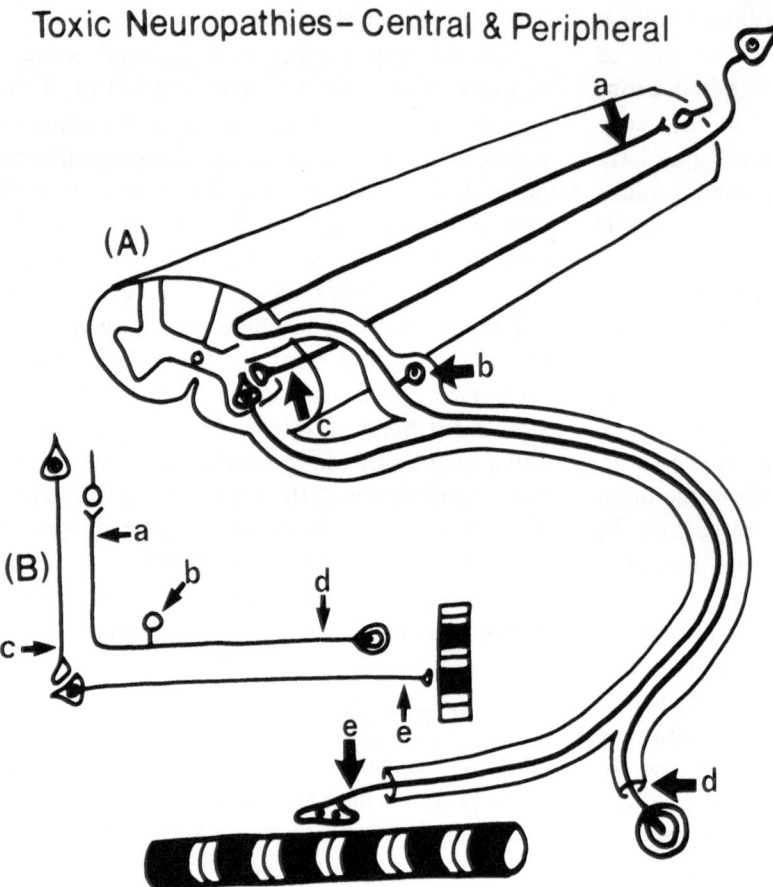

Fig. 16.13. Patterns of damage in toxic neuropathies. **A** The distal ends of the gracile tracts (*a*) and the cortico-spinal tracts (*c*) in the spinal cord together with the distal ends of motor (*e*) and sensory (*d*) fibres in peripheral nerves are the most common sites of degeneration in toxic axonopathies. Sensory neurons in the dorsal root ganglia (*b*) may be damaged in neuronopathies.
B Diagrammatic form of **A** used in Fig. 16.14. Symbols *a–e* are the same as in **A**.

Axonopathies—dying-back neuropathies

In the majority of toxic neuropathies it is only the distal ends of the axons which are damaged. Some toxins such as thallium, arsenic and the nitrofuran drugs appear to interfere with pyruvate metabolism and thus mimic thiamine deficiency. These substances cause a distal axonopathy (Fig. 16.14C) in which the terminal portions of sensory and motor axons degenerate, particularly in the hands and feet. Other toxins, particularly hexacarbons, acrylamide and organophosphorus compounds, cause degeneration not only of the distal ends of the peripheral axons but also the distal ends of axons in the spinal cord. Thus the terminal portions of the axons in the gracile tract of the posterior columns and the corticospinal tracts are damaged (central–peripheral–distal axonopathy) (Fig. 16.14D).

Some drugs may affect only central tracts. Clioquinol, for example, causes a central–distal axonopathy (Fig. 16.14B) affecting long fibres in the spinal cord and in the optic tracts; this drug causes subacute myelo-optico neuropathy (SMON).

Clinically, toxic axonopathies present with a glove and stocking sensory loss and a slowly evolving distal motor impairment as it is the longest, largest axons which are first affected. Because the affected axons undergo retrograde degeneration (dying-back phenomenon) the course of the illness is predictable. Clinical signs ascend the limbs and involve shorter nerves if the intoxication continues, but almost complete recovery of the neuropathy may occur if intoxication ceases. CNS signs of spasticity and ataxia due to dying-back of the axons in the long ascending and descending tracts in the spinal cord may be masked by the peripheral neuropathy, but as the neuropathy recovers, the CNS signs become prominent and may be the major residual disability. Removal of the toxin often carries an excellent prognosis for the peripheral nerves, as the cell body remains intact and regeneration of the distal axons occurs with reconnection to target organs. Recovery of function takes place in the proximal–distal gradient as the shorter axons are last to be affected and have less distance to regenerate. Little, if any, axonal regeneration occurs in the CNS tracts in the spinal cord, so spasticity and ataxia may remain unresolved.

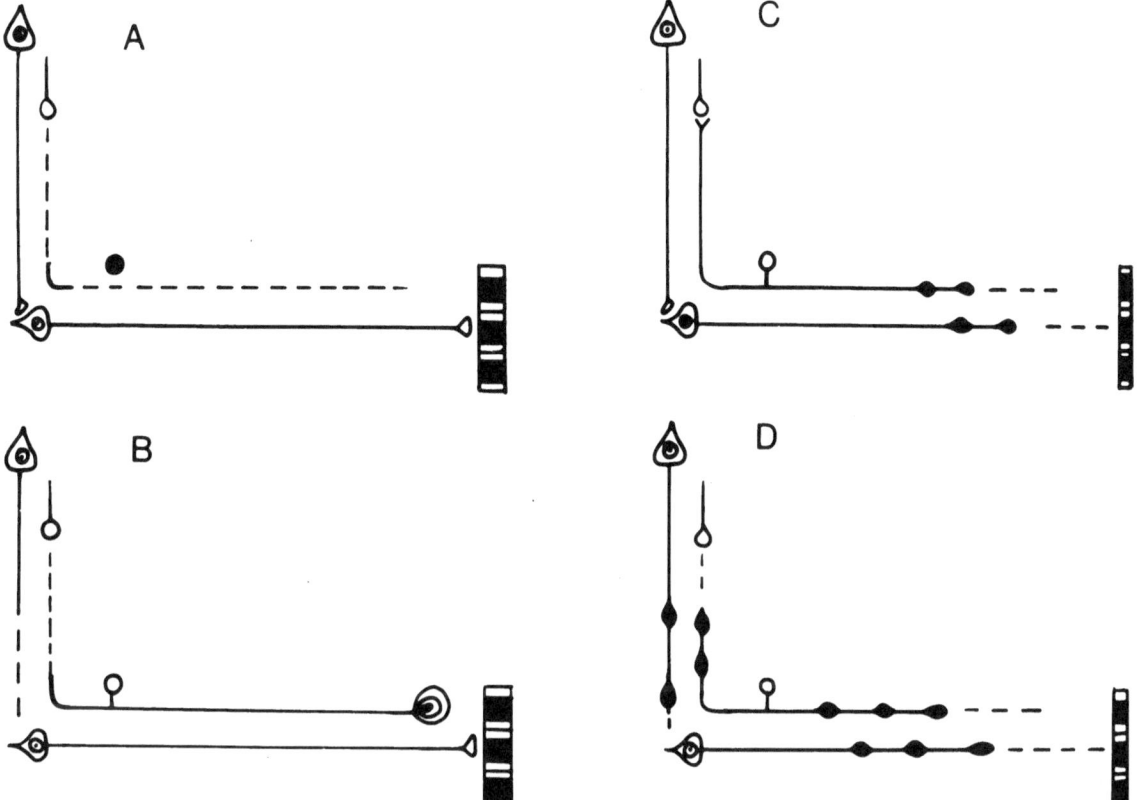

Fig. 16.14. Toxic neuropathies—central and peripheral.
A Neuronopathies with destruction of sensory neurons in dorsal root ganglia and degeneration of distal and central sensory axons, e.g. Doxorubicin disrupts DNA synthesis; mercury—action unknown.
B Central–distal axonopathy: degeneration of long tracts in the spinal cord, e.g. Clioquinol (SMON)—action unknown.
C Peripheral–distal axonopathy affecting the long distal sensory and motor fibres, e.g. thallium—disturbance of pyruvate metabolism; Isoniazid—disturbance of pyridoxal metabolism.
D Central–peripheral–distal axonopathy. Degeneration of long central and peripheral fibres, e.g. hexacarbons—inhibit glycolysis; acrylamide—action unknown; organophosphorus compounds—phosphorylation of esterases; carbon disulphide—inhibits oxidative phosphorylation. The actions of these toxins may cause local disturbance of axoplasmic flow.

The precise *metabolic* lesion is known in very few cases of toxic neuropathy but, with a number of substances, the structural changes in the axons may reflect either a generalised or localised defect in axoplasmic transport. There are two main components of axoplasmic transport. Fast transport at 400–450 mm per day is probably associated with the smooth endoplasmic reticulum within the axons. Slow axoplasmic transport has two main components. One component moves at 1–2 mm per day and transmits neurofilaments, most tubulin and some actin. The other component moves at 2–5 mm per day and conveys actin, some tubulin and other proteins.

One of the features of a number of toxic neuropathies is the appearance of *axonal swellings*, particularly in the regions proximal to nodes of Ranvier (Fig. 16.15). In hexacarbon intoxication, as for example in 'glue sniffers', focal enlargement occurs in the long peripheral and central axons.

Each enlargement contains a mass of 10-nm filaments similar to neurofilaments; mitochondria and other axonal organelles are displaced to the periphery of the axon and the myelin sheath surrounding the fibre is thin and attenuated. The distal axon becomes shrunken and atrophic and eventually degenerates. Another form of focal axon swelling is seen in large diameter, long central and peripheral axons in tri-ortho-cresyl phosphate poisoning, but in this case the axon swellings contain large numbers of angulated, vesicular profiles similar to smooth endoplasmic reticulum. In both these intoxications, the pathological changes seen in the nerves may represent local disturbances of axoplasmic flow but the metabolic lesion may be different in each case.

In addition to toxic neuropathies due to direct intoxication, distal axonopathies may be a feature of *alcoholism* and *vitamin deficiencies*.

Little useful clinical information may be gained

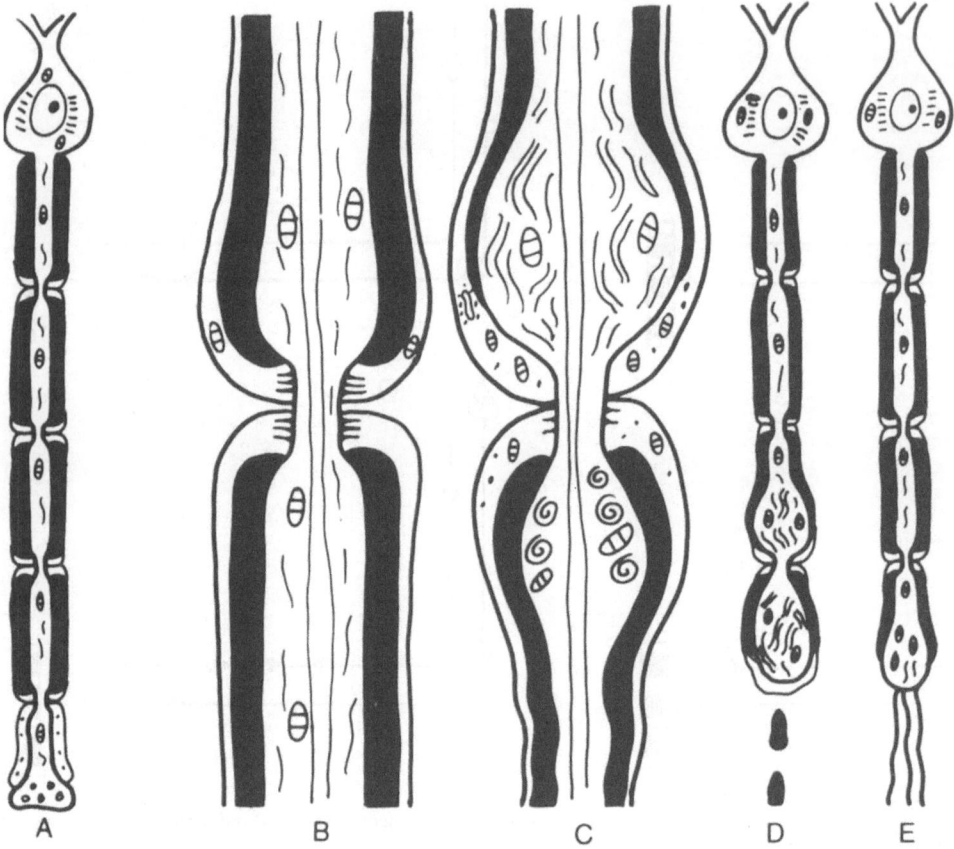

Fig. 16.15. Diagram to show the features of hexacarbon (toxic) neuropathy
A Normal neuron and axon.
B Normal node of Ranvier.
C Swelling of axon proximal to the node of Ranvier with intra-axonal accumulation of neurofilaments. The distal axon is atrophic.
D Degeneration of the axon distal to the swelling.
E Regenerative axon sprouting seen particularly following cessation of intoxication.

from nerve biopsies in patients with toxic axonopathies although muscle biopsies from distal parts of the limbs may show degeneration of the fine intramuscular nerves. However, the *pathological* findings at autopsy may be valuable in evaluating the pattern of neurological damage and possibly in identifying the toxic agent. Examination of the distal ends of the gracile tract in the medulla and the distal ends of motor and sensory nerves in the limbs should reveal the pathological pattern of a distal axonopathy. If degeneration of axons is seen throughout the ascending tracts in the dorsal columns and throughout the sensory nerves, then a neuronopathy affecting the posterior root ganglion cells is more probable.

Demyelination in toxic neuropathies

The action of some toxic agents may be due to their effects upon myelin sheaths both in the central and peripheral nervous systems. Hexachlorophene, for example, causes vacuolation and destruction of myelin sheaths in the brain and in the peripheral nerves, whereas systemically administered diphtheria toxin appears to act directly on the Schwann cells and induces segmental demyelination confined to the peripheral nervous system. Lead, on the other hand, appears at act upon endothelial cells in the brain and peripheral nerves causing disruption of permeability barriers and oedema. In lead intoxication there may be widespread segmental demyelination in the peripheral nerves.

Metabolic neuropathies

Peripheral neuropathy is a feature of a number of metabolic disorders, especially diabetes, uraemia and porphyria.

Most *diabetics* develop a symmetrical distal polyneuropathy but it is only clinically troublesome in about 5% of patients; these are usually the diabetics who are poorly controlled. When the neuropathy is mild, there is slowing of nerve conduction velocities and segmental demyelination is detectable in nerve biopsies. In the more severe cases there is axonal degeneration. Some diabetics also develop an autonomic neuropathy characterised by impotence, bladder and bowel disturbances and postural hypotension. Autonomic neuropathies are usually associated with a distal sensory neuropathy. The metabolic disorder which causes these neuropathies is not known. A symmetrical mononeuropathy also occurs in diabetics, affecting either the cranial nerves or the limb nerves; this type of neuropathy usually occurs in elderly patients with mild diabetes and is characterised by sensory loss and pain. Axonal degeneration in the nerves probably results from ischaemia due to disease of the small vessels in the nerves. A motor neuropathy may also be seen in diabetes with wasting and weakness in the thighs (diabetic amyotrophy). Muscle biopsy in such cases may reveal changes of denervation.

Patients with *uraemia* may develop a chronic distal symmetrical neuropathy which is predominantly sensory but may have a significant motor component; the neuropathy is often improved with adequate treatment by dialysis. Pathological studies show that the neuropathy is due to axonal degeneration in the distal portions of the sensory nerves particularly involving large fibres.

Apart from diabetes, the predominant lesion seen in most metabolic neuropathies is a distal axonopathy.

Amyloid neuropathy

A number of different types of protein are deposited in tissues in the various forms of amyloidosis. Peripheral neuropathy is associated with (a) autosomal dominant *hereditary* forms of amyloidosis particularly the Portuguese (Andrade) type and (b) *non-hereditary* amyloidosis due to monoclonal gammopathies when a serum-M-component or Bence-Jones proteinaemia is present.

In neuropathies associated with B-lymphocyte dyscrasias, the amyloid is related to immunoglobulin light chains whereas in familial amyloidosis the deposits are unrelated to immunoglobulin. Amyloid may be deposited in extraneural connective tissue and thus cause a compressive neuropathy, particularly carpal tunnel syndrome; or the amyloid may accumulate within the endoneurium

and be associated with a generalised polyneuropathy. Finally, the amyloid may be deposited in the walls of the intraneural vessels and lead to an ischaemic neuropathy.

Clinically, patients with both familial and nonfamilial polyneuropathy due to amyloid present with early impairment of pain and temperature sensation and autonomic disturbances.

Examination of nerve biopsies from such patients (Fig. 16.16) shows a severe reduction or absence of non-myelinated fibres, a variable loss of small myelinated axons and relative preservation of large myelinated fibres. The reasons for the selective loss of non-myelinated axons is unclear. Amyloid may be seen in the walls of endoneurial vessels and as blobs or diffuse lakes within the endoneurium. By light microscopy, the amyloid can be identified by its apple-green birefringence in polarised light and by its positive staining with Congo red. Electron microscopically, the 7–10-nm amyloid fibrils can usually be identified (Fig. 16.17).

Inflammatory disorders of peripheral nerves

Inflammation in peripheral nerves may be due to the spread of suppuration to involve local nerves, or due to virus infections such as varicella zoster with involvement of the dorsal root ganglia as described above. Direct invasion by bacteria and inflammation also occur in leprosy. Sarcoidosis and the immunological reactions observed in postinfective polyneuropathy (polyradiculopathy) (Guillain–Barré syndrome) are other types of inflammatory disorder seen in peripheral nerves.

Guillain–Barré syndrome

Guillain–Barré syndrome is the commonest cause of an acute paralytic illness in Western countries. There is a sudden onset of polyneuropathy developing in severity over a few days so that the patient may require artificial ventilation. A history of a previous viral or other infection may or may not be present. After 1–4 weeks, the patient begins to recover; the course of the disease and the completeness of recovery depend upon the severity of the original neuropathy, which is indicated clinically by the time course of recovery rather than by the severity of the paralysis. Provided that the phase of clinical deterioration is succeeded by the phase of clinical recovery within 7 days, complete clinical recovery can be expected, however severe the paralysis. Once the weakness has remained at its

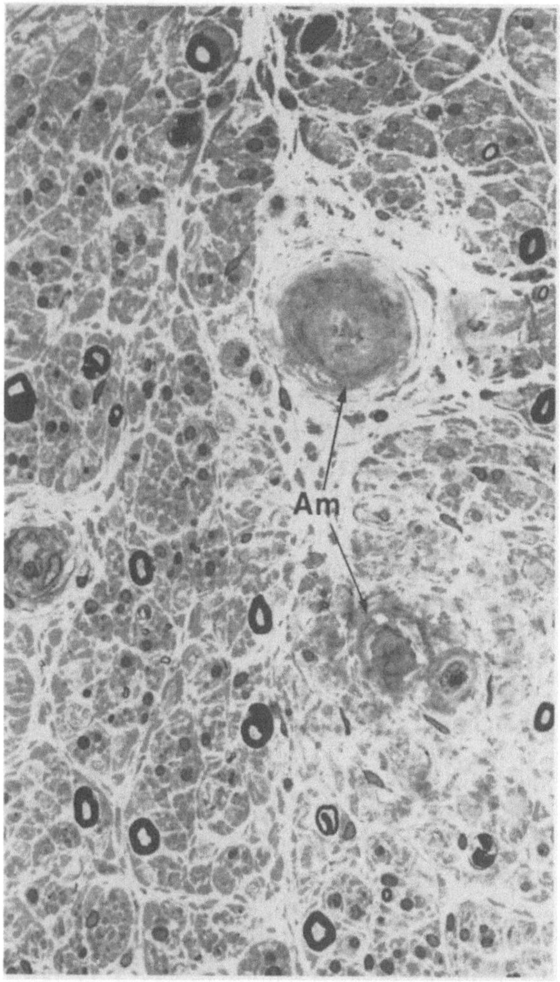

Fig. 16.16. Amyloid neuropathy: sural nerve biopsy showing amyloid (*Am*) around a vessel and in the endoneurium. There is gross loss of myelinated and non-myelinated axons. (1-μm resin section stained with toluidine blue, ×415)

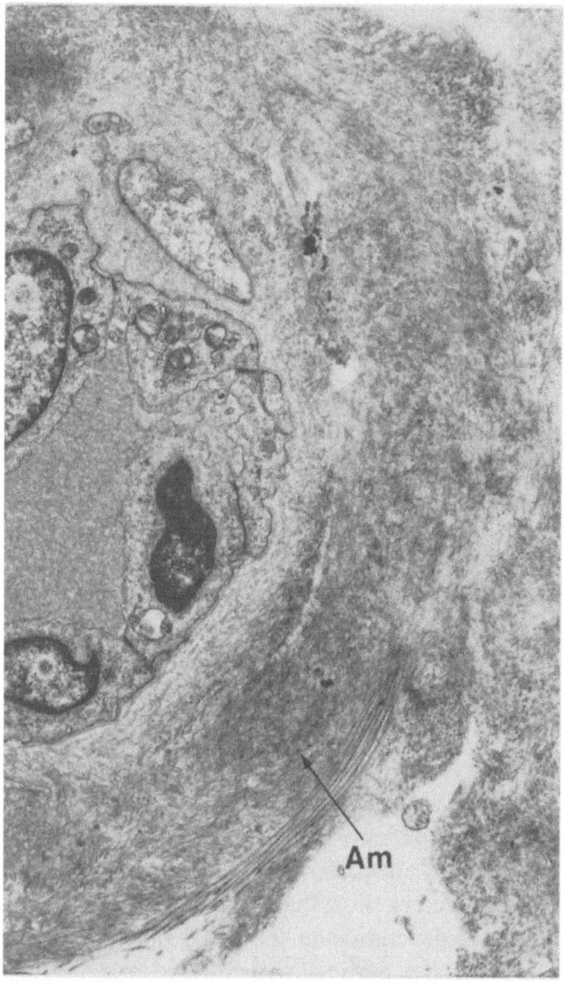

Fig. 16.17. Amyloid neuropathy. An endoneurial blood vessel (*left of picture*) with a mass of amyloid fibrils (*Am*) forming a layer around it. (EM ×7750)

most severe for 10 days or more, complete recovery becomes less likely. The prospects for recovery tend to worsen the longer its onset is delayed. The disease is fatal in about 5% of cases. Occasionally this type of neuropathy enters a chronic relapsing stage. Steroids do not improve the outcome in the acute stages, although patients who enter the relapsing phase may become steroid dependent. Plasma exchange has recently been shown to provide temporary resolution of the clinical symptoms in some cases and the dialysate can induce a polyneuropathy when it is injected into the nerves of animals.

The CSF in Guillain–Barré syndrome shows the characteristic changes of a high protein level but with few cells. Electrophysiological studies during the acute stages have shown that the neuropathy is due to *segmental demyelination* and this has been confirmed by pathological studies. Nerve biopsy is rarely required for diagnosis in the acute stages of the neuropathy. A number of important pathological studies have been performed, however, in patients dying from the disease.

In the acute stages of the disease there is perivascular accumulation of lymphocytes and macrophages in the spinal cord and in the peripheral nerves, especially in the anterior spinal nerve roots. The basic pathological process is that of allergic segmental demyelination in which macrophages strip the myelin from the axons; the Schwann cells appear to play little part in the demyelinating process but undergo mitosis and rapidly begin the process of remyelination. Pathologically, Guillain–Barré syndrome bears many similarities to experimental allergic neuritis induced in animals by sensitisation to peripheral nerve myelin.

Leprosy

Widespread in subtropical and tropical zones throughout the world, leprosy probably affects 15 000 000 people or more. The disease is caused by an acid-fast bacillus, *Mycobacterium leprae*, and is expressed as two major forms, lepromatous and tuberculoid leprosy, and as various intermediate or borderline types.

Peripheral nerves are affected in all types, but in *lepromatous leprosy* the mycobacteria are more numerous and widespread throughout the body. In the skin, the bacilli are present in foamy macrophages within the dermis; in peripheral nerves. groups of mycobacteria can be seen electron microscopically within Schwann cells, especially those associated with non-myelinated fibres. Bacilli are also present within axons. Axonal degeneration is a prominent feature and may result from the infection of Schwann cells and axons by mycobacteria.

In *tuberculoid leprosy*, granulomatous lesions, resembling sarcoid, form within the nerve and axonal degeneration occurs. Few lepra bacilli are seen but the nerves are gradually destroyed and replaced by granulomatous tissue. The resulting denervation leads to anaesthesia in the peripheral parts of the limbs with ulceration and ultimate loss of digits.

Peroneal muscular atrophy and hypertrophic neuropathy

Although not particularly common, patients with this group of diseases have characteristic clinical, electrophysiological and pathological features. The commonest type of peroneal muscular atrophy (*Charcot–Marie–Tooth disease*) has an autosomal dominant inheritance pattern and presents in the first or second decade with progressive atrophy of muscles particularly in the distal parts of the legs. Sensory signs are also present and electrophysiological studies may show gross slowing of conduction in motor and sensory peripheral nerves. Gross hypertrophy of the nerves is rarely seen but biopsies of sural and other sensory nerves reveal a characteristic pattern of onion-bulb whorls (Fig. 16.11). In the early stages of the disease,

evidence of segmental demyelination and thinly myelinated remyelinating fibres may be seen. The onion-bulb whorls at this stage are often small and are only visible in 1 μm resin sections or by electron microscopy as they consist of only one or two layers of Schwann cells surrounding a myelinated axon. Much larger onion-bulb whorls are seen in the later stages of Charcot–Marie–Tooth disease; some whorls are empty whereas others have myelinated fibres at their centre. Myelin sheath thickness varies, indicating that remyelination has followed the recurrent segmental demyelination. The whole cross-sectional area of the nerve is usually increased partly by the presence of whorls and partly by an expansion of the endoneurial connective tissue. There is a marked loss of myelinated axons in the later stages of the disease although occasional regenerating clusters may be seen at the centre of the whorls.

The results of studies in which short lengths of nerve from patients with Charcot–Marie–Tooth disease have been transplanted into immunodeficient mice, suggest that there is a basic Schwann cell defect in this type of hypertrophic neuropathy which leads to recurrent segmental demyelination and remyelination. Loss of axons, particularly in the distal parts of limbs, eventually leads to extensive muscle denervation and atrophy.

Dejerine–Sottas disease is a recessive inherited neuropathy also characterised by recurrent segmental demyelination and hypertrophic neuropathy but the muscle wasting is more widespread than in Charcot–Marie–Tooth disease. The onset of the disease is in infancy or childhood and the patient may be severely disabled as a young adult with muscle wasting, weakness and contractures in the limbs, and spinal deformity. Diagnosis can be confirmed by demonstrating thickened nerves, slowing of nerve conduction velocities and onion-bulb whorls on nerve biopsy.

Disorders of lipid metabolism

In most of the sphingolipidoses, which includes the gangliosidoses, abnormal amounts of lipid accumulate within the CNS due to deficiencies in specific intracellular enzymes (Chaps. 11 and 13). Peripheral nerves are particularly affected in two lipidoses in which there is a defect in the metabolism of myelin lipids, although even in these diseases the CNS damage overshadows the peripheral neuropathy.

Metachromatic leukodystrophy (sulphatide lipidosis)

Metachromatic leukodystrophy has a recessive inheritance pattern and derives its names from the accumulation of cerebroside sulphate (sulphatide) in the white matter of the brain and peripheral nerves. This lipid shows brown metachromasia when stained with cresyl violet or thiamine. In the infantile form of the disease, children present at the age of 2–3 years with progressive paralysis and intellectual deterioration and may die within 2 years. Juvenile and adult forms are later in onset and run a more benign course. There is slowing of nerve conduction velocities and extensive *segmental demyelination* in motor and sensory nerves. The disease is characterised by a deficiency in the enzyme arylsulphatase A and the sulphatide accumulates in brain, nerves, and in renal tubular cells. The diagnosis can be confirmed by examination of early morning urine deposits for metachromatic granules derived from renal tubular cells, and by the demonstration of arylsulphatase A deficiency in peripheral blood leukocytes, or in cultured fibroblasts. Peripheral nerve biopsies reveal extensive segmental demyelination in teased preparations and globules of sulphatide within the nerve are stained orange in frozen sections by Holländer's technique. One-micron sections of resin-embedded nerve (Fig. 16.18) reveal many thinly myelinated fibres and osmiophilic lipid inclusions in Schwann cells and macrophages. A distinctive lamellated pattern of stacked discs with a 6-nm periodicity (Fig. 16.19) is seen when the lipid inclusions are examined by electron microscopy.

Krabbe's leukodystrophy

Krabbe's globoid leukodystrophy is also inherited in an autosomal recessive pattern. Patients present at 2–6 months of age with convulsions, restlessness and irritability, followed by progressive rigidity and ultimate bulbar paralysis. Extensive demyelination is seen in the brain with the accumulation of large globoid cells 20–30 μm in diameter containing galactocerebroside. Segmental demyelination occurs in peripheral nerves where there is a similar accumulation of globoid cells and the presence of cytoplasmic tubular and angulated crystalloid inclusions. The disease is due to a deficiency of the enzyme galactocerebroside beta-galactosidase, a defect seen in the twitcher mouse which mimics

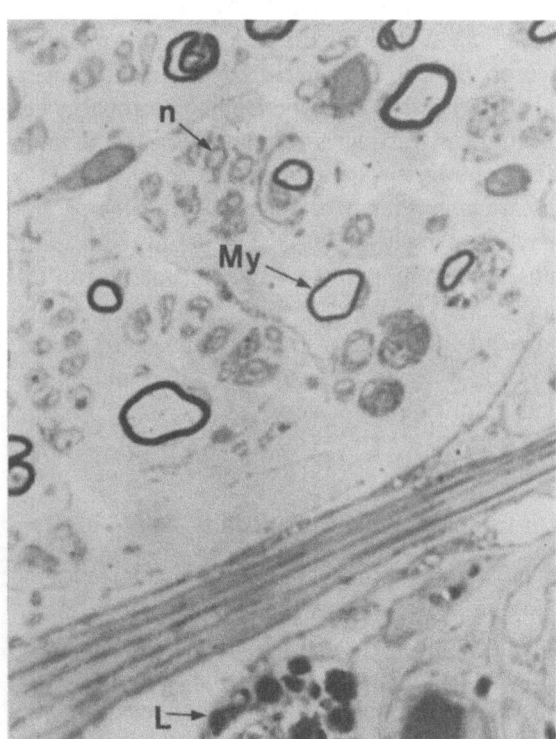

Fig. 16.18. Metachromatic leukodystrophy. TS of sural nerve showing thinly myelinated remyelinating nerve fibres (*My*) and preserved non-myelinated fibres (*n*). Sulphatide lipid inclusion in macrophage (*L*). (1-μm resin section, × 1575)

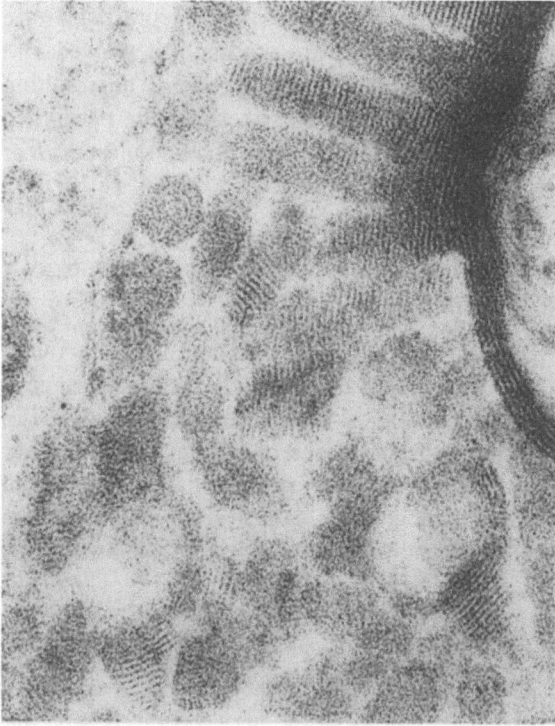

Fig. 16.19. Metachromatic leukodystrophy. EM of sulphatide lipid deposit showing 5 to 6-nm periodicity. (× 167000)

many of the pathological aspects of Krabbe's disease.

Refsum's disease

Patients with Refsum's disease (heredopathia atactica polyneuritiformis) also develop a characteristic peripheral neuropathy. This disease is inherited as an autosomal recessive trait, and presents with retinitis pigmentosa, cerebellar ataxia, ichthyosis, nerve deafness and a chronic progressive peripheral neuropathy. There are raised levels of the fatty acid, phytanic acid, in the serum and in the tissues, probably due to a failure of alpha-oxidation of phytanic acid. Improvement in symptoms has been obtained by a dietary control of phytols. There is segmental demyelination and hypertrophic neuropathy with onion-bulb whorl formation in the peripheral nerves; there may also be a severe reduction of myelinated fibres due to axonal degeneration.

Fabry's disease

Painful peripheral neuropathy occurs in Fabry's disease (angiokeratoma corporis diffusum), a disease with an X-linked recessive inheritance pattern and a deficiency of the enzyme ceramide trihexosidase. There is widespread deposition of ceramide trihexoside throughout arteries in the skin and in the kidney. Similar lipid deposits are seen in the perineurium of peripheral nerves and there is a moderate reduction in myelinated fibres.

Lipoprotein disorders

Inherited disorders where there is a deficiency of lipoproteins may also be complicated by peripheral neuropathies with axonal degeneration and the accumulation of lipids within Schwann cells.

Neuropathies in malignant disease

Peripheral nerves may be focally invaded by malignant tumours, particularly carcinomas. Cranial and spinal nerve roots may be infiltrated by malignant cells in carcinomatous meningitis and in leukaemic involvement of the meninges. Such invasion by neoplastic cells usually results in axonal degeneration.

Encephalopathies and peripheral neuropathies may also present as *non-metastatic complications of malignant disease*. Death of neurons and perivascular lymphocytic infiltration may be seen in the brain, spinal cord and posterior root ganglia. Peripheral neuropathies are most commonly seen in patients with carcinoma of the bronchus, stomach, breast, pancreas and colon and may be associated with a myopathy. The neuropathy can be mild or a severe, sometimes relapsing, crippling, sensorimotor polyneuropathy. Histologically, the nerves show varying loss of axons and lymphocytic infiltration.

Autonomic neuropathies

Involvement of the autonomic nervous system is seen in a number of diseases such as diabetes, Guillain–Barré syndrome, Fabry's disease, familial amyloidosis and dysautonomia. Other lesions of the autonomic nervous system are rare and only sometimes limit the life span of the patient. Cases of acute pandysautonomia have been described with postural hypotension and loss of thermoregulator reflexes and sudomotor activity. Pathological investigation of these patients is difficult due to the inaccessibility of the autonomic nervous system but in some cases degeneration of the intermediolateral columns of the grey matter in the spinal cord has been found at autopsy. A more severe condition is seen in the Shy–Drager syndrome where there is postural hypotension, defective sweating and sphincter disturbances linked with signs of basal ganglia disease and parkinsonian features (Chap. 14). Autopsy investigation of such patients should include examination of the sympathetic chains, the splanchnic nerves, and autonomic ganglia in the gut wall as well as a full study of the brain and spinal cord.

Further reading

Asbury A K, Johnson P C (1978) Pathology of peripheral nerve. Saunders, London, Philadelphia

Cavanagh J B (1979) The 'dying back' process. A common denominator in many naturally occurring and toxic neuropathies. Arch Pathol Lab Med 103: 659

Dyck P J, Thomas P K, Lambert E H (eds) (1975) Peripheral neuropathy. Saunders, London, Philadelphia

Ludwig J (1979) Current methods of autopsy practice (2nd edn). Saunders, London, Philadelphia

Prineas J W (1981) Pathology of the Guillain–Barré syndrome. Ann Neurol 9 [Suppl.]: 6

Spencer P S, Schaumburg H H (eds) (1980) Experimental and clinical neurotoxicology. Williams and Wilkins, Baltimore, London

Weller R O, Cervós-Navarro J (1977) Pathology of peripheral nerves. Butterworths, London, Boston

World Federation of Neurology: Research Group on Neuromuscular Disorders. (1968) Classification of the neuromuscular disorders. J Neurol Sci 6: 165

Chapter 17

Diseases of Muscle

The development of new techniques for the histological study of muscle has led to fresh concepts of the pathogenesis and classification of neuromuscular disorders. In this chapter a general account of the pathological reactions of muscle will be given, particularly in relation to biopsy material, although some attention will also be given to autopsy findings. The features of individual disorders will be summarised.

Muscle biopsy technique

In recent years fixation in formol-saline, with subsequent paraffin-embedding, has been superseded by the use of unfixed, frozen material since a variety of enzyme histochemical and immunohistological methods can be applied to the latter.

Subcellular organelles can thus be studied by light microscopy, and different fibre types can be identified. In addition, the classic histological stains, adapted for unfixed tissue, can still be used. Many of these newer histochemical techniques produce permanent results so that slides can be stored for future study. The blocks of frozen tissue can themselves be stored indefinitely in liquid nitrogen.

Fresh muscle obtained at biopsy must be snap-frozen in liquid nitrogen. This is best done at the time of the biopsy although it can be delayed for a few minutes without detriment to the histological results. However, for electron microscopy fixation of small pieces of the biopsy in cold, buffered 2 % or 4 % glutaraldehyde must be carried out at once in order to avoid artefactual swelling of mitochondria and sarcoplasmic tubules. Fixation in glutaraldehyde should be allowed to continue for about 4 h;

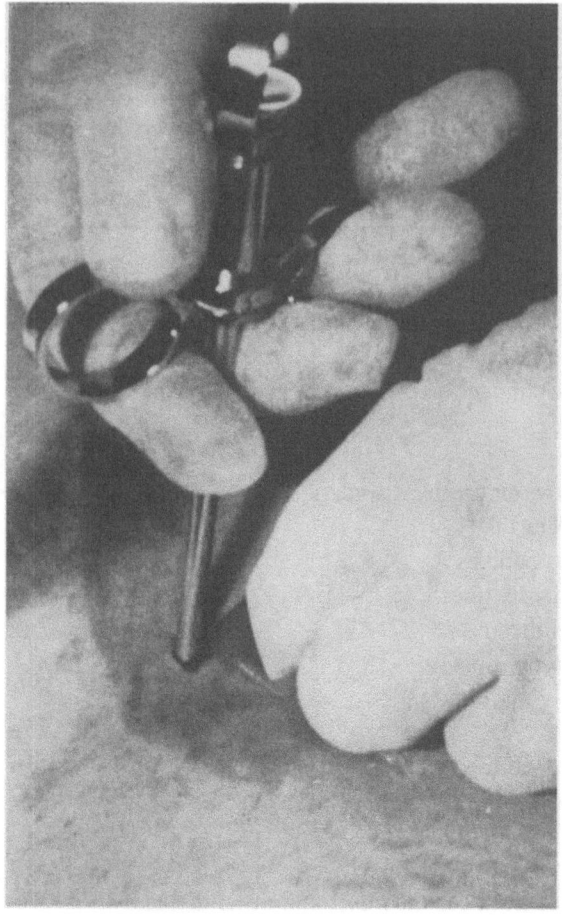
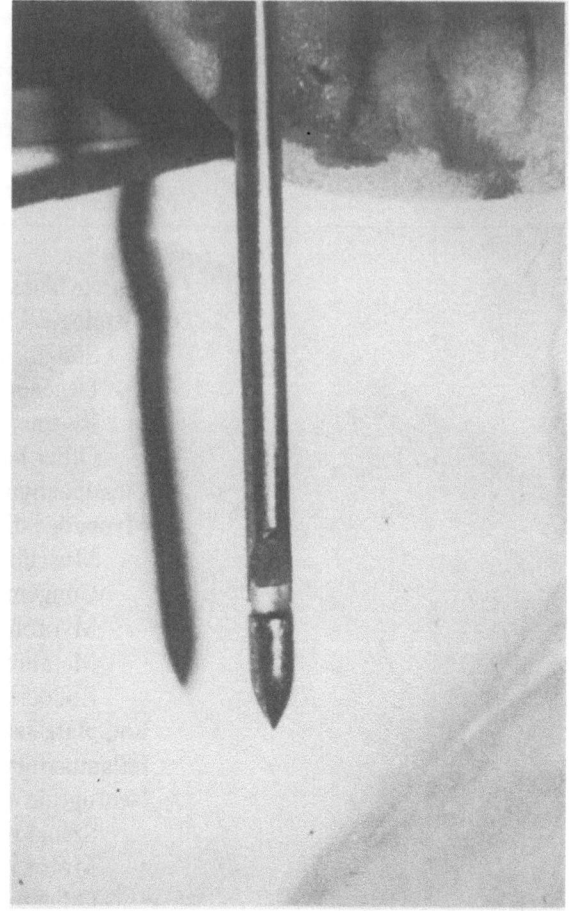

Fig. 17.1. Needle biopsy.
a The modified Bergstrom muscle biopsy needle is pushed into the muscle, usually the vastus lateralis of the thigh, through a small nick in the skin, under local anaesthesia.

b The biopsy specimen seen here close to the cutting edge of the needle is sufficient both for enzyme histochemical and ultra-structural studies.

the tissue can then be placed temporarily in buffered saline before dehydration and embedding in resin.

Ice crystal artefact is often difficult to eliminate in laboratories unused to handling fresh tissue for snap-freezing. It is important to take particular care to prepare small cylindrical blocks of tissue (3 × 2 mm) from the fresh biopsy specimen. The muscle should be kept moist with a few drops of buffered saline or Ringer's solution to avoid drying artefact. A sharp new knife-blade should be used when cutting tissue into smaller pieces since the muscle quickly becomes sticky and contracts when touched. Blunt knives cause disruption of the tissue and lead to difficulty in interpreting the biopsy. Open biopsy allows study of relatively long fascicles of muscle so that well-orientated serial blocks can be taken. In needle biopsies (Fig. 17.1), however, smaller pieces are available. These can usually be accurately orientated before freezing, but it is

sometimes useful to use a dissecting microscope for this purpose. With practice quite large pieces of tissue can be obtained with this needle or punch biopsy technique.

The tissue block is attached to a small disc of cork by a blob of Tissue-Tek, and then snap-frozen in isopentane cooled nearly to its freezing point in a thermos of liquid nitrogen. Snap-freezing directly in liquid nitrogen causes explosive boiling of the nitrogen. This can be largely prevented by coating the tissue in talc, if the isopentane technique is not used. Gaseous nitrogen is a relatively poor conductor of heat and this leads to slow and differential cooling of the tissue and so to the formation of ice crystals within the fibres. Similarly, when cutting sections in the cryostat, a warm knife, or warm slides, must be avoided. Ice crystal artefact can sometimes be cleared from a block of tissue by allowing it to thaw at room temperature and then re-freezing. However, this manoeuvre results in the loss of some enzyme activity, and in some rounding and enlargement of the fibres.

A series of 6–12 consecutive sections should be cut, each 5–8 μm thick. Good longitudinal sections are difficult to produce because of imperfect orientation of muscle fibres in most blocks, but they can be very useful.

Histological methods and fibre typing

The H & E stain provides general information about the biopsy, particularly in recognition of the presence of degeneration or regeneration of muscle fibres, of the presence of inflammatory cell exudates and of studies of the nucleation of individual fibres. The elastic–van Giesen stain is particularly useful in assessing connective tissue changes. The modified Gomori trichrome stain has become popular since it enables delineation of nuclei, fibrous tissue, myofibrillar material (bluish) and inter-myofibrillar substance (red). The H & E and trichrome stains may also differentiate two fibre types, the red and pale fibres of older workers, but this is not always very obvious.

A large number of enzyme histochemical reactions are available and in most laboratories a routine series is used (Fig. 17.2). This series should provide a clear differentiation of fibre types and should yield a variety of organelle-specific reaction products so that mitochondria, sarcoplasmic lipid droplets, myofibrils, cell membranes, sarcoplasmic glycogen, and perhaps also ribonucleic acid and acid phosphatase can be identified. The nicotine adenine dinucleotide tetrazolium reductase (NADH) technique is particularly useful as it produces a permanent preparation of good contrast, which allows fibre type differentiation to be recognised approximately. The reaction product is localised in mitochondria and also, non-specifically, in the tubular system of the inter-myofibrillar sarcoplasm. Succinic dehydrogenase (SDH) is located only in mitochondria but the reaction product is often less easily visualised than in the NADH technique.

Fibre typing (Table 17.1) is performed, by convention, in myofibrillar adenosine triphosphatase (ATPase) preparations. This reaction produces different results depending on the pH of the pre-incubation; this property is utilised in classification of subtypes of type 2 fibres. Pre-incubations are carried out at pH 9.4, 4.5 and 4.3. In good preparations there should be a pattern reversal between the pH 9.4 and pH 4.3 pre-incubations, fibres which are dark in the former being pale in the latter (type 2 fibres). In the pH 4.5 pre-incubations some type 2 fibres show an intermediate reaction (type 2B fibres). Type 2 fibres react more strongly for myophospharylase, located at the cross bridges of the active component of the myofilament, but this method does not produce permanent results.

Table 17.1. Classification of fibre types in human muscle (Swash and Schwartz 1981)

	Type 1	Type 2A	Type 2B
ATPase pH 9.4	Pale	Dark	Dark
ATPase pH 4.5	Dark	Pale	Dark
ATPase pH 4.3	Dark	Pale	Pale
NADH-tr	Dark	Intermediate	Intermediate
Glycogen	Pale	Dark	Intermediate
Myophosphorylase	Pale	Dark	Dark
Neutral lipid	Plentiful	Sparse	Sparse
Physiological characteristics	Slow	Fast: fatigue resistant	Fast: rapidly fatiguing
Metabolic characteristics	Oxidative	Oxidative/ glycolytic	Glycolytic

Neutral lipid droplets are most satisfactorily demonstrated by the Oil-Red-O method; a counterstain of Ehrlich's haematoxylin enables basophilic fibres and sarcolemmal nuclei to be recognised. A number of other methods for neutral lipid, e.g. Sudan black, can be used but they are generally less satisfactory. Glycogen granules and cell membranes, together with other membranous structures, can be shown by the periodic acid Schiff (PAS) method. Predigestion with diastase allows verification of the presence of glycogen in the untreated sections. The sections should be fixed on the slides with alcohol for the most uniform results. Acid phosphatase, located in lysosomes, can be demonstrated in abnormal fibres, particularly in those undergoing autolysis. Basophilia in regenerating fibres is a useful indication of regenerative activity, and this can be confirmed by specific reactions for RNA, such as bright fluorescence with acridine orange.

Other less routine methods applicable to frozen tissue include immunohistochemical techniques utilising the immunoperoxidase reaction for the demonstration of immunoglobulin and complement in blood vessels and in abnormal muscle fibres, or mononuclear inflammatory cells.

Motor end-plates can be visualised by methods for acetylcholinesterase, and this can be enhanced

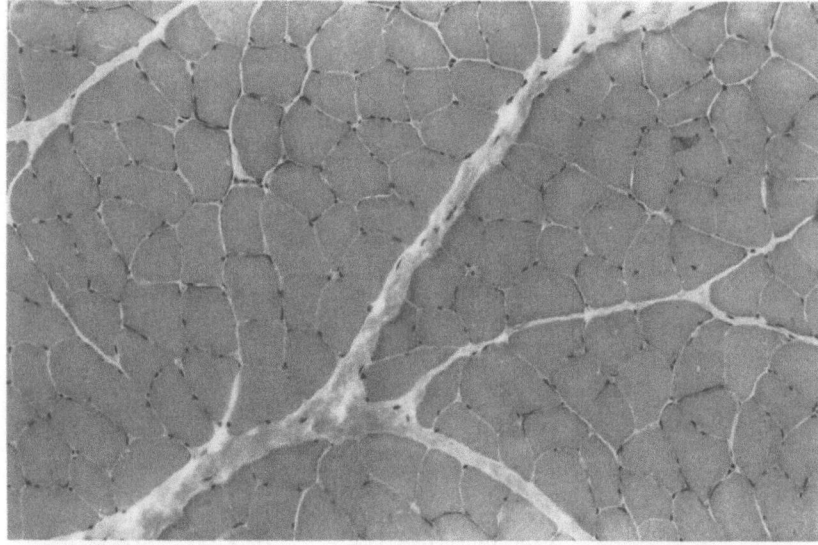

Fig. 17.2. Normal muscle
a H & E TS. The fascicular pattern is well marked, and the muscle fibres are smoothly curved, show only slight variation in size and shape, and are separated from each other by endomysial connective tissue and capillaries. Very few fibres contain central nuclei. (× 140)

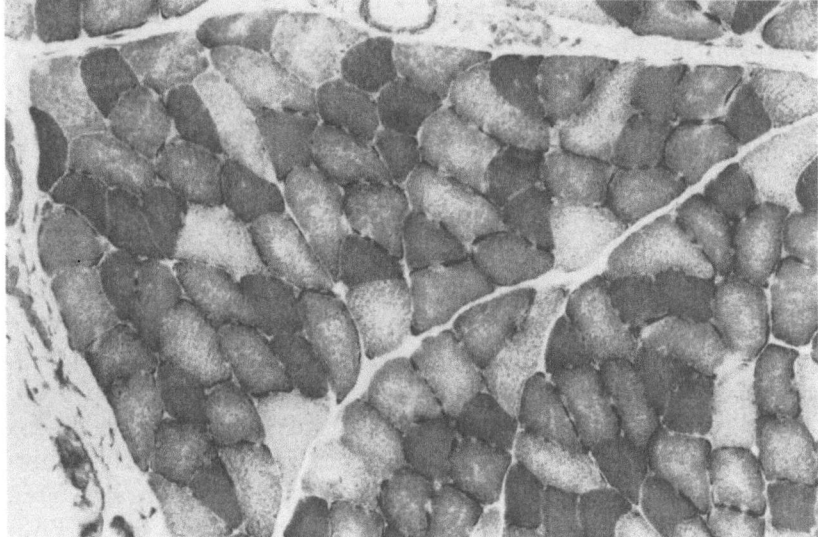

b NADH TS. There is a mosaic arrangement of fibres of various intensity of reaction. Type 1 fibres are dark and type 2 fibres pale but this distinction is often uncertain since type 2A fibres tend to react more darkly than type 2B fibres. The intermyofibrillar reaction product gives a finely granular appearance in normal muscle fibres. Arteriolar walls also react positively. (× 140)

with a silver impregnation technique which enables the terminal innervation to be studied in sectioned material. The supravital methylene blue method is a more capricious technique for examination of muscle innervation which can be applied only to blocks of fresh tissue (Fig. 17.3).

Electron microscopy is not often used in routine diagnosis, although semi-thin sections of plastic-embedded muscle, stained with toluidine blue or paraphenylene diamine, provide a useful adjunct to light microscopy of frozen sections. Electron microscopy itself can then be used to examine specific points in relation to various organelles in abnormal fibres.

Histological features of neuromuscular disease

In neuromuscular disease muscle fibres may be damaged or destroyed. This causes atrophy of muscle if compensatory processes of repair and regeneration are inadequate. Function can be restored only if muscle fibres regain their innervation, and if interfascicular and endomysial connective tissue planes do not interfere with the processes of contraction and relaxation. In addition, the arteriolar and capillary circulation must be maintained. In chronic or progressive disorders there may be considerable distortion of the fasci-

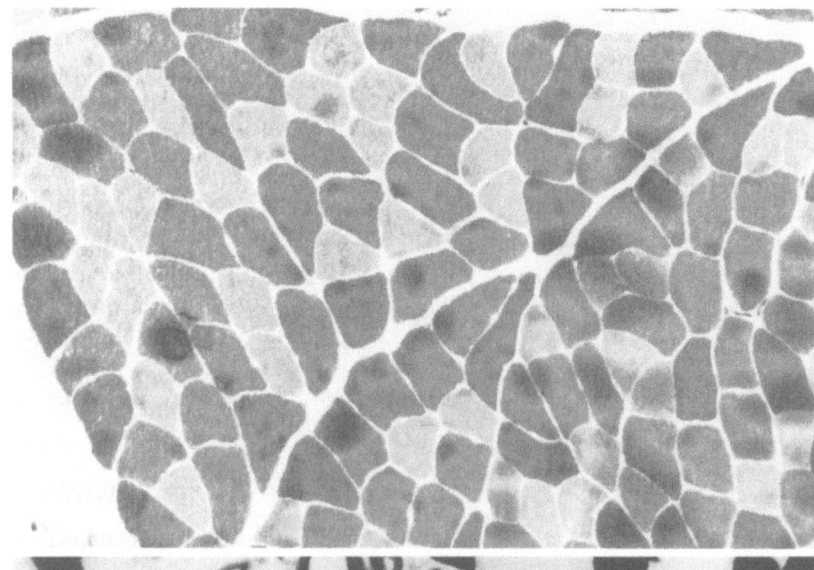

c ATPase, pH 9.4 Type 1 fibres are
  pale and type 2 fibres dark. (× 140)

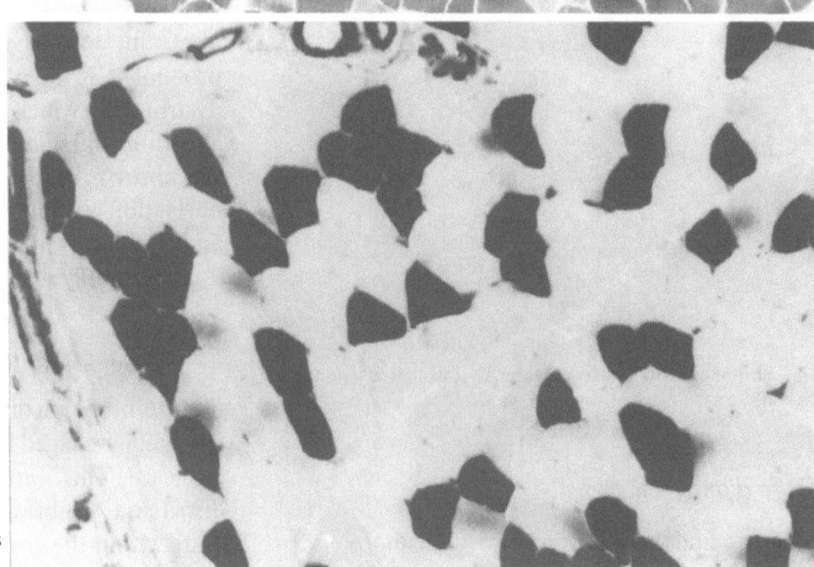

d ATPase, pH 4.3. The mosaic
  pattern is reversed. Type 1 fibres
  are dark and type 2 fibres pale.
  (×140) (b, c and d are serial sections
  from the same area of muscle).

cular organisation of a muscle, so that normal functional capability may become disturbed even though muscle bulk is relatively preserved.

Statistical methods

Changes in the distribution and size of type 1 and type 2 fibres can be described by simple statistical methods. These give information about selective involvement of fibre types which is important in diagnosis.

Fibre-type predominance

The proportion of fibres of each histochemical type varies in different muscles. For example, tibialis anterior normally contains a majority of type 1 fibres. However, in the three muscles most commonly selected for biopsy, quadriceps (vastus lateralis), biceps brachii and deltoid, type 2 fibres are found in greater number than type 1 fibres. In these three muscles there is an approximately even proportion of type 1, type 2A and type 2B fibres. A change in the proportion of a fibre type is termed *fibre-type predominance*; type 1 fibre predominance is present when more than 55% of fibres in one of these three muscles are type 1 fibres, and type 2 predominance when more than 80% of fibres are type 2 fibres.

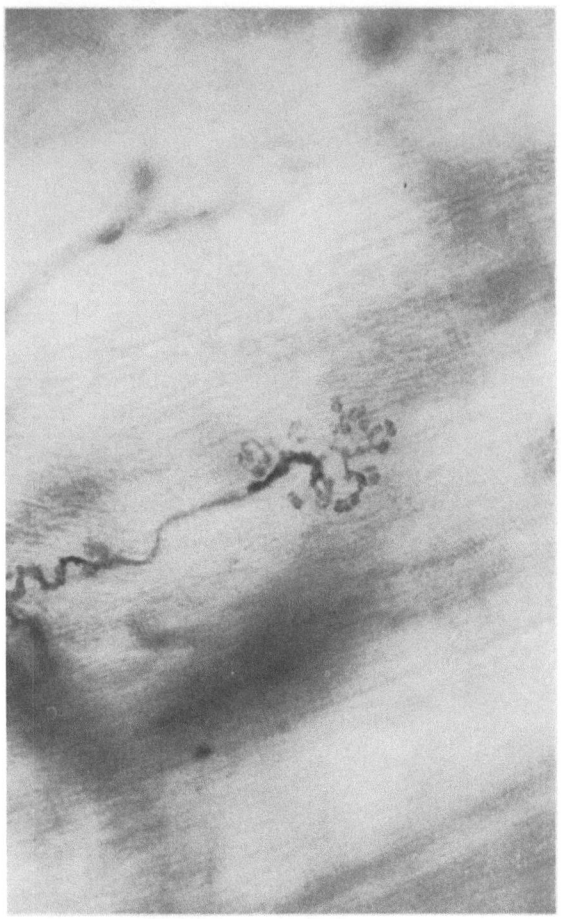

Fig. 17.3. Supravital methylene blue. Rat motor end-plate. (× 350)

Fibre diameter

Atrophy and hypertrophy are difficult to assess subjectively and it is useful to calculate the mean of the lesser diameters of at least 100 fibres in the biopsy, including fibres of both types, in order to compare these with normal values (Table 17.2). Since muscle fibres in children are smaller than those of adults, and vary at different ages, these measurements are most useful in adults. Selective atrophy of type 1 or type 2 fibres may be important in diagnosis.

Table 17.2. Mean muscle fibre diameter in normal adults (biceps muscle)

	Men	Women
Type 1	65 μm	60 μm
Type 2	75 μm	50 μm

Selective type 2 fibre atrophy is common. It is a feature of diffuse atrophy of any cause; for example

after immobilisation of a limb in a plaster cast, in cachexia, in corticospinal tract lesions, in myasthenia gravis or in arthropathies. It may also occur in collagen–vascular disease, in steroid myopathy and in osteomalacia. *Type 1 fibre atrophy* is less common. It is a particular feature of myotonic dystrophy but also occurs in myotubular myopathy, nemaline myopathy, and in congenital fibre type disproportion. In collagen–vascular disorders affecting muscle, such as dermatomyositis or rheumatoid arthritis, selective atrophy of fibres of both histochemical types may occur at the periphery of muscle fascicles. This is probably due to capillary shut-down leading to ischaemia of the periphery of affected fascicles.

Central nucleation

Centrally placed nuclei are found in less than 3 % of fibres in normal muscle. Central nucleation is prominent in myopathies, especially in myotonic dystrophy in which long chains of central nuclei are a feature, and in centronuclear myopathy, in which the fibres resemble early fetal myotubes. Central nucleation is a general feature of regenerating fibres and also occurs in hypertrophied fibres. In addition, it is commonly associated with fibre splitting.

Fibre-type grouping

Muscle fibres of different histochemical types are normally arranged in a random distribution within fascicles. This random distribution reflects the dispersion of fibres belonging to individual motor units within the cross-sectional area of the muscle. The motor unit is a functional concept and consists of an anterior horn cell, its axon and terminal axonal branches, its motor end-plates and the muscle fibres which are thus innervated. All the muscle fibres innervated by a single motor unit are thus of identical histochemical and physiological type. If there is damage to an axon or its branches destruction of all or some of the muscle fibres innervated by this axon may occur. Reinnervation of the denervated muscle fibres occurs by axonal sprouting from nearby motor end-plates or terminal axonal branches, or by regrowth from the muscle fibres' original innervation. In the former case the muscle fibres may change their histochemical type if their new innervation represents a motor unit of different histochemical type from their original innervation. If this process is continued, or is extensive enough *fibre-type grouping* may occur

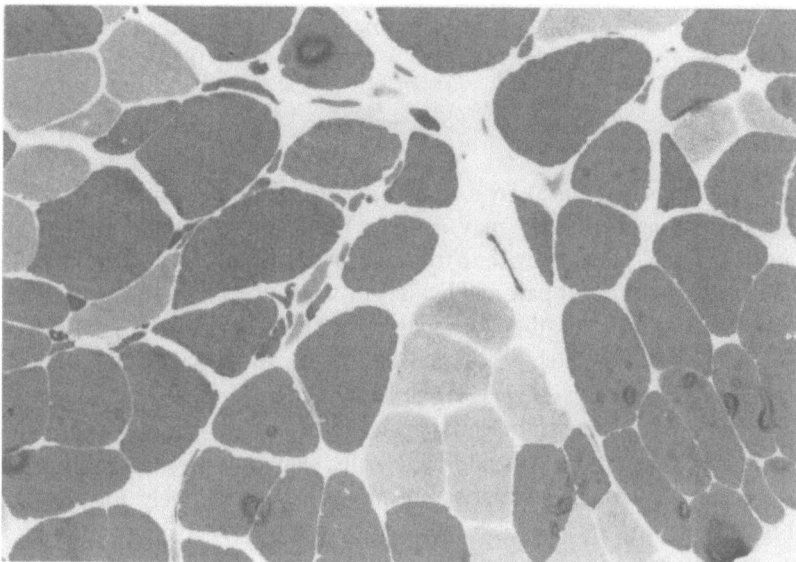

Fig. 17.4. Fibre-type grouping in Kugelberg–Welander disease. ATPase pH 4.3. Type 1 fibre-type grouping is present, and small pointed denervated fibres of both fibre types can be seen: disseminated neurogenic atrophy. There is type 1 fibre hypertrophy. (× 140)

(Fig. 17.4). Fibre-type grouping thus indicates effective functional compensation by reinnervation in a neurogenic disorder of some chronicity. By convention, it is said to occur when *two or more* fibres of the same histochemical type are enclosed at all points on their circumference by other fibres of the same histochemical type. This usually means that there are at least ten fibres in the group (Fig. 17.4), but clearly this depends on fibre size, and on the shape of the fibres. When there is fibre-type predominance, enclosed fibres will become more frequent without necessarily implying that fibre-type grouping is present and it is therefore important to establish that fibre-type grouping affects both type 1 and type 2 fibres before accepting it as evidence of a neurogenic disorder. Nonetheless, fibre-type predominance is itself a factor which should lead to suspicion of a neurogenic disorder.

If collateral reinnervation is ineffective, either because of disease of anterior horn cells or axons, or because it has reached its biological limit in the remaining healthy axons in a neurogenic disorder, irreversible denervation atrophy will occur. Such muscle fibres appear small, narrow and pointed. They often contain prominently basophilic, dark, pyknotic nuclei, and react unusually intensely for NADH. In rapidly progressive, or acute denervating disorders, such fibres are scattered singly or in clusters: *disseminated neurogenic atrophy* (Fig. 17.4). In chronic disorders, when there has been opportunity earlier in the illness for collateral reinnervation of isolated denervated fibres resulting

in fibre-type grouping, the group of denervated fibres may be very large, even occupying whole fascicles: *grouped denervation atrophy*. This is particularly characteristic of motor neuron disease and of the spinal muscular atrophies.

Fibre-type grouping and the presence of small, pointed, NADH-dark fibres are thus the cardinal features of a neurogenic disorder (Table 17.3).

Degenerative changes

Degenerative and regenerative activities in single

Table 17.3. Histological features of myopathic and neurogenic disorders (Swash and Schwartz 1981)

Myopathic	Neurogenic
1 Prominent degenerative and regenerative changes in individual fibres	1 Fibre-type grouping
2 Increased variability in fibre size	2 Fibre-type atrophy
3 Fibrosis may be prominent	3 Clusters of small pointed fibres, often dark in NADH and non-specific esterase preparations
4 Architectural changes prominent	4 Target fibres or core fibres
5 Various specific morphological abnormalities	5 Fibre-type predominance
6 Type 2 fibre atrophy	6 Type 1 fibre hypertrophy
7 Perifascicular atrophy	7 Only rare degenerative changes
8 Blood vessels abnormal in inflammatory myopathies	8 Rare architectural changes
9 Fibre-type grouping uncommon	9 Little fibrosis
	10 Blood vessels normal

muscle fibres are the main diagnostic features of myopathic disorders (Table 17.3). These changes occur in a variety of different forms, some of which are specific to certain disorders.

Necrotic fibres

Necrotic fibres (Fig. 17.5) are a common feature of the myopathies, but they may also be found in biopsies from patients with chronic neurogenic disorders. They appear pale and hyaline or vitreous in H & E stains. Later, they lose their eosinophilic character, become patchily stained, and begin to undergo phagocytosis (Fig. 17.5) or liquefaction. Sometimes an endomysial cellular reaction occurs around them, composed of endothelial cells, sparse round cells, macrophages and sarcolemmal nuclei (Fig. 17.5). Necrotic fibres usually contain prominent patches of acid phosphatase–positive material. If the blood supply to a fascicle is interrupted, fibre necrosis will occur, but the endomysial tubes and basal lamina scaffold may remain intact, producing an appearance of rings of empty endomysial tubes: *subendomysial necrosis*. This appearance is seen particularly in polymyositis and in other acute necrotising myopathies. Large, rounded hyaline fibres are particularly characteristic of Duchenne muscular dystrophy. In longitudinal section the zone of hyaline change is seen to be of limited extent, and to consist of hypercontraction and smudging of the cross-striations of the fibre.

Moth-eaten fibres

Moth-eaten fibres are fibres in which the normally regular intermyofibrillar network seen in the oxidative enzyme reactions, e.g. NADH, is disturbed. This architectural change preferentially affects type 1 fibres. The abnormality often takes the form of a whorled appearance; areas of non-reactivity with NADH are often present near these whorls and these areas are usually slightly basophilic. This change is not specific to any single disorder but is particularly associatd with inflammatory myopathies, when it is most marked at the periphery of a fascicle (Fig. 17.6).

Fibre splitting

Splitting of muscle fibres is common in chronic disorders. It is a feature of chronic neurogenic muscle diseases, such as spinal muscular atrophy, when it particularly affects the hypertrophied type 1 muscle fibres, but similar splitting occurs in Duchenne muscular dystrophy, in limb-girdle myopathies and in polymyositis. It may be important in functional compensation for loss of muscle fibres in these disorders. Fibre splitting is a normal phenomenon near musculo-tendinous insertions. Further, it must not be confused with subendomysial regeneration since in the early stages of the latter several discrete myotubes may be found with a single endomysial cylinder.

Splitting usually begins from the periphery of a fibre (Fig. 17.7), the line of separation marked by newly formed plasma membrane extending towards a centrally placed nucleus and often consisting of a sarcoplasmic cleft within the depth of the fibre. The cleft appears slightly basophilic, and stains positively for RNA. It is associated with ribosomes, glycogen granules and mitochondria (Fig. 17.8), indicating that the process of fibre splitting involves increased local metabolic activity. Sometimes a fibre may be seen, in serial sections, to split into multiple fragments some of which, having become separated from their parent fibre, undergo irreversible denervation atrophy. In chronic neurogenic disorders splitting may lead to fibre necrosis and regeneration, with variability in fibre size and increased central nucleation: *secondary myopathic change*.

Ring fibres

In many chronic neuromuscular disorders ring fibres occur, but they are particularly associated with myotonic dystrophy (Fig. 17.9). A displaced strand of one or more myofibrils takes up a spiral position around the periphery of the fibre; these myofibrils are thus fractured and in this sense the ring fibre can be regarded in the general category of split fibres. Ring fibres in myotonic dystrophy are often associated with sarcoplasmic masses, which consist of peripheral zones of sarcoplasm, devoid of myofibrils and of other organelles.

Target fibres

Best seen in NADH and ATPase preparations, target fibres consist of fibres in which a central pale, unreactive zone is surrounded by a densely reactive intermediate zone and a third, relatively normal, outer zone which extends to the periphery of the fibre. Sometimes there may be a darkly reactive spot within the pale central zone. Most target fibres are type 1 fibres. The abnormality is particularly

Fig. 17.5. a Necrotic fibres, TS. In this H & E preparation of an acute toxic myopathy occurring in a patient treated with epsilon aminocaproic acid there is extensive necrosis of muscle fibres with early regeneration, and a sparse lymphocytic endomysial reaction. The necrotic fibres contain macrophages. (× 350)
b Necrotic fibre, TS. EM. Disorientated A bands are seen in the necrotic muscle fibre at the bottom of the picture. A macrophage is present within this fibre and parts of other macrophages and of a fibroblast and a capillary can be seen outside the basal lamina of the fibre. (× 10000)

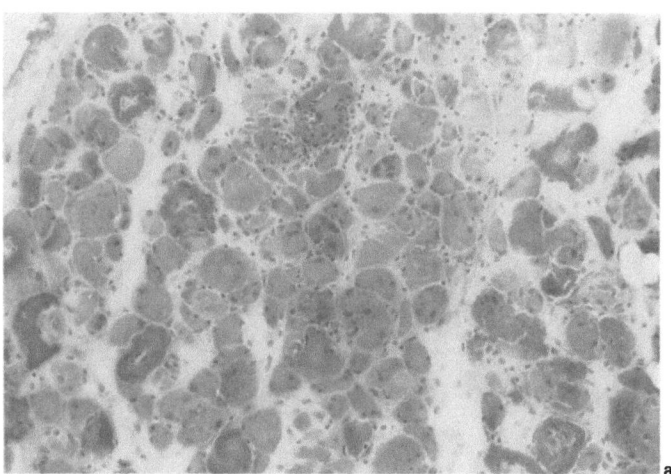

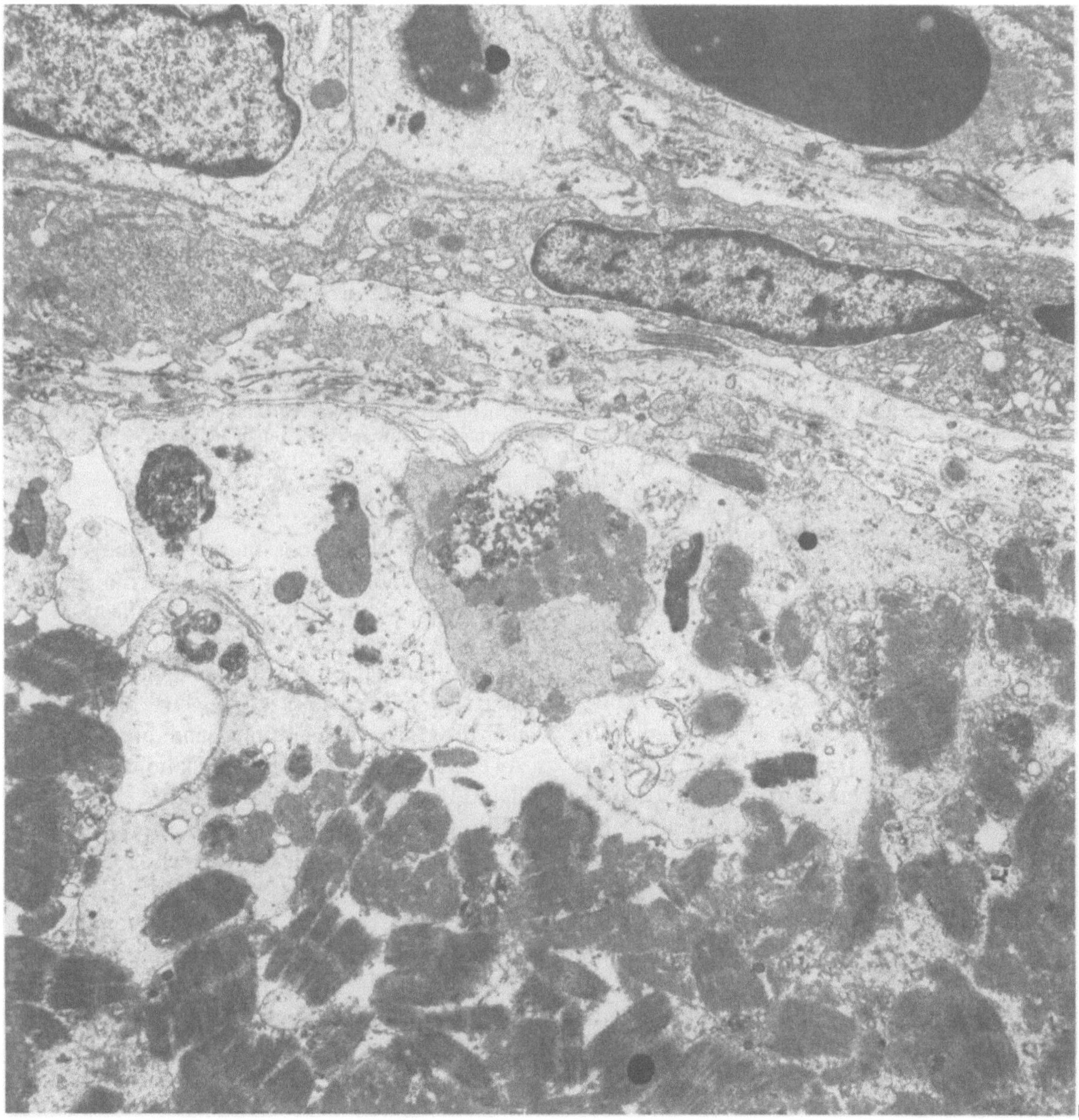

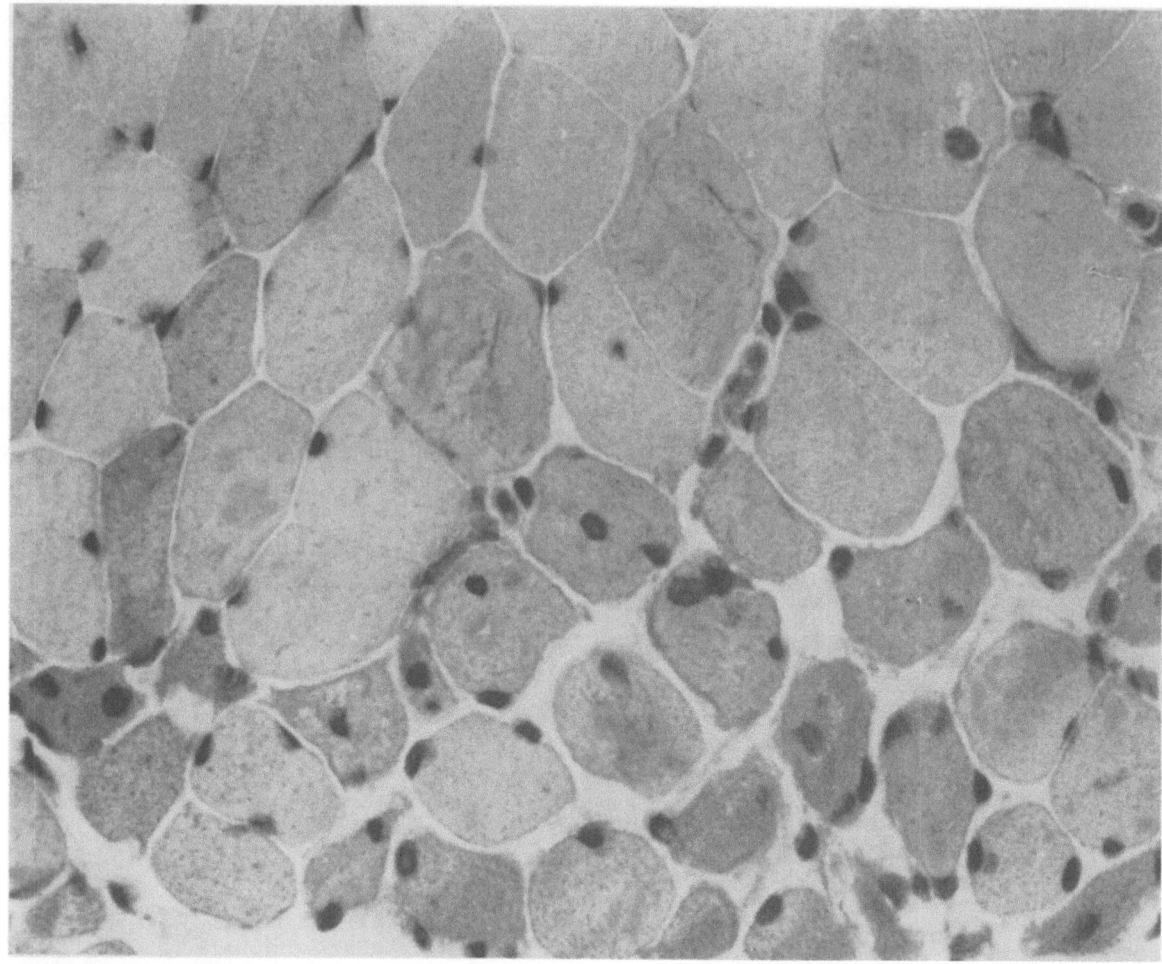

Fig. 17.6. Polymyositis. Haematoxylin and oil red O. TS. At the periphery of the fascicle the muscle fibres are smaller, and show irregular basophilic sarcoplasm, often with centrally placed enlarged nuclei. These are moth-eaten fibres; the basophilia is indicative of regenerative activity. (× 140).

common in denervated muscle, especially in acute neuropathies or in other rapidly progressive disorders such as nerve injuries or motor neuron disease (Fig. 17.10) but it has also been noted in disuse atrophy following tenotomy.

Central cores

Fibres showing central cores may sometimes be difficult to distinguish from target fibres. A distinction has been drawn between fibres with structured cores in which the central NADH-unreactive core reacts positively for ATPase, and unstructured cores, which are unreactive both for NADH and ATPase, but which lack the intermediate dense zone. The latter are sometimes termed core-targetoid fibres, a term which exemplifies doubts about the specificity of the abnormality. Central cores have been associated particularly with a rare congenital myopathy, central core disease.

Ragged-red fibres

In H & E preparations ragged-red fibres appear coarsely granular. The granular material is faintly basophilic and is particularly prominent at the periphery of affected fibres. The abnormal zones (Fig. 17.11) stain brightly red in Gomori trichrome preparations, are dark in NADH and succinic dehydrogenase preparations, and unreactive for ATPase. They contain accumulations of neutral lipid. Almost all ragged-red fibres are type 1 fibres. With the electron microscope (Fig. 17.11) the abnormal zones are seen to consist of accumulations of enlarged, bizarrely shaped mitochondria which often contain osmiophilic granules and paracrystalline inclusions. Ragged-red fibres are a feature of limb muscle biopsies of patients with familial 'ophthalmoplegia plus', a disorder which may be associated with a mild proximal myopathy, cerebellar ataxia and retinitis pigmentosa (Kearns–

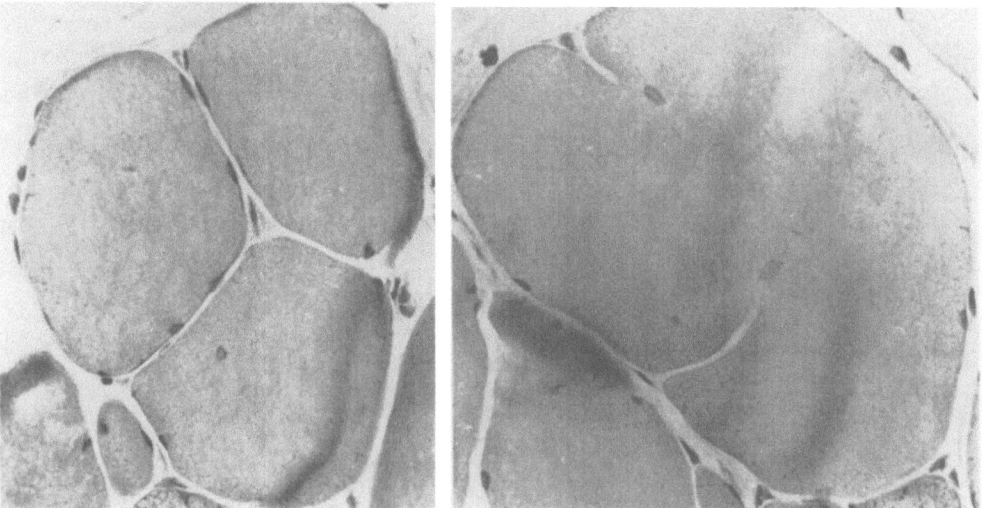

Fig. 17.7. Kugelberg–Welander disease. H & E. TS. These two sections are of the same fibre, 80μm apart. The relation between centrally migrated nuclei and the clefts of fibre splitting is well shown. (× 350)

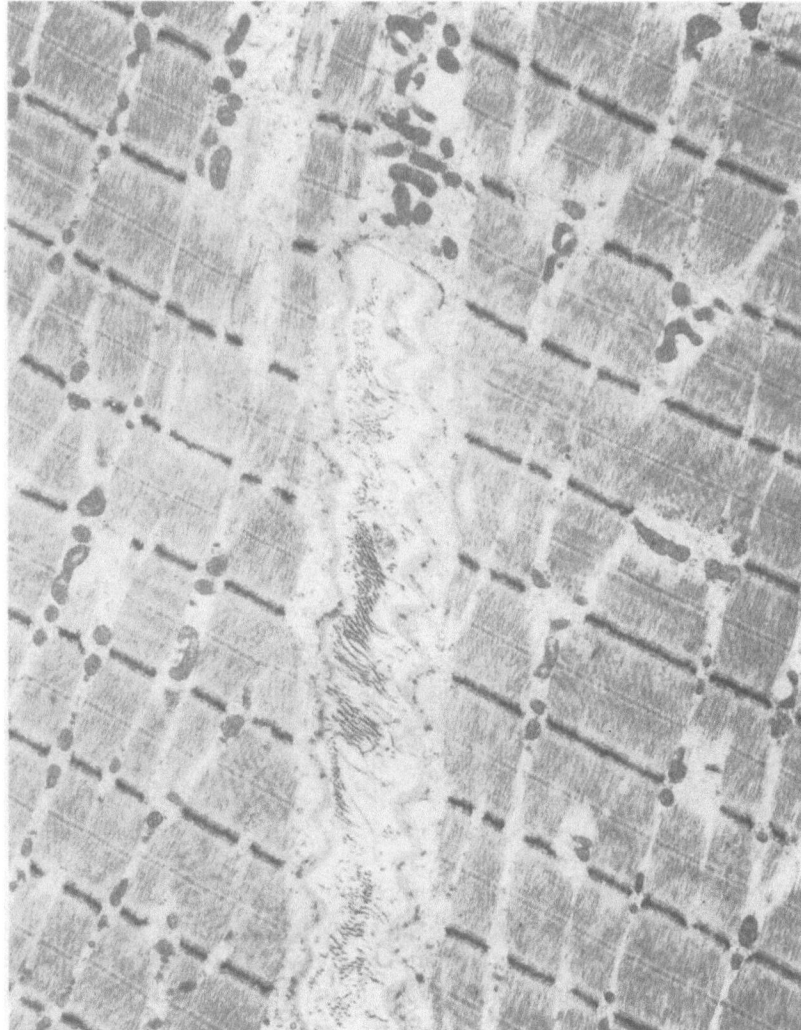

Fig. 17.8. Kugelberg–Welander disease. EM. Fibre splitting. The apex of the split is marked by a trail of mitochondria extending through the sarcoplasm of the fibre. The register of Z bands, and of sarcomeres, is preserved in this slightly oblique section. (× 15000)

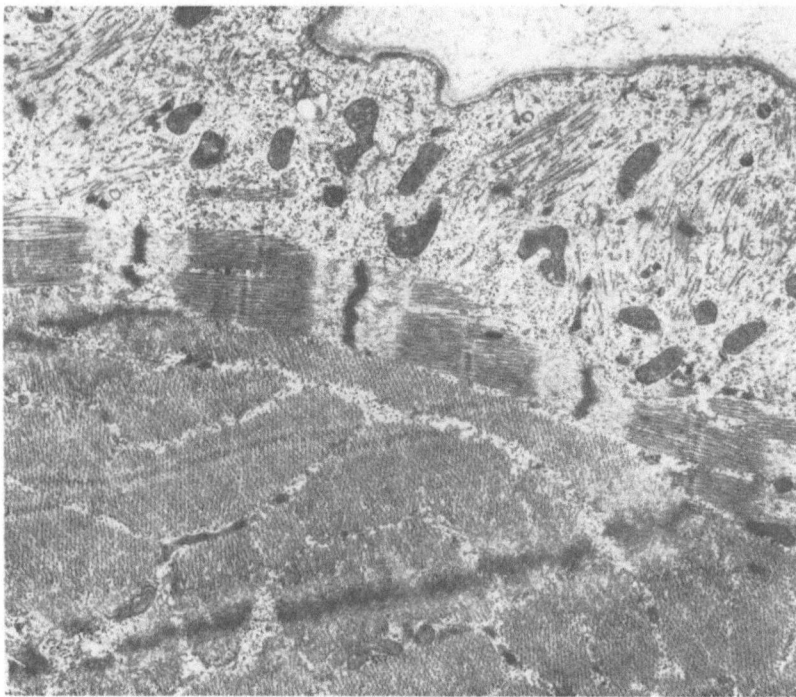

Fig. 17.9. Myotonic dystrophy. EM. Ring fibre with sarcoplasmic mass peripheral to it. (× 5000)

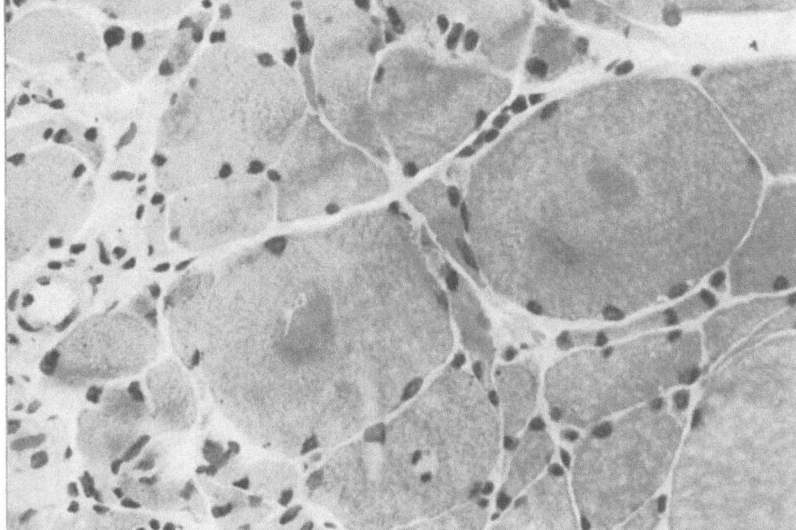

Fig. 17.10. Target fibres in acute denervation from motor neuron disease. H & E. TS. Although more clearly seen in NADH preparations target fibres can often be recognised in H & E. The larger fibres show a homogeneous central target zone. There are many small denervated fibres, a number containing dark pyknotic nuclei. (× 350)

Sayre–Shy syndrome) (see Chap. 14 and Table 14.3), but they have also been described in a variety of other neuromuscular disorders, including a number of cases of myopathies associated with defective mitochondrial oxidation.

Tubular aggregates

Aggregates of sarcoplasmic tubules do not produce fibres of a generally granular appearance, but resemble ragged-red fibres in that the abnormal zones are red in Gomori preparations, positive for

NADH and unreactive in ATPase preparations. However, affected fibres are nearly always type 2B fibres. The abnormality can be confirmed by electron microscopy. It is a non-specific change, but has been particularly associated with the periodic paralysis.

Rod bodies

Best seen in Gomori preparations (Fig. 17.12), rod bodies are small red, rod-like structures scattered in the sarcoplasm of affected fibres, especially in the

Fig. 17.11. Ragged-red fibres
a H & E. The peripheral parts of the affected fibres are faintly basophilic and the central parts appear granular or 'ragged'. (× 350)
b Succinic dehydrogenase. The abnormal parts of the ragged-red fibres react strongly in this mitochondrial enzyme preparation. (× 140)

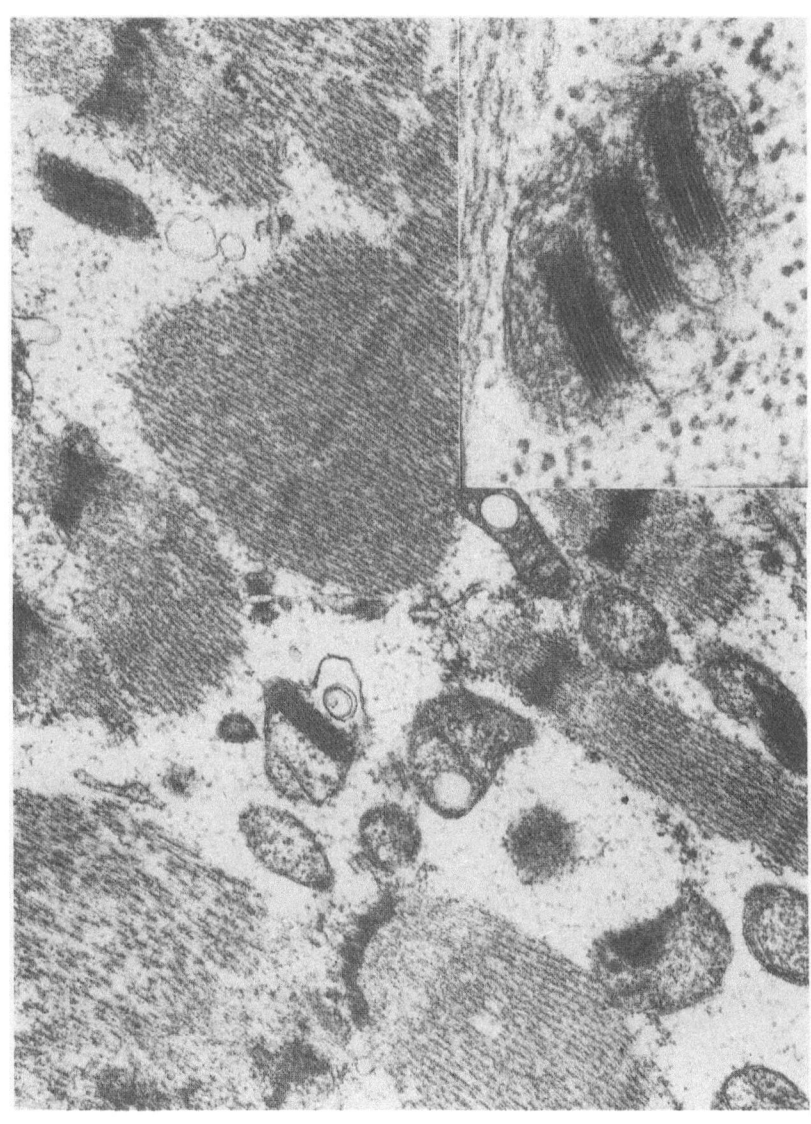

c Electron microscopy. The mitochondria show a variety of morphological abnormalities, particularly in the pattern of their cristae, and they contain typical paracrystalline inclusions. (× 10000) (inset × 35000)

Fig. 17.12. Rod bodies.

a Gomori trichrome. Multiple rod-like bodies are found in otherwise normal fibres. (×350)

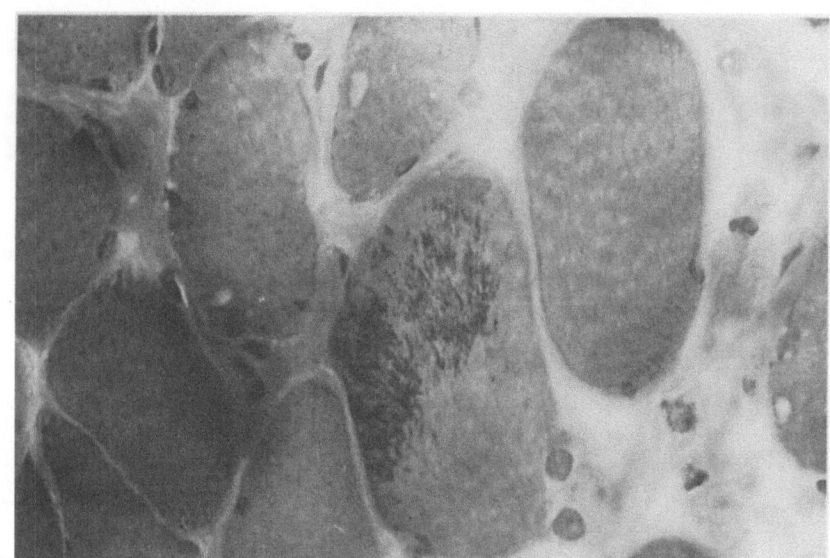

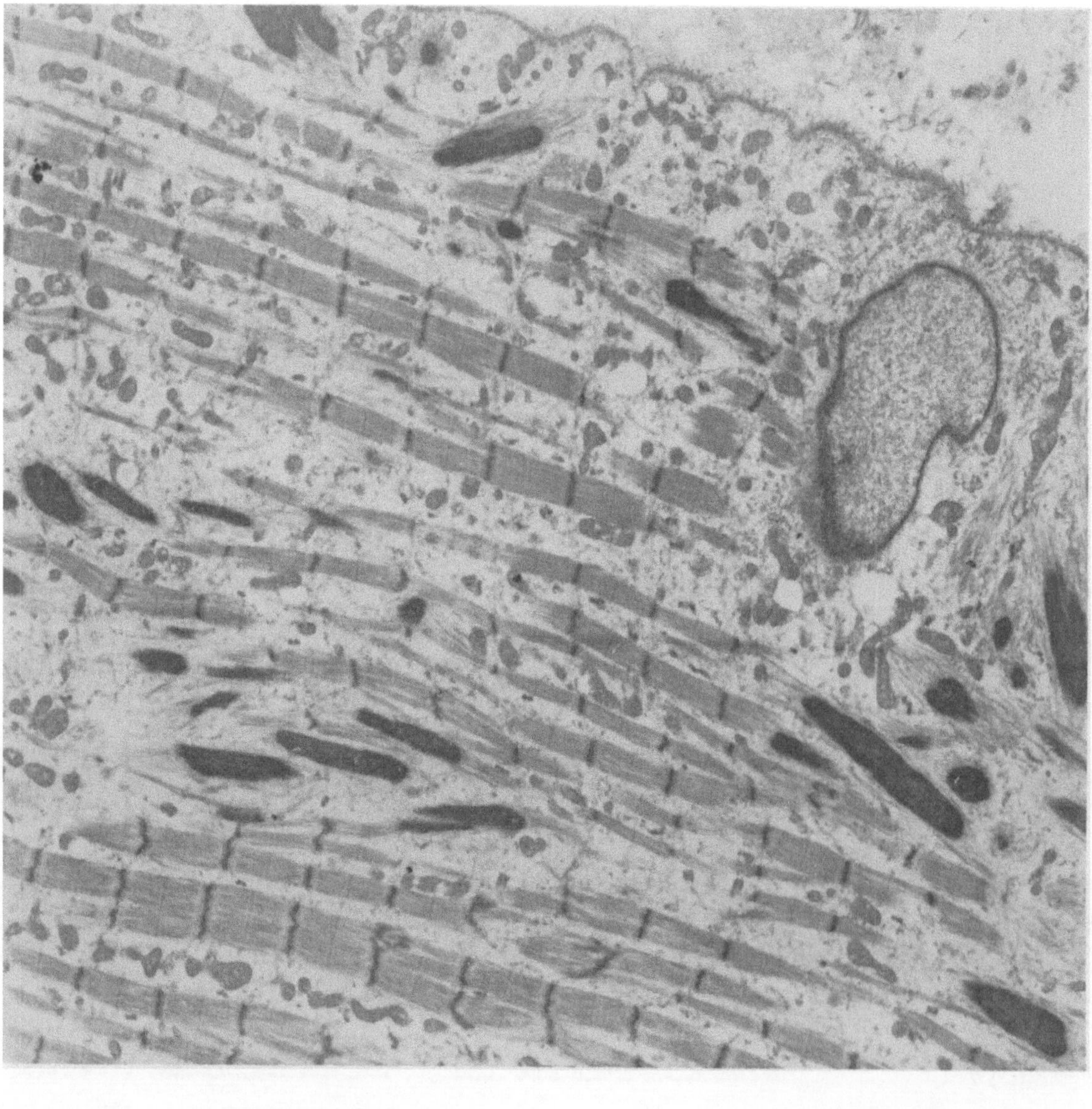

b EM. Rod bodies are often associated with zones of myofibrillar abnormality. They arise from Z band material. (×7500)

sarcolemmal region. They are faintly basophilic and are red with PTAH in paraffin-embedded muscle. Their origin from Z band material can be recognised by electron microscopy. They were first described in a familial, non-progressive myopathy with hypotonia, termed nemaline myopathy, but have since been recognised in benign, adult-onset limb-girdle myopathies, and in a variety of other disorders.

Cytoplasmic bodies

Small, eosinophilic, PAS-positive zones within otherwise normal muscle fibres have been particularly associated with collagen–vascular diseases, such as dermatomyositis, but when present in small numbers their significance is uncertain. These cytoplasmic bodies appear reddish in Gomori preparations.

Lymphorrhages

Focal accumulations of lymphocytes in the interstitium are non-specific, but occur particularly in myasthenia gravis and in motor neuron disease.

Regenerative changes

Muscle has considerable regenerative potential after injury. After fibre necrosis, which may be limited to a segment of a muscle fibre, regeneration can occur either in continuity with the undamaged portions of the fibre ('continuous' repair) or from myoblast formation in the necrotic segment itself ('discontinuous' repair). The former is likely to occur when necrosis in an abnormal segment is partial. The latter represents a form of subendomysial regeneration, discussed above. Regeneration begins at a stage after injury or necrosis when phagocytosis of necrotic material is still incomplete. At this stage, mononucleated cells are abundant in the interstitium around the necrotic fibre.

Regenerating fibres are usually smaller than neighbouring normal fibres. Their sarcoplasm is basophilic and may appear foamy because it contains many tiny lipid droplets (Fig. 17.13). They usually contain multiple, centrally located, vesicular, enlarged nuclei with prominent nucleoli and a dispersed chromatin pattern. Cytoplasmic RNA can be demonstrated with special stains and this is accompanied by an abundance of ribosomes, polyribosomes and rough endoplasmic reticulum, prominent Golgi apparatus, and immature, poorly orientated, thick and thin filaments. In discontinuous regeneration repair proceeds initially from mononucleated myoblasts which are derived partly if not wholly from activation of satellite cells. These myoblasts enlarge to form long, basophilic, multi-nucleated, ribbon-like cells, which later fuse, thus forming a new fibre. Attention has recently been drawn to the importance of programmed cell death in this process of 'fusion' of myoblasts to form a single reconstituted fibre.

Satellite cells, found in normal muscle, consist of a subsarcolemmal nucleus, surrounded by sparse granular sarcoplasm containing free ribosomes, Golgi apparatus, endoplasmic reticulum and mitochondria, but devoid of myofilaments. The satellite cell is limited by plasma membrane and is situated beneath the basement membrane of the muscle fibre. The number of satellite cells in a muscle is increased after injury, during regeneration, and after denervation.

Other features

Motor-end plates are seen uncommonly in most biopsies, but can be studied in motor-point biopsies. Proliferation of the pre-terminal apparatus, with simplification of the synaptic folds, accompanied by deposition of IgG and C3 in the synaptic cleft, occurs in myasthenia gravis, a disease characterised by the presence of a circulating IgG antibody to acetylcholine receptor protein.

Blood vessels, including arterioles, veins and capillaries, are difficult to examine systematically in muscle biopsies. In polymyositis and polyarteritis, necrosis of the arteriolar wall with hyaline change, thrombosis and, more frequently, infiltration of the wall by small round cells and plasma cells, may occur. Capillary necrosis or shut-down may lead to peri-fascicular atrophy, and filamentous or tubular inclusions have been reported in endothelial cells in childhood-type dermatomyositis. In the latter disorder deposits of IgG and C3, representing immune complexes, have been reported in capillaries and arterioles.

Endomysial connective tissue is increased in most myopathies and in some chronic neurogenic disorders but marked fibrosis is an especially characteristic feature of Duchenne dystrophy.

Small *nerve fascicles* are often found in muscle biopsies and it is occasionally possible to recognise abnormalities such as segmental demyelination or axonal dying-back changes in patients with neuropathies.

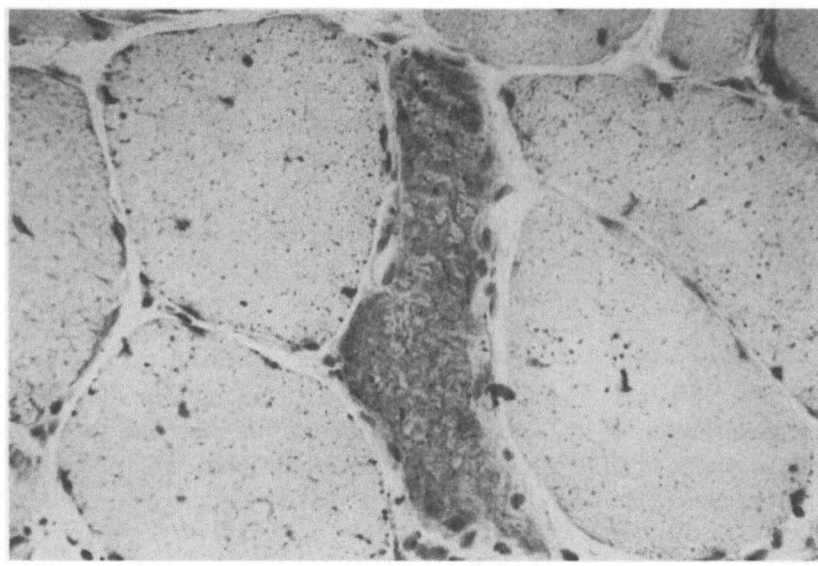

Fig. 17.13. Oil red O haematoxylin. TS. The regenerating fibre is smaller than its neighbouring fibres. Its sarcoplasm is basophilic and foamy. (× 350)

Muscle spindles are found fairly frequently. Normal muscle spindles consist of a capsule of perineurial cells, fibrocytes and collagen which encloses a periaxial space filled with mucopolysaccharide and containing several small intrafusal muscle fibres, the nuclear bag and nuclear chain fibres, a bundle of small nerve fibres and a few capillaries. There are normally at least two nuclear bag fibres and three to ten nuclear chain fibres. These fibres receive a complex motor and sensory innervation. Characteristic abnormalities occur in myotonic dystrophy, consisting of fragmentation of the intrafusal muscle fibres and proliferation of their associated innervation. Abnormalities also occur in Duchenne dystrophy and in motor and sensory denervation.

Golgi tendon organs and pacinian corpuscles are rarely seen in muscle biopsies.

Classification of neuromuscular disorders

Neuromuscular diseases are broadly classified into myopathic and neurogenic disorders. The classification shown in Table 17.4 includes most of the disorders likely to be encountered, but omits some very rare disorders.

Myopathic disorders

Muscular dystrophies

The term muscular dystrophy refers to a group of genetically determined diseases characterised by progressive degenerative changes in muscle fibres, without primary abnormality in the lower motor neuron. They are classified (Table 17.4) according to their clinical, morphological and genetic characteristics.

Duchenne muscular dystrophy

A progressive myopathy, Duchenne muscular dystrophy is inherited in a sex-linked recessive pattern, so that it is carried by females and expressed only in males. It presents in infancy, with delay in the achievement of motor development, especially with delay in walking. It is often characterised by hypertrophy and hardness to palpation of calves and shoulder muscles. Weakness is principally proximal at first but as the disease progresses, weakness becomes generalised, although distal muscles are always relatively spared, and the external ocular muscles are apparently never affected. Scoliosis, dysphagia and cardiomyopathy develop and there is often a degree of mental retardation. Affected boys never learn to run, and death usually occurs before the 18th year. The blood creatine phosphokinase level is greatly raised, often to values several hundred times the normal

Table 17.4. Classification of neuromuscular disorders

Myopathic disorders

A *Genetically determined myopathies*
   1 Muscular dystrophies
        (i) Duchenne muscular dystrophy
        (ii) Becker muscular dystrophy and other X-linked dystrophies
        (iii) Limb-girdle muscular dystrophy
        (iv) Facio-scapulo-humeral muscular dystrophy
        (v) Scapulo-peroneal syndrome
        (vi) Ocular myopathy
        (vii) Oculo-pharyngeal muscular dystrophy and the mitochondrial myopathies
   2 Myotonic syndromes
        (i) Myotonic dystrophy
        (ii) Myotonia congenita
        (iii) Paramyotonia congenita
        (iv) Other myotonic syndromes
   3 Benign myopathies of childhood
        (i) Central core and multicore disease
        (ii) Nemaline myopathy
        (iii) Myotubular (centronuclear) myopathy
        (iv) Congenital fibre-type disproportion
        (v) Congenital muscular dystrophy
        (vi) Others
   4 Metabolic myopathies
        (i) Glycogenoses
        (ii) Periodic paralysis
        (iii) Disorders of lipid metabolism, e.g. carnitine deficiency
        (iv) Malignant hyperpyrexia
B *Endocrine myopathies*
   1 Thyroid myopathies
   2 Parathyroid disorders and osteomalacia
   3 Pituitary disorders (acromegaly)
   4 Steroid myopathy
C *Inflammatory myopathies*
   1 Idiopathic
        (i) Polymyositis
        (ii) Dermatomyositis
        (iii) Childhood dermatomyositis
        (iv) Polymyositis and dermatomyositis associated with carcinoma
        (v) Polymyositis and dermatomyositis associated with collagen vascular disease
        (vi) Granulomatous polymyositis (sarcoidosis)
   2 Infections
        (i) Viral
        (ii) Bacterial
        (iii) Parasitic infestations
D *Drug-induced myopathies*
Disorders of neuromuscular transmission (end-plate disorders)
   1 Myasthenia gravis
   2 Myasthenic syndrome (Eaton-Lambert syndrome)
   3 Botulism, and other toxins.

Neurogenic disorders

A *Disorders of anterior horn cells*
   1 Spinal muscular atrophies
        (i) Severe (infantile) spinal muscular atrophy (Wernig–Hoffman disease)
        (ii) Intermediate spinal muscular atrophy
        (iii) Mild (juvenile) spinal muscular atrophy (Kugelberg–Welander disease)
   2 Motor neuron disease
   3 Poliomyelitis and other viral disorders
   4 Other anterior horn cell disorders
B *Disorders of motor nerve roots*
C *Peripheral neuropathies* (see Chap. 16).
   1 Genetically determined polyneuropathies
        (i) Type 1 (peroneal muscular atrophy)
        (ii) Type 2 (neuronal type of peroneal muscular atrophy)
        (iii) Type 3 (hypertrophic neuropathy of Dejerine and Sottas)
        (iv) Type 4 (hypertrophic neuropathy with phytanic acid storage—Refsum's disease)

Table 17.4. (*continued*)

    (v) Type 5 (neuropathy with spastic paraplegia)
    (vi) Others, e.g. metachromatic leukodystrophy, etc.
    (vii) Acute intermittent porphyria
    (viii) Amyloid neuropathy
2 Acquired neuropathies
  (a) Mononeuropathies
      (i) Traumatic
      (ii) Entrapment and compressive
      (iii) Brachial neuritis (neuralgic amyotrophy)
  (b) Polyneuropathies
      (i) Inflammatory polyradiculoneuropathy (Guillain–Barré syndrome)
      (ii) Metabolic, e.g. diabetes mellitus, renal and hepatic disease, vitamin deficiencies, alcohol
      (iii) Toxic and drug-induced neuropathies
      (iv) Associated with malignant disease
      (v) Infections, e.g. diphtheria and leprosy
      (vi) Associated with connective tissue disease
      (vii) Others

range; this abnormality is present in affected boys before the disease is recognisable clinically. Female carriers of the gene for Duchenne dystrophy usually also show slightly raised levels of creatine phosphokinase in their blood, both at rest and after exercise, and this may be useful for detection of the carrier state in genetic counselling.

Muscle biopsies (Fig. 17.14) show the typical features of a myopathy, but these abnormalities vary in severity according to the stage of the disease and the muscle biopsied. In the early stages there is abnormal variation in fibre size with prominent focal areas of small, basophilic regenerating fibres. The muscle fibres generally appear unusually rounded. Even at this stage of the disease there may be increased interfascicular and endomysial fibrous tissue. As the disorder progresses fibrosis becomes more evident and large, rounded, darkly staining fibres (hyaline fibres), which are prominently eosinophilic and stain reddish in trichrome preparations, are a prominent feature. Scattered necrotic fibres undergoing phagocytosis, and small clusters of regenerating fibres are also present and fibre splitting may be prominent at this early stage of the disease. In severely affected muscles the fascicular pattern of the muscle becomes destroyed, and the remaining muscle fibres become arranged in irregular bundles surrounded by adipose and fibrous tissue. Nerve fascicles are relatively spared, but muscle spindles are involved, and eventually destroyed. In the early stages it is not uncommon for regenerating clumps of fibres to form small

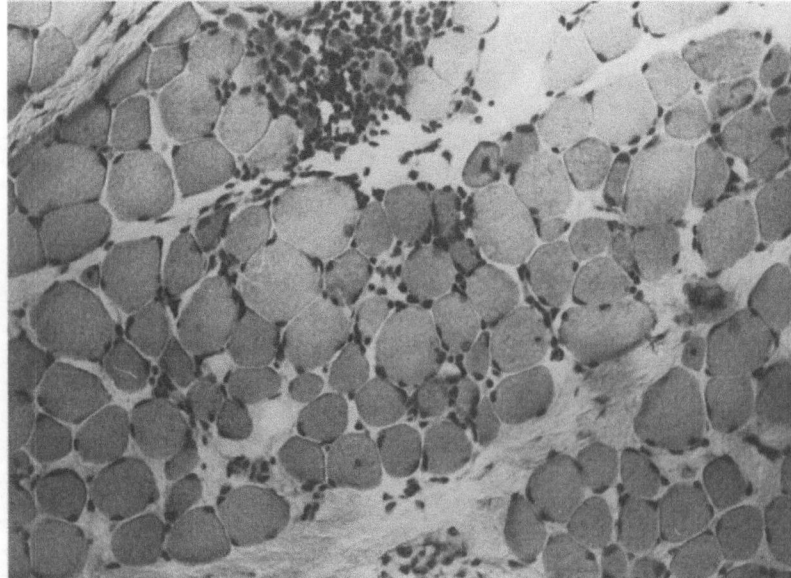

Fig. 17.14. Duchenne muscular dystrophy. TS. H & E. There is increased variation in fibre size with clusters of basophilic regenerating fibres surrounded by a prominent cellular response. The muscle fibres are unusually rounded and there is interfascicular fibrosis. (× 140)

groups of fibres of similar histochemical type, but fibre-type grouping is not a feature of the disease. Biopsies usually show type 1 fibre predominance and the normally clear differentiation of type 1 and type 2 fibres in the ATPase reaction at pH 9.4 is impaired so that many fibres appear to be of intermediate histochemical type.

Electron microscopy shows non-specific degenerative and regenerative changes. However, the plasma membrane of necrotic and of apparently normal muscle fibres in Duchenne dystrophy is defective, allowing abnormal permeability and thus leading to swelling and focal necrosis of fibres. This abnormality may be the cause of the focal 'hyper-contraction bands' found in some muscle fibres in this disorder, an abnormality which seems to underlie the formation of the darkly staining hyaline fibres. Studies using the freeze-fracture technique to visualise the details of membrane ultrastructure have shown a reduction in the number of intramembrane particles in the two faces of the fractured membrane from dystrophic muscle fibres, and extensive areas in which only a few particles can be seen. In particular, the number of 'square array' pits in the membrane is reduced. It has been suggested that this abnormality, which may be distributed more widely than in muscle alone, may be the primary defect in Duchenne muscular dystrophy.

At *autopsy* the proximal muscles are largely replaced by fat and fibrous tissue. The peripheral nerves and spinal cord are normal and there is no reduction in the number of anterior horn cells, evidence that the electrophysiological finding of reduced numbers of functioning motor units in Duchenne muscular dystrophy is due to the abnormality in the muscle, rather than to a primary neurogenic phenomenon. However, in the brain abnormal patterns of gyral development, pachygyria or microscopic heterotopias have been observed and the weights of brains from boys with Duchenne dystrophy are less than those of normal controls.

The *carrier state* can be detected by muscle biopsy in some instances. In addition to elevation of the serum creatine phosphokinase level, there may be slight myopathic changes consisting of slight variability in fibre size, excess central nucleation and, more rarely, focal necrosis and regeneration of single fibres. These findings have been taken as evidence in support of the hypothesis that expression of the gene for Duchenne dystrophy in females depends on variations in the degree of inactivation of paternal or maternal X chromosomal material (Lyon's hypothesis).

Becker muscular dystrophy

A disorder similar to Duchenne dystrophy, Becker muscular dystrophy is of lesser severity, so that survival into adult life, with preservation of the ability to walk, is a criterion for diagnosis. Like Duchenne dystrophy, it is inherited as an X-linked recessive disorder. It has been associated with deutan colour blindness and the Xg blood group, suggesting that it is genetically distinct from Duchenne muscular dystrophy. The muscle biopsy generally shows similar features to those of Duchenne dystrophy, but the abnormalities may be less severe, and there may be large numbers of small fibres, some of which appear pointed and resemble denervated fibres.

Limb–girdle muscular dystrophy

Muscular dystrophy in a limb–girdle distribution, with proximal weakness affecting legs more than arms, is not a common disorder. It is inherited in an autosomal recessive pattern. The disease may progress rapidly or slowly and it is probable that this pattern of muscular weakness does not represent a specific disease entity but, rather, results from a number of different biochemical disorders. In the past patients with spinal muscular atrophy were often misclassified as limb–girdle dystrophy but modern enzyme histochemical methods have eliminated this problem. The creatine phosphokinase is usually moderately raised.

The muscle biopsy shows fibres of varying size, with increased central nucleation, a few scattered necrotic or regenerating fibres and striking hypertrophy of some fibres. Fibre-type grouping is absent. Oxidative enzyme preparations show fibres, particularly larger fibres, with a whorled appearance indicating an abnormal distribution of lipid and mitochondria and, therefore, an abnormal pattern of myofibrils. PAS preparations show a similar abnormality. Electron microscopy shows no specific abnormality.

Facio-scapulo-humeral muscular dystrophy

The shoulder girdle and facial muscles are principally affected in facio-scapulo-humeral muscular dystrophy. The syndrome probably results from a number of different causes, including muscular

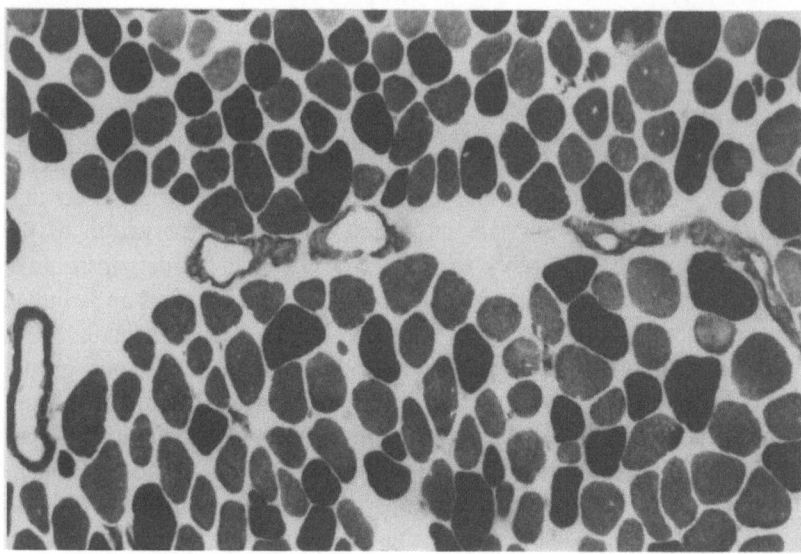

Fig. 17.15. Congenital muscular dystrophy. TS. ATPase, pH 9.4. The muscle fibres are small, unusually rounded and separated from each other by dense, but unstained, fibrous connective tissue. Areas of fatty infiltration are evident. (× 140)

dystrophy, myasthenia gravis, various congenital myopathies, polymyositis and chronic neurogenic disorders. Cases due to idiopathic dystrophy form a minority and in these cases changes found in biopsies of affected muscles are often surprisingly slight. *Scapulo-peroneal myopathy* forms a rare subgroup of this disorder in which weakness principally affects peri-scapular and peroneal muscles; the extensor digitorum brevis muscles are strikingly spared. This latter syndrome also has a neurogenic form.

Congenital muscular dystrophy

The syndrome of congenital muscular dystrophy presents from birth with hypotonia and generalised weakness. Contractures develop; there may be associated mental retardation. In some cases improvement occurs with increasing age. The muscle biopsy may show mild or quite striking myopathic changes with marked endomysial fibrosis and accumulations of adipose tissue. The muscle fibres are often strikingly small (Fig. 17.15). This syndrome is one of the causes of arthrogryposis multiplex.

Muscular dystrophy with involvement of external ocular muscles, and the mitochondrial myopathies

Cases of progressive external ophthalmoplegia with ptosis, of oculopharyngeal myopathy associated with some skeletal muscular weakness, and of external ophthalmoplegia associated with limb–

girdle weakness, cerebellar ataxia, retinitis pigmentosa, heart block and a raised CSF protein form a distinct but rare group of syndromes. External ophthalmoplegia is a rare occurrence in most other myopathies or dystrophies; it occurs in some childhood forms of multicore myopathy, and is a major feature of myasthenia gravis.

In these syndromes biopsy of a proximal upper limb muscle may reveal ragged-red fibres. Other myopathic features, including slightly increased variability in fibre size, increased central nucleation and increased endomysial fibrous tissue may be seen. Ultrastructural studies reveal mitochondrial abnormalities similar to those found in other 'mitochondrial myopathies' (see also p. 312). Ragged-red fibres also occur in a number of other neuromuscular disorders, including limb–girdle myopathies with defects of mitochondrial oxidation, uncoupled oxidative phosphorylation leading to weight loss, hypothyroidism, facio-scapulohumeral weakness, carnitine deficiency and polymyositis. More than 1 % of type 1 fibres should be affected by ragged-red fibre change before the abnormality can be regarded as significant. It has been suggested that ragged-red fibre change can occur as one aspect of regeneration or degeneration, thus accounting for their occurrence in conditions other than the myopathies associated with progressive external ophthalmoplegia.

Congenital myopathies

The congenital myopathies present at birth or in early infancy as the 'floppy infant' syndrome, or later in childhood as proximal or generalised muscular weakness. In most instances these disorders are non-progressive, or only very slowly progressive, and the creatine phosphokinase level is often normal.

Central core disease

In typical examples central core disease is a non-progressive congenital myopathy beginning shortly after birth, but cases of later onset have been described. Congenital dislocation of the hip may occur. Hypotonia is a prominent feature, but weakness is not severe. The disorder is usually dominantly inherited.

The muscle biopsy shows poorly differentiated fibres but there is usually type 1 fibre predominance. In most fibres a core is seen which is devoid of enzyme reactivity in oxidative enzyme preparations (Fig. 17.16). Electron microscopy shows that these cores contain few mitochondria and little sarcoplasmic reticulum (Fig. 17.16). Various myofibrillar abnormalities including streaming of the Z line, occur in this region. The cores have a predilection for type 1 fibres and should be distinguished from target fibres, an abnormality found in denervated muscle. This distinction is not always easy however and the term 'core-targetoid fibre' is sometimes used. Cores may be 'structured', retaining their myofibrillar pattern and thus being demonstrable in ATPase preparations, or unstructured, losing their myofibrillar and intermyofibrillar structure.

In *minicore (multicore) disease*, a similar but sporadic or autosomal recessive disorder, the muscle biopsy shows multiple areas of focal decrease in mitochondrial oxidative enzyme activity, usually associated with focal degenerative changes in myofibrils. These areas, unlike the cores of classic central core disease, do not extend very far through the length of affected fibres but are relatively sharply circumscribed. Central nucleation is usually prominent.

Nemaline myopathy (rod body myopathy)

In this myopathy rod-like structures occur in the muscle biopsy. Clinically the main feature is floppy muscular tone, usually noted at birth. Weakness, if present, affects the arms more than the legs. Respiratory difficulties are common in infancy. The severity of the disorder varies greatly from case to case. This disorder is probably identical with Krabbe's universal muscular atrophy. The disease is probably inherited as an autosomal dominant characteristic. The nosological position of nemaline myopathy has become particularly controversial since reports of the occurrence of similar nemaline bodies in a variety of other disorders, including denervation, psychosis, experimental tenotomy, myotonic dystrophy, polymyositis and Adie's syndrome. In some cases of nemaline myopathy, apart from the presence of the rods, the biopsy has been normal but in many instances there is increased variability in fibre size, the rod bodies being more prominent in the smaller fibres, and increased central nucleation. In oxidative enzyme preparations whorled fibres may be seen. The rod bodies are usually predominantly subsarcolemmal in location. Either or both fibre types may be affected. With the electron microscope the rods can be seen to be derived from Z band material (see Fig. 17.12). Rod bodies have been reported to co-exist with central cores and there may thus be similarities between these two disorders.

Myotubular myopathy

Also known as centronuclear myopathy, myotubular myopathy is a rare disorder characterised by hypotonia with delayed motor milestones in infancy, followed by a slowly progressive myopathy, involving facial and sometimes external ocular muscles. Adult onset cases, usually women, have been reported. In one family there was an association with diabetes mellitus. Central nucleation is found in nearly all the fibres in the biopsy. In the central regions of affected fibres oxidative enzyme activity is absent or abnormally intense, and myofibrillar ATPase is absent in these regions. In some cases type 1 fibre hypertrophy has been described.

Congenital fibre-type disproportion

The characteristic feature of congenital fibre-type disproportion is only evident on muscle biopsy. Clinically, affected infants are floppy or even very weak from birth but after 2 years of age there is usually some improvement. The disorder is associated with congenital dislocation of the hip, low body weight and short stature, kyphoscoliosis, a highly arched palate, and foot deformities. The biopsy shows small type 1 fibres and normal or enlarged type 2 fibres. No other abnormality is present. Differential diagnosis must be made from severe infantile spinal muscular atrophy, a disease with a much poorer prognosis, from congenital

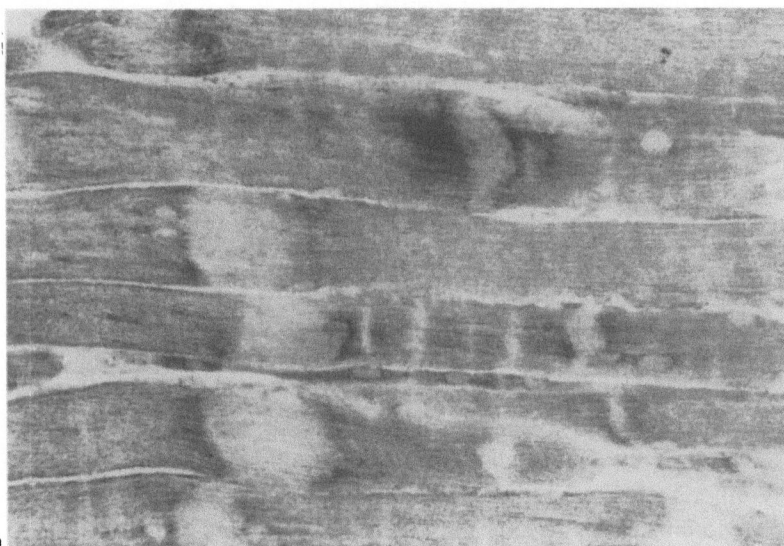

Fig. 17.16. Multicore disease with focal loss of cross-striations.
a LS. NADH. Several non-reactive core-like zones of varying size are present. These zones are also non-reactive for ATPase. ($\times 350$)
b EM. In this oblique section the abrupt transition between the disorganised core and the neighbouring normal myofilaments is clearly seen. ($\times 15000$)

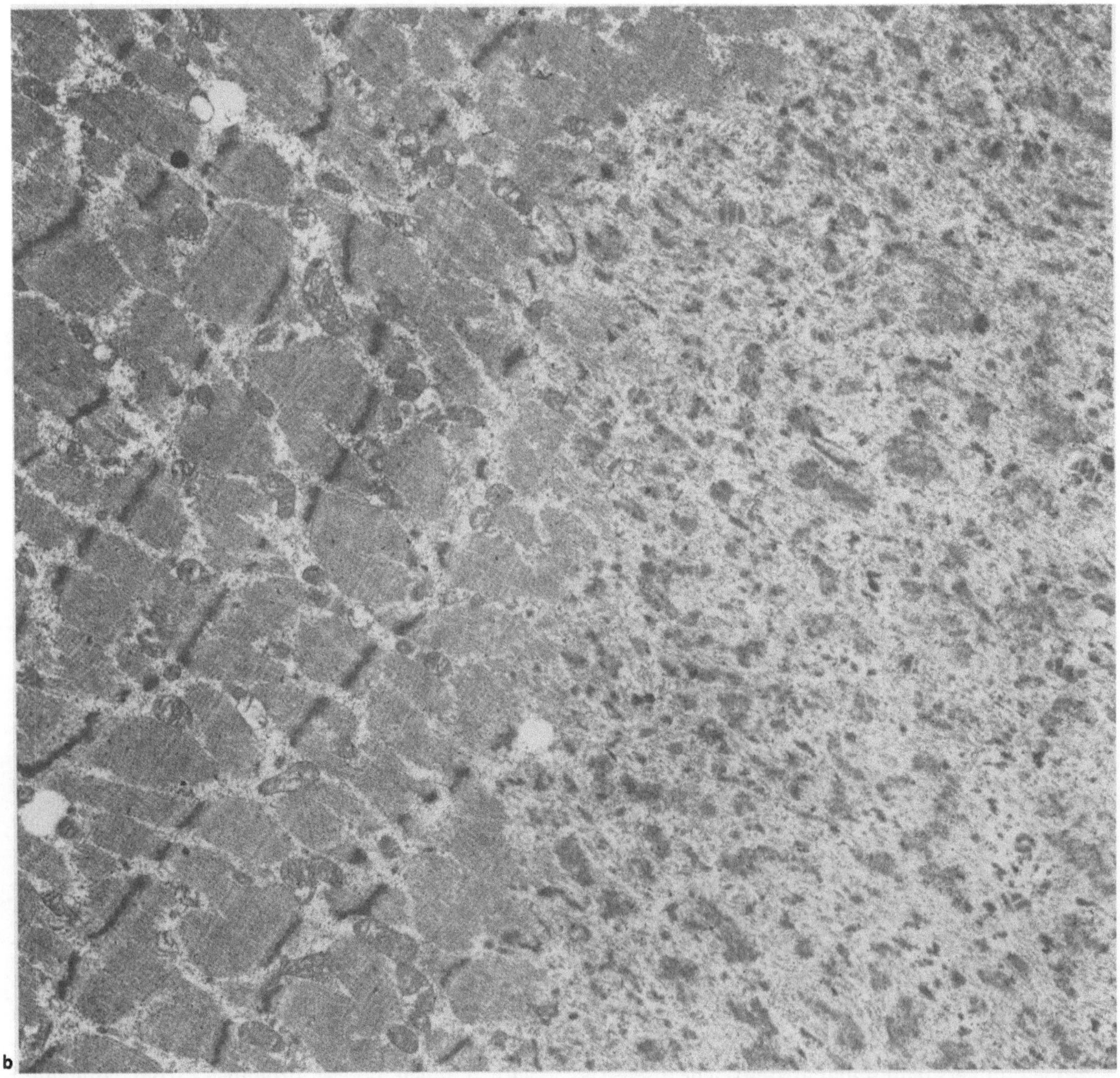

myotonic dystrophy, and from myotubular myopathy with type 1 fibre hypotrophy. The pattern of inheritance is variable.

Other congenital myopathies

In a number of reports, individual cases or families have been described in which myopathies beginning in infancy have been associated with abnormalities in muscle fibres which are, as yet, unclassified. These include myopathies with subsarcolemmal 'fingerprint' inclusions, myopathies with abnormal sarcotubular systems, zebra body myopathy and myopathies with cytoplasmic bodies or tubular aggregates. The term 'minimal change myopathy' has been used to describe cases such as these, in which the muscle biopsy shows only minimal myopathic abnormalities without more specific features.

Floppy infant syndrome

A syndrome of weakness and hypotonia in infancy, due to any of a number of congenital or acquired myopathies, neurogenic disorders or brain diseases of infancy, is referred to as floppy infant syndrome. It may also be caused by disorders of elastic tissue, such as Ehlers–Danlos disease. It is not a disease entity.

Arthrogryposis multiplex

Another syndrome of varying causation is arthrogryposis multiplex. The term refers to a complex clinical deformity, usually due to a progressive disorder, consisting of muscular wasting and joint and skeletal deformities. The onset is in infancy and leads to inability to stand or walk. The syndrome may occur in a number of progressive, congenital myopathies, in spinal muscular atrophy or in chronic, infantile polyneuropathies.

Myotonic syndromes

This group of disorders includes patients in whom myotonia, a state of delayed relaxation of muscle fibres, occurs alone or in association with myopathic muscular weakness. Myotonia, although recognisable clinically, must be differentiated by electromyographic criteria from other forms of persistent contraction of muscle fibres. It is probably due to an abnormality in ionic conductance in the muscle fibre membrane.

Myotonic dystrophy

In myotonic dystrophy myotonia is associated with muscular weakness and wasting, frontal baldness, testicular atrophy, ptosis, dysphagia and cataract. Cardiomyopathy and diabetes mellitus and some degree of mental retardation are common. The disease usually begins in adult life or in adolescence and the weakness is most evident in facial, sternomastoid, neck extensor and distal limb muscles. The tendon reflexes are usually absent. In childhood the disease may also present with these features but in the congenital form of myotonic dystrophy the clinical manifestations are somewhat different. There is hypotonia and failure to thrive, with respiratory difficulties in the perinatal period. Facial weakness is very prominent but myotonia is usually absent. If the infant survives, cardiomyopathy and mental retardation become evident. This form of the disease is particularly common in children of mothers with the disease. Myotonic dystrophy is inherited as a Mendelian dominant characteristic.

In both adult- and congenital-onset cases the creatine phosphokinase is usually normal. Abnormalities in IgC and IgM concentration and metabolism have also been reported. In the adult-onset type, muscle biopsies show marked changes. There is increased variability in fibre size with type 1 fibre atrophy, and some degenerative changes in single fibres, consisting both of fibre necrosis and of patchy myofibrillar degeneration, often with the formation of peripherally placed masses of granular sarcoplasm free of myofibrils. Fibrosis is a feature only in very wasted muscles. There may be a number of other abnormalities, including fibres with a moth-eaten appearance in NADH preparations, and a variety of inclusions are seen in ultrastructural studies. Rod bodies have also been reported in myotonic dystrophy. A striking feature is central migration and proliferation of muscle fibre nuclei resulting in the occurrence of long chains of centrally placed vesicular nuclei in longitudinal sections. Displaced myofibrils, forming ring fibres are also common in this disease.

The muscle spindles show a characteristic abnormality consisting of fragmentation of intrafusal muscle fibres (Fig. 17.17), more marked in their polar than their equatorial regions, with proliferation of the motor and sensory innervation. The muscle spindle abnormality is not uniformly distributed, some spindles being more affected than others.

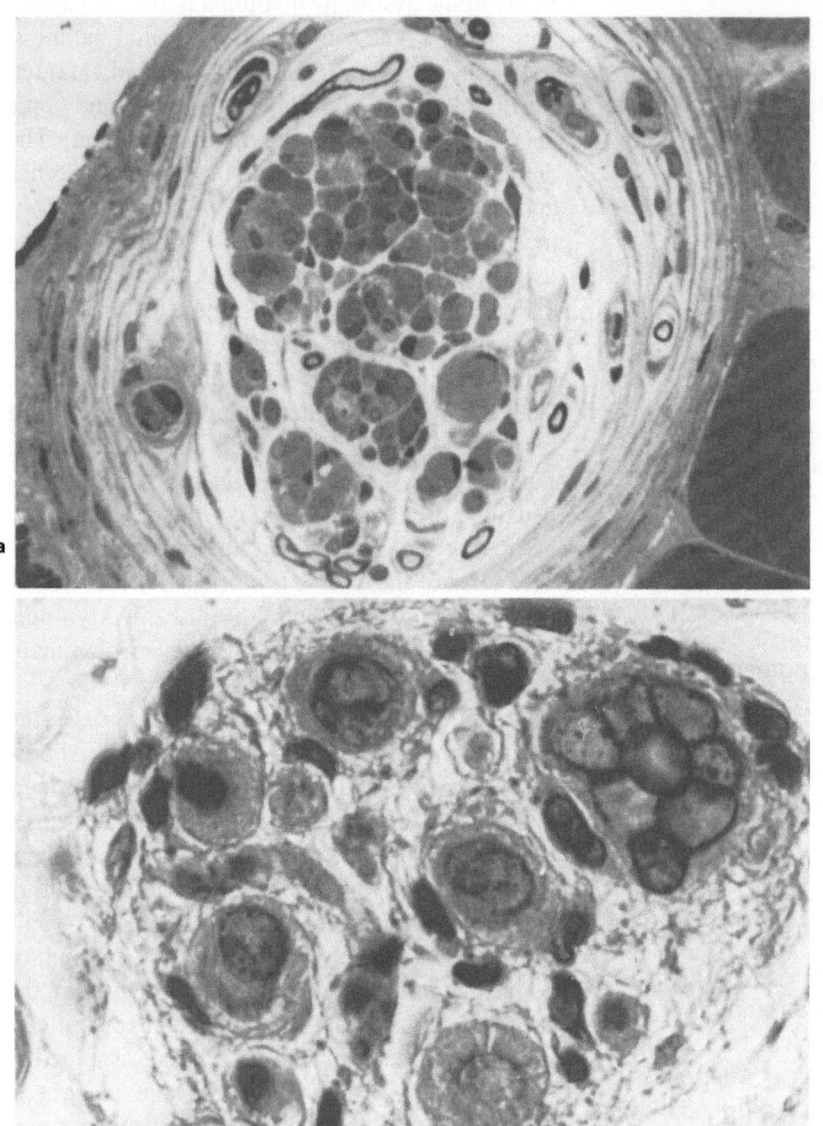

Fig. 17.17. Muscle spindle in myotonic dystrophy. TS.
a There is fragmentation of the intrafusal muscle fibres. (×350)
b Normal muscle spindle. Note the presence of a multinucleated nuclear bag fibre, and of several nuclear chain fibres. (×1400)

Small pointed fibres, strongly positive for NADH and for non-specific esterase, containing pyknotic nuclei, are commonly found in myotonic dystrophy, suggesting that denervation occurs in the disease. Histological studies of the innervation of the extrafusal muscle fibres in myotonic dystrophy have revealed abnormalities. Motor end-plates show proliferative changes, with extensive subterminal axonal branching and expansion of the end-plate zone but there is doubt whether these abnormalities are primary, or secondary to the dystrophic changes in the muscle fibres themselves.

In the less common congenital form of myotonic dystrophy the muscle biopsy shows similar abnormalities but the main feature is the presence of small round fibres with central nuclei, type 1 fibre atrophy, and sarcoplasmic masses. The latter are faintly basophilic, NADH-positive and ATPase-negative peripheral zones of sarcoplasm which are empty of myofibrils. They are reddish-brown in Gomori preparations.

Myotonia congenita

Also known as Thomsen's disease, myotonia congenita begins in childhood and is aggravated by cold and fatigue, or by sudden voluntary muscular contraction. It may be disabling and painful and is associated with marked muscular hypertrophy, but weakness is uncommon. The disease may be

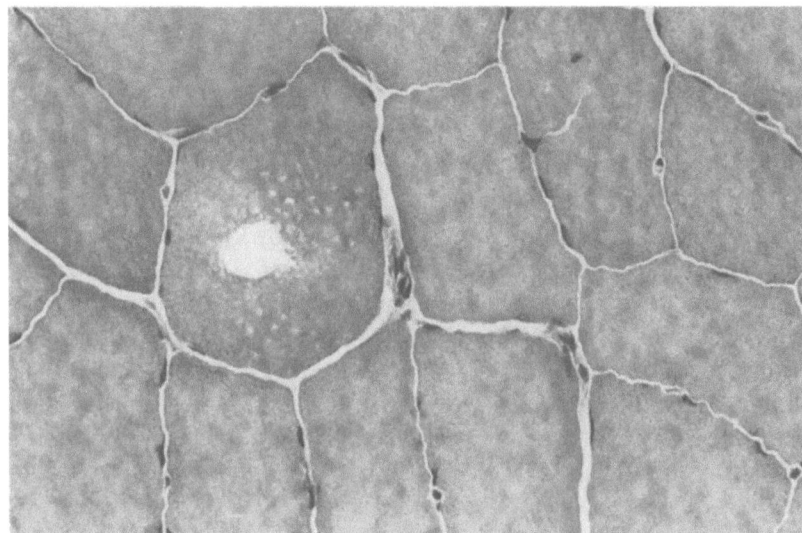

Fig. 17.18. Myotonia congenita (dominant type). TS. H & E. There is fibre hypertrophy with fibre splitting (note the central nucleus) and rare fibres show necrotic features. (× 140)

inherited as a recessive or dominant trait, and the recessive form is more likely to be accompanied by muscular weakness, although this is rarely severe. Muscle biopsies show hypertrophy without myopathic changes, but absence of type 2B fibres has been reported and a few scattered necrotic fibres may occur (Fig. 17.18).

Paramyotonia congenita

Eulenberg's disease consists of myotonia induced or aggravated by cold. There is controversy whether this syndrome is a distinct disorder since reports of patients with paramyotonia congenita have shown features overlapping with those of Thomsen's myotonia congenita and with hyperkalaemic periodic paralysis.

Other myotonic syndromes

Myotonia is a minor feature of some patients with periodic paralysis, in whom it is particularly evident in the upper eyelids. Myotonia is also a feature of the Schwartz–Jampel syndrome, consisting of myotonic lid-lag, muscle weakness, dwarfism and a characteristic facies.

Metabolic myopathies

The metabolic myopathies comprise those myopathies, of varying severity, associated with biochemical defects. In some, a fixed or progressive myopathy develops but in others there are recurrent episodes of muscular weakness often associated with transient myoglobinuria and muscular pain.

Glycogenoses

The glycogen storage diseases are all uncommon and muscular involvement does not occur in all of them (see Chap. 12). Myopathy is prominent, among other manifestations, in acid maltase deficiency (type 2 glycogenosis), in amylo 1–6 glucosidase deficiency (type 3 glycogenosis), in myophosphorylase deficiency (type 5 glycogenosis— McArdle's disease) and in phosphofructokinase deficiency (type 7 glycogenosis), but only in the latter two diseases are muscular symptoms the major manifestation.

In the infantile, autosomal recessive variety of acid maltase deficiency proximal weakness, often associated with enlargement of the heart, liver and tongue, develops. Death usually occurs from cardiorespiratory failure before the age of 1 year. A milder form of the disease, leading to death in the second decade, resembles Duchenne dystrophy in its clinical manifestations. An adult-onset form has also been reported.

In acid maltase deficiency the creatine phosphokinase is slightly raised and muscle biopsy shows a marked vacuolar myopathy. The normal histological pattern of the muscle is destroyed by glycogen-containing, PAS-positive vacuoles. These vacuoles are also strongly reactive for acid phosphatase. The autophagic nature of the vacuoles is confirmed by electron microscopy which shows glycogen granules packed free in the sarcoplasm, in whorled, membrane-bound glycogen bodies, and in autophagic vacuoles. In type 3 glycogenosis liver and muscle are involved. Although muscular involvement is relatively slight the muscle biopsy shows a prominent vacuolar myopathy. The vacuoles contain glycogen but, unlike those found in type 2 glycogenosis, these vacuoles are not lysosomal in origin and are negative in stains for acid phosphatase.

In myophosphorylase (type 5) and phosphofructokinase (type 7) deficiencies easy fatiguability is followed, in late childhood or adolescence, by severe muscular cramps with weakness on exertion. Adult-onset cases also occur. Transient myoglobinuria may occur in these episodes. Later mild permanent proximal weakness may develop. Although an autosomal recessive pattern of inheritance is usual, McArdle's syndrome is commoner in boys than girls. The blood creatine phosphokinase levels are raised after exertion in both syndromes, and during ischaemic exercise the venous lactate fails to rise. The muscle biopsy shows only minor histological changes. The PAS reaction shows an excess of sarcoplasmic glycogen and some small PAS-positive subsarcolemmal vacuoles. Necrotic or small fibres occur and internal nucleation is common. Histochemical stains for phosphorylase demonstrate no reaction product in McArdle's disease and a similar absence of phosphofructokinase activity has been demonstrated in type 7 glycogenosis. Ultrastructurally, glycogen deposition is prominent both in intermyofibrillar sarcoplasm and in subsarcolemmal vacuoles.

Abnormalities of lipid metabolism

These myopathies are characterised by the accumulation of neutral lipid in muscle fibres and by a variety of degenerative changes, including ragged-red fibres, in individual fibres. Carnitine deficiency and carnitine palmityl transferase deficiency are the best documented examples. These two disorders are also classified as mitochondrial myopathies because they are due to defects of mitochondrial metabolism and are accompanied by characteristic morphological changes in mitochondria in affected fibres. Weakness and myoglobinuria, with muscular pain, occur after exercise. In systemic carnitine deficiency plasma, muscle and hepatic carnitine levels are low and hypoglycaemia may occur. There is gross wasting and cachexia. A form in which this deficiency is restricted to muscle has also been recognised. In carnitine palmityl transferase deficiency cachexia is not a feature. Fasting may induce attacks of weakness and myoglobinuria together with a rise in blood triglycerides. The

muscle biopsy in carnitine palmityl transferase deficiency is usually normal, but in systemic or muscle carnitine deficiency there is a destructive myopathy of variable severity with prominent lipid-containing acid phosphatase-positive vacuoles (Fig. 17.19). In addition, a number of disorders of the respiratory enzyme chain in muscle mitochondria have been recognised, for example, cytochrome b deficiency; these can often be suspected from the presence of ragged-red fibres in the biopsy. Diagnosis of these disorders rests on demonstration of the primary biochemical disorder by quantitative biochemical studies, although it may be possible to suggest the likely defect from the clinical, biochemical and histological features.

Other causes of myoglobinuria

Myoglobinuria may occur whenever there is acute necrosis of muscle, as in polymyositis, acute toxic myopathies etc. (Table 17.5).

Table 17.5. Classification of myoglobinuric myopathies

Metabolic	e.g. glycogenoses, lipid storage myopathies, malignant hyperpyrexia
Toxic	e.g. carbon monoxide poisoning, alcohol, certain drugs
Traumatic	
Ischaemic	(anterior tibial compartment syndrome)
Post-infection	
Idiopathic rhabdomyolysis	

Periodic paralyses

Inherited as autosomal dominant traits, the periodic paralyses are characterised by attacks of flaccid paralysis of varying severity associated with a low, normal or high serum potassium in the attacks. The term adynamia episodica hereditaria has been used to describe the normokalaemic variety. In some patients attacks of weakness have been observed with either normal or raised serum potassium levels. The clinical features of these three forms of periodic paralysis overlap. In hypokalaemic periodic paralysis weakness often begins in sleep although, like hyperkalaemic periodic paralysis, a period of rest after vigorous exercise may also induce attacks. Weakness may be provoked in the hypokalaemic variety by a heavy carbohydrate meal, cold, anxiety or by a glucose load. Insulin will also induce an attack. The attacks

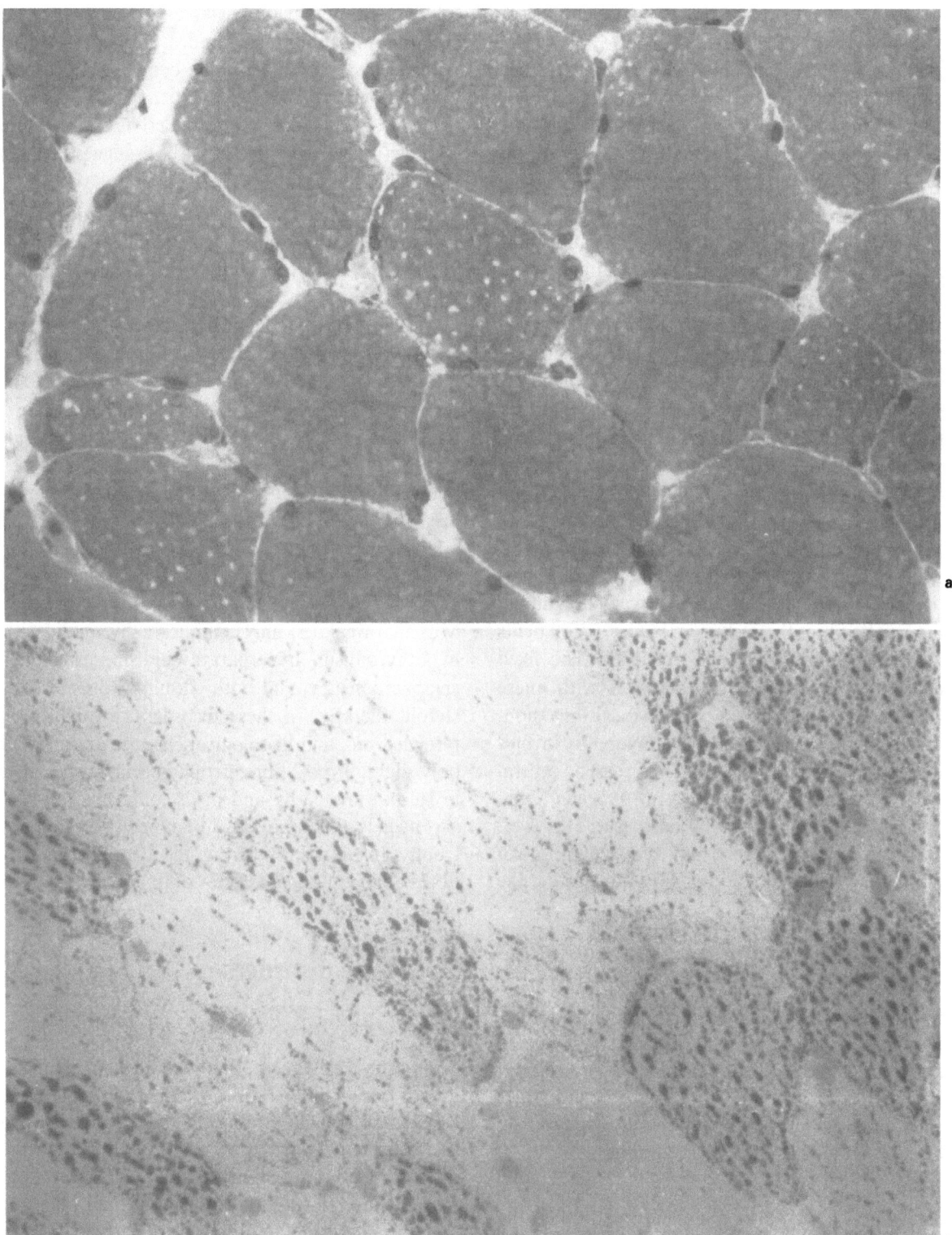

Fig. 17.19. Lipid storage myopathy due to muscle carnitine deficiency. TS.
a H & E (× 200)
b Oil red O. The muscle fibres contain vacuoles, which consist of neutral lipid droplets. (× 200)

of weakness in hypokalaemic paralysis are usually more severe and more prolonged than in the other forms of periodic paralysis, but death in an attack is uncommon. The disease usually begins in infancy or childhood and after several attacks of severe weakness it may become apparent that there is some fixed or even progressive proximal weakness. This is often asymmetrical. Myoglobinuria is obvious only in severe attacks. In Oriental races a form of hypokalaemic paralysis may be a presenting feature of thyrotoxicosis.

Biopsies taken between attacks of weakness may show little or no abnormality, but in attacks there are often large vacuoles in muscle fibres. In severe attacks some fibres become necrotic and the typical sequence of necrosis, ingestion by macrophages and basophilic regeneration, usually subsarcolemmal, then occurs. Although the vacuoles appear empty in H&E stains they usually contain traces of PAS-positive material. However, electron microscopy reveals that the vacuoles are membrane-bound and continuous with the sarcomplasmic reticulum and T-tube system. Other, non-specific, tubular abnormalities have also been described. Calcium salts (hydroxyapatite) may occur in the vacuoles, and in the muscle fibres themselves, in biopsies of patients with long-standing periodic paralysis. The fixed myopathy found in some patients with these syndromes is associated with typical but non-specific histological features of a myopathy including variability in fibre size, increased central nucleation, single fibre necrosis and regeneration, and increased endomysial fibrous tissue. However, even in these cases there may be vacuolation of fibres and this is thus an important clue to the diagnosis.

Other forms of hypokalaemic paralysis

Severe hypokalaemia of any cause may induce muscular weakness with typical vacuolar changes in the muscle biopsy. For example, hypokalaemia from excessive diuretic therapy, renal disease, alcoholism or liquorice ingestion may occasionally be sufficiently severe to induce weakness.

Malignant hyperpyrexia

In this disorder a mild or even subclinical myopathy, dominantly inherited, is associated with a tendency for fatal hyperpyrexia to develop during general anaesthesia. The hyperpyrexia seems to result from heat produced by intense and general-ised muscular rigidity. Tachycardia, tachypnoea, cyanosis and a severe metabolic acidosis accompany the hyperpyrexia. Extensive muscular necrosis follows with myoglobinuria, a very high serum creatine phosphokinase and, sometimes, renal failure. Recovery is usually complete in those patients who survive the hyperpyrexia, hyperkalaemia and acidosis. The underlying metabolic disorder is ill-defined, but it has been suggested that most anaesthetic drugs release sarcoplasmic and sarcotubular calcium ions, causing muscular contraction. Susceptibility can be recognised by an in vitro provocation test using muscle tissue obtained by biopsy.

Muscle biopsies taken after an attack of hyperpyrexia show extensive muscle fibure necrosis, followed by regeneration. Biopsies taken from susceptible subjects not otherwise affected show minor abnormalities consisting of slightly increased variability in fibre size with increased central nucleation. The serum creatine phosphokinase may be slightly raised in these patients.

Endrocrine myopathies

Muscular weakness may complicate thyrotoxicosis, hypothyroidism, hyperparathyroidism, osteomalacia, acromegaly, and both Cushing's disease and steroid therapy. In these disorders, myopathy is rarely severe, and histological changes are usually only slight. Type 2 fibre atrophy occurs, especially in steroid myopathy and in osteomalacia, and in acromegaly there may also be type 1 fibre hypertrophy. In steroid myopathy, the atrophic type 2B fibres often contain an excess of lipid droplets.

End-plate disorders

Myasthenia gravis

Characterised by fluctuating weakness, myasthenia gravis particularly affects cranial muscles. It consists principally of abnormal fatiguability after sustained activity, with improvement after rest. The disease is commonest in young adults, affecting women three times more frequently than men. In addition, several childhood forms exist (Table 17.6). A quarter of all patients with myasthenia gravis present before the age of 20 years but less than 5% present before the age of 10 years. Myasthenia beginning before the age of 2 years is usually termed 'congenital myasthenia'. Although

Table 17.6. Classification of myasthenia gravis

1 Adult-onset myasthenia

2 Juvenile myasthenia, a disorder similar to the adult disease

3 Congenital (or infantile) myasthenia

4 Transient neonatal myasthenia in infants born to myasthenic mothers

the clinical features of infantile and juvenile myasthenia may be similar, patients with congenital myasthenia tend to have a benign, non-progressive course. Ocular manifestations may be prominent. The term infantile myasthenia is better reserved for cases of *severe* myasthenia, beginning before the age of 2 years, since this disorder may present with bulbar and respiratory problems. In both congenital and infantile myasthenia siblings are also commonly affected, an uncommon feature in adult or juvenile myasthenia. About 70% of patients with juvenile or adult myasthenia show HLA-B1, HLA-B8 and HLA-DW3 haplotypes but this association does not occur in the congenital or infantile forms of the disease. Neonatal myasthenia is a transient disorder. About 15% of infants born to myasthenic mothers are floppy and weak, requiring anticholinesterase therapy during the first month after birth. Adult onset myasthenia is occasionally associated with thyrotoxicosis and with polymyositis.

Lymphoid hyperplasia and an increase in the number and size of germinal centres occur in the thymus in about two-thirds of patients with adult or juvenile myasthenia. Thymoma occurs in about 20% of these cases but is very rare in infants and children. In congenital and infantile myasthenia the thymus is usually normal. Muscle biopsies in myasthenia, of any type, reveal little abnormality in most cases. Lymphocyte accumulations (lymphorrages) are common but are not specific for myasthenia, having been reported in neurogenic disorders and in polymyositis. Type 2 fibre atrophy occurs in about half and lymphocyte accumulations in about a quarter of patients with myasthenia gravis. This type 2 fibre atrophy is often irregularly distributed within the biopsy, suggesting that it is not necessarily a non-specific phenomenon. Scattered small pointed fibres, or even fibre-type grouping have also been reported, suggesting that denervation and reinnervation occur during the course of the disease. Denervation is usually due to myasthenic damage to motor end-plates. Characteristic abnormalities occur in the motor innervation in myasthenia gravis, consisting of elongated motor endings without evidence of axonal sprouting (dysplastic pattern) and of increased collateral ramification of motor axons (dystrophic pattern) with the formation of multiple end-plates. Ultrastructural studies of motor end-plates in myasthenia have shown that the post-synaptic region is smaller than normal, with loss (simplification) of the post-synaptic folds. The mean nerve terminal area is also smaller in myasthenic end-plates, but the numbers of synaptic vesicles are normal. In myasthenia gravis the number of functional acetylcholine receptors in the post-synaptic membrane at the motor end-plates is reduced due to an interaction between the receptor protein itself and a circulating antibody to acetylcholine receptor protein, found within the IgG fraction of the serum proteins. Such antibodies to extracted human acetylcholine receptor protein can be demonstrated in 90% of patients with myasthenia gravis. Receptor degradation is thus accelerated in the disease. This process is complement dependent, the deposition of immune complex leading to macrophage activation and so to destruction of the motor end-plate. End-plate and nerve terminal proliferation results from regeneration.

The site of synthesis of acetylcholine receptor antibody in myasthenia gravis, and the role of the thymus, or of thymus-dependent lymphocytes in this humoral disorder, are uncertain. However, it has been shown that preparation of lymphocytes from germinal centres in the thymus glands of patients with myasthenia gravis can synthesize this acetylcholine receptor antibody.

Passive transfer of immunoglobulin G from myasthenic patients to the mouse causes myasthenic weakness in the recipient mouse, and neonatal myasthenia, which is associated with gradually declining levels of acetylcholine receptor antibody in the serum of affected infants, may result from a similar passive transfer mechanism. However, the severity of myasthenic weakness in myasthenia does not correlate readily with levels of circulating acetylcholine receptor antibody, suggesting that other host factors may be important. Further, in congenital myasthenia, acetylcholine receptor antibody may not be demonstrable. These newer concepts of myasthenia gravis have led to rationalisation of the role of anticholinesterase drugs, of immunosuppressant therapy, and of thymectomy in the management of the disease.

Inflammatory myopathies

The inflammatory myopathies have been classified into four subgroups (Table 17.7). In adults polymyositis may occur alone, or in association with a heliotrope discoloration of the skin, especially in areas exposed to sunlight. In many patients there are associated features of multiple system involvement, especially polyarthropathy, necrotic ulcers of digits, and renal or cardiopulmonary involvement. In older patients, especially those over the age of 50 years, dermatomyositis or polymyositis is associated with cancer, particularly bronchogenic carcinoma. The incidence of this association is probably about 10% to 20%. Polymyositis complicating connective tissue disease is usually relatively benign, but it may be severe, especially in patients with rheumatoid arthritis or polyarteritis nodosa and in these there is usually pathological evidence of an active vasculitis.

Table 17.7. Classification of idiopathic inflammatory myopathies

---

1 Polymyositis, beginning in childhood (aged less than 16 years) or in adult life, and acute, subacute or chronic in course

2 Polymyositis, with some skin changes, or with associated features of other connective tissue disorders, e.g. polyarthropathy

3 Severe connective tissue disease with slight muscular involvement

4 Polymyositis or dermatomyositis associated with malignant disease

---

Dermatomyositis of childhood is a distinct but uncommon disorder, presenting with muscular weakness, skin lesions and systemic symptoms. Muscular weakness is usually proximal, may be very severe and usually also involves facial muscles. The skin lesion, as in adult polymyositis dermatomyositis, may be florid or quite inconspicuous. It is more prominent in exposed skin. There is usually muscular pain and tenderness, with fever and weight loss. Hepatosplenomegaly, fleeting polyarthropathy, cardiac involvement, calcification of muscle and skin, and ulceration of skin and gastro-intestinal tract may also occur.

The creatine phosphokinase and the ESR are usually, but not always, raised. In patients with widespread muscular damage the creatine phosphokinase may be raised even to several hundred times the normal value.

The *muscle biopsy* in polymyositis of any type shows a number of typical features. There is increased variability in fibre size with atrophy of both fibre types. Fibre hypertrophy is uncommon but in chronic cases there may be some hypertrophy of type 1 fibres, and fibre splitting may occur in these cases. Scattered small angular fibres, intensely reactive for NADH, are usually present, indicating that denervation has occurred. This results either from damage to the peripheral nerves, as in polyarteritis nodosa, or from infarction of small nerve twigs in the muscles themselves. Fibre type grouping is frequently found but the numbers of fibres within these groups are small when compared with biopsies from neurogenic disorders. Necrotic and basophilic regenerating fibres are common, especially in patients with a subacute course, and central nucleation is frequent. These abnormalities are characteristically patchily distributed.

In patients with an acute onset there may be patchy, but widespread, subendomysial necrosis, often in a fascicular distribution, suggesting a vascular causation (Fig. 17.20). Architectural changes in individual fibres are common, particularly at the periphery of a fascicle. These changes include loss of ATPase reaction in the centre of a fibre and patchy loss or accentuation of the NADH and PAS reactions causing a pronounced 'moth-eaten' appearance, or even a 'ghost' fibre unreactive in all enzyme preparations. Cytoplasmic bodies and ring fibres also occur. Inflammatory changes, often predominantly perivascular, occur in about 75% of biopsies in polymyositis. Fibrosis occurs as the disease progresses.

These inflammatory cell exudates may be widely distributed in the endomysial spaces, or may be quite focal. In some cases they are closely associated with arterioles, and in others with larger vessels, and they may then infiltrate the wall of the vessel. Fibrinoid necrosis and thrombosis of affected vessels is sometimes seen. The inflammatory cells consist mainly of small lymphocytes, but macrophages, plasma cells and eosinophils may be identified. In one form of the disease a peripheral blood eosinophilia is associated with prominent involvement of muscular fascial planes; *eosinophilic fascitis*. It is important to recognise however, that inflammation may be absent from the biopsy.

It has been suggested that the *childhood form* of dermatomyositis is due to a vasculitis affecting arterioles, small veins and capillaries in affected muscles and other organs. The finding of extensive perifascicular atrophy and architectural changes supports this concept. Deposits of immunoglobulin

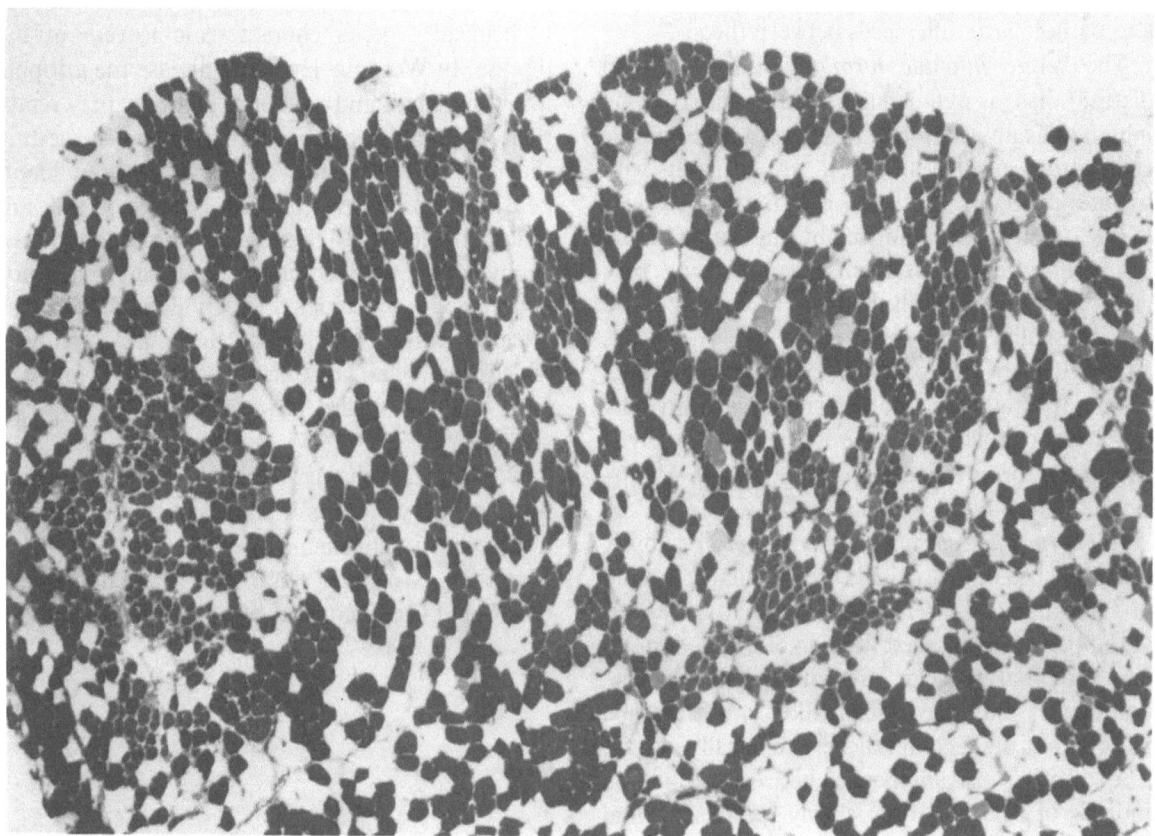

Fig. 17.20. Acute polymyositis. TS. ATPase, pH 4.3. There are several fascicular zones of subendomysial regeneration, consisting of small fibres of intermediate histochemical type, corresponding to infarcts in the muscle. (× 80)

and complement in small blood vessels, particularly in veins, can sometimes be found but the possible role of humoral and cell-mediated mechanisms in the pathogenesis of the disorder remains undetermined. Muscle capillary endothelial cells contain undulating tubular cytoplasmic inclusions, are thicker than normal and are often surrounded by reduplicated basal lamina and it has been suggested that capillary necrosis is the primary lesion in the childhood form of dermatomyositis, leading to the characteristic perifascicular distribution of the changes in muscle fibres in this disease. Undulating tubules and evidence of capillary necrosis have not been reported in the adult form of polymyositis, but capillary damage does occur in adult onset polymyositis, and in polymyositis associated with connective tissue disorders, such as rheumatoid arthritis.

Although a viral aetiology has been suggested only a few cases associated with high antibody titres, especially for Coxsackie B virus and myxovirus, have been reported. In addition, in some cases the disease seems to be triggered by a preceding viral infection.

Neurogenic disorders

Diseases involving the motor unit cause denervation of muscle. The motor unit is the lower motor neuron, consisting of anterior horn cell, motor nerve fibre, motor end-plates and of the individual muscle fibres innervated by these structures. The neurogenic disorders can be grouped into those due to disease of the anterior horn cells themselves, and those in which the motor nerve fibres are primarily affected, the *motor neuropathies*. In the latter group, there may be damage to axons, or to Schwann cells, and in many there may be associated involvement of sensory nerve fibres. These peripheral neuropathies are discussed in Chap. 16.

Spinal muscular atrophies

The spinal muscular atrophies, affecting only the lower motor neuron, are common. Although subclassification of these cases into severe infantile, intermediate, adolescent and adult-onset types seems arbitrary, since the age of onset of these groups overlaps and classification can only be finally determined by the outcome, there are clinical and pathological differences between them.

The *severe infantile form* (Werdnig–Hoffman disease) has a well-defined genetic basis, being inherited as an autosomal recessive trait. Sporadic cases also occur. Severe generalised weakness with hypotonia becomes evident during the first few days of life, or may even be noticed by the mother before birth since fetal movements may become progressively weakened. Bulbar palsy develops and death usually occurs before the age of 1 year, although survival to about 3 years sometimes occurs. In a rare variant of spinal muscular atrophy the bulbar nuclei may be selectively involved causing a progressive bulbar paralysis (Fazio–Londé syndrome).

In *intermediate spinal muscular atrophy* disability is less marked but the child is usually unable to walk or stand unaided. Weakness is symmetrical and is accompanied by marked wasting of affected muscles. Proximal muscles are almost always predominantly affected. Fasciculation is not a usual feature, but the tendon reflexes are usually absent. The disorder usually begins between 3 and 15 months of age. It is only slowly progressive and survival into adolescence is common; some patients may improve a little. Cardiac muscle is not involved. Both autosomal recessive and, less frequently, dominant forms occur.

Mild spinal muscular atrophy (*Kugelberg–Welander disease*) begins after the age of 2 years. Indeed, it usually begins in late childhood or adolescence. The course is only very slowly progressive and the ability to stand and walk is usually retained. Weakness is predominantly proximal and is often asymmetrical. Sometimes there is a striking distal predilection, but the presentation is often similar to that of muscular dystrophy. Rarely, this disorder may present in a *scapulo-peroneal distribution*. The scapular weakness and the characteristic sparing of the extensor digitorum brevis muscles excludes Charcot–Marie–Tooth syndrome. Scapulo-peroneal weakness may also be myopathic in origin. An *adult-onset form* of the disease, beginning after the third decade is uncommon. It has a benign outcome.

Muscle biopsies in spinal muscular atrophy show somewhat similar features in the severe and intermediate varieties. There is atrophy of both type 1 and type 2 fibres and the atrophic fibres are usually arranged in large groups of identical histochemical type, even affecting whole fascicles (Figs. 17.4,

17.21). Some fascicles contain isolated or small groups of hypertrophied fibres of uniform histochemical type, a characteristic feature of the disease. In Werdnig–Hoffman disease the atrophic fibres are small and rounded, and they may retain their mosaic histochemical distribution, suggesting that denervation has occurred without compensatory reinnervation, or that they are undifferentiated 'fetal' fibres. Interpretation of atrophy of this type, without fibre-type grouping or hypertrophy in a biopsy, is very difficult. Because atrophy can be very severe the muscle spindles, which show changes due to denervation only in more chronic disorders, may be unusually conspicuous.

Degenerative changes in single muscle fibres are not a primary feature of these severe forms of the disease but in chronic, milder forms, especially in Kugelberg–Welander syndrome, such changes are common. These consist of increased interstitial

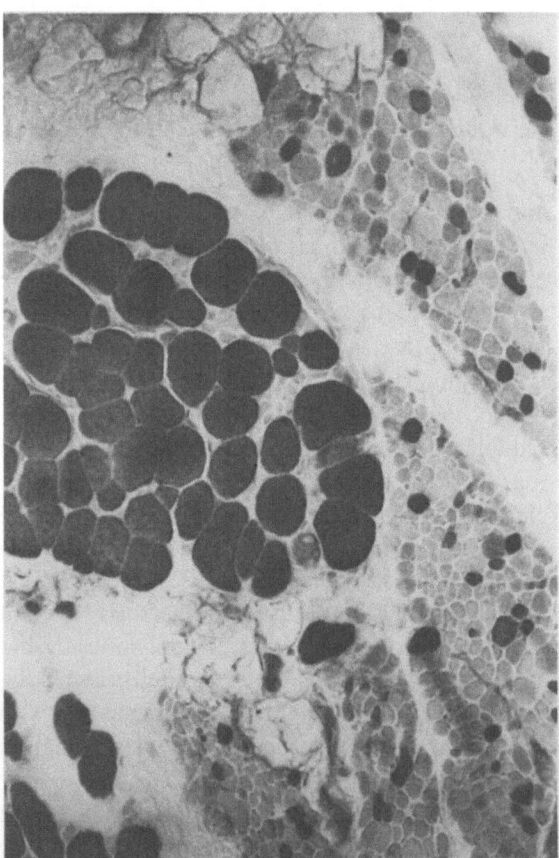

Fig. 17.21. Werdnig–Hoffman disease. TS. ATPase, pH 4.3. Sheets of small fibres of indeterminate histochemical type occupy some fascicles. Occasional type 1 fibres are seen in these abnormal fascicles. An adjacent fascicle consists of large type 1 fibres. The interfascicular planes are thickened. (× 140)

fibrosis, degenerative and regenerative changes in single muscle fibres, fibre hypertrophy, especially affecting type 1 fibres, fibre splitting, increased central nucleation, and fibres containing whorls and a moth-eaten myofibrillar pattern in NADH preparations. In H & E preparations these secondary 'myopathic' changes may be so prominent that an erroneous diagnosis of primary myopathy may be suggested. However, ATPase preparations show fibre-type grouping.

Clusters of narrow pointed fibres are relatively uncommon in spinal muscular atrophies except in the later, less well compensated stages of the disorder (Fig. 17.4) although this is a characteristic feature of other acquired and more rapidly progressive forms of denervation. In mild spinal muscular atrophy supravital methylene blue stains reveal terminal axonal branching and sprouting, illustrating the effectiveness of the collateral reinnervation associated with fibre-type grouping. In the CNS many anterior horn cells are lost. Remaining anterior horn cells and somatic motor neurons in the bulbar nuclei show chromatolysis and degenerative changes, consisting of pyknosis, neuronophagia and gliosis.

Motor neuron disease

In motor neuron disease (amyotrophic lateral sclerosis) there is clinical evidence of involvement of both upper and lower motor neurons. The disorder is quite variable in presentation and course. It is most frequent in the fifth and sixth decades. The main features include progressive weakness and wasting, often beginning asymmetrically, with involvement of the bulbar and respiratory musculature, but with sparing of ocular muscles and of urinary and anal sphincter muscles. Fasciculation is a prominent feature. Pseudo-bulbar palsy, progressive atrophy and marked corticospinal signs are present to varying degrees. Survival beyond 5 years from diagnosis is uncommon. About 5%–10% of cases are familial and there is a clinical association with a mild dementia in about 20% of cases. The cause of motor neuron disease is unknown.

The muscle biopsy shows fibre-type grouping (Fig. 17.22) affecting both type 1 and type 2 fibres. Fibre-type atrophy is unusually prominent and there are many scattered, pointed, NADH-reactive denervated fibres, containing dark, pyknotic nuclei. There may be type 1 fibre hypertrophy so that increased variability in fibre size may develop later in the disease with other features of secondary myopathic changes, although these features are not prominent. Axonal degeneration can sometimes be recognised in intramuscular nerve fibres, but sensory nerve endings in muscle spindles are unaffected. Marked terminal axonal sprouting is a feature of the earlier, relatively well-compensated stages of the disease.

At *autopsy* there is striking, often almost total, loss of anterior horn cells, except in the sacral segments innervating the sphincter musculature and in the ocular motor nuclei. The crossed and uncrossed corticospinal tracts are atrophic and gliotic with extensive loss of axons and myelin. The ventral roots are atrophic due to axonal degeneration but the posterior roots are normal. There may be similar abnormalities in fibres efferent from the motor cortex. Remaining anterior horn cells appear

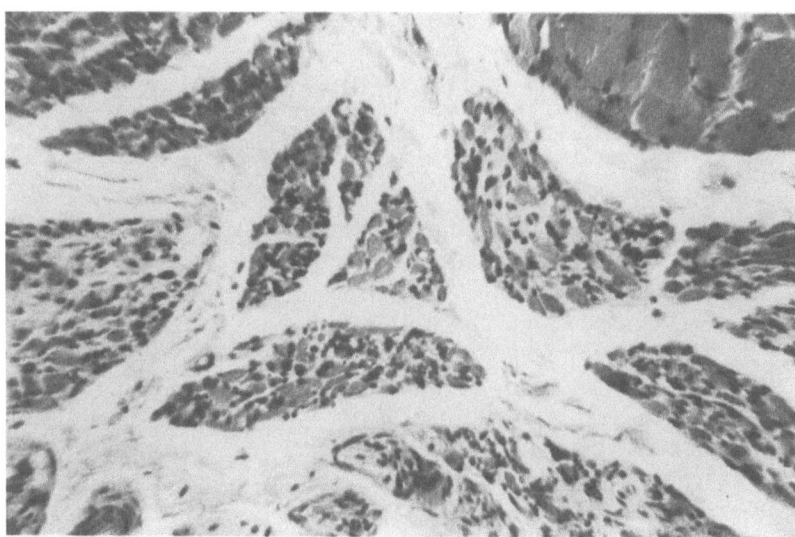

Fig. 17.22. Motor neuron disease. TS. H & E. In this autopsy specimen there is advanced grouped denervation atrophy, affecting whole fascicles. (×140)

small and pyknotic. Chromatolysis is uncommon but neuronophagia may be seen. Loss of anterior horn cells, and of motor neurons from cranial nerve nuclei is patchy, asymmetrical and variable at different levels in the cord. The neurons of the third, fourth and sixth cranial nerve nuclei, and in Onuff's cell group in the S_2 and S_3 ventral horns, related to urinary and anal sphincter innervation, are always spared. The Betz cells of the motor cortex are usually reduced in number, and the degeneration of the corticospinal tracts observed in the cord extends up through the brain stem into the middle thirds of the crura of the cerebral peduncles, and into the posterior parts of the posterior limbs of the internal capsule. Gliosis of these abnormal corticospinal pathways, and of the diseased anterior horns of the spinal grey matter is usually a prominent feature. Alzheimer plaques and neurofibrillary tangles are often present in increased number in the neocortex.

Other anterior horn cell disorders, and other diseases causing denervation of muscle

Denervation, with fibre-type grouping from collateral reinnervation, occurs in other diseases of anterior horn cells, including poliomyelitis, syringomyelia, herpes simplex myelitis and spinal cord trauma or infarction. Similarly, denervation of muscle occurs in disorders of anterior nerve roots,

and of motor nerves, as in the peripheral neuropathies. The latter disorders are discussed in Chap. 16.

Further reading

Drachman D B (1979) Myasthenia gravis—a disorder of acetylcholine receptors. In: Aguayo A J , Karpati G (eds) Current topics in nerve and muscle research. Elsevier, Amsterdam, p 87

Dubowitz V (1978) Muscle disorders in childhood. Saunders, London

Dubowitz V, Brooke M H (1973) Muscle biopsy—modern approach. Saunders, London

Emery A E H, Burt D (1980) Intracellular calcium and pathogenesis and antenatal diagnosis of Duchenne muscular dystrophy. Br Med J 280: 355

Engel A G (1981) Metabolic and endocrine myopathies: In: Walton J N (ed) Disorders of voluntary muscle. Churchill Livingstone, Edinburgh, p 665

Morgan-Hughes J A (1982) Metabolic myopathies. In: Matthews W B and Glaser G H (eds) Recent advances in clinical neurology. Churchill Livingstone, Edinburgh p 1

Pearn J (1980) Classification of spinal muscular atrophies. Lancet i: 919

Rowland L P (1980) Biochemistry of muscle membranes in Duchenne muscular dystrophy. Muscle and Nerve 3: 3

Schwartz M S, Sargeant M S, Swash M (1976) Longitudinal fibre splitting in neurogenic muscular disorders: its relation to the pathogenesis of 'myopathic' change. Brain 99: 617

Swash M, Schwartz M S (1981) Neuromuscular diseases: a practical approach to diagnosis and management. Springer-Verlag, Berlin Heidelberg New York

If we shadows have offended,
Think but this and all is mended,
That you have but slumber'd here
While these visions did appear.
And this weak and idle theme,
No more yielding but a dream,
Gentles, do not reprehend:
If you pardon, we will mend.

A Midsummer Night's Dream,
Act V, Scene 2.

Appendix

The Advisory Group of the Department of Health made several recommendations on Creutzfeldt–Jakob disease (CJD) which included the sterilization procedures set out below. [Abstracted from: Report of Advisory Group on the management of patients with Spongiform Encephalopathy (Creutzfeldt–Jakob Disease) (CJD). HMSO, London, November 1981.]

Sterilization procedures

There is evidence that CJD agent will resist standard methods of disinfection and sterilization using heat, formaldehyde, 70% alcohol, ultra violet and ionising radiation. For a number of other methods, eg ether, chloroform and iodophors, there is no evidence either way and we do not recommend their use. Autoclaving infected equipment at 121°C for one hour has been recommended, but experiments have suggested that at least one strain of scrapie agent is resistant to this. Further investigations on sterilization procedures are in progress.

As an interim measure, we recommend that one of the following autoclave procedures should be employed.

    i.   a single cycle 121°—124°C (15 lb pisi) for 90 minutes holding time at temperature (HTAT)

    ii.   a single cycle 126°—129°C (20 lb psi) for 60 minutes HTAT

    iii.   a single cycle 136°—138° (30 lb psi) for 18 minutes HTAT or
    6 separate cycles
              136°—138°C (30 lb psi) for 3 minutes HTAT

To achieve these cycles, autoclaves should be calibrated by a suitably qualified person. All apparatus should then be washed thoroughly and autoclaved again as necessary.

Limited evidence suggests that exposure to hypochlorite should act as a disinfectant. Therefore, as an interim measure until work in progress provides more reliable information, the use of a 1% dilution of hypochlorite containing 10,000 ppm available chlorine (freshly prepared dilute sodium hypochlorite BP) is recommended for use on contaminated surfaces leaving it for half an hour. For decontamination of laboratory equipment, other than metal (which is corroded by hypochlorites) soaking for 18 hours in a 1% dilution of hypochlorite containing 10,000 ppm available chlorine is advised.

Subject Index

a selection of new and recent titles of related interest

Craniocerebral Computer Tomography
Confrontations with Neuropathology
With collaboration of D. Baleriaux, D. Crolla, J. Dietemann, R. Dom, J. Flament, N. Heldt, Y. Palmers, J. Termote
1980. 112 figures in 498 separate illustrations. X, 130 pages (Atlas of Pathological Computer Tomography, Volume 1). ISBN 3-540-09879-8

Computed Tomography in Intracranial Tumors
Differential Diagnosis and Clinical Aspects
Editors: E. Kazner, S. Wende, T. Grumme, W. Lanksch, O. Stochdorph
Authors: G. B. Bradač, U. Büll, R. Fahlbusch, T. Grumme, E. Kazner, K. Kretschmar, W. Lanksch, W. Meese, J. Schramm, H. Steinhoff, O. Stochdorph, S. Wende
Translated from the German by F. C. Dougherty
1982. 693 figures. XI, 549 pages. ISBN 3-540-10815-7

R. Nieuwenhuys, J. Voogd, C. van Huijzen
The Human Central Nervous System
A Synopsis and Atlas
2nd revised edition. 1981. 154 figures. VIII, 253 pages. ISBN 3-540-10316-3

W. Seeger
Atlas of Topographical Anatomy of the Brain and Surrounding Structures for Neurosurgeons, Neuroradiologists and Neuropathologists
1978. 258 figures. VII, 544 pages. ISBN 3-211-81447-7

J. Lang
Clinical Anatomy of the Head
Neurocranium – Orbita – Craniocervical Regions
Translated from the German by R. R. Wilson, D. P. Winstanley
1982. 388 four-colored figures und 189 diagrams. XIV, 492 pages. ISBN 3-540-11014-3

The Cranial Nerves
Anatomy Pathology Pathophysiology Diagnosis Treatment
Editors: M. Samii, P. J. Jannetta
1981. 410 figures. XVII, 664 pages. ISBN 3-540-10620-0

E. Braak
On the Structure of the Human Striate Area
1982. 44 figures. VI, 87 pages (Advances in Anatomy, Embryology and Cell Biology, Volume 77). ISBN 3-540-11512-9

F. G. Zak, W. Lawson
The Paraganglionic Chemoreceptor System:
Physiology, Pathology, and Clinical Medicine
1982. 225 figures. 583 pages. ISBN 3-540-90621-5

W. Seeger
Microsurgery of the Spinal Cord and Surrounding Structures
Anatomical and Technical Principles
1982. 201 figures. VII, 410 pages. ISBN 3-211-81648-8

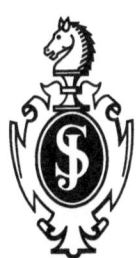

Springer-Verlag
Berlin
Heidelberg
New York

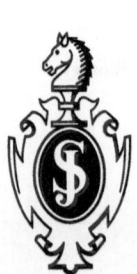